Fauci-Topian Vaccine Sacrifice and Lockdown of the Innocents

HISTORIC TIMELINE & SCIENCE OF COVID-19, VACCINES, VIRUS TESTING LOCKDOWNS, PAST EPIDEMICS & PANDEMICS, HIV, & VACCINE CANCERS

ANDREW MANIOTIS, PHD

30 N Gould St Ste R Sheridan, Wyoming 82801

ISBN: 978-1-7378077-3-5
Contact@AlfredRWallace.com

This 1802 colored etching, included on the cover of this book, "The Cow-Pock—or—the Wonderful Effects of the New Inoculation!" by James Gillray, a British political cartoonist, depicts humans turning into cows after receiving smallpox vaccinations which at the time were made from the pus of infected cow sores. Depicted in the center of the picture delivering the vaccination is Edward Jenner, credited with starting modern vaccination as a practice, using his lancet to pierce the arm of a seated working woman.

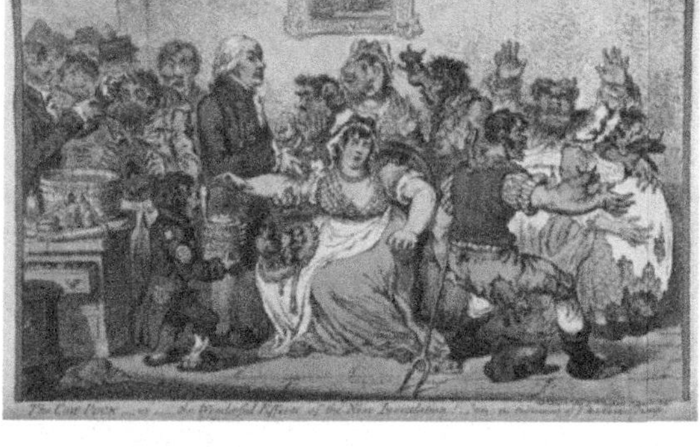

This book is dedicated to all the people ever harmed by medical errors and pharmaceutical side effects, which a recent 2016 study from Johns Hopkins suggests kill over 250,000 Americans a year making medical errors and pharmaceutical side effects the third leading cause of death in the United States. See https://hub.jhu.edu/2016/05/03/medical-errors-third-leading-cause-of-death/.

This book is also dedicated to the Americans who may have died and may die in the future from side effects from the Covid-19 injections. The US Vaccine Adverse Reporting System (VAERS), launched in 1990, created by the National Vaccine Childhood Injury Act signed by Ronald Reagan into law in 1986, reports that over 25,000 reports have been submitted to VAERS of deaths quickly following and potentially related to Covid-19 shots. See the US federal government Vaccine Adverse Event Reporting Data here for Covid-19 vaccines: https://vaers.hhs.gov/data.html.

According to a US federal government Health and Human Services report, less than 1% of vaccine adverse event reports are submitted to the federal government Vaccine Adverse Event Reporting System (VAERS):

https://digital.ahrq.gov/sites/default/files/docs/publication/r18hs017045-lazarus-final-report-2011.pdf.

VAERS COVID Vaccine Adverse Event Reports

Reports from the Vaccine Adverse Events Reporting System. Our default data reflects all VAERS data including the "nondomestic" reports.

All VAERS COVID Reports US/Territories/Unknown

1,168,892 Reports
Through March 4, 2022

25,158 DEATHS	138,247 HOSPITALIZATIONS	122,734 URGENT CARE
179,952 DOCTOR OFFICE VISITS	9,400 ANAPHYLAXIS	14,544 BELL'S PALSY

4,279 Miscarriages	12,953 Heart Attacks	35,913 Myocarditis/Pericarditis	46,515 Permanently Disabled
5,890 Thrombocytopenia/ Low Platelet	28,698 Life Threatening	40,716 Severe Allergic Reaction	12,852 Shingles

ABOUT THE AUTHOR

Dr. Andrew Maniotis and his team at Harvard Medical School's department of pathology and surgical research pioneered and established the new science of cellular tensegrity and chemically defined and functionally demonstrated the self-assembling properties responsible for genomic continuity and mechanical integrity of the genomes of vertebrate cells by using microsurgical techniques under chemically defined In Vitro conditions. See this article on cellular tensegrity Dr. Maniotis' Harvard team published in the Proceedings of the National Academy of Sciences of the United States (PNAS). https://www.pnas.org/content/94/3/849.

Maniotis later designed the most accurate malignant melanoma cancer lab test in the world at the time because of his discovery of Vasculogenic Mimicry.

These articles published in Science Magazine include detailed descriptions by editors, other scientists and doctors of some of Dr. Maniotis' teams' breakthrough contributions in cancer diagnostics, including coverage of "Vasculogenic Mimicry" in malignant cancers, a term first coined by Dr. Maniotis, and also the field cellular tensegrity which Dr. Maniotis worked on while working as a research scientist at Harvard Medical School: https://www.science.org/action/doSearch?AllField=maniotis;

In 1998, Dr. Maniotis' Harvard team's work on cellular tensegrity was distinguished by The Royal Society, and Royal Chemical Society, London, and an invited article written about cellular tensegrity was published in Scientific American, found here: http://time.arts.ucla.edu/Talks/Barcelona/Arch_Life.htm.

A simplistic definition of **Vasculogenic Mimicry** which defines malignant cancers first described by Dr. Maniotis in 1999, can be found in Wikipedia here: https://en.wikipedia.org/wiki/Vasculogenic_mimicry.

Because of his discovery of Vasculogenic Mimicry in malignant cancers, Dr. Maniotis was invited to serve on Grant Review Study sections at The National Cancer Institute on multiple occasions: 1998 & 1999, National Cancer Institute Invited Grant Reviewer. "Therapeutic Modulation of Angiogenesis in Disease." Washington, D.C. Fall 2000; National Cancer Institute Invited Grant Reviewer: "APA, Screening Technologies Branch DTP, DCTD," Washington, D.C., Fall 2008; Invited National Cancer Institute Grant Reviewer, "Melanoma Program Project Review," National Cancer Institute, Bethesda, Maryland.

Approximately 941 of the primary research articles that discuss Vasculogenic Mimicry since Maniotis' discovery have been published in what the field considers top-tiered, critically peer-reviewed science and medical journals, with no peer-reviewed report since 1999 (when Maniotis first described vasculogenic mimicry) that vasculogenic mimicry is not a diagnostic hallmark of all malignant cancers: https://www.ncbi.nlm.nih.gov/pmc/?term=vascolugenic+mimicry.

At the University of Iowa during his first Assistant Professorship where he researched the biology of cancer, Maniotis discovered and named the phenomenon of "VASCULOGENIC MIMICRY" (**VM**) in malignant cancers, which over the next 20 years has essentially replaced the anti-angiogenesis anti-cancer paradigm that had spawned a 4.9-billion-dollar industry, and which in 1999 was promised to cure cancer non-toxically in two years, but which shortly thereafter was abandoned because anti-angiogenesis failed in 4 human cancer clinical trials. An article was written in the Chicago Tribune in 1999 about Dr. Maniotis's then recent breakthrough VM cancer discovery which contradicted the anti-angiogenesis cancer paradigm:

https://www.chicagotribune.com/news/ct-xpm-1999-09-17-9909170133-story.html

Dr. Maniotis also served as Associate Professor at the University of Illinois at Chicago where Dr. Maniotis created and served as Program

Director of "The Efficient Causes and Designs Consortium" in the department of bio-engineering, and in The Department of Pathology. Dr. Maniotis created and developed the program; "the Cell Biology of Cancer." Since leaving the University of Illinois, Chicago Medical School, Dr. Maniotis has been engaged in developing a combination of hyperbaric and nutritional medicine aimed at the non-toxic therapeutic treatment of cancers and other syndromes that are unresponsive to current medical standards of care and protocols of treatment.

Maniotis co-authored, researched, and published multiple scientific articles with two members of the National Academy of Sciences including Dr. Mina Bissell, the longtime head of life sciences at Lawrence Berkeley National Laboratory and endosymbiotic evolutionary biologist Dr. Lynn Margulis who developed the GAIA hypothesis. Maniotis also authored a chapter called "Heredity: From Bacterial Genophores to Human Chromosomes" in a book organized and edited by Dr. Lynn Margulis called: "Chimeras and Consciousness: Evolution of the Sensory Self."

By August, 2021, and 20 years after the discovery of vasculogenic mimicry, The National Library of Medicine's (PUBMED) NCBI's website listed 3801 PUBMED Central (PMC) journal articles, 14 books, and 19 protein databases that have archived the developing science of vasculogenic mimicry. Top tier journals that have featured work on VM are listed on the National Library of Medicine's website here: https://www.ncbi.nlm.nih.gov/pmc/?term=vascolugenic+mimicry

The Encyclopedia of Cancer has a definition of Vasculogenic Mimicry: https://link.springer.com/referenceworkentry/10.1007/978-3-642-16483-5_6165.

Although the biological function of Vasculogenic Mimicry continues to be an active area of biological and medical investigation throughout the world, Dr. Maniotis no longer agrees with these definitions written in Wikipedia and The Encyclopedia of Cancer. He did not write them. Despite one of his mentors at Harvard (Judah Folkman) and his group having been the world's most passionate advocates, researchers, and developers of tumor anti-angiogenesis as a non-toxic, and non-mutable cancer therapeutic target, with the goal of finding non-toxic host proteins that might block tumor-stimulated angiogenesis and its corresponding ability to perfuse and oxygenate a growing tumor, and thus tumor growth and spread, Dr. Maniotis now believes that Vasculogenic Mimicry channels have nothing to do with a functional perfusion and oxygenation conduit to a growing tumor, or that the Vasculogenic Mimicry patterns represent a pseudo tumor-made vasculature.

Instead, according to Dr. Maniotis, his view of cancer today points to work studying the process of the formation of Vasculogenic Mimicry "channels" together with work in which the reversion of malignant tumors to benign tissue is experimentally manipulated suggests that VM represents a tumor biofilm. This "tumor biofilm" does not form until cancer becomes malignant and metastatic. This new hypothesis regarding the primary significance of VM in malignant metastatic tumors has been the result of twenty years of research with Maniotis' own group at The University of Illinois Medical School following his initial characterization of Vasculogenic Mimicry as tumor-made vascular channels at the University of Iowa. In support of this idea, he cites a wealth of evidence exists, and in fact this information has existed for decades, that malignant tumors switch to an anaerobic (glycolytic) metabolism, and do not require oxygen or a blood perfusion system to provide oxygen. These ideas were inspired by Otto Warburg's insightful early 1900's work on glycolysis and tumors that was published between the 1930's and 1950's, which was then followed by Richard A. Malmgren and Clyde C. Flanigan's 1955 demonstration that tetanus spores can germinate only in tumor-bearing mice but never in non-tumor bearing mice or their embryos, which validated Warburg's anaerobic cancer environment hypothesis. With the well-established knowledge that tetanus spores only can germinate in an anaerobic (oxygen-lacking) tissue environment, or in malignant tumor-bearing animal models, the case for malignant cancer being a disease of anaerobic metabolism was experimentally demonstrated, supporting Warburg's lactic acid measurements (anaerobiosis) of ALL cancers. Dr. Maniotis is now attempting to determine if this is the case in the context of VM.

Dr. Maniotis' education and postgraduate research:

1992-1997. Fellow in Surgical Research, Laboratory of Surgical Research and Tumor Angiogenesis, Dr. Judah Folkman, Director. Department of Surgical Research and Pathology, Harvard Medical School, Boston MA.

1991-1992. NIH-post-doctoral Fellow in Cell biology, Cell Biology Group, Worcester Foundation For Experimental Biology, Shrewsbury, MA.

1986-1991. Ph.D., Cell Biology, Cytoskeletal Biology. Departments of Cell, and Molecular Biology, University of California, Berkeley, CA.

1986. Graduate stipend for evolutionary studies, Museum of Vertebrate Zoology, University of California, Berkeley CA. Pre-graduate education and research: 1985-1986. Research Technician, Bioengineering of Functional Muscle. Department of Zoology, University of California, Berkeley CA.

1983-1985. Research Technician, Neuroexitotoxicity, and Developmental Neurobiolgy. McDonnell Center For Higher Brain Function, Departments of Psychiatry, Anatomy Cell Biology, Washington University School of Medicine, St. Louis, MO.

1980-1983. A. B., Physical Anthropology, Human Osteology, Primatology, Population Genetics. Department of Anthropology, Washington University, St. Louis, MO.

Finally, it is worth mentioning that in 2004, Maniotis was recruited to The Board of Directors and Advisor, World Association for Vaccine Education, and The Doctors for Emergency preparedness have posted his articles on multiple occasions.

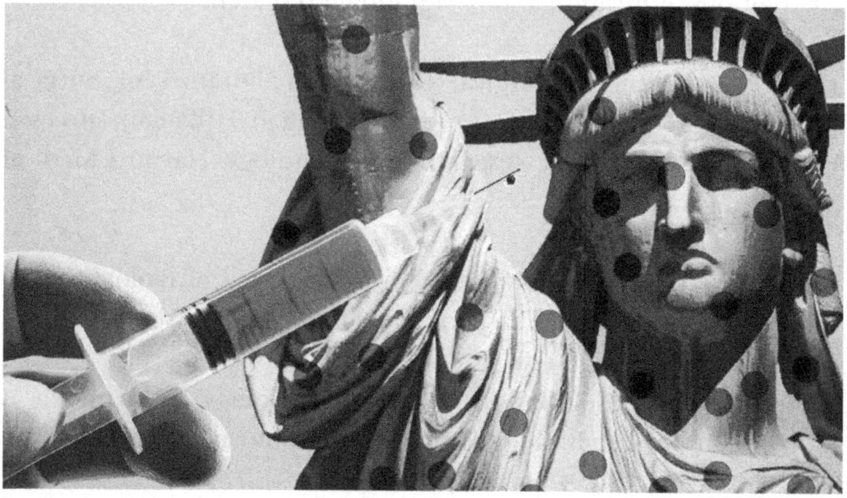

The Statue of Liberty receiving a measles vaccine during New York Governor Mayor De Blasio's reign of terror which threatened religious, orthodox Jews with a fine if they did not get vaccinated with the MMR vaccine and could prove it. The image above was produced during the April 15, 2019 Mayor de BLASIO-declared measles "public health emergency" in ultra-orthodox Jewish communities in Williamsburg, Brooklyn, New York.

"Under the mandatory vaccinations, members of the city's Department of Health and Mental Hygiene will check the vaccination records of any person who may have been in contact with infected patients. The city can't legally physically force someone to get a vaccination, but those who have not received the MMR vaccine or do not have evidence of immunity may be given a violation and could be fined $1,000."

https://abc7news.com/new-york-measles-brooklyn-mandatory-vaccine-yeshiva/5240261/

TABLE OF CONTENTS

About The Author V

Introduction: Science is Not About the Prizes – It is About the Surprises 1
- Paralysis Epidemics 9
- Sars Coronaviruses 12
- Population Growth Control Vaccines? 14
- Rumor Viruses & Virus Testing 15
- Sars 35
- The Great Reset 37
- Testing 50

Chapter I: Vaccines, Covid and the Sacrifice of Common Sense – Forecasts and Auguries of Sorcerers, Witches, and Doctors 59
- Inoculations and Vaccines as Selective Forces on the Human Immune System 69
- Immunization, Inoculation, And Vaccination 70
- Question: Which Immunity Producing Mechanisms Do Vaccines Alter to Produce Immunity? Is it Really as Worked Out as the Medical and Biological Textbooks Say? 75
- Sars Begins in 2003 and Vaccines Roll-Out in February 2021 93

The Evolution of the Early Vaccination Paradigm and the Real Story of Polio – Since the Dawn of Vaccination there has Been a War of Disinformation and False Narratives 96
The Rotovirus Vaccine Roll-Out of Paul Offit 111
The Gifts of Insanity, How Vaccines Began, and How Car Wax Can Save Your Life 116
Can a Polio Vaccine Help Stop the Coronavirus, or Would It Be More Effective to Stop Covid-19'S Reign of Terror Simply by Removing Leading Public Health Officials Who Have Been Given Leadership Roles and Have Invented Other Past Hoaxes?.................................127
Healthy Carriers/Asymptomatics 129
Sars Cov-2 Covid-19 Rhetoric is Based on "Hiv" Testing Rhetoric and Treatment Catastrophes and Other "Challenger-Sized Disasters"................140
References 158
Vaccines and Brain Damage 163
Indictments..167
Epidemic, Endemic, and Herd Immunity 173
Evolution Does Not Anticipate Future Events..........175
Cdc Admits That "Nearly All Polio Outbreaks Since 1961 Were Caused by the Oral Polio Vaccine" 184
No Vaccine Ever Has Been Rigorously Safety Tested for Carcinogenic Potential in Humans However Ample Animal Studies Indicate Vaccines Cause Cancers in Mammals 188
Vaccine Induction of Cancer and the Science of Vaccine Damage: Vaccine Injection Site Spacial and Temporal Associations with Malignant Cancers and Other Maladies..................................190

Irrefutable Scientific Evidence of Vaccine-Induced Cancers in Dogs and Cats at their Vaccine Injection Sites 199
What Causes Vaccine Induced Cancer: Vasculogenic Mimicry as a Tumor Tissue-Produced Biofilm and an "Apogenetic" Controlling Element Suggests a Mechanism to Explain How Damage by Vaccination Occurs Via Dysregulation of Fibronectin and Laminin 210
Tissue Mimicry is Conrolled by Fibronectin and Laminin-A Clue as to How Both Viruses and Vaccine Injuries or Vaccine Inductions of Cancers Lead to Fibrosis 211
A Wide Range of Vaccine-Induced Diseases Besides Cancers in Dogs and Cats 216
With Anthony Fauci and Others Leading the Charge, Perhaps the Largest Failure of the Aids Era Was Published in 2009 in the Nejm: A 3% Rate of Protection (Over Background Levels without the Vaccine) 220
Religious Terminology, Football Strategies, Aids Research, and Original Antigenic Sin 221
Rumor Biology 223
Four Axioms Regarding Vaccines, Genetics, and Epidemics 226
Symptoms and Types 243
Causes 243
Diagnosis 243
Now We Enter the Wonderful World of Sars-Cov-19. What Do the Preliminary Studies with Sars Vaccines Show? 245
Abstract Background: 246
Genetic Engineering, Molecular Biology, Gain of Function Mutants, and Bio-Warfare 251

A Solution to the 12 Hour Sars-Cov-2 Crisis Window that Has Shown Nearly 100% Success Rates 258
Hyperbaric Oxygen Therapy (Hbot) 258
Analysis of the Possible Effects Of Hbot On Ncp 266
Advantages of Hbot 267
Limitations of Hbot 268
Slow Virologists 287
The Human Consequences of False-Positive Diagnoses 291
The Threshold for Establishing Herd Immunity For Sars-Covid-19 Is Not Yet Clear 299
Lab Testing Epidemics, Prevalence, and False-Positives and Negatives have Precedents in "Hiv" Testing and the Human Consequences of False-Positive Diagnoses 308
If Pcr Test Kit Inventor & Nobel Prize Winner Kary Mullis Were Alive Today 314
The Real Fly in the Ointment of Sars-Cov-2 Testing is Christian Drosten 320
External Peer Review of the Rt-Pcr Test Advanced by Drosden Reveals 10 Major Scientific Flaws at the Molecular and Methodological Level: Consequences for False Postive Results: Review Report Corman-Drosten Et Al, Eurosurveillance, 2020 325
The Problems and Consequences that are Emerging with False Positive and False Negative Covid-19 Testing have Precedents in "Hiv" Testing 327
A Solution To The Testing Madness 349
Inaccurate Viral Lab Tests Create and Inflate the Illusion of a Pandemic by Creating Millions of False-Positives 354

The Healthy Sick People 357
The Accuracy Problems with Covid-19 & All Other Viral Testing: Multifactorial Singularities And 20,000 Birds 360
Lockdowns 365
Chapter II The Great Timeline of Vaccine Experimentation On Human Beings: Specific Data From Many Sources 372
Smallpox Travels to the Americas 376
The Conditions Under Which the Anti-Compulsory Vaccination League was Formed in Britain, and When "The Small-Pox" was Introduced from San Francisco 377
Paralysis Outbreaks Began to Occur in Vermont, and it was Non-Contagious in Families, and it was Associated with Cotton Farming, Apple Farming, and Arsenate Residues 386
The Baffling Nature of Tuberculosis Ignites the Public Health and Safety Eugenicists to Begin their Coordinated Efforts to Control Citizens and Parents Via Medical Terrorism 390
The Supreme Court Hands Down its Ruling In The Jacobson Case: Jacobson Vs Commenwealth of Massachusetts Docket 197 Us 11 in 1905 392
The Duration of Immune Bodies in the Blood after Anti-Typhoid 397
The Cause of The Greatest Disease in Human History: 20,000,000 Lives are Estimated to Have Died, But the "Spanish Flu" wasn't from Spain and is Now Believed to Have Been Partly Caused by an International Vaccination Campaign, War, and Not Pfeiffer's Bacterial Baccilis 402

Prevention, Social Distancing, and Lockdown Control of the Great Flu Didn't Work 411
Great Epidemics of Deadly Disease, in Animals and Mankind, Caused by Vaccination: Letters...... 417
Vaccination Both a Theoretical and a Proved Cause of Epidemics and Now Pandemics.............. 418
Grave Nature of Recent Epidemic of Influenza and Pneumonia.. 418
Epidemics are Actually Caused by Vaccination 421
Vaccine Factories a Possible and Proved Source of Epidemics and Should be Investigated by Congress and the Government (In a Democracy, the People-Us-Are the Government) 422
1918 – Epidemics and High Death Rates in the Army Probably Caused by Wholesale and Repeated Vaccinations. Death Rate of Army from Disease Much Greater than that of Civil Population 423
West Nile Virus is Said to Originate from a Healty Black Woman in 1937 before Electron Microscopes Could Confirm it was a Virus............ 430
One Particle from a Turd Launches the Polio Era .. 434
Between the 1950'S and 1980'S, 12 Million Vaccines Cause Yaws, "Hiv," Shistosomiasis, and Hepatitis C.. 435
The Days of Innocence are Over: How Cervical Cancer Cells Changed the World and Helped Win the Biological Arms Race............................... 436
Cdc Changes the Rules for Defining Polio Again 443
Birds Start Swapping Genes with Humans after about 100 Million Years 446
The Era of "Hepatitis B, "Aids," "Slow" Virologists, and Beliefs Regarding Blacks as the Origins of all Pandemics Begins While Dr. Robert Gallo Thinks Viruses Cause Cancers and not Atomic Bombs.. 448

The Pre-Aids Rumor Virus Era Formally Begins 459
Summary 468
Smallpox Vaccine Triggers Aids? 473
Autism Explodes in the United States 479
Blumberg's Frankenstein and-The Homicide of Hepatitis B Vaccine 485
How "Original Antigenic Sin" has Come about During the Era of "Hiv-Aids" Vaccines 507
1995 – Survey of Competing Theories of Aids: A Brief History 509
Disease Progression Despite Antibodies 522
Hepatitis B Vaccine Actually Caused More Illness than the Disease by a 20 to 1 Ratio 526
Birds Catch Cold Flus Too, But it isn't Passed from Person to Person and the Entire Chicken Population of Hong Kong is Slaughtered: The Bird Influenza Era Begins 529
The Bird Flu Era Starts Cashing Out 530
Division of Aids (Daids) Says Everybody's Got "Hiv's" Capsid Protein in their Cells, But to Convict Only Those with More than 30pg/Ml P24 Protein. 533
"Hiv's" Most Important Molecule, Reverse Transcriptase is Found in Chicken Vaccines, And Is Destroyed With Dnase (Reverse Transcriptase is a Protein, not a Nucleic Acid that would be Sensitive To Dnase) 534
How to Read "Aids" Science: Determining Seroconversion from Vaccines Versus True "Hiv" Infection Depends on What Size Your City is, Communication, and Emergency Phone Numbers538
Because the U.s. Vaccine Programmes Couldn't Make Anthrax Vaccine, George Bush Threatened Canada Not to Bust Bayer's Patent Rights on Cipro During the Events Surrounding 9/11 572

More Success with Animal Models of "Hiv/Aids" 619

Children Who Get Flu Vaccine Have Three Times Risk of Hospitalization For Flu, Study Suggests 635

How Did My Daughter, 10, Get Hiv in 2009? 638

Summary of Uk Safety Experience 661

Experts Suggest That Smallpox Vaccine Would Protect Against Hiv (Instead of Cause it as They Said Before) 673

Background: 678

Conclusions: 678

Chapter III The Timeline of the Sars-Covid 19 Great Reset 694

Final Thoughts on Covid-19 Vaccines and Issues with Lab Tests 754

Genetic Determinism in Part has Made Possible the Current Covid-19 Crisis and the Orwellian Lockdown Experience it has Engendered Must be Abandoned and Replaced with an Appreciation of the Dynamic Reciprocity Taking Place in Living Systems 758

Chapter IV Irreconcilable Differences and Historical Distortions 763

Pro-Vaxers and Anti-Vaxers and Seven Outcomes of Vaccine Campaigns 770

The Seven Outcomes of Vaccine Campaigns 776

Vaccines as a Selective Force on the Human Immune System 780

Chapter V Conclusion 788

Generalizations, and Predictions Diagnostics, Aetology, and Causation Regarding Our Present Crisis and the Futures of "The Healthy Sick People" and the Science of Vaccine Damage 788

There is a Solution: The Invention of the Toilets and Development of the Concept of Hygienge Probably has Been More Valuable than Vaccines and Probably Constitutes the Best Public Health Measure You Will Ever Find Anywhere 796
"Let The Food Be Thy Medicine" -Seizures Can be Controlled 800
Appendix I: Reference List for Christine Johnson's Article, "Whose Antibodies are they Anyway? 803

References 803

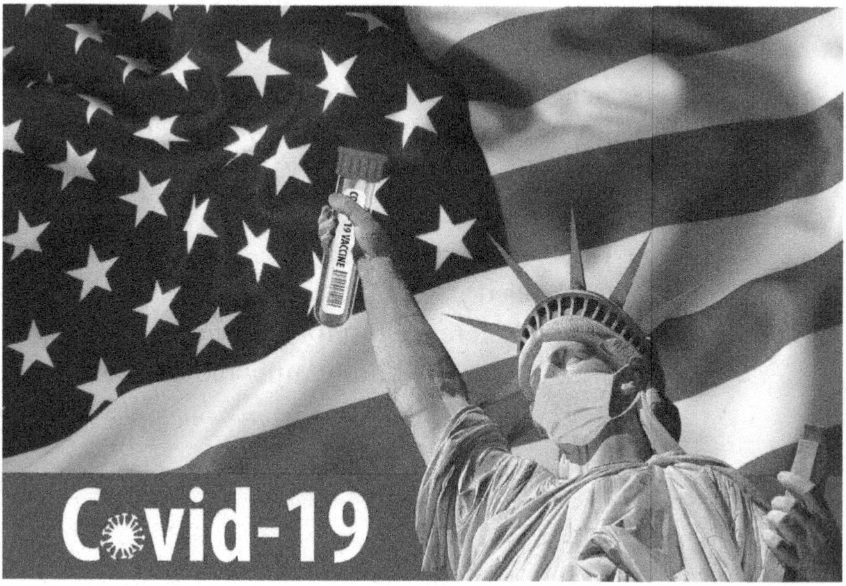

Fourth Amendment

The right of the people *to be secure in their persons*, houses, papers, and effects, against unreasonable searches and seizures, *shall not be violated*, and no Warrants shall issue, but upon probable cause, supported by oath or affirmation, and particularly describing the place to be searched, and the persons or things to be seized.

INTRODUCTION

SCIENCE IS NOT ABOUT THE PRIZES – IT IS ABOUT THE SURPRISES

As a research scientist, as a teacher, and as a human being interested in improving the lives of my children, my students, my friends, families, and our society, my training in science has forced me to question accepted facts and assumptions that I was taught. One of the great lessons of education is to teach others to question their assumptions, especially those things that are of critical importance, such as the health and well-being of a society.

Authentic science is about aggressively trying to disprove hypotheses and theories. Rigorous testing and transparency is the best way to elucidate the truth. In this manner of disproof, science always is expanding its vision and knowledge and in effect is forever striving toward "The Good." According to some of the ancient Greeks, striving toward the good meant that a "good teacher" was rated as a good teacher if their students knew more than they knew. Another way of viewing the nature of science is that it is like a ship that sets sail yet never reaches its distant shore.

History is a critical tool to unravel our current crisis of SARS-COVID-19. Yet only a limited and fragmentary knowledge about homologies of DNA or RNA sequences have been used to justify a global lockdown. This limited and fragmentary knowledge of comparative genetic sequences may be shown in the future to be irrelevant to the current pandemic because knowledge about sequence homologies has been worthless regarding past epidemics and pandemics, or has proven to be not even descriptive of the causal basis of many disease syndromes and their assumed "genetic" causes.

Dogma and a static worldview have no place in science. When we are faced with such modern phenomena as growing rates of pediatric cancers on a national scale, increasing levels of children with learning disabilities, increasing environmental toxins and pollutants and their consequent largely unexplored health effects on populations, or global pandemic influenzas, we are at a place in time like the Wright Brothers were situated in the history of aviation – in a situation much like when they flew their rickety plane for the first time at Kitty Hawk only a few hundred meters. During these primitive beginnings of aviation, did the Wright brothers imagine that humans would be able to someday fly around the entire earth in a few hours in jets, or travel into space?

It takes considerable skill to ask scientifically disprovable questions that will yield information regardless of the answers that a question engenders, and it requires considerable patience to make a habit of separating information from our trust or distrust of the sources of authority of that information.

The problem of origins has always been problematic in biology as it is in all sciences because we rarely see when the origin of a thing or a process happens in complex, exceptionally large, or slow, or amazingly fast, or very small contexts: The origin of The Universe? The origin of life? The origin of vertebrates? The origin of humans? The origin of the chemical elements? And similarly, the real first causes of most diseases? These are but a few examples where time frames, scale sizes, and in the context of living systems and disease, complexity itself has confounded our understanding of origins.

Is all the talk about animal origins of viruses for human epidemics or pandemics factual, or is it completely unsubstantiated (monkey to human in the case of HIV, camel to human in the case of MERS, or bat or pangolin or fish to human in the case of SARS-COVID-19)? Or are these assertions simply more of the same molecular sequence-based propaganda?

With viruses and virus-like particles, which are not living things, but byproducts of healthy and diseased cells, we do know that their origins always occur within the cells that make them. We do not know however, the causal relationship of viral-like particles to most disease pathologies because of complex responses of the immune system to the presence of viral-like particles and the complex changes those tissues exhibit when viral antigens are present in the organism. SARS-COVID-19 presents a good example of this practical gap in our knowledge about viruses and the immune system, in addition to their interactions with the vascular, nervous, or other systems.

In this regard, and with a blind faith in molecular reductionism that worships the DNA or RNA sequence, and which worships and pays homage to Watson and Crick's "secret of life," Anthony Fauci and his friends presently have shut down the entire human race. Fauci and his friends at NIH and CDC and in some state governments have destroyed countless lives, kept children out of school for a year and a half, denied the elderly visitation by their children, ruined myriads of careers and jobs and millions of small businesses, on the basis of a sequence homology of RNA/DNA.

By contrast, Kristi Noem of South Dakota never has shut down her state, and it appears that South Dakota's economy, and the positivity of its citizens has remained intact. Although South Dakota is not a very populated state, it is thriving better than any other state in the union because it (and Governor Noem) has met SARS-COVID-19 rationally. During the height of the SARS-COVID-19 crisis, South Dakota, and Florida under Governor Ron DeSantis, both rationally focused their efforts on the elderly or already sick who had symptoms or were in risk groups rather than "jailing" everybody. Should South Dakota Governor Kristi Noem and her team be given a Nobel Prize? Should Florida Governor DeSantis be maligned by the corporate media pundits, Fauci, and the Biden White House as a "villain" that wouldn't listen to these Fauci-topian dictates, when Florida's SARS-COVID-19 health outcomes are far better than most of the country without all of the collateral economic and psychological damage of mandated masks and lock-downs? In a recent independent study by Dr. Atlas, a SARS-COVID-19 frontline physicians has demonstrated that lockdowns have recently been shown by SARS-COVID-19 physicians to be an independent variable for causing increased morbidity and death (The SARS Pandemic: Will the Truth Prevail? **https://www.youtube.com/watch?v=t6kmm70ji5c)**

Culturing and transmission experiments with masks and mask-wearing have shown in numerous studies to trap pathogenic microbes and make no difference in incidence of SARS-CoV-2 acquisition. What do "cases" mean if the people being tested are asymptomatic? Should we instead focus on hospitalizations and total all-cause mortality rather than just PCR lab positive "cases"?

Why does the current COVID-19 crisis appear to be permeated with "HIV=AIDS" era thinking (***"do you know your status, have you been tested, have you taken your meds, have you gotten your vaccine"***)? These mantras repeated during the HIV-AIDS era remind me of what we hear today about SARS-COVID-19. Are there any similarities between the immune suppression of so-called AIDS victims and SARS-COVID-19 victims? Or is it that the same people who created the AIDS debacle still are working currently in positions of great influence since the AIDS era of the 1980's, such as that cadre of folks that may be best described as "the rumor virologists" (Anthony Fauci, Robert Gallo, Debora Birx, Robert Redfield, and the CDC and the NIH)?

Why hasn't the horrendous air pollution of the atmosphere over the first two epicenters of SARS-COVID-19, which were Wuhan, China, and Bergano, Italy been discussed by the corporate media? There were even televised Chinese citizen protests shown on corporate media illustrating excessive levels of eye-watering and choking air pollution in Wuhan, China immediately preceding the beginning of the 2019 SARS-COVID-19 pandemic. Also, why hasn't the widely disseminated information about the two mandated and legally enforced H1N1 and Hep C experimental vaccine campaigns in fall of 2019 in Bergano, Italy that preceded the Italian SARS-COVID national lockdown and vaccine mandates been more widely acknowledged and discussed?

By analogy, in the context of medicine and the primitive state of development (a "medical dark ages") which it now occupies, we might ask ourselves a hypothetical question: will we someday be able to effectively prevent or ameliorate the deadly disease of cancer and other diseases and do no harm to normal non-tumor cells in the process through non-toxic therapeutics? This was the dream and reasoning of one of my late mentors at Harvard Medical School, Dr Judah Folkman, and he believed that in the cancer context, the non-toxic inhibition of tumor growth could be achieved if he developed what is now the abandoned field of tumor anti-angiogenesis.

Although Dr. Folkman's strategy of non-toxic tumor anti-angiogenesis did not work for human cancers in 4 human clinical trials, the strategy and substances discovered in the process of attempting but failing to block the vascular growth and its provision of oxygen has worked in the contexts of other diseases such as diabetic retinopathy. A possible reason for the failure in the cancer context was an assumption: that tumors, like all tissues are fueled by aerobic respiration (oxygen), when much evidence had been overlooked regarding glucose as being the fuel of tumors which switch to a partial anaerobic (lacking oxygen) existence.

(See: Editorial: When a drug fails. New York Times, July, 2010 **http://www.nytimes.com/2010/07/26/opinion/26mon1.html**)

SARS-COVID-19 is often compared to "The great Spanish Influenza of 1918," yet clinical trials conducted during the 1918 influenza years do not support this claim. First of all, it should be realized that just because some medical historians have surmised that the Great Spanish Flu was caused by a virus that afflicted people with flu-like symptoms, that this statement is a completely unsubstantiated assumption, and in fact it is probably incorrect.

At that time, Pfeiffer's bacillus (a bacterium) discovered toward the end of the 1800's was thought to be the causative agent of several epidemics between the late 1800's and also the Great Spanish Influenza of 1918, and a two decade-long search by Dr. Milton Rosenau and others to find Pfeiffer's bacillus and to show it caused the influenzas during the first and second decades of the 1900's utterly failed to show it caused influenza, or even was associated with it.

In Dr. Milton Rosenau's era, electron microscopes had not yet been invented, nor were they even a thought on a physicist's blackboard before the late 1920's which launched the development of electron microscopy into the mid-1930's. The first fully functional and useful electron microscope (EM) became operational around 1939. **Therefore, there was no lab instrument or device available with which any virus could have been clearly seen and visualized until 1939.**

In Dr. Rosenau's day, while he chased Pfeiffer's bacillus during the first two decades of the 1900's, and instead of any direct visualization of any virus being possible (since EM's weren't yet invented in 1918-19), a variety of ingenious filter types were used to strain out any and all potentially pathogenic microbes in order to provide information about the size of a potential infectious entity, and thus determine at least the dimensions of any agent(s) transmitted that might be responsible for an infection.

Dyes with known pH and other affinities also were used to assess chemical nature of cellular parts and pathologies. Rosenau's characterization of The Great Influenza's causative agent involved tests for both infectivity and transmissibility from sick victims of influenza to more than 100 healthy volunteers in at least 6 human experiments using volunteers. In at least 5 of the smaller volunteer clinical trials that Dr. Rosenau organized to assess infectivity and transmissibility of influenza showed that even when direct exposures of infected sera and lung aspirates of dying or dead patients were collected and then were exposed to healthy volunteers in the form of IV injections, shaking hands, talking 2 inches from a face, coughing of an infected person to a healthy one, **NO** influenza or illness in any of the multiple (6 different) human clinical experiments he organized and carried out occurred (Milton Rosenau, M.D. Experiments to determine mode of spread of Influenza. Journal of The American Medical Association. Vol 73, No 5, pps 311-313, Aug 2, 1919). Dr. Rosenau supervised these experiments that were carried out with the help of the Public Health Service and the U.S. Navy on Gallops Island, the quarantine station in Boston Harbor, and on Angel Island, its counterpart in San Francisco.

Recently, an elegant review paper appeared describing the work of Jeffery Taubenberger, Johan V Hultin, and David M. Morens regarding what a viral genome sequence of The Great Spanish Influenza microbe of 1918 might have been, which they pieced together using modern molecular reverse genetics techniques from material obtained from permafrost's in Canada (Discovery and characterization of the 1918 pandemic influenza virus in historical context. Antivir Ther. 2007; 12 (4 Pt B): 581-591, 2007).

I am not aware of any electron micrographs that documented any virus from these permafrost samples that Taubenberger et al. uncovered: all of their reconstruction is based only upon biochemical (molecular) comparisons. Therefore, it is an unsubstantiated assumption to claim that these permafrost samples contained any coronaviruses, and we are left with the same situation we were placed in historically when Rosenau attempted to determine the pathological agent responsible for the Great Spanish Influenza almost 40 years before the technology of electron microscopy was even invented and reliable and could be used to visualize 120 nM-sized coronaviral crown-shaped particles.

By contrast, Rosenau's 100-year-old 1919 infectivity and transmission experiments may be arguably far more informative in understanding SARS-COVID-19 today than Taubenberger et al.'s 2007 reverse genetic approach to reconstruct a "Great Spanish Flu" genome from an assumed infectious and pathogenic viral cause. This is because Rosenau unequivocally and experimentally demonstrated that in living human beings that there probably was no infective or transmissible agent responsible for "The Great Spanish Influenza" of any kind-not a Pfeiffer's bacillus bacterium, not a fungus, not a mycoplasma, or not even an assumed virus.

Postulating that when influenza is transmitted in a society, the normal transmission routes by which influenza is transmitted are through casual exposures, and to simulate how it was believed influenza may be naturally passed between infected persons and healthy persons, Dr. Rosenau first attempted to transmit the postulated influenza agent through measured experimental casual exposures that involved shaking hands, handling objects, an influenza victim coughing 2 inches away from a healthy person's face, and talking at close proximity. When these casual attempts at transmission did not infect or sicken the healthy, direct injections of lavages of dying or dead persons lung or respiratory fluids was attempted. All attempts to transmit the influenza failed. Perhaps there was another much more likely explanation regarding why so many became ill to account for the projected numbers of 50 million calculated and assumed dead during the Great Influenza?

As it turns out, evidence was later discovered that further supports the conclusion that the Great Spanish Flu probably had nothing to do with an infectious or transmissible microbe.

This evidence instead provides compelling evidence that the 1919 influenza was most likely the result of pre—WW1 over-vaccination, first on military bases, and then in the general civilian population. It appears it was mostly incompetence, rather than malice, that led to these vaccine-deaths during the Spanish-Flu. These Spanish-Flu era vaccines were originally funded and developed by the Rockefeller Institute for Medical Research, which had been established by John D. Rockefeller using his oil wealth in 1901 to support intensive scientific research in medicine, especially infectious diseases.

Similarly, Covid-19 testing and Covid-19 vaccine policy advocacy today has been largely funded by the same Rockefeller Foundation which coincidentally helped finance the World War 1 vaccination campaign that coincided with the so-called Spanish Flu. Why are the same oligarch families involved over the last 100 years in creating our society's pandemic and vaccine policy? How can any of this so-called "philanthropy" benefit the world's peasants and plebeians when the historic and contemporary scientific evidence clearly contradicts their medical policy positions? Which shareholders in which pharmaceutical and testing companies benefited the most from this "pandemic philanthropy" over the last 100 years?

This conclusion that a global vaccine campaign contributed to the deaths attributed to Spanish Flu was arrived at because US military physician and vaccination records of that Spanish-Flu period together with military records of influenza outbreaks in over-vaccinated military bases compared to similar vaccine and prevalence records obtained from the civilian population revealed the fact that those military inductees were essentially pelted with vaccines, and that when the 1918 influenza began, deaths from what was called "Spanish Flu" were 1/4th more prevalent at first on military bases than in the civilian population.

The so-called "influenza" cases of 1918 radiated out from military bases to the general public after the inductees were vaccinated.

The reality is that there is far more that we do not know about the unintended consequences of medical interventions than we do know.

Other relevant documents, sources, and observations regarding the origins of the Great Spanish 1918 influenza from over-vaccination also have been provided by Eleanor McBean in her book, Vaccination the Silent Killer (p28, Source: Dr. Rebecca Carley) where she provides evidence that among the civilian population that was not vaccinated, there was no influenza, and where there was vaccination, there was much morbidity from Spanish Influenza vaccination.

PARALYSIS EPIDEMICS

Epidemics other than influenzas (and pandemics) also have occurred many times during the 1900's, although global lockdowns or even national lockdowns or quarantines were not implemented during these health crises. Probably one of the most feared and widely known of these "epidemics" were the epidemics of paralysis, or what later was named as "polio" epidemics. However, again the documented medical and scientific histories of "epidemic paralysis" or polio epidemics are accompanied by many verifiable facts which argue against the paralysis syndrome being either infectious or contagious or due to some transmissible microbe.

For example, during the latter part of the 1800's, epidemics of paralysis were recorded when New England orchards were sprayed with calcium arsenate, and again during the 1950's when the "polio epidemic" everybody has heard about occurred again, as DDT was sprayed everywhere including in family kitchens and on food. These ubiquitous DDT pesticide sprays were accompanied during those times with pictures in prominent magazines of sinister houseflies landing on babies in their cribs, which was believed to be the feared source of acute flaccid paralysis.

It appears perhaps that the largest shareholders of the world's largest chemical companies developed a sophisticated PR campaign to divert attention away from DDT towards an elusive virus as the cause of polio. It is interesting that these same chemical company shareholders also were the largest funders of virology and vaccine research.

Additionally, during these early smaller paralysis epidemics, nobody could figure out how one person in a large family would become paralyzed without spreading the paralysis to their siblings and close contacts. **Celebrated physicians such as the head of the poliomyelitis society and others during and after the 1950's also had noted that the anterior horn cells of the spinal cord of assumed microbe-induced paralysis during that paralysis epidemic were identically damaged in paralysis cases that had been poisoned by pesticides.**

In addition, reports of these small paralysis epidemics greatly *increased* following the Salk polio vaccine era of the mid-1950's, as documented for instance by some of the first cases that were admitted to Michael Reese hospital in Chicago. For instance, on April 16,

1955, an infant with paralysis was admitted to Michael Reese Hospital in Chicago, IL. The patient had been inoculated in the buttock with "Cutter's" polio vaccine and a week later, on April 24, had developed flaccid paralysis of both legs.

A month later, in May, ninety-nine cases of polio became eventually attributed to Cutter vaccine in California, with the incidence of polio among other cutter vaccinees exceeding the textbook definition of a wild polio epidemic in Idaho by nearly 3-fold, with eighty-eight cases attributed to Cutter vaccine, which was an incidence that was fifteen times greater than pre-vaccine paralysis cases.

Before it was over, the "Cutter incident," as it was called in scientific circles, resulted in 260 people contracting polio and almost 200 cases of paralysis, with eleven deaths. This was why the Salk vaccine was immediately halted in most places round the world where it had been rolled-out in in the previous weeks. This "Cutter incident," as it was called, was one reason why perhaps the Sabin oral polio vaccine was then promoted and still is promoted so vigorously. But in 1972, Jonas Salk, who became a bitter critic of Sabin (the inventor of the IPV-inactivated polio vaccine), testified before a Senate subcommittee, and exclaimed that: ***"nearly all polio outbreaks since 1961 were caused by the oral polio vaccine."***

And by 1992, America's Centers for Disease Control (CDC) in Atlanta admitted that the polio live-virus vaccine had become the main cause of polio in the United States. Specifically, the CDC asserted that:

"From 1973 to 1983, **87%** of all (non-imported) cases of polio resulted directly **from vaccine administration**. Even more amazingly, it was asserted that **every** non-imported case of polio in the United States from 1980 to 1989 was vaccine-induced." (Strebel, P. M., et al., Epidemiology of Poliomyelitis in the U.S., One Decade after the Last Reported Case of Indigenous Wild Virus Associated Disease, Clinical Infectious Diseases, CDC, February, pp. 568-579, 1992). Currently, there have been many allegations that the oral polio vaccine appears to be creating small paralysis epidemics in India and in Nigeria, as part of the WHO's and Gates Foundation's drives to promote polio vaccines in these Nations.

During this polio epidemic of the 1950's (there have been many this last Century), at least in the US, and although an alarm went off internationally, the most draconian consequence of the "epidemic" was that people were temporarily banned from theaters and schools. Yet no paralysis epidemic or any other one of these "declared" paralysis epidemics, or other transmissible disease epidemics have been accompanied with the moniker of "pandemic," or by a global response of similar even National lock-down mandates, or by voluntary or mandated global quarantines for any other infectious disease as we have seen with COVID-19.

Regarding pathological behavioral epidemics, a growing "suicide epidemic" is now said to be claiming returning veterans of "the Freedom Operations" of the Middle East, and an opioid epidemic nationwide is said to be in full swing. Epidemics of violence in economically depressed areas in all our major cities has become commonplace. **Still again, nothing like even a national lockdown has occurred for any of these behavioral "epidemics."**

SARS CORONAVIRUSES

SARS coronaviruses were first isolated, and high-resolution electron micrographs of SARS coronavirus-like particles were documented by Tyrrell and Bynoe in 1966. The crown-shaped SARS coronavirus-like particles also were shown to be associated with the transmission of a significant number of colds. Although these SARS-CoV-2 viral-like particles were isolated, photographed, were crown-like in appearance, and are associated with colds and occasional pneumonias, the mechanism of their pathogenicity is still not clear. One fact is certain though: coronaviruses are real viruses and not cellular garbage that simply look like viruses.

Morphologically, the crown-shaped SARS coronavirus particles which have been isolated and elegantly photographed using EM have not been experimentally transmitted to volunteers during SARS-COVID-19 to produce the feared atypical massive cytokine storm-associated pneumonia symptoms, or the crown particle-associated vascular and coagulation problems which tend to be a primary cause of death in SARS-COVID-19 atypical pneumonia victims. This is probably because it would be deemed unethical, and potentially fatal to any voluntary recipients who might harbor cryptic pre-existing conditions, and the incredibly old and those with one, two, three or more underlying health conditions.

It is worth noting in addition for such a thought experiment that would involve infecting volunteers with SARS-CoV-2, since the beginning of the SARS-COVID-19 pandemic there have been developed curative protocols to manage current victims with mild, atypical pneumonia symptoms before they require hospitalization or die, but these protocols have not been widely publicized until recently because of the "promise" of universal vaccination, and all the politics that goes with a vaccination solution.

The experiment of David Tyrell and Mark Bynoe involved exposing volunteers to a nasal swab from a boy with a mild cold in 1960. This original "B814" nasal swab sampling and transmission was supplemented by repeating the procedure later using other volunteers who had developed colds.

A number of In Vitro and chemical experiments also were performed on the samples, which revealed that the agent associated with the induction of colds wasn't influenza A,B, C viruses, parainfluenza 1,2,3,4 viruses, respiratory syncycial viruses, adenoviruses, cytopathic enteroviruses, herpes simplex viruses, rhinoviruses, or mycoplasma pneumonae. None of these were found.

Filter experiments lent further evidence that the agent was a virus because the agent could pass through a bacteria-tight filter, was inactivated by ether, and could induce colds in volunteers that in preparation as recipients, were given sufficient antibiotics to cure a fully developed infection with the "Eaton agent" (M. pneumonia) (Elizabeth Mahase, BMJ, 396, 2020). The agent was then imaged on an electron microscope and dubbed a coronavirus by June Alemeda and David Tyrell.

Another critical fact is that in a vast majority of "cases," and as Rosenau's 1919 experimental transmission studies showed, when and if transmission did or does not occur, symptoms (influenza symptoms) tend to be mild rather than deadly.

This fact supports the likelihood that it is the relative health or robustness, or the relative infirmity or pre-existing health conditions of the infected person (or population) which determines the severity of disease symptoms: not the infectious agent itself. Apparently this was true during the SARS and MERS epidemics, as it does today with SARS-COVID 19. It is the health of the host rather than the pathogen that determines outcome.

POPULATION GROWTH CONTROL VACCINES?

By 1974, a NSS Memorandum 200 [National Security Study Memorandum 200] had already been drafted by Henry Kissinger, and was based on a classified memo sent by Kissinger to select cabinet officials of the Nixon Administration titled: Implications of Worldwide Population Growth for US Security and Overseas Interests (THE KISSINGER REPORT), it wasn't until 1976 that information became generally known about the design and implementation of human sterilization vaccines that were being tested on human subjects with the addition of HCG concealed in tetanus toxoid vaccines to induce anti-HCG antibodies to thwart pregnancy. The motion by Kissinger and others was to be modeled after PIP which is a legal term which describes eugenic sterilization of a person who is either mentally ill or mentally defective and will either severely handicap any future offspring through heredity or is unable to properly care for a child.

"Antibody response to Pr-beta-HCG-TT vaccine in human subjects Contraception 1976 Feb;13(2):237-43. doi: 10.1016/0010-7824(76)90037-8. G P Talwar, S K Dubey, M Salahuddin,C Das https://pubmed.ncbi.nlm.nih.gov/1245129/"

Abstract

PIP: Antibody response to processed beta human chorionic gonadotropin tetanus toxoid vaccine (Pr-beta-HCG-TT) was investigated in 4 human subjects who were in reproductive age and of proven fertility and had undergone tubal ligations. The subjects responded by producing detectable anti-HCG antibodies after a lag period of 6-8 weeks and plateau levels at about 5 months after primary immunization with the vaccine. Anti-HCG antibody titers were still high in 3 subjects after nearly 11 months of immunization. The titers declined to near 0 after 16 months in 1 subject indicating the reversibility of antibody response with this vaccine. The antibodies reacted immunologically with the HCG molecule and were competent to neutralize the biological activity of HCG in the radioligand receptor assay.

In 2014, a report appeared with the following title:

"A mass sterilization exercise': Kenyan doctors find anti-fertility agent in UN tetanus vaccine."

https://www.lifesitenews.com/news/a-mass-sterilization-exercise-kenyan-doctors-find-anti-fertility-agent-in-u

I cannot conceive of a better way of preventing illnesses, epidemics, or vaccine-associated endemically growing syndromes than by preventing fertilization, can you?

RUMOR VIRUSES & VIRUS TESTING

The "HIV-AIDS" era also forms the basis our current COVID-19 crisis because a high-ranking appointee named Robert Gallo still runs the National Institute of Health's Institute for Human Virology, supported by Anthony Fauci, and with the highest biomedical budget of them all, brokered by under Trump by the lead White House strategist of the Global coronavirus "pandemic," Debora Birx, with help from former appointed head of the CDC, Robert Redfield. All three, Gallo, Birx, and Redfield, were veterans of the HIV-AIDS era in the 1990s and strategy/policy for HIV-AIDS. HIV-AIDS brought us sexual distancing, whereas the opportunity of Covid-19 brought us social-distancing. Additionally testing asymptomatic people during Covid gets its precedent in HIV testing, with many scientists, including the inventor of PCR testing, Nobel Prize winner Kary Mullis, and Dr. Rodney Richards, creator of the very first HIV tests for Amgen, and myself all in disagreement with NIH and CDC guidance about the utility or accuracy of asymptomatic virus testing.

Robert Gallo, Anthony Fauci, Barbara Birx, Robert Redfield, the CDC, the NIH, and many others foisted the "HIV" testing and AZT hoax upon a generation of gay men (most of the early AIDS deaths were from side effects from AZT, the drug used to treat AIDS). Additionally, we proved in landmark court cases that the test kits used to determine if someone had "HIV" were defective and giving off false-positives much of the time and ruining countless lives. Just look up the case of Audrey Serrano, who I was chief scientific advisor to, who was awarded $2.5 million by a court for a false HIV diagnosis. Her life was ruined by mistakes made by people influenced by Gallo, Fauci, and Birx.

Audrey Serrano was the first diagnosed "AIDS" patient I consulted with as her unpaid lead scientific advisor. I performed this work at night and on the weekends while working as a full-time medical school researcher and associate professor at the University of Illinois at Chicago Medical School. We proved in court that Audrey Serrano was wrongly diagnosed with HIV/AIDS and Audrey was awarded $2.5M. Audrey stopped taking AZT and her quality of life improved dramatically and she went on to lead a healthy and normal life, although she still had lingering health issues related to her past consumption of AZT. This is the first court case in the USA of an AIDS patient successfully overturning their diagnosis in a court in the United States. There were **hundreds of thousands** of other

AIDS patients who could have proven the same and overturned their HIV/AIDS diagnosis in court due to defective HIV test kits if they had the benefit of the right scientific experts in virology and lab tests helping them. Here you can read a CBS article about Audrey Serrano's successful court case: https://www.cbsnews.com/news/woman-misdiagnosed-with-hiv-awarded-25m/

This important video interview is with me, Audrey Serrano, and Dr. Rodney Richards who worked as a lead scientist at AMGEN on developing the very first HIV test kits. This is a must-watch explanation from the developer of the first widely-used HIV tests in the US of the scientific problems with using leading mainstream lab tests to confirm HIV/AIDS viral status (as well as other viral infections): https://www.bitchute.com/video/dIpw3moUXTKZ/ What is contained in this video could be said about Covid-19 testing.

Leaping forward in time from the era of the 'polio epidemic" of the late 1950's to the late 1960's to Nixon's and Johnson's war on cancer, what may be most aptly described as an extended iatrogenic catastrophe took place and which still is taking place today, with the huge, failed effort to prove that postulated cancer viruses caused cancers in humans without confounding co-factors or without permissive carcinogenic experimental conditions. In effect, an enormous, failed effort was unleashed by the biomedical community in and following this era to demonstrate that viruses caused cancer.

These assumed cancer viruses included Rous's sarcoma virus, SV-40, or Simian Virus 40 and various cancers associated with its molecular signature, Baruch Blumberg's hepatitis B virus and liver cancers, HTLV-1, HTLV-II, and leukemias, which was repurposed and renamed by Robert Gallo HTLV-III", then LAV by the French Nobelist's Montagnier's group, and then which then later was renamed "HIV" by the Varmus committee.

Even though Payton Rous protested and wrote begrudgingly in his Nobel acceptance speech lecture that there was never any proof a cancer virus in his studies, or in any other studies that could directly link tumor viruses to any cancer, but much evidence implicating a soluble toxin, the biomedical community ignored him because they wanted to believe there was a cancer virus. **For instance, in his 1966 Nobel acceptance speech, Rous argued that his Sarcoma causing agent he had discovered was never shown to cause cancer in humans, nor had any other virus, yet his observations and concerns were and are still completely ignored.**

In the context of "HTLV-I," "HVLV-II," and "HTLV-III which was named "LAV" then "HIV," during the late 1970's, Robert Gallo and others failed to show any causal connection or even a convincing association (which is not proof of causation) between his assumed cancer viruses HTLV-I and HTLV-II, HTLV-III and leukemias. Instead of accepting that no virus was directly linked to a cancer, including those viral ghosts Robert Gallo was trying to push on the world, Gallo first tried to promote popular survey data he had acquired of Japanese residents who had lived near Nagasaki and Hiroshima during the atomic bombings who had contracted leukemia some years after the US terrorized their civilian city populations instead of their armies with atom bombs.

Within weeks to months of Robert Gallo's claims which at first attempted to link three new viruses to leukemia, the biomedical community dismissed them, and his cancer-virus ideas were totally discredited. Dr. Peter Duesberg, the National Academy of Sciences Member, Semmelweis National Award Member, and the discoverer of retroviruses always has maintained that "HIV" is nothing but a harmless molecular passenger that does no harm. For this view, Duesberg has been persistently and constantly vilified by the AIDS establishment for 35 years.

But NIH's Robert Gallo, a close professional colleague of NIH's Anthony Fauci, wanted his picture in The Big Picture Book of Viruses next to a first cancer virus cartoon picture or photograph of a viral-like particle, and when the biomedical community laughed at him and told him to go home, and when the early 1980's sexual revolution hit, he invented or transformed "HTLV-III into "the AIDS virus."

The result of these numerous failures to demonstrate that any cancer virus was the likely direct cause of cancer in human leukemias despite Robert Gallo's & the biomedical establishment's initial zeal to do so, and as a result of Gallo's failure and everyone else's failure to link a virus to leukemia or to any other cancer, HTLV-III/"HIV" was eventually fully accepted as being the so-called "AIDS" virus after it was renamed "HIV."

Not only that, "HIV" was promoted as being the single agent responsible for the first two AIDS-defining syndromes, Kaposi's sarcoma, and Pneumocystis carinii pneumonia because "HIV" supposedly allowed normally harmless and ubiquitous pathogens to take hold in the "HIV" infected persons (it is not yet established whether P. carinii is a fungus or a protozoan)./span>

During the late 1980's after the biomedical world eventually realized that Gallo's 3rd imagined cancer-virus association he named HTLV-III was another mistaken molecular association of a virus with cancers, and these molecular signatures were renamed "HIV," which now was linked to the cancers and immune suppressive spectrum of diseases associated with AIDS (including the cancer, Kaposi's sarcoma). Then, "HIV" was accused of being the probable cause of AIDS by the Varmus committee while he was director of the biomedical research establishment.

For example, Gallo believed that "HIV" caused the normally indolent Kaposi's lesion associated with another viral signature (Herpes virus VIII) to behave aggressively only in "HIV" immunocompromised people. Similarly, he believed that "HIV" caused a normally harmless and ubiquitous microbe called Pneumocistis carinii which normally is present and does no harm in immunocompetent people, caused fatal pneumonias in "HIV" immunocompromised victims.

Gallo propagandized these interpretations even after the noted tumor anti-angiogenesis guru, Harvard Medical School's Dr. Judah Folkman who was my chairman and boss, rejected the idea and data that aggressive Kaposi's sarcomas could be caused by "HIV" while I worked for Dr. Folkman at Harvard. Despite these exchanges between

Dr. Folkman and Dr. Gallo in the hallways where I worked at Harvard Medical School's 9th floor in The Ender's building, Gallo persisted in his propaganda that "HIV" caused the immunosuppressed conditions which allowed Herpesvirus VIII to cause a malignant form of Kaposi's sarcoma, and Pneumocistis carenii to cause fatal pneumonia.

But it was still a mystery how a normally indolent Kaposi's lesion that had been seen on the ankles of Mediterranean males **for 100 years before the AIDS era** and named by Moritz Kaposi a Century before could be the result of the same pathogen that caused the aggressive form which became malignant, and often metastatic to the lungs and other vital organs, and life-ending in the immunologically suppressed victims (IV drug users, transfusion recipients, etc.).

The obvious answer for everyone seemed to be that immune suppression itself could lead to cancer, that is, until Dr. Folkman reminded everyone that the child's immune system is far less developed than an older person's immune system, yet cancer is predominantly a disease of old persons.

The initial 1984 AIDS "pandemic" by press release was presented to the American public and to the world by a sun glass-wearing Robert Gallo with HHS Secretary Margaret Heckler standing by his side while announcing, "the probable cause of AIDS has been found, to be a **variant of a known cancer virus**." An effective "HIV" vaccine was promised to be forthcoming in 2 years (by 1986).

In the context of both past and current "HIV" test kits, and in the context of the continued failure for modern diagnosticians to 1) properly isolate "HIV" on a sucrose density gradient since the 1980's and then employ electron microscopic verification of the isolated band at 1.16 grams/sucrose/liter (**an identification test for retroviruses**), or 2) show that the particles from the 1.16 sucrose gradient band could cause AIDS in an experimental animal (**fulfilling Koch's postulates**), and 3) **the utter failure to demonstrate "HIV" viremia in an "HIV" positive infected person said to harbor "HIV" viral loads in the millions even once (not "SIV" signatures in monkeys which constitutes a different molecular signature or entity than "HIV")**, or 4) demonstrate infection in any animal model infected with human mythical "HIV" purified particles, the existence of "HIV" has remained a fiction, if not a lie throughout the entire AIDS era. Not only that, the relationship between "HIV" and any of the dozens of clinical diseases the "experts" said "HIV" causes never has been demonstrated.

Now some 37.9 million people are said to have been claimed by AIDS world-wide, which qualifies it at least as a theoretical pandemic that has been far more destructive than other so-called pandemics and epidemics. However, just as with Covid-19 vaccines are causing tens of thousands of deaths today, many of the deaths attributed to AIDS were actually caused by the toxic, off-label chemotherapy drug AZT and other comorbidities including lack of clean water, clean food, and exposure to medical industry chemical toxins. As with Covid-19 testing, HIV tests were abused to create an illusion people were dying of AIDS that were in fact dying of other illnesses including iatrogenic (medically-caused) illnesses. According to a recent study out of Johns Hopkins medical errors and pharmaceutical side effects are the third leading cause of death.

Importantly, and relevant to what currently is going on with SARS-COVID-19 and the initial stigmatization of it being "a Chinese disease," the AIDS syndrome was highly politicized during the Reagan Administration because of homophobia and stigmatization of the gay community to such an extent that Reagan himself wouldn't even use the word "gay," or AIDS publicly.

A few years into the "AIDS epidemic," Luc Montagnier's group at the Pasteur Institute claimed to have isolated "LAV" or "lymphadenopathy-associated virus" in 1983 (later renamed "HIV") from a homosexual male who had been treated for gonorrhea and syphilis several times in the preceding years (which was the first case among many that led to the "sexual distancing" recommendations of those times-see Papadopulos-Eleopulos E, Turner VF, Papadimitriou J, Page B, Causer D, Alfonso H, Mhlongo S, Miller T, Maniotis A, Fiala C. A critique of the Montagnier evidence for the HIV/AIDS hypothesis. Med Hypotheses 63(4):597-601, 2004).

After several famous movie stars and other high profile, white, "innocent" American victims became ill with profound immune suppressive illnesses or PCP pneumonia, such as the actor Rock Hudson, a boy named Ryan White who then was accused of generating a positive "HIV" test while presenting clinically with various non-specific symptoms came to the attention of the nation, AIDS became more mainstream and accepted as a paradigm by the establishment. Ryan White's crisis as was Kimberly Bergalis' crisis, were relatively non-specific health crises in young, white, non-gay victims of the "HIV" tests (prone to false positives just like modern Covid-19 tests), and like many others their high-profile plights became politicized which ultimately led to The Ryan White Act which still is in place today.

Ryan White's demise and death was likely caused likely by his intake of the AIDS pharmaceutical AZT. "Shortly after, Ryan began taking AZT, a failed cancer drug that was the first anti-HIV medication. And shortly after, he started his journey to becoming a worldwide spokesman for AIDS education." https://eu.indystar.com/story/news/health/2020/04/07/ryan-white-would-48-inside-his-life-and-death-aids-30-years-ago/2907636001/

A great article about the unethical use and fast-tracking "Warp Speed" introduction of AZT as an AIDS treatment during the AIDS era is this classic article by Celia Farber in Spin Magazine: https://www.spin.com/featured/aids-and-the-azt-scandal-spin-1989-feature-sins-of-omission/

Here is what Bob Guccione Jr., the founder of Spin magazine, wrote in 2015 about Celia Farber's reporting in the 1989 on AZT:

> ***"At the end of 1989****, two years after we had started the highly controversial AIDS column in SPIN, we published an article by Celia Farber called "Sins of Omission" about the truly bad and corrupt science surrounding promoting AZT as a treatment for the syndrome of diseases.*
>
> *Celia was the editor and frequent writer of the column and unearthed hard evidence of the cold-bloodedness of the AIDS establishment pushing a drug that was worse than the disease and killed*

faster than the natural progression of AIDS left untreated. AZT had been an abandoned cancer drug, discarded because of its fatal toxicity, resurrected in the cynical belief that AIDS patients were going to die anyway, so trying it out was sort of like playing with the house's money. Because the drug did not require the usual massively expensive research and trial processes, having gone through those years earlier, it was insanely profitable for its maker, Burroughs Wellcome. It was a tragically perfect storm of windfall profits, something to pacify AIDS activists and the media, and a convenient boom to the patent holders for HIV testing.

Celia — who should get the Congressional Medal of Honor for her brave and relentless reporting, here and throughout the ten years we ran the column — exposed the worthlessness of the drug, the shady studies and deals to suppress the negative findings, and its awful and final consequences. This piece very literally changed the media's view of AIDS and sharpened their discerning and skeptical eye. And soon after, AZT was once again shelved, hopefully this time forever.

Many times over the years since, people have come up to me and said that reading this article saved their lives, that they either stopped taking the drug and their health improved vastly, or they never took it because of what we reported. Nothing ever made me prouder."

— Bob Guccione Jr., founder of SPIN Magazine, October 3, 2015

Kimberly Ann Bergalis (January 19, 1968–December 8, 1991) was the first to allegedly contract "HIV/AIDS" from a medical appointment (the Dentist David Acer) and was the first alleged case of clinical transmission of HIV. Her death was likely caused, like Ryan White's, by the side effects of AZT, a failed chemotherapy drug that was so lethal it was not allowed by the FDA to be used for cancer patients but was fast-tracked for use on "AIDS" patients with the help of people like NIH's Anthony Fauci and Robert Gallo. This 1991 Seattle Times article describes Kimberly's AZT side effects prior to her death: *Her pain: "I have lived to see my hair fall out, my body lose over 40 pounds, blisters on my sides. I have lived to go through nausea and vomiting, continual night sweats, chronic fevers of 103 to 104 that do not go away anymore. I have cramping and diarrhea… . I have lived through the torturous acne that infested my face and neck – brought on by AZT."* See: https://archive.seattletimes.com/archive/?date=19910620&slug=1290084

Wikipedia's account of Kimberly Ann Bergalis case: *"The incident prompted The CDC to conduct a phylogenetic analysis of the DNA sequences of the viral envelope gene, and the analysis revealed that the viral sequences from five patients, including Bergalis, were more closely related to the dentist's viral sequences than to those from local controls. Later analyses identified another HIV-positive patient with a viral sequence closely related to Acer's. Independent review of the CDC tests strengthened the case that Bergalis' HIV infection was linked to Acer…The Florida Department of Health and Rehabilitative services subsequently tested over 1000 patients, discovering two additional HIV-positive patients. The CDC would eventually identify a total of ten HIV-positive former Acer patients and link the infections of six to Acer… During the last months of her life, Bergalis' case was cited by some politicians and journalists as an example of a 'blameless' HIV infection that had been allowed to happen due to the CDC and the healthcare industry being overly responsive to the concerns of AIDS activists and the gay community."*

Many other AIDS deaths, however, were most likely due to doctors' poisoning the "HIV-positive" **accused victims** of the diagnostic tests with the so-called AIDS drug AZT given at exceptionally high doses, as was also the case with the entire "HIV" positive gay community between the mid 1980's and early 90's, until the lethal drug concentration was eventually reduced enough in AIDS patients in the late 90s to enable the AZT drugged to survive a few years longer than only one or two years after starting AZT. Yes, many of the salacious side effects of AIDS including pneumonia, weight loss, and reduced immunity, were exact side effects of taking the cancer chemotherapy drug AZT.

The "AIDS" cases among "innocent," non-homosexual, and white victims like Ryan White and Kimberly Bergalis with the help of the Reagan administration and homophobia eventually led to terrorizing the nation and the world with panic-porn, and to the justification and the [false] belief and mandate that "everyone was at risk," that "you should know your status" ("HIV" status), and that "even asymptomatic people should be tested" (similar to what is going on today with SARS-Covid-19). The mandates for "HIV" testing were also fueled by the damaging slogan "AIDS does not discriminate" mantra that we have all came to love and to know during the AIDS era

The precedence for today's failed social-distancing during Covid-19, and the failed testing of asymptomatic people for Covid-19 and failed "Warp-Speed" therapeutics and vaccines, can be traced back to the same exact people and failed policies during the failed HIV/AIDS era and all can be traced back to Anthony Fauci and Robert Gallo at NIH.

Such National treasures as Arthur Ashe, the tennis legend, Rudolph Nureyev,the epitome of ballet perfection, and the two-time Heavyweight Champion of the world, Tommy Morrison (at the height of his boxing career) were all "HIV" tested and accused of having "the AIDS virus." But it was the test itself, and dangerous AIDS treatments, and not "HIV" itself that led to each of their professional and health destruction.

I knew Tommy Morrison as a good friend over a several year period after his false-positive HIV diagnosis. Tommy Morrison was a 1993 world heavyweight champion WBO boxer who starred in the Rocky V movie. Tommy was "HIV" tested during a pre-fight physical causing the destruction of his professional and personal life due to a false-positive HIV virus test result due to a faulty, inaccurate virus test. Between 1989 and 1996 during his pre-fight physicals, Tommy always was found in perfect health by every measure by the physicians the boxing commission had hired, and by his own personal physicians. Tommy was perhaps one of the healthiest humans I have ever met, but after 1989, he was shamed by the stigma so he hid from the world the fact that he had tested "HIV"-positive because he had loved boxing so much. The stigma of a positive test could disqualify him from the blood sport. **He also had had a son and several wives of many years who had sex with Tommy who all were tested and found to be "HIV" negative.**

Don King had somehow found out about Tommy's "status," and demanded that the Nevada Boxing Commission force Tommy to take a pre-fight "HIV test" before his 1996 fight with Mike Tyson. My guess is King did this to disqualify Tommy from being able to fight Mike Tyson because of both his successes and defeat to Ray Mercer in previous fights.

When the results of that test came back positive, Tommy then told the press and his fans that he had lived a promiscuous lifestyle for many years, not only in Hollywood when he made Rocky V with Sylvester Stallone, but during his entire teenage and adult life. Everyone became concerned about many of Tommy's bloody fights they had witnessed between 1989 and 1996, and that Tommy may have transmitted "HIV" to many of his opponents. The Nevada Boxing Commission, and everyone else suggested "HIV" testing each and every fighter Tommy had faced during those years.

However, surprisingly, NIH's Anthony Fauci made one of his signature flip-flop statements and came to Tommy's rescue and defense and stated to the media that: "one study showed that the likelihood of transmitting the AIDS virus in a football game, with much contact, was "astronomically low — one in about 80 million." Fauci cited as extremely beneficial the professional and college basketball rule requiring a player who is bleeding to come out of a game so that the wound can be covered.

(https://www.washingtonpost.com/archive/sports/1996/02/13/morrison-confirms-hiv-result/c108319f-74fb-4821-a130-dcb6a336c793/).

I hold no resentments or grudges towards any of these people. I pray they eventually wake up, look at new scientific evidence with a fresh perspective, apologize, and speak the truth, and help us reform the medical system and dark ages we now find ourselves in. We are all flawed, and everyone can change and reform. Sometimes we are blinded to the truth. As a scientist I respect anyone who changes their opinion in light of new scientific evidence more than someone who holds the same opinion regardless of what new "disproving" evidence has shown them.

Tommy did not die of AIDS but instead he died at the age of 44 from harm caused by his doctors (iatrogenocide) because of septicemia, septic shock, multi-system organ failure and, ultimately, cardiac arrest as the result of a botched surgery he had received for an infected spider bite under his right pectoralis muscle. The surgeons left 20 feet of gauze in the surgical wound they debrided because they forgot to remove it, and it became infected over the course of a week before his wife found a tip of the 20-foot bandage sticking out of his chest one morning, took him to the hospital, and then called me.

Tommy Morrison died in agony and with a touch of pugilistic syndrome, but not of "HIV" infection. During the AIDS era, I had witnessed approximately 50 similar tragedies due to the belief in a phony molecular test that has no prognostic value.

There were many other high-profile people also who were similarly sacrificed on the altar of "the AIDS virus," and also were killed by the toxicity of AZT or other iatrogenic interventions following their positive "HIV" tests that condemned them all to the failed cancer drug arsenal of the AIDS establishment, or other toxic treatments. But it did not really matter what these folks actually died from.

The "HIV"-positive test result immediately placed them in the "HIV/AIDS" death camp. In fact, all of the iatrogenic drug deaths after the first AZT Fischl trial in 1987 were blamed on "HIV" and AIDS rather than the rank poison drugs the victims were given. If victims, victim's families or the friends of a person exhibiting a positive "HIV" test, or even many highly respected doctors such as Alfred Hassig (who was head of the European blood bank) or scientists who'd discovered retroviruses such as Peter Duesberg, protested the fake "HIV" tests or the fake pathogenesis believed to be specific to "HIV," or if they protested the drug iatrogenocide of the nucleoside analogs or the toxicity and worthlessness of the protease inhibitors, they were silenced, marginalized, fired, shunned, threatened, and summarily destroyed by the AIDS establishment monster led by persons such as Robert Gallo, Anthony Fauci, Deborah Birx,

Robert Redfield, the CDC, NIH, and many other promoters of the "HIV=AIDS" paradigm and the toxic cancer drug solution.

It took the Ryan White Act following his death from the so-called AIDS drug AZT to codify the mandates that "everyone was at risk," "do you know your status," slogans that we have all come to love and know during the AIDS era. All of the iatrogenic drug deaths after the first AZT Fischl trial in 1987 were blamed on "HIV" and AIDS.

It did not (doesn't) matter to them that p24, another protein once thought to be unique to "HIV" is known to be expressed in the thymus glands of **HIV-negative** children (Dura WT, Wozniewicz BM. Expression of antigens homologous to human retrovirus molecules in normal and severely atrophic thymus. Thymus 22 (4):245-54, 1994).

Nor did it matter to them that other studies show that goat and cow milk that is unpasteurized induce positive "HIV" tests (Willman et al., Heterophile Antibodies to Bovine and Caprine Proteins Causing False-Positive Human Immunodeficiency Virus Type 1 and Other Enzyme-Linked Immunosorbent Assay Results. Clinical and Diagnostic Laboratory Immunology, p. 615-616, Vol. 6, No. 4, July 1999).

It did not give them pause when the work was published that showed that fifty percent of dogs also exhibited "HIV" structural proteins but did not develop "AIDS" (Strandstrom et al., Studies with canine sera that contain antibodies which recognize human immunodeficiency virus structural proteins Cancer Res 1990 Sep 1;50 17 Suppl: 5628S-5630S). It was and still is of no concern to them that chromosome reconstitution experiments testing the hypothesized ability of "HIV" integrase to interact with normal chromosomes in order to integrate the "HIV" genome into the infected cell's genome revealed that the enzyme had no activity when compared side by side with histone H1 or polyamines, or the topoisomerases, and thus constituted a negative control for the minor groove-binding of the topoisomerases (Bojanowski, K., Maniotis, A., Ingber, D. DNA topoisomerase II can control chromatin topology and drive chromosome condensation without enzymatically modifying DNA. J. Cellular Biochem. Vol. 69:127-142, 1998).

Most importantly perhaps in the context of this analysis because it is so frequently given and given early in life, that the hepatitis B vaccine is known to cause positive HIV test results (Lee, D, Eby W, Molinaro, G. HIV false positivity after Hepatitis B vaccination. Lancet 339: 1060, 1992). This is a similar fraud to the manner by which influenza vaccines cause "HIV" positive test results in all age groups (Simonsen L, Buffington J, Shapiro CN, et al. Multiple false reactions in viral antibody screening assays after influenza vaccination. Am J Epidemiol 141:1089-1096,1995).

The first large-scale HIV vaccine trial was undertaken in 1998. The VaxGen trial was initiated as a Phase 3 trial of a vaccine called AIDSVAX (VAX004) in North America and the Netherlands involving more than 5,400 volunteers. It failed utterly to protect a single vaccine recipient from acquiring an "HIV-"positive lab test. In 1999, NIAID began the first African preventive HIV vaccine trial in Uganda, and the first large-scale HIV vaccine trial in a developing country began, and it ended without a single vaccinated person protected from acquiring a positive "HIV" test or AIDS.

VaxGen then initiated a Phase 3 trial of AIDSVAX (VAX003) involving over 2,500 volunteers in Thailand. By 2004, all VaxGen candidate vaccines had failed to exhibit protection against acquiring HIV in multiple Phase 3 trials. All of these trials were resounding failures. In 2007, NIAID halted the Phase 2 Step and Phambili studies due to safety concerns. The STEP Study was a Phase II b clinical trial intended to study the efficacy of an experimental "HIV" vaccine based on a human adenovirus 5 (HAdV-5) vector. The study was conducted in North and South America, the Caribbean, and Australia. The final assessment of the results of the aborted STEP trail, according to Robert Gallo, was that it was a "challenger-sized disaster".

A related study, the "Phambili trial", used the same experimental vaccine that was used in the STEP trial and was conducted at the same time as the STEP trial, but on a different population of vaccine recipients in South Africa. These trials were co-sponsored by Merck, the HIV Trials Network (HVTN), and the National Institute of Allergy and Infectious Diseases (NIAID). In South Africa, the trial was overseen by the South African AIDS Vaccine Initiative. All of them failed to prevent a single "HIV"-positive test result or the development of AIDS. And some of these trials were eventually terminated before their scheduled conclusion, when the Data Safety Monitoring Board determined that the vaccine was not preventing HIV infection and was possibly enhancing susceptibility to HIV "infection" in some of the study participants (it was inducing false positive "HIV" tests). This phenomenon of prematurely stopping vaccine trials has happened many times in the past, and not only with "HIV" vaccines.

In 2005, Newsweek reported that VaxGen, a little-known California biotechnology company at that time, would start its first delivery of its anthrax vaccine to the government and military for Bush's war in Iraq six months later than originally slated. The company was awarded an $877.5 million contract to produce and manufacture the anthrax vaccine, which was developed by the U.S. Army Medical Research Institute of Infectious Diseases (USAMRIID), and it was issued as a reward for the company's vaccine failure to protect a single individual from acquiring an "HIV"-positive test result in their previous "HIV"-vaccine trials.

Seventy-five million doses of VaxGen's vaccine were then procured for the Strategic National Stockpile under Project Bioshield, a joint Department of Homeland Security (DHS) and Department of Health and Human Services (HHS) initiative to stimulate the creation of a domestic biodefense industry. Five million doses of Vaxgen competitor Bioport's vaccine were also procured in response to Bioport's aggressive lobbying and anti-VaxGen campaign. VaxGen's vaccine was never approved by the Food and Drug Administration. Bioport's vaccine, which has been used by the Defense Department, has been controversial because of its side effects and its FDA approval has been disputed (Project on Government Oversight, Vera Hassner Sharav).

Results of the Phase 3 "HIV" Thai vaccine Trial (RV144) at first claimed that the vaccine combination demonstrated a modest preventive effect in humans. The trial, which enrolled more than 16,000 volunteers, was the first, and to date, the only (up to 2009), large clinical study (of the more than 225 failed trials) that has claimed any kind of efficacy for an investigational HIV vaccine.

This large Military-Thailand "HIV" vaccine trial, which deployed its "HIV" vaccine dud in 8 thousand arms and resulted in only a fraudulently statistically arrived at significance compared to placebo controls injected only with an aluminum-containing solution to mimic the experimental vaccine's contents was claimed as "a success." However, if you look at the numbers published regarding this "HIV" vaccine trial carefully involving 8,000 recipients injected with the "HIV" envelope protein GP160 and aluminum, and 8,000 controls injected only with aluminum but lacking GP160 glycoprotein, a difference in "true seroconversion" between the two groups was reported as 0.6% (of 8,000) experimental "HIV" vaccine: versus 0.8% with aluminum only controls. This is what is called "a modest effect" of a vaccine, according to the AIDS establishment.

Here is the outcome of that trial more graphically:

Aluminum boosted Aluminum without Background "HIV" detection:

-gp120 "background"-	-gp120 Military-	-Thailand trial aluminum-
1.3%	0.6%	0.8%

The numbers would make it appear that it is a good idea to inject everybody with aluminum only because it is cheap-and will reduce the levels of "HIV" detection by 0.5% in the absence of co-injected and expensive to acquire and manufacture gp120 (1.3 is the background level, -0.8=0.5% over background).

According to Anthony Fauci in recent statements, the Military-Thailand "HIV" trail was a dazzling success! This trial cost 101 +

million. One might ask the question: "What benefit was gained for that expenditure and what benefits will be obtained for the 500 million a year spent for the 172 vaccines that have been in 'the pipeline' since then?"

According to what was understood two decades ago about man's immune system, it was assumed that a vaccinated individual would develop antibodies against those molecules that are foreign to the human body. This would mean, in the case of an "HIV/AIDS" vaccine, and whether "HIV" was isolated and purified to homogeneity or not, the vaccinated would need to carry around a letter to prove their "HIV-positive status" was caused by a vaccine, rather than from "risky" behaviors, or from being in an "at risk" group (from sex, dirty needles, exposure at the time of birth, breast-feeding, transfusions, being of African descent, being gay, being a drug addict, being pregnant, from having an autoimmune disease, or for dozens of other reasons).

But after more than 224+ failed "HIV" vaccine trials, letters as proof of "HIV" vaccination have not been needed. The few who have exhibited an "HIV-positive" test result (the expected outcome after vaccination) have been told their "HIV-positive" status was due to their own "risky" activities (drugs, sex), and not due to the vaccine. These individuals are now regarded and treated as AIDS patients, regardless of their health status, and despite the fact they received an "HIV" vaccine. The repeated failure of "HIV" vaccines to produce an appropriate immune response (conversion from a negative to a positive "HIV" test result) or to confer protection from "HIV" or AIDS in those vaccinated after so many "HIV" vaccine trials except perhaps in a tiny number of recipients (e.g., 0.6%) strongly suggests some measure of urgency or alarm is in order.

Failure to seroconvert to a positive "HIV" test result after vaccination can mean one of two things: either the principles underlying immunology, biochemistry, genetics, epidemiology, virology, cell biology, pharmacology, neonatology, and cancer biology simply do not apply to "HIV/AIDS," or it means that the hypothesized "HIV" causation of "AIDS," and the imagined and false molecular biological causal basis of AIDS AND several other "molecular diseases" have generated catastrophic disasters.

The high death rate of victims given the rank AIDS drug poisons was really no surprise because AZT toxicity blocked DNA synthesis and human cell division as proven during the drug's development. In the 1960's it was tested as a cancer drug in rats harboring implanted tumors, but it was shelved for its toxicity to save rats from being poisoned to death and ruining experiments. Yet for some reason, Sam Broder was appointed by President Ronald Reagan to be Director of the National Cancer Institute in 1989, and he decided to dust off AZT, and use it to poison a generation of gay men, and pregnant mothers in Africa and elsewhere. Broder was a cancer and biomedical researcher who became Director of the National Cancer Institute from 1989 to 1995 where he had co-developed the nucleoside DNA replication inhibitors (zidovudine (AZT), didanosine (ddI) and zalcitabine (ddC) which were all highly immunotoxic, neurotoxic, and liver-toxic failed and often deadly cancer drugs.

In Vitro experiments of cancer cells with AZT and indirect biochemical tests indicated that AZT possibly inhibited cancer cell proliferation but it was deemed too deadly to use on cancer patients. However insanely, AZT became licensed for the treatment of AIDS, which is a disease characterized by a lack of cells instead of like cancer, wildly dividing cells. After the 4-month Fischl Human AZT trial was abruptly and prematurely halted after a record 4 months, AZT was then insanely repurposed for AIDS and for those exhibiting an "HIV"-positive test, or symptoms of immune collapse. Normally DNA terminators (inhibitors of DNA replication) when used in cancer are cycled because they are so toxic, and the body cannot replace its normal cells as long as the drug is taken and for a largely unknown period after the drug is stopped. Yet the "HIV" AIDS protocol ignored this decades acquired knowledge and replaced it instead with these phrases, "be compliant and take your meds," "hit hard and early," and "you aren't entitled to taking a "drug holiday," which would come to characterize the AIDS-drug era. Other phrases were, "because your virus will mutate and kill you if you stop the drug, you must be forever compliant."

As long as the fact that AIDS never has left its original risk groups is ignored, no science can be accomplished regarding this anergic immune suppressive states that are diagnosed as AIDS. Regarding the original risk groups during the AIDS era, starvation was and still is one of the most certain ways of acquiring the helper-T-cell ratios characteristic and diagnostic of AIDS in places like Africa (and elsewhere). Meanwhile, and during the massive drug liberation of the 1980's in developed countries, illicit IV drug use (as well as the prescription use of certain drugs) constituted and remains still today the other primary risk group for the development (not infection) of AIDS, because of the antigenic mayhem shooting drugs and certain prescriptions drugs cause, not because of any effects of an infectious, transmitted virus, fungus, or mycoplasma.

In Los Angeles in 1981, Dr. Michael Gottlieb reported that cytomegalovirus (CMV) causes AIDS because he found CMV in 100% of his first 5 sick patients. A decade later in 1991, it was reported that 22/34 AIDS victims harbored Mycoplasma incognitis infections whereas 0 (zero) patients that were not sick with anergy and without AIDS showed evidence of Mycoplasm incognitis infection (Lo SC, Hayes MM, Wang RY, Pierce PF, Kotani H, Shih, JW. Armed Forces Institute of Pathology: Newly discovered mycoplasma isolated from patients infected with HIV. Lancet. Dec 7; 338 (8780):1415-8, 1991).

As long as the non-transmissibility co-factors such as starvation and IV drug use in the context of AIDS is ignored, the reality of an infectious agent in AIDS will remain a fable. Non-infectiousness and non-transmissibility was unequivocally shown to be the case in the case of the mythical "HIV" by the failure to transfer of a positive RT-PCR+ test result between any of 150 positive/negative sexual partners as the Padian study clearly showed with that study's recorded transmission rate of zero among 150 discordant couples having protected and unprotected sex over a 10-year period (Padian, et al. Heterosexual Transmission of HIV in Northern California: Results from a Ten-Year Study." American Journal of Epidemiology. August, 1997). This result was reminiscent of Rabinau's 6 failed infectivity and transmission experiments published in 1919 where he even injected sera and lung aspirates taken from dying or dead victims of influenza into volunteers without transmission of influenza, yet the finding has been persistently ignored by the AIDS establishment.

And as long as AZT and similar toxic protease inhibitors are used to irrationally block some mythical viral replication in AIDS victims, the bodies will continue to pile up. Even the theoretical effect of an "anti-viral" is biologically irrational because viruses are made by cells, and to impede or block viral production necessitates interfering with some normal cellular metabolic processes, not by directly "killing" or incapacitating a virus. Basic virology has long established that the exterior of viruses, as are all of its molecules, made by the cells they infect. Both AZT and the protease inhibitors not only are failed and highly toxic cancer drugs that block cell division and other essential cellular processes such as DNA synthesis, but they have also been shown to be directly cytotoxic and neurotoxic. No improvements will be made to reverse the profound anergy and immune suppression of nutrition-AIDS or drug-induced AIDS as long as this "HIV=AIDS" hypothesis is not demolished. It is hoped that this type of insanity will not be used again to manage SARS-COVID-19, although in some respects it is in the context of the new vaccines, and despite the medical leadership of SARS-COVID-19 being comprised of the same leaders that led the AIDS era: Anthony Fauci, Debora Birx, Robert Redfield, Robert C. Gallo, the CDC, and the NIH, not to mention the contributions of some of the same globalists (who funded AIDS and are now funding the vaccine development of SARS-COVID-19).

SARS

This same scenario that happened during the AIDS era is now being repeated over and over again with SARS-COVID-19. People die of car accidents, of old age, of complications of diabetes, of complications of obesity, of cancer. Yet if they receive a positive test result on Drosden's PCR test for SARS-COVID-19, they are said to have died of COVID-19. In the context of SARS-COVID-19, it is important to realize that it has been known since 2017 that the seasonal influenza vaccine not only causes many false positive SARS-CoV-2 tests, but it also induces military inductees receiving their typical flu shot upon recruitment to suffer from coronavirus respiratory pathogenicity 30% more often than from other respiratory viruses. For the Department of Defense study see: Greg G Wolf. Influenza vaccination and respiratory virus interference among Department of Defense personnel during the 2017-2018 influenza. Vaccine 38, 350-354, 2020 and: https://www.sciencedirect.com/science/article/pii/S0264410X19313647?via%3Dihub).

In 2003, SARS viruses associated with colds were again isolated to relative purity and the initial purification validated at electron microscope resolution again, and these isolates were shown to cause disease in a macaque animal model, as published by Ron A. M. Fouchier, Thijs Kuiken, Martin Schutten, et al in 200 which was presented in a Nature paper (Koch's Postulates Fulfilled for SARS Nature, VOL 423, p. 240, 2003) confirming Tyrell and Bynoe's and others' earlier 1960's work on the association of colds and SARS-CoV-2 crown shaped viral-like particles. Although these particles in the Fouchier et al. study were isolated from a total of 4 sick macaques (two initially, then two experimentally infected), this did not mean that the SARS viral particles directly caused their illness. The exact mechanisms of pathogenesis of these particles today are still an active area of investigation (their pulmonary versus vascular tropisms and perturbation of clotting, etc.), and Fouchier et al. appropriately provided the following caveat about assuming SARS virus particle pathogenesis is fully responsible for SARS with the statement: "*SARS-associated coronavirus (SCV) fulfils all of Koch's postulates as the primary aetiological agent of SARS. This does not exclude the possibility that other pathogens, including human metapneumovirus*

(HMPV) and Chlamydia pneumoniae, may have exacerbated the disease in some SARS patients."

THE GREAT RESET

Confusingly, and frightfully, we then arrived at the wonderful psychedelic light show of COVID-19 in 2019-20, and allegations and even official investigations began to emerge that appeared surreal. These allegations argued that the origin of SARS-COVID-19 was man-made as a result of Dr. Fauci and the NIH funding to the Wuhan Institute of Virology to make sinister and life-ending "gain of function" (GOF) constructs on a harmless bat coronavirus, and that somehow, that viral construct escaped or was released on the world to cause millions of deaths.

Instead of a story about elegant volunteer transmission and ultrastructural characterization studies as we had been accustomed to hearing about since Tyrell and Bynoe's 1966 experiment, or instead of reading about elegant animal transmission experiments as Fouchier et al's 2003 elegant macaque transmission and pathology experiments had shown, we were presented with a kind of surreal pseudo-scientific apocalyptic nightmare that featured the destruction of civilizations throughout the entire planet.

Although some of the pious molecular sequencers swore that "Gain-of-Function" constructs were in fact what constituted the new deadly coronavirus through comparisons of sequence analyses, it goes to show how far we have departed from science being about the surprises and strayed from science's utility as a tool to know.

All we were left with was extreme speculation, fear, and uncertainties regarding SARS-COVID-19, which served only to accomplish an avoidance of any truly scientific discussion, honest inquiry, or in earnest scientific investigation, which persists to this day.

The entire human race and all of the enlightenment it had acquired over the past 2000 years, and civilization itself was "reset"

and became guided by sorcery and a Faucitopian nightmare of a lock-down and vaccine-induced iatrogenocide instead of science.

In addition, and initially, in both of the worlds of SARS-COVID-19 atypical pneumonia case epicenters, Wuhan, China, and Bergano, Italy, environmental air pollution had been a serious concern as a co-factor in the development of the SARS-CoV-2 associated atypical pneumonias. For instance, before SARS-COVID-19 was ever announced, air pollution had been the topic and the focal point of loud protests in China before SARS-COVID-19 was announced. Between December, 2019-through March 2020, satellite cameras orbiting the earth over Italy clearly documented thick cloud banks of air pollution floating over Bergano, Italy, and they clearly showed that this Northern region of Italy for some reason harbored some of the worst air pollution in Europe.

However, and in addition, and also part of the Bergano SARS-COVID-19 experience, a more likely trigger than air pollution for SARS emergence in this SARS-COVID-19 epicenter had been set into motion. It was the consequence of what has now become the familiar specter in the history of epidemics of over-vaccination by a rabid Italian Health Ministry whose mantra and divine mission was to vaccinate every Italian who breathed during the previous decade.

In the fall of 2019, a new experimental H1N1 flu vaccine was jabbed into some 400,000 Italians through a new draconian vaccine mandate, followed in December 2019 by a new, experimental hepatitis C vaccine given to some 40,000 of the of those same 400,000 thousand Italians who had previously received the experimental H1N1 flu vaccine in September.

This was beyond criminal conceptualization, because hepatitis C never has been isolated in the first place, or convincingly photographed with an electron microscope, and the so-called hepatitis C liver disease, detected of course only through surrogate markers (no hepatitis C virus has ever been isolated), always has predominantly been a disease of IV drug addicts, and early during the so-called AIDS pandemic it was claimed, "affected persons (with AIDS) eat too many peanuts and drink too much hard booze" – not Northern Italians eating their pasta with goat cheese. Another way of illustrating the wisdom of mandating the hepatitis C vaccine is to ask, "are Northern Italians all IV drug addicts deserving of a hepatitis C vaccine?" Or to ask, did the coming weather-frosted coming of an ordinary seasonal flu epidemic warrant the jabbing of 400,000+ Italians upon threat of fines?" Such threats were levied at the Italian people. Whether the Chinese in Wuhan also were playing around with vaccines pre-SARS-COVID-19 is unknown, but possible.

Perhaps it is no coincidence that we are faced with the same ethical and public health crisis policy conundrums today that Americans of the early decades of the late 1800's and early 1900's had to navigate through:

Americans had to navigate the yellow fever "epidemic" in which blood-letting and mercury was still being applied for its victims. Americans also navigated the New England paralysis "epidemic" that later became associated with the late 1800's calcium arsenate poisonings of the tree orchards in New England and elsewhere. Calcium arsenate is an important environmental pollutant still today, and dominates much of the modern ground water pollution and contamination literature, because iron, lead, and calcium carbonate-rich rocks absorb arsenic, as did New England residents at the time, who consumed a lot of fruit and developed paralysis. Americans navigated the rapids of the Great Spanish Flu "epidemic" of 1918 that followed the first mandatory vaccinations of WWI soldiers. Americans navigated the closing of all movie theaters, schools and swimming pools during the 1950's and 1960's polio era "epidemic" during the height of the DDT era when the polio disease was said by corporate media to be spread by flies, and when in fact DDT, which causes paralysis, was being sprayed even in kitchens and on food.

Why were not some or all of these similar large-scale "epidemics" throughout history accompanied by global or even national lock-downs or quarantines of healthy, asymptomatic people to the extent that warranted the declaration of a global pandemic as we are currently experiencing, or even culture-specific or country-wide lock-downs implemented during various national epidemics?

Or have these "global lock-downs" happened before, and the history books have lost track of them? South Dakota led by Kristi Noem never had a lockdown since the beginning of SARS-COVID-19, and they managed the elderly or elderly and infirm victims only, and that state has shown financial and health prosperity like few other states in recent months, and also, they have experienced no excessive mortality compared to states that have insisted on draconian "Faucitopian" lockdown measures for its citizens and businesses.

These well documented facts do not mean that the SARS-CoV-2 virus-like particles are not a necessary co-factor in the SARS-COVID-19 syndrome. However, the South Dakota experience suggests that there are alternative ways to reduce mortality risk from SARS-COVID-19 that do not include lockdowns and Covid-19 vaccines and ventilators.

Also, regarding the emergency lockdown and vaccine responses to SARS COVID-19, Dr. Russell Blaylock, a board-certified neurosurgeon, college professor, and renowned author of many books regarding medicine, has asserted that vaccines are not necessary for Covid-19, and this is Dr. Blaylock's reasoning:

A) SARS-COVID-19 doesn't meet the criteria of a pandemic because all age groups aren't equally or lethally affected as they are each year mildly by the seasonal world-sweeping flu (only the extremely aged or those harboring one, two, and three or more pre-existing morbid conditions tend to show symptoms of SARS-COVID-19) whereas all age groups exhibit a sensitivity to seasonal flu, which he argues does qualify as a pandemic disease because it sweeps through the world, although it is a mild disease in the vast majority of cases.

To this Dr. Blaylock adds, "When examining the death rate by age, it is seen that this virus is hardly the 1918 flu virus authorities are implying it to be. Official data shows that the non-institutionalized fatal infection ratio for all age groups is 0.26%. For those less than age 40, the risk of dying from this virus falls to 0.01%, meaning these people have a 99.99% chance they will recover should they become infected. In Italy, which had the highest death rate from this virus in the world, found that over 98% of the case fatalities occurred among those over age 80 years who had at least two prior major medical conditions;"

B) the death rate from SARS-COVID-19 is vanishingly low (in agreement with most government and independent sources), and only those of extreme age (like the Bergano experience) and those harboring one, two, and three or more pre-existing medical conditions die of SARS-CoV-2;

C) when effective treatments are available for those morbidly ill with an infectious disease, such as hydroxychloroquine, ivermectin, steroids, and anti-coagulants, there is no need to vaccinate everybody;

D) the latest VAER's figures suggest that more than 4,200 people have died in connection with the vaccines. Of these 943 died from Covid vaccines that were aged 12 to 17 years old.

For a published analysis one must go back to an earlier date, as it was used in a calculation for comparison — vaccine deaths vs COVID infection deaths. At the time of that study, 1,551 Covid-19 vaccine-related deaths were reported to VAERS (today that VAERS # is about 20,000 COVID-19 vaccine deaths). That would be a death rate of 0.0028%. If we correct for the poor reporting, we will see there were most likely 155,100 deaths or 0.28% death rate for all the vaccinated. The death rate from the infection itself was 0.01% for those under age 40 years. That would mean that the death rate from the vaccine was approximately 28 times higher than the death rate from the virus itself. The numbers of adverse events so far tallied by VAERS and other vaccine adverse effect monitoring mechanisms in place now suggest that in a noticeably short few months, the SARS-COVID-19 vaccines will create hundreds of thousands and probably millions of permanently vaccine-damaged people in 2021.

Interestingly, Dr. Blaylock also pointed out that we have no idea concerning the safety of these vaccines, or how long the spike proteins continue to be made by our vaccinated cells, since no studies on what happens to the spike proteins once they have been injected have been done, and most important, there is no information about how long the mRNA will keep producing the spike proteins that are introduced via the vaccines have been conducted. The mRNA introduced via the vaccine produces large amounts of the spike protein for an undetermined period of time, which accumulates in the brain and several other organs for what could be a prolonged period. And because it is known that the spike protein is highly immunogenic and toxic, it is possible the spike protein will act as a continuous source of inflammation and excitotoxicity (immunoexcitotoxicity) in the brain and result in several neurodegenerative diseases, such as Alzheimer's dementia, Parkinson's disease, and ALS, among others in the long run.

Other celebrated physicians, such as cardiologist Dr. Peter McCullough of the Heart and Vascular Institute in Dallas have been treating SARS-COVID-19 victims successfully since the beginning of the pandemic by using a medical strategy that first dampens the effects of the virus-like particles using an anti-viral, followed by managing the explosive and highly deregulated and unusually severe immune response of the spike proteins of SARS-CoV-2 with hydroxychloroquine, ivermectin, and steroids, following by a regimen of anti-coagulants which he claims blocks the actual terminal phase of the disease in those harboring one, two, or three or more pre-existing conditions or who are very old.

He and his colleagues refer to this approach as Sequential Multi-drug therapy. He has been reporting near 100% success rates at treating SARS-COVID-19 of these victims without vaccination, as he has testified before congress, and written about in two of the most cited papers currently published in the peer-reviewed literature that describe his protocol of Sequence Multi-drug therapy. He is perhaps one of the few physicians in the US who is treating SARS-COVID 19 patients early to avoid two outcomes: hospitalization and death. https://www.foxnews.com/politics/dr-peter-mccullough-tells-tucker-carlson-today-the-world-has-gone-off-the-rails-with-treating-covid-19.

The fact that McCullough's Sequence Multi-drug therapy works, or any other protocol that improves the resistance and rehabilitation and cure of SARS-COVID-19 victims works would threaten the FDA Emergency-Use-Authorization (EUA) approval of vaccines. This is because a condition for approval of an Emergency Use Authorization is stated in legal language in the following way:

> *"Under an EUA, FDA may allow the use of unapproved medical products, or unapproved uses of approved medical products in an emergency to diagnose, treat, or prevent serious or life-threatening diseases or conditions when certain statutory criteria have been met,* ***including that there are no adequate, approved, and available alternatives.*** *" McCollough's Sequential Multi-drug therapy would be such an adequate, approved, and available alternative that would keep people out of hospitals, treat SARS-COVID-19 victims, and prevent death."*

Meanwhile, in Queensland, Australia, they are jailing physicians for 6 months if they treat early with hydroxychloroquine, and reports are news-flashed around the globe from Australia threatening to round people up and incarcerate them in quarantine camps for at least 14 days until they test RT-PCR-negative for SARS-CoV-2. The entire United States University System is now threatening to require vaccination and proof of vaccination for all students to return to school next term without exemptions of any kind being granted, although faculty are not under this same threat currently.

Despite the well-established knowledge that SARS-CoV-2 vaccines have been shown to cause what is known as life-threatening pulmonary "enhancement" or exacerbation of pulmonary disease resembling SARS-COVID-19 itself as well as cardiomyopathies in humans and in animal models, and publications by the army have shown that that a number of routine vaccines can enhance the detection of coronaviruses to a detection level that is 1/3 higher than any other virus (a phenomenon called viral interference), the pharmaceutical criminals and the world are pitched on universally administered untested vaccines, and they are committed to ignoring existing therapeutics which are already proven safe, and which work, such as Sequential Multi-drug Therapy.

These SARS-CoV-2 vaccines are known by government vaccine adverse event reports also to cause hypoxemia (an inability to breathe or dissolve oxygen into the bloodstream), in addition to autoimmune diseases of all kinds, clotting disorders, bleeding disorders which usually constitutes the proximal cause of death.

A short listing of known Covid-19 vaccine-adverse events compiled during the last several months from VAERS, the US federal government's Vaccine Adverse Event Reporting System, and patient testimony presented recently by renowned, and accomplished neurosurgeon, Professor, & author Dr. Russell Blaylock includes:

- **Persistence of an intense immune reaction producing continuous tissue and organ destruction.**
- **Induction of autoimmunity involving a number of tissues and organs (we know that the spike protein cross-reacts with over 28 human tissues and cell components.)** ***(EG: in other words, the antibodies we produce will attack any one or all of those 28 tissues – we will be attacking ourselves)***
- **Induction of swelling of various tissues (edema).**
- **Problems with coagulation, which can include bleeding and/ or blood clots.**
- **Induction of immune cell priming, which can set the stage for widespread inflammatory tissue destruction and agonizing death.** ***(EG: or pathogenic priming or antibody-dependent enhancement).***

- **Triggering of neurodegenerative disorders, such as Alzheimer's dementia, Parkinson's disease and especially ALS.**
- **Triggering transverse myelitis with permanent paralysis—either paraplegia or quadriplegia.**
- **Triggering of multiple sclerosis.**
- **Worsening of reactions to wild type virus in vaccinated individuals, leading to severe immune reactions or death.**
- **Myocarditis and sudden cardiac death or progressive heart failure.**

It has been reported by many front-line medical sources that ventilators have killed off many of the sickest patients after they are utilized during the last breathless stages of SARS-COVID-19 morbidity. Ventilators simply cannot provide enough oxygen for the atypical pneumonia syndrome that is experienced by SARS-COVID-19 victims during the last morbid stages of their illness. This, like vaccines, is a form is iatrogenocide, meaning death by medical intervention.

This fact invites a suggestion regarding the best and least toxic possible therapeutic for the sickest atypical pneumonia patients. Hyperbaric oxygen therapy has shown a success rate of nearly 100% recovery rate in most small trials, and in most HBOT-SARS-COVID-19 trials so far, a success rate of 100% during even the fatal stages of disease progression (with HBOT, the PaO2/FiO2 ratio is adjusted such that the available oxygen- (PAO2) is forced into the blood and becomes blood-dissolved oxygen-FiO2). Numerous clinical trials of HBOT currently are being conducted using hyperbaric oxygen therapy in China, Texas, New York, NIH, and elsewhere.

This technology of treating people with pressurized air began 300 years ago as a treatment for altitude sickness, and because oxygen wasn't discovered until the mid-1800's, it wasn't combined with pressure for any therapeutics. The familiar use of modern hyperbaric oxygen was an essential tool for divers experiencing the bends, smoke inhalation victims (who work predominantly in fire departments), poisoning victims, infections unresponsive to drugs (because the pressurized oxygen oxidizes everything including viruses), healing wounds that will not heal, and many other indications.

These are but a few of its 16 FDA approved uses in the US for hyperbaric oxygen, whereas Russia employs HBOT for 73 conditions that do not respond to current standards of medical care. With all of hyperbaric oxygen's alphabet list of other non-toxic benefits which will be presented in detail, and which will be a major topic covered in one of the earlier chapters, it is not only rational for those who are the most severe atypical pneumonia victims, but it works, and there are many ongoing small clinical trials of hyperbaric oxygen and SARS-COVID-19 victims that are currently in progress.

In this regard, and as a related topic, it has been established that a local or systemic hypoxic state occurs in various tissues during disease syndromes such as cancer and SARS-COVID-19, and also following vaccinations, as has been shown in the past happening to brains after vaccination by brain-injury and neurology expert Dr. Andrew Moulden. The hypoxic damage either can be local or systemic. Researchers in March, 2021 at Columbia University Irving Medical Center published an article in the journal Brain looking for SARS-CoV-2 were looking at the brains of 41 individuals who had succumbed to SARS-CoV-2 and using multiple techniques could not detect virus in neurons but found traces of viral RNA in brain blood vessels. However, they did find small pockets of hypoxic damage particularly in the brain stem, which they explain as being the result of hypoxia. They argue that these pockets of hypoxia-damaged neurons activate glia to attack and eat them, which then occurs leaving the victim with permanent damage.

https://academic.oup.com/brain/advance-article/doi/10.1093/brain/awab148/6226391?searchresult=1

Hyperbaric oxygen safely, effectively, and rapidly reverses these hypoxemias with as few as only 5 "dives" in a hyperbaric chamber. Of course, it goes without saying that early treatment would prevent this kind of damage. HBOT is used extensively for stroke patients with hypoxic brain damage, cerebral palsy with great success, autism spectrum disorders, and many other neurological maladies. In addition, in the context of therapeutically "bringing back" stroke patients with HBOT, it has been found, that although neurons die in stroke patients as they do in all severe hypoxic brain damage, often a penumbra of neurons surrounding the dead neurons are only "crippled," and not dead. These penumbral areas can be "brought back to life" with HBOT "dives," and significant amount of function if not complete function is restored. The same might be true with the hypoxic permanent brain damage brought about by the hypoxemia created in the brain and brain stem by SARS-CoV-2.

In its 300-year-old history, only 2 people and a horse have been killed with hyperbaric oxygen before guidelines were set into place to avoid sparks in the chamber from horseshoes or articles attached to clothing. Twenty-five-million-dollar Kentucky racehorses enjoy hyperbaric oxygen frequently when they damage or injure their legs because HBOT induces their wounds or breaks to heal twice as fast.

As the data in this book will prove and demonstrate, there never has been a vaccine in all of history that has been rigorously scientifically safety tested in the same way as standard medications or food products and no vaccine in history has scientifically been proven to be effective by any scientific measure in all of history using scientific methods and evidence rather than public relations.

Having been written about or mentioned in Science Magazine numerous times and worked in the world's leading scientific research labs at Harvard Medical School, UC Berkeley, Washington University Medical School, the University of Illinois at Chicago Medical School, and having reviewed grants for the National Cancer Institute, I can say with professional certainty as a leading cancer scientist and biologist that almost all vaccine science and virology science is 100% junk, garbage science and vaccine science for some odd reason abides by a different set of rules from the more rigorous science practices required in other areas of biology and other scientific fields like physics or chemistry. Corruption by money and special interests seems to be the reason. Vaccine narratives about efficacy and safety are more of a product of medicine-by-press release public-relations than of scientific method. They are neither safe, nor effective as this book will prove.

Regarding a natural source of SARS-CoV-2 (the non-Gain of Function natural acquisition of SARS-CoV-2 hypotheses), currently, nobody has reported seeing a leaping virus, although many "authorities" initially speculated, based on zero scientific evidence, that it leapt from bats, and pangolins, and out of fish markets. God knows what other innocent critters have been accused. Both alpha and betacoronaviruses have been linked to rodents, birds, and market civits.

Similarly, during MERS (the Middle Eastern Respiratory Syndrome) debacle, it was believed at that time, based on zero scientific proof or evidence, that SARS leapt off of camels to humans.

For the initial acquisition of AIDS, it has been argued for decades that "HIV" leapt off of monkeys to humans during the 16th Century slave trade, as Dr. Robert Gallo once argued using art work from the 1600's as evidence, and reinforcing once again, the AIDS establishment's racially motivated theory of a monkey to black man disease origin of AIDS, which had precedent from the other unscientific, medicine-by-press release, narratives from the hepatitis B and hepatitis B vaccine era of the 1970's, and other vaccine eras as well.

It also should be emphasized in the context of vaccines and cancer that no vaccine, especially the new cadre of Pfizer's, Moderna's, J&J's, and AstraZeneca's (or any other vaccine of the past designed to prevent diseases other than seasonal influenza) has been tested for its carcinogenic potential on the eggs of the women they are given to.

It was widely reported in the leading journals and newspapers during the cancer era of the 1960's, that mothers who imbibed a tranquilizer known as DES (Diethylstilbestrol) gave birth to daughters that had ovarian cancers. In other words, because the drug affected cells of the ovary of the female fetus, the affects were not seen until the next generation of women had matured.

It can take sometimes two generations before genetic damage and adverse impacts of medicines are seen in future generations. Rather than study a new vaccine or medicine for 12 months or 10 years, we should be analyzing population impacts from medications over multiple generations. While this may sound overly-cautious, one only needs to review the history of DES (Diethylstilbestrol) to see how future generations can be biologically maimed by the decisions of our parents and grandparents.

Also, in the context of vaccines and cancers, there has been decades of well- established science analyzing vaccine carcinogenicity initiated by groups of veterinarians. Veterinarians and veterinary schools have demonstrated with numerous population studies and case studies that vaccines cause malignant cancers in dogs and cats that predictably occur at the site or near the site of vaccinations, prompting veterinarians to adopt a tail-administered vaccine protocol.

Their reasoning derives from their clinical experience that if and when cancer develops at the vaccine-injection site due to a vaccine, the tail can be removed, and the more central vital parts of the body are spared. This has been written about by the University of Florida school of veterinary medicine, and numerous prominent veterinarians and professors of veterinary medicine from places like Purdue University, by The Feline Sarcoma Society, Britain's Canine Health Concern, and by veterinarians world-wide.

Vasculogenic mimicry may hold clues as to the mechanism of how vaccines often induce malignant cancers in both animals and humans. It appears vaccine-induced cancers involve the matrix proteins fibronectin and laminin which are dysregulated by vaccines, and this explains how these cancers form concomitant with, and spatially proximate to the vaccine administration site. This will be discussed in detail in the section entitled "The Science of Vaccine Damage."

If it is not clear enough yet, we are living in the dark ages of medicine right now. **A recent study out of Johns Hopkins reported**

that medical errors and pharmaceutical side effects are the 3rd leading cause of death in the USA. I think this underestimates the reality.

Everything we are told about SARS-COVID-19 has been derived from a blind faith in molecular reductionism of the DNA or RNA sequence which worships and pays homage to Watson and Crick's DNA and RNA sequences constituting the "secrets of life." For almost two generations now, this religion, or as some might assert, this reductionist mental illness has afflicted many scientific and medical minds, and this reductionist thinking has dominated much of the biological sciences. As its God, DNA and RNA sequences are the cause and creator of everything living. Molecular reductionism of this kind has essentially destroyed the sciences of biology, physiology, and bio-mechanics and replaced them with a chemistry of "dead, dissociated molecules." What is unique about living systems is their organization, not their parts.

TESTING

Nobel Prize winner and chemist Dr. Kary Mullis discovered the underlying science and technology used today in all RT-PCR testing, which has been widely used to detect SARS-COVID-19 cases, in science, medicine, law, and a variety of other fields where identification applications are essential tools (missing persons, etc.), and because RT-PCR has changed so many fields of human endeavor, Kary Mullis received the Nobel Prize. Our relationship began and grew through online science and medical forums on which both of us shared information and efforts in helping AIDS patients confirm or reject the accuracy of their positive HIV laboratory protein and nucleic acid tests (RNA or DNA).

Dr. Kary Mullis persistently warned the scientific and medical communities and the world that in the scientific literature, there is not a single proof that "HIV" causes AIDS, and he invented the RT-PCR tests that indict both "HIV" positive victims and SARS-COVID-19 victims, although his test was in recent years adulterated by Christian

Drosden whose current modifications of Mullis's RT-PCR are now used to accuse and convict people of harboring SARS-CoV-2 viruses today. In both contexts of "HIV-AIDS" and the SARS-COVID-19 "pandemic," RT-PCR testing is the entrance through the gates of hell to a potential life-time in medical hell and healthcare purgatory. As victims of positive testing, those who test positive often must look forward to a lifetime of medical interference and 4th amendment, Nuremberg, and Helsinki Accord violations of their lives. Their "disease diagnoses," detected by an indirect PCR test (with its majority of false-positives) becomes their prison cell. This phenomenon happened in both the "HIV-AIDS" era and is happening again in the era of SARS-COVID-19, and many of the same people have led both international responses to "HIV" and "SARS-COVID-19" propaganda (Tony Fauci, Deborah Birx, Robert Redfield, and behind the scenes, Robert Gallo with his rumor viruses).

Most of the current COVID-19 lab testing centers are currently using Dr. Mullis's RT-PCR tests, along with several modifications of RT-PCR that have arisen in recent years, but nobody has tested them along with EM confirmation of viremia in asymptomatic "cases," which are overwhelmingly in the high 99+% range, and the false positive rates of the RT-PCR tests have been legion since the AIDS era. Therefore, it may be prudent to investigate if at least one SARS-CoV-2 viral-like particle can be detected at the level of electron microscopy in an asymptomatic RT-PCR-positive person. When this question was asked during the era of "HIV" for a rather high-profile legal case (the Tommy Morrison case – a former WBO heavyweight boxing champion who once fought George Foreman and appeared in the Rocky V movie with Sylvester Stallone), an electron microscopy (EM) viral load comparison revealed that in a clinical healthy "positive" extremely healthy man harboring a RT-PCR-detected viral load of 4 million, that not one "HIV" particle could be found in his blood, or lymph nodes at the level of ultrastructural resolution (EM).

The EM studies were carried out in parallel with the same blood samples sent to be RT-PCR tested, and the EM was carried out at Mass General's EM diagnostic lab, Kansas City's Medical School, and MD Anderson. This study which I directed is unpublished but available upon request. None of these diagnostic centers of EM testing for viruses could find a single "HIV" viral particle (despite high RT-PCR-detectable viral loads in each of 5 cases that were blinded and sent to each testing facility). As SARS-CoV-2 is a real virus, unlike "HIV," it would be of great interest to learn if ultrastructural visualization of SARS-CoV-2 particles could be visualized with EM in any of the 99.7% of the asymptomatic RT-PCR-positive victim's lung lavages, or blood.

And now with SARS-CoV-2, whether we have viruses supposedly naturally "jumping off" bats, and pangolins and various small carnivorous mammals as sources of "jumping viruses," or instead, we have viruses escaping from NIH/Fauci-funded Wuhan laboratories, it would save countless lives to document at the level of electron microscopy the ubiquitous presence of crown-shaped particles, and also, to expose lavages and lung samples to ether, to first inactivate, and then transmit "the infectious and pathogenic agent", to an experimental animal such as a macaque to ignite influenza symptoms.

As of June 10, 2021 we now hear Dr. Fauci announcing the new delta variant of SARS-CoV-2 now infects children, blowing away the well documented fact that the atypical COVID-19 pneumonia has been manifested on MRI's from the beginning of the pandemic almost exclusively in one risk group; the extremely aged, and those harboring one, two, or three or more preexisting morbid conditions like diabetes, obesity, heart disease, respiratory problems, and cancers. Are we going to tolerate "all of us now being at risk, even our 3-year olds" now with Dr. Fauci's new "delta variant?" Or is this simply more propaganda, junk science, and lies?

In other words, instead of only enjoying "sexual distancing" bought to us by our friendly Robert Gallo and Anthony Fauci AKA Faucitopia during the 1980's, now we have "social distancing" with COVID-19, and masks, along with the mental stress and psychotic mental duress these worthless behaviors foster. Humans are social primates.

For the criminals behind this fiasco, SARS-CoV-2 is so much more of an effective and equal opportunity pathogen than "HIV" (the existence of which has not been proven via Electron Microscopy lab tests in 35 years) don't you agree?

To have an endogenous, ubiquitous, and harmless gastrointestinal virus, such as SARS-CoV-2 and many other coronaviruses that all are typically characterized as being normal intestinal subcellular passengers in a variety of mammals including man and man's best friend, the dog, the opportunities seem endless in social engineering based on fear tactics.

And although the little blue masks are currently worn over the face, it may be possible in the future if the fear mongers get their way, that a second "mask" ought to be wrapped around the buttocks like a diaper, as coronaviral-like particles have been characterized for decades now as typically being asymptomatic, intestine localized entities in most contexts that have been well characterized. Therefore, perhaps a blue diaper worn outside the pants, in addition to a mask should become part of an educated, responsible, and politically correct person's wardrobe for some time, lest they face incarceration or fines or quarantine camps?

These small, so-called "epidemics" raise critical questions about herd immunity and about disease definitions. Yet, the same degree of hysteria and panic used to scare governments and the public into a global lock-down because of COVID-19 panic-porn by the corrupt media and corrupt politicians apparently did not escalate into global lock-downs in most if not all of these past or other declared epidemics including some of the several plague epidemics that have occurred since around the time of Christ, several leprosy epidemics, the British smallpox epidemics in the late 1800's, or the non-contagious paralysis (polio) epidemics of the last Century.

Vaccinations and inoculations are incredibly complex practices, that touch all aspects of our modern lives and our children's lives, and through a historical lens approach, and with a little deduction and luck, a firm prehistorical and early historical light on the past illuminates the "how's," "what's," "when's," "where's," and the most important question – **why** have we inoculated and vaccinated for centuries, **even before any germ theory was in place**, and **why do we vaccinate today**? Are vaccines really any more scientifically validated than leeches were centuries ago? The truth is after reading the primary-sourced data in this book the reader may see that centuries-old practice of using leeches to bleed the sick may have a better, historic cost-benefit than the centuries-old practice of vaccination.

Why should we continue to mandate vaccines in the future to attend schools, to obtain honest work as a health care provider, to travel abroad, etc.?

Are vaccines more akin to sorcery than to any recognizable science? This is the question every reader should ask as they read this book and the historic primary-sourced, scientific evidence.

From an early age, most of us as small children were told that vaccinations and inoculations are perhaps one of humanity's greatest achievements, or are, in fact, our greatest achievement. Yet when we are hauled off to our family doctor's office as small children and we are old enough to be aware that on that day we will receive that painful "shot" in a medicinal-smelling office from a man or woman wearing a long white coat, and as we try to talk ourselves into mustering the resolve to not burst out in tears when that "stuff" is injected, do we really think that vaccines are humanity's greatest accomplishment (what 4-10 year-old accepts and does not fear vaccinations)?

What does the actual primary-sourced data and evidence show us regarding "Man's greatest achievement?"

When entire nations or a planet of organisms are exposed to a foreign protein via injection, inoculation or vaccination, the intervention qualifies as a selective force on our future evolutionary path, and natural selection does not anticipate future events.

When a vaccine is rolled out nationally or globally, it is critically important to address **Natural Selection** regarding the topic of pandemics, epidemics, and endemic disease in the context of both vaccinations and inoculations (such as TB).

The topic of so-called "herd immunity", so often discussed carelessly in the media, press releases, and by celebrity doctors, will be clarified in many of the following chapters.

For instance, a fundamental scientific question to ask is do we know, or can we ever know if "herd immunity" is actually something that is desirable in the first place for a species, or might it be something to fear and avoid because "herd immunity" may indicate a loss or lack of natural immunological diversity or "species-wide heterogeneity."

In the biological sciences, the genetic and physiological diversity of all traits that have been carefully studied have been fundamentally characteristic of living systems that have insured survival.

This fact has been repeatedly encountered with the undeniably successful hybrid strategies of selective breeding in agriculture and animal husbandry in which diversity constitutes the foundation of successful agricultural practices, and most likely, the most basic biological foundation for the continued natural evolution of all living systems.

Immunological diversity in populations is also more adaptive or "fit" than immunological homogeneity in the Darwinian sense of the word, meaning that populations, not individuals, are more robust or "fit" to their environment(s) due to immunological heterogeneity, as opposed to being forced to face their immunological environments via universally mandated vaccines with immunological sameness or homogeneity artificially engineered by means of population-wide vaccination with the same antigen. Immunological diversity constitutes the basis of natural immunological resistance.

What information should be believed about Covid-19 vaccines and what should we teach our children to be true? What does the evidence tell us about the risk and reward of Covid-19 vaccines? VAERS (the US government's vaccine adverse event reporting system) tells one story and the press releases of the CDC and Pfizer tell us another story. The problem is, we as a society and scientific community are being prohibited from now completing the proper, transparent, non-corrupted, scientific Covid-19 vaccine risk analysis, Covid-19 vaccine cost-benefit-analysis, and now our children are being denied an actual university education without genuflecting before the Covid-19 Vaccine Church. Our children will be denied entrance into many colleges this coming 2021 fall without proof of Covid-19 vaccines.

Dr. Robert Gallo, Anthony Fauci's colleague at NIH, famous for his work with HIV, recently advocated an oral "polio vaccine" for COVID-19 as a stop-gap measure until we allow ourselves and our children to accept the non-safety tested and unknown efficacy producing COVID-19 vaccines that are now being "rolled-out."

COVID-19 is permeated with AIDS thinking, and the same people who created AIDS policy are working currently on COVID-19.

When you read the critically important historic vaccination and pandemic timeline included in this book, THE GREAT TIMELINE OF VACCINE EXPERIMENTATION ON HUMAN BEINGS: SPECIFIC DATA FROM MANY SOURCES you may notice a pattern repeated throughout the past two hundred years of epidemics and vaccine campaigns since the time of Edward Jenner and smallpox: that after mass vaccination campaigns certain things occur that are rather surprising to those of us that had a different understanding of how vaccines work. The "certain thing(s) to occur, are an enhancement of epidemic and endemic diseases (from cancers to brain disorders to autoimmune diseases to infertility).

Certainly, as a former medical school associate professor and Harvard research scientist and NIH post-doctoral fellow and NIH-funded cancer researcher, I was surprised that the primary-sourced 240+ year history of vaccinations demonstrate this fact so clearly. I expect you will be equally shocked after reviewing the timeline I organized of 240+ years of vaccine history from primary sources.

As I wrote earlier in this introduction, we seem to be living in the latter phase of the medical dark-ages era. My hope is that with proven "open-source", non-patented, medical technologies like hyperbaric oxygen we can exit these medical dark-ages and initiate a new medical renaissance.

I hope that the widely varied primary-sources of information presented in this analysis and timeline will enable the reader to arrive at their own thoughtful and well-considered conclusions about vaccine history comfortably and peacefully, even if the reader's conclusions differ from mine. If this result is realized, then the many lifetimes of work documenting historic and modern vaccine and pandemic history that this book represents will have been more than worth the effort.

CHAPTER I

VACCINES, COVID AND THE SACRIFICE OF COMMON SENSE – *FORECASTS AND AUGURIES OF SORCERERS, WITCHES, AND DOCTORS*

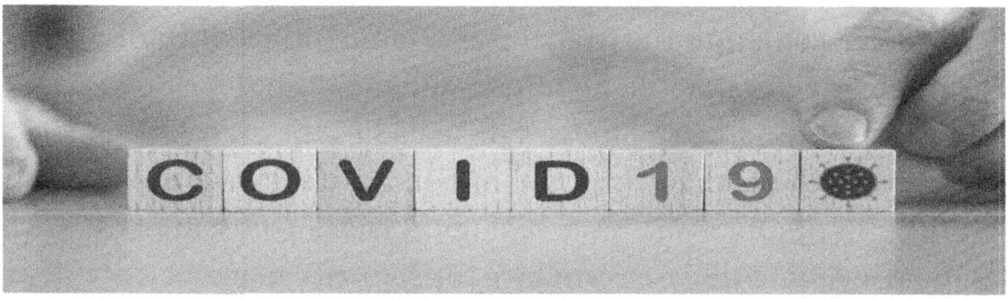

THE WORD "PHARMACEUTICAL" (ΦΑΡΜΑΚΕΙΑ) OR pharmacy derives from the Greek word "pharmakeia," which translates: "sorcery," "witchcraft." Since ancient times and through the middle ages, potions, drugs, and other types of concoctions have been associated with witches or sorcerers. Modern virologists and epidemiologists are constantly prophesying about the emergence of new epidemics, "pandemics," or deadly new viruses we hear about daily in "breaking news" reports, and the prescription for any illness, infirmity, and aging and death itself, has become typically "pharmaceutical" in nature in the form of a vaccine or drug.

As we sit in a global "pandemic" lockdown the likes of which has never been seen and recorded in human history to the extent and degree of uncertainty with which it has currently expanded globally, a unique opportunity has presented itself with the coming and the passing of this SARS COVID-19 global terrorist alert. One's decision to obtain a vaccine or avoid one for oneself or for one's child can be a fiercely turbulent mental brainstorm and malady, and when faced with mandates of forced medical procedures such as to test or not to test, or to vaccinate or not to vaccinate, to obtain a "vaccine passport," to wear a "sheep nose" mask for a year or more over your nose and mouth, to travel on an airplane and pass airport security and risk testing "positive," to travel to another state without proving you have not tested "positive," or have had a Moderna or Pfizer-BioNtech vaccine against SARS-C0V-2 during the previous 3 days thanks to Bill Gates and the Globalists, and to be threatened to be thrown into a quarantine camp until you test RT-PCR-negative for 14 days, this kind of fear, and the decision to act or behave according to that fear can become quite paralyzing. Without sufficient information, it can be difficult to evaluate inter-epidemic or in the case of SARS-COVID-19, "pandemic" illnesses or maladies, or even familiar sicknesses such the familiar seasonal influenzas that occur endemically every year, without some basic biological facts first set in place, such as the concept of disease resistance, or species variations.

One reason that it can be daunting to analyze a complex issue such as the emergence of a pandemic illness such as SARS-COVID-19 or "The Great 1918-19 Great Spanish Influenza" which was not really due to a contagious disease, is because these panics occur periodically, and unpredictably. What is even more baffling, is that the causality of previous epidemics or indeed this pandemic are not really known. In at least several cases in the context of influenza, these epidemics appear to have occurred concomitantly with cholera epidemics. This fact begs the question about "the seed" versus "the soil" hypothesis that Pasteur first wrote about.

Yet, during almost every television show, on most networks, there is the constant clamor of unrelenting lawsuits and warnings about each drug's or vaccine's side-effects, while showing hopeful pictures of what are depicted as very sick people climbing mountains or playing sports with children with smiles on their drug managed faces, always followed, for purposes of liability, with that advertised drug's caveats and sudden withdrawals and recalls of what were supposed to be "scientifically-proven" drugs that are marketed and fed to millions of other "healthy inherently sick folks" like candy (who are not yet aware they are sick so they must be taught that they are sick).

The medical and scientific priests and ministers who sermonize about our inevitable deaths without a lifetime of pharmaceutical management no longer wear long dark robes and promulgate to us about our inherent "sinfulness" by nature, or our fall from some Divine grace, as was the case during the Western Christian eras of superstition and witchcraft. Now, the medically pious are obedient to a clergy of men in long white "sterile" robes, whose medical school vow is to convert a pious congregation to the belief that they are inherently physically, mentally, and psychologically "sick" from birth, when we first require vaccination within several minutes to months of our lives, and again when we are admitted to schools upon threats of parental incarcerations and stiff fines for non-vaccine compliance.

Most importantly, it may surprise many to learn that the deontology associated with whether to allow vaccine mandates or not may not be a simple pro or con, for or against, decision, but may involve as many as at least 7 different types of decisions, or ***7 Deadly Sins***, with many associated results:

- **A. vaccines do damage to individuals;**
- **B. vaccines do nothing to most individuals in a population (harming only a few), as would a shot have filled with water administered correctly (without any air bubbles or impurities);**
- **C. vaccines cause small outbreaks/harm small populations;**

D. vaccines do nothing to prevent diseases, so disease definitions are changed as evidence for vaccine effectiveness (e.g., smallpox-leprosy; polio era-encephalitis);

E. vaccines can spread the disease vaccinated against to non-vaccinated people;

F. vaccines cause different diseases in humans than vaccines are supposed to immunize against;

G. vaccines may alter the natural resistance of populations and obscure the evolution of immunologic diversity in an attempt to instill artificially, a kind of homogenization of the human response to a suspected pathogen which "may" arrive... in the future.

This last of the **Seven Deadly Sins**, result "**G**," is the most problematic and difficult to understand, or rectify at this point when entire populations of some countries are currently being vaccinated.

The concept of "herd immunity" may be a conceptual violation of everything biologists and life scientists of all disciplines know, that runs contrary to how populations through geological time periods have remained "non-extinct" or "extant"? (extant being the technical term for "still here among the thriving-not extinct"). Heterogeneity, be it genetic or physiological, is the bedrock of robust population responses to a universe of unknown pathogens, and not only of individual organisms, but of populations.

Biologists have been aware of the benefits of natural variation in natural populations, and agriculturalists and animal breeders have depended on a phenomenon called hybrid vigor for uncounted centuries to produce better livestock and crops. In almost every if not all examples of natural variation in nature, and in artificial selection during animal breading or crop farming known, natural variation in nature and hybrid vigor in animal husbandry and crop diversity (poly-culture) yields more vigorous, robust, hearty, and fit offspring or more resistant plants in every measurable way compared to the offspring or progeny that arise from crosses through matings between homozygous or genetically similar individuals.

Genetic or physiological homogeneity in populations of animals or plants or crops used in agriculture that are 'homogenized' genetically are less apt to survive if an unexpected plague or if a blight should descend, which can kill the entire population because there are not any variants permitted that will at random, resist that specific assault on the population simply because they are different.

Whether intentional or not, by injecting an identical antigen (foreign agent) directly into the blood circulation of every member of a vaccinated population, it is theoretically possible that the immune systems of entire populations, or indeed, entire cultures will become uniform or "homogenized" to respond in the same way to that antigen or invader when it appears in the future, and the population will be unable to neutralize that antigen if it does appear, because the diversity of natural variation (and or natural immunological variation) has been intentionally (or unintentionally) destroyed or compromised via vaccination of the same foreign antigen in every member of that population in advance (of the unwanted future encounter with it).

For example, several times in recorded history it has been reported that the abatement or cessation of widespread (not universal) vaccinations resulted in an almost immediate and nearly complete eradication of normally-experienced cases seen before the vaccine was discontinued. As mentioned before, in 1886-1892 in Australia when a few children died as a result of smallpox vaccinations, the government abolished compulsory vaccination in that country and smallpox suddenly declined to the vanishing point. Australia had only three cases of smallpox in 15 years as compared with Japan's record of 165,774 cases and 28,979 deaths from this cause in only 7 years under compulsory vaccination and re-vaccination. This intention to "immunologically homogenize" or "train" the immune system via delivery of the same antigen to entire populations has never been achieved. Vaccines have instead wreaked disaster: in the confines of islands or in one or two nations where records have been kept, for instance, between December 2020, and January 2021, Italy experienced a massive outbreak of SARS-CoV-2 in late December following an H1N1 vaccine in September of more than 400,000 Northern Italians followed by an "experimental" hepatitis C vaccine in early December, 2020.

Many in the biomedical community see the disconnect that is happening currently with the emerging and growing population of SARS-COVID-19 asymptomatics which is to be expected, because the death rates continue to decline to the point that overall death rate of 0.6% claimed recently by ER MDs in California to be that states current figure, which means that the survival rate is in the range of 99.4%!

In other words, as it has been with most if not all successful responses to natural epidemics, it appears to be "the soil," and not "the seed" that is of the most need of attention. In other words, the nutritional and overall health of the symptomatic over 75 year old populations should be attended with vitamin C and D. When presenting with atypical pneumonia, the atypical pneumonia victim should be given non-ventilator-mediated therapies such as hyperbaric oxygen treatment and ivermectin, that have both individually been shown to deliver nearly 100% curative therapeutic responses to atypical pneumonia. And consistent with this are the age breakdown categories of the elderly or people with preexisting conditions who are being most heavily impacted by COVID-19 [despite the constant noise heard about the occasional younger cases).

It is most decidedly an issue of "soil" and not the "seed" (the SARS-CoV-2 SARS virus being the seed, and the incredibly old or those with preexisting conditions being the "soil" of the "pandemic)."

These issues have been voiced and supported by many whose scientific opinions should matter most. As far back as 1966, the cancer virologist, Payton Rous made this issue crystal clear when he said in his 1966 Nobel Prize acceptance speech that "no human cancer has ever been linked to a viral cause." As Kaposi's sarcoma was one of the first two "AIDS-indicator" illnesses, and the fact that Robert Gallo and Anthony Fauci have been agents and architects of the "virus-AIDS" hypothesis already had opposed, and then dismissed by the scientific community for trying to link viral cancers due to another virus, HTLV-1 and then other viruses-HTLV-II and then HTLV-III to human leukemias of Japanese who lived near Nagasaki and Hiroshima,it remains a fact consistent with Rous's assertion that no virus ever has been convincingly linked to a human cancer.

When it is tacitly assumed that some kind of unfounded faith in biological causality exists in sequence identity comparisons, and the unbridled and undeserved faith in molecular testing warrants anything resembling certainty of function, there clearly has not been sufficient skepticism to be of much use to guide diagnostic interpretations, not to mention therapeutic decision making based on those interpretations. This delusion about the reality of sequence homology and sequence identity, rather than direct electron microscopic verification and validation never was demonstrated as lunacy as much as it was during the era of "HIV" and AIDS. Are we condemned now to repeat this testing insanity with SARS-CoV-2?

As you will hopefully discern, the field of "HIV/AIDS" has departed from the "scientific and medical consensus" that had advanced the notion that Acquired Immune Deficiency Syndrome was caused by ("LAV") and "HIV," and the field has moved toward the recent 2009 documented claim made by Luc Montagnier, the Nobelist who is credited for the initial discovery of "HIV" (LAV) and who now points to many co-factors and causes of AIDS other than "HIV." Some of these new beliefs were articulated by Dr. Montagnier in an excellent award winning documentary made by Brent Leung called "House of Numbers:"

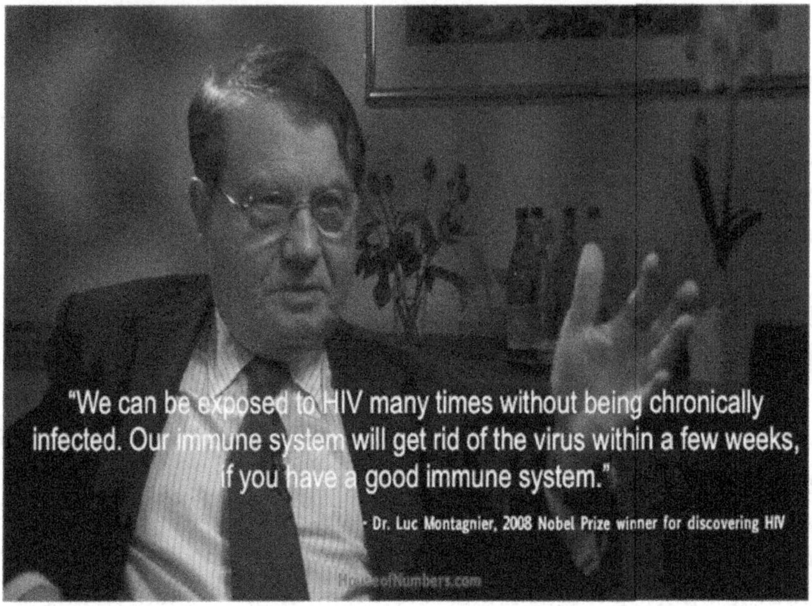

Dr. Luc Montagnier: "We can be exposed to HIV many times without being chronically infected. Our immune system will get rid of the virus within a few weeks, if you have a good immune system."

Interviewer (Brent Leung): If you have a good immune system, then your body can naturally get rid of HIV?

Dr. Luc Montagnier: Yes.

Interviewer: If you take a poor African, who's been infected and you build up their immune system, is it possible for them to also naturally get rid of it?

Dr. Luc Montagnier: I would think so.

Interviewer: That's an important… Dr. Luc Montagnier: It's important knowledge which is completely neglected. People always think of drugs and vaccine.

Interviewer: There is no money in nutrition, right?

Dr. Luc Montagnier: There is no profit, yes

Visit "HouseofNumbers.com" for review, biographies, and more video, where his interview can be heard in its entirety in the film "House of Numbers:" https://www.youtube.com/watch?v=PyPq-waF-h4

HOW THE CONCEPT OF "ORIGINAL ANTIGENIC SIN" IN THE CONTEXT OF FAILED "HIV" VACCINES HAS COME ABOUT DURING THE ERA OF "HIV/AIDS."

Gallo's and Heckler's 1984 press release was entirely forgotten or overlooked by the Nobel Committee, and toward the end of a Congressional document prepared by the Government Office of Technology Assessment, we find that the term "original antigenic sin" was advanced to describe why 30 "HIV" vaccines had failed to prevent "HIV" positive tests or AIDS-associated syndromes by 1995.

However, it should be emphasized that the most recent tally of the number of "HIV" vaccines and human vaccine trials that have been declared "duds" (and often abruptly terminated mid trial) number in the 200's, yet this information has been removed from NIH's website in recent years.

What is "original antigenic sin, in the context of vaccines?

A) When a vaccinated individual is exposed to a non-cross-reactive strain of HIV that induces the production of antibodies specific for the vaccine strain, that are unable to neutralize the newly encountered strain (in plain words, when an "HIV" vaccine doesn't work-prevent the acquisition of a positive "HIV" molecular signature or AIDS-indicator diseases).

B) The fixing of an immune response in a "non-adaptive pattern."
C) When vaccinated individuals may be no worse off than

unvaccinated individuals, because non-vaccinated individuals also have a lag in generation of antibody to HIV, because their immune response has not been "primed" by vaccination.

The conclusions of The Office of Technology Assessment Book were presented to the 1995 Congress of the United States by the AIDS Research Advisory Committee (ARAC) of the National Institute of Allergy and Infectious Diseases (NIAID).

From these conclusions, it was recommended that Phase III clinical trials with enveloped vaccines should not proceed in the United States because of scientific, political, and ethical issues, and because of the significant level of scientific uncertainty about the wisdom of immediate trials" (1995 Congress of the United States: Office of Technology assessment. Adverse Reactions to HIV Vaccines: Medical, Ethical, and Legal Issues. Roger C. Herdman, Director).

INOCULATIONS AND VACCINES AS SELECTIVE FORCES ON THE HUMAN IMMUNE SYSTEM

The vaccinologists, whether they realize it or not, by proposing to jab 100's of millions of humans with the same antigen, or 4.9 Billion humans as the WHO has proposed, is in effect an attempt to homogenize the human immune response.

In effect, perhaps a better way of discussing this issue is to evoke the evolutionary biological terms directly. Industrial melanism was a phenomenon that was documented at the height of England's industrial revolution when there were enormous quantities of smoke being belched out of chimneys during their industrial revolution for the first time. A white species of moths was known to populate the birch trees in British forests, but Naturalists noted that as the pollution increased, the birch trees the white moths inhabited began to turn a dingy gray due to the pollution, and the moths stood out like sore thumbs on the graying background. As a result, these moths became easy pickings for birds and other predators, but one observant entomologist noted that a "mutant" gray moth clone began to expand. This in effect was one of the earlier confirmations of Darwin's Natural selection process.

Although it is only theoretical at this point, it is possible that vaccinations of entire populations are akin to industrial melanism in so far as the "soot" being the vaccines is "selecting" a particular immune response among populations of humans in this case. The selective force, being the vaccine, in effect, is altering the entire immunological futures of our species. Do they really have that right?

Natural immunological and genetic diversity, empirically supported the successes of hybrid vigor in agricultural contexts, has formed the basis of some of the best achievements and discoveries in human history, as well as in making social decisions toward "the good" for the simple practical reason that diversity of all kinds better and naturally ensures a larger set of potential successful, robust resources upon which future success can draw from. In other words, many possible sources of vigor rather than only one or several "selected" "founder" types is a richer wellspring of possible resistance in the face of unknown future challenges to a species.

IMMUNIZATION, INOCULATION, AND VACCINATION

The terms inoculation, vaccination, and immunization often are used interchangeably, but for the purposes of this analysis, clear distinctions must be made between vaccinations and inoculations, which typically refer to the manner by which foreign molecules are introduced into the body. In the case of inoculations, this shall refer to the manner by which tuberculin inoculation is administered shallowly under the dermis. The terms vaccines or vaccinations shall refer to the injection of solution into large muscles of the buttocks or upper arm.

Immunization is a conceptual absolute or a desired goal in the future, and it is arguable if perfect immunization ever has been achieved, because as we will see, there are examples where many types of vaccines, given early in life, wear off in a few years, which is why certain vaccines are administered many times or as boosters, and why among the innocents who receive vaccinations and inoculations, schedules are maintained. Our understanding of how immunity works is at its infancy. The word immunization is not descriptive of what inoculations or vaccines do, because the hopes and predictions of "herd immunity" have so far never been achieved, as there is ample evidence to support that 100% vaccinated groups have become sick with a variety of different contagions immunized against, despite lack of vaccine hesitancy or non-compliance in situations where forced or mandated vaccination of 100%, such as crews aboard Navy ships. This same imperfection extends and can be generalized also to larger populations of entire countries, including those vaccine roll-outs where records of revaccinations have been kept.

Often, when medical interventions do not work as they are proposed that they should work, or are in theory supposed to work, the "EXPERTS" always say the same lame thing: "Oh, the reason why our drug or vaccine didn't work is because "it mutated" around the drug or intervention, as if the thing causing the malady were a moving target!!! This leaves the impression of the microbial world we are surrounded by as being something like a Las Vegas card sharp shuffling a deck of "genetic cards."

But as we will review later, these failures are largely due to human arrogance, more than a result of "mutation" or change. If an organism is constantly mutating its genomic instructions which store the raw materials for building living cells, and they are constantly mutating, then how on the earth do things remain as distinct recognizable lions, or tigers, or bears, or E. Coli, or any of the assorted "rumor viruses," or "viral-like particles" that the cells of organisms (and even bacteria) produce by the trillions? These so-called viruses are nothing more than a nucleotide molecule wrapped inside of a shell of protein shell. When the viral particle enters the cell by whatever means, it is assumed that the protein shell is removed or dissolved by a cell that takes it in, and the genetic molecule of the virus-like particle is exposed and chemically then reacts with the cells' synthetic machinery to begin replicating that genome to make and assemble more like particles.

In 1889, Alfred Russel Wallace, who was Darwin's collaborator and the co-discoverer of Natural Selection perhaps more than anyone else changed the practice of forced vaccine compliance to the centuries-old superstition of inoculations and the vaccination that was ushered in a century before by The Jennerian paradigm of vaccination, by publishing two extensive volumes in 1889 that he first submitted to The British Parliament entitled: **"VACCINATION-PROVED USELESS AND DANGEROUS FROM FORTY-FIVE YEARS OF REGISTRATION STATISTICS"** (The Reese Collection), and in another that followed, entitled, **"THE ARMY AND NAVY: A DEMONSTRATION OF THE USELESSNESS OF VACCINE."**

This second volume Wallace wrote clearly demonstrated a synthesis of follow-up results from the forty-five years of registration statistics along with the newer anecdotal reports of both uselessness, and **how vaccines spread diseases they are designed to prevent.**

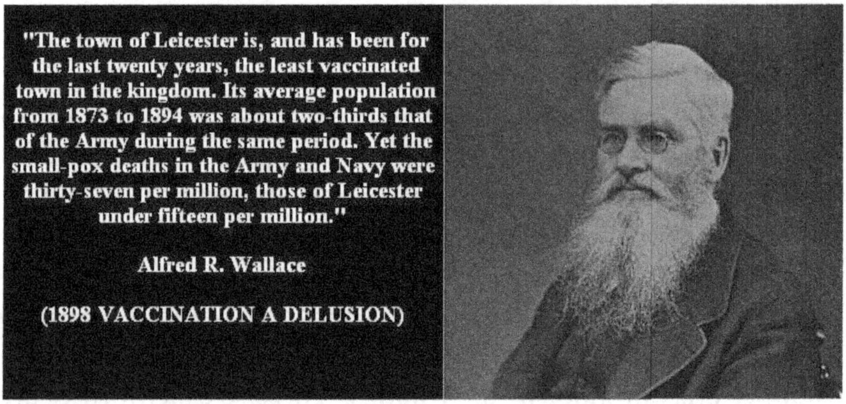

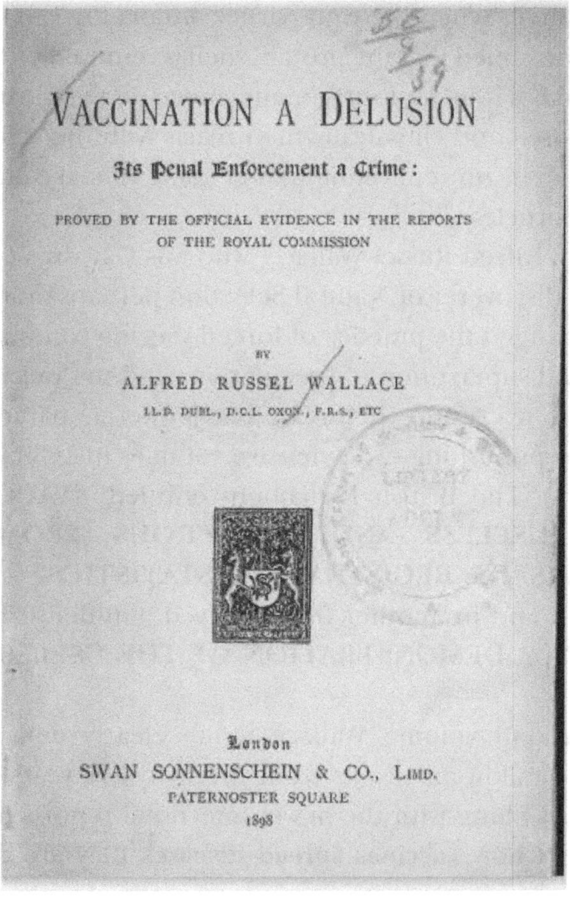

VACCINATION A DELUSION

Its Penal Enforcement a Crime:

PROVED BY THE OFFICIAL EVIDENCE IN THE REPORTS
OF THE ROYAL COMMISSION

BY

ALFRED RUSSEL WALLACE

LL.D. DUBL., D.C.L. OXON., F.R.S., ETC

London
SWAN SONNENSCHEIN & CO., LIMD.
PATERNOSTER SQUARE
1898

Another example where military records show us that vaccines cause harm are the **United States Navy military records** of the so-called "Spanish Flu" at the time:

– *In 1917, U.S. soldiers were vaccinated prior to going overseas to fight in WW I. They soon begin to "drop dead by the thousands" on both sides of the Atlantic from a strange syndrome that preferentially attacked young adults.*

– *In the Army over a million men were hospitalized for influenza and pneumonia, and of these there were more than 44,000 deaths. There were approximately 5,000 deaths among Navy personnel. Hospital admission rates and death rates for American troops stationed in Europe were lower than for troops in the United States. The large number of recruits concentrated in close quarters probably accounted for higher rates in the latter. In the camps having the larger numbers of recently vaccinated trainees incidence and mortality was highest, and in all camps the rates were higher in recruits than in seasoned troops... When appropriate adjustments are made for differences in the age and sex distribution of military and civilian populations, it appears that the death rate was about one-fourth higher in the Army than in the civilian population of the United States. The incidence and mortality of influenza in military personnel in 1918-19 has been described in great detail in Epidemiology and Public Health by Vaughan, and in Volume 9 of the history of the Medical Department of the United States Army in the World War.* ***[See also the Surgeon General's account in Annual Report of the Secretary of the Navy, 1919*** *— Miscellaneous Reports*

– In Osler's book, "**Modern Medicine**," (1913, Vol. I, pages 32 and 33), and also in his "**Principles and Practice of Medicine**"(8th edition, 1918, page 330, see also pages 135 and 139 in the Supplement) Osler wrote:

Another most significant fact in this connection is the high death rate from disease in the Army, as compared with the civil population, which I will now consider:

... the death rate of the Army in the United States from disease for the year ending August 30, 1918, is given as 6.4; that is, about 6 l/2 deaths for every thousand men in the Army. The age-groups composing the Army are, of course, on the general average, between twenty and forty, inclusive. In the same Report it is admitted that the male civilian death rate for the same ages as in the Army (twenty to forty) was about 4.7, which is a difference of 1.7 or nearly 2 per 1000 in favor of the civil population or civilian males!

This civil death rate is thus, actually and relatively, much lower than the army death rate...The figures 6.4 per thousand for the Army and 4.7 per thousand for the civil population of the same ages is a great actual difference, but, of course, means, relatively, a much greater total difference against the Army because the army population is made up of "hand-picked" men selected for their nearly perfect health and physique and the absence of all serious constitutional diseases such as tuberculosis and others, which are all excluded from the army group. On the other hand, the civil population of the same age-group of twenty to forty includes the healthy and diseased, and particularly those afflicted with tuberculosis, which constitute a big fraction, and which disease is most prevalent and fatal in this very age-group of twenty to forty! Yet this civil population, containing all the diseased at the most fatal adult ages, has a much lower death rate than the "hand-picked" physically perfect army group!

Now what is the cause of this much higher death rate in men of the most physically perfect class, and who are now treated with the best sanitary and hygienic living conditions, and where the death rate should be the lowest? What is the cause of this difference if it is not that extraordinary medical practice, or malpractice, which deliberately impregnates the bodies of these exceptionally healthy and "hand-picked" men with a whole series of the worst type of disease infections known that is, septicemic infections, like the typhoid and the variolas, etc.? And should anyone wonder, therefore, if the death lists of the army should show plainly in the blood poisoning diseases of pneumonia, meningitis, etc., ***which are known to follow frequently after vaccination?***

QUESTION: WHICH IMMUNITY PRODUCING MECHANISMS DO VACCINES ALTER TO PRODUCE IMMUNITY? IS IT REALLY AS WORKED OUT AS THE MEDICAL AND BIOLOGICAL TEXTBOOKS SAY?

To immunize means to generate immunity or attenuate disease if a harmful microbe is encountered in the future either naturally, or when introduced artificially (again). Coulter cogently makes a strong case for vaccines constituting a **homeopathic practice by default because nothing about the procedure or consequence of that procedure is about directly attacking the pathogen**: vaccination is a homeopathic procedure because the approach is attempting to alert the organism's natural defenses. During the process of artificially inducing immunity with most inoculations or vaccines, one is presenting "like" or a disarmed facsimile to the recipient and is not attempting to kill or incapacitate the [future] pathogenic entity thought to be causing the disease or illness, other than to alert the body as to its presence, and without allowing the infectious agent to unleash its full potential for harm. Ever ask yourself why Western Medical physicians and establishment folks hate homeopaths so much, while they jab your daughter or son? Irrational. Insanity. Vaccines are the King Midas story–feed 'em a little poison, and they be protected.

Many mechanisms through the Centuries regarding the attainment of immunity have been proposed in different contexts:

The 46 observations of Thucydides who noted in a 430 BC plague epidemic, that: "those who recover from a [natural] disease is never attacked twice?"

Or Rhazes (930 AD) belief that: "smallpox may be due to a fermentation of blood which is expelled from the body during the first attack of the pox?"

Or Girolamo Fracastoro's conclusion he arrived at in 1553 about acquired immunity that: "acquired immunity to smallpox results from the expulsion during the first illness of the menstrual blood contaminant without which clinical disease could not recur?"

Or Paul Ehrlich's side chain hypothesis of acquired immunity that posited that: "antitoxins represent nothing more than side-chains reproduced in excess during regeneration, and therefore [they are] pushed off from the protoplasma, and so coming to exist in a free state?" (P. Ehrlich, Proc. R. Soc. Lond. 66, 424-448, 1899);

Or perhaps they are convinced by the "instructionists' theories of immunity which were expressed variously as: A) "an antigen acts as a template which instructs the cell as to what antibody it has to form?" (Breinl, F. & Haurowitz, F., Z. Physiol. Chem., 192:45, 1930); or that B) "the completed antibody molecule will possess to some degree a stereochemical correspondence with the antigen for the reason that each structural unit has been selected and oriented, at the moment of synthesis into the antibody molecule, to fit the local configuration and affinities of the antigen surface?" (Mudd, S.,J., Immunol. 23,423-427, 1932).

Or Linus Pauling's idea that "It is assumed that antibodies differ from normal serum globulin only in the way in which the two end parts of the globulin polypeptide chain are coiled, these parts, as a result of their amino-acid composition and order, having accessible a very great many configurations with nearly the same stability; under the influence of an antigen molecule, they assume configurations complementary to surface regions of the antigen, thus forming two active ends. After the freeing of one end and the liberation of the central part of the chain this part of the chain folds up to form the central part of the antibody molecule, with two oppositely-directed ends able to attach themselves to two antigen molecules?" (L. Pauling, J Am Chem Soc. 62: 2643-2657, 1940,) and who received Nobel Prizes in 1954 and again in 1962).

"Once an antigen is introduced into the body, that antigen would find its way into the cells of the reticuloendothelial system [of living cells], where contact with local proteinases would result in adaptive modification of the enzymes during the dissolution of the antigen molecule. These newly adapted enzymes would then be able to synthesize a globulin molecule specific for the antigen in question.

Moreover, these adaptive enzymes would not only replicate within the antibody forming cell itself, but the information for antibody specificity which they carried would be perpetuated also within any daughter cells that might result from proliferative activity. Such an expanded population of specifically adapted antibody forming cells (later called a clone) would account well for the heightened secondary or booster antibody response upon subsequent re-exposure to antigen" (Silverstein, A.M, Cellular Immunology 91, 263-283, 1985).

Similar ideas of the cellular mechanisms of immunity were later elaborated to include the presence of a functional template, and expressed as "the indirect template theory" by F.M. Barnett, and F. Fenner in 1953: (i) "To account for the non-antigenicity of body components these were assumed to carry ' selfmarkers '; at some point in the antibody-producing sequence a 'recognition unit' was postulated to act as a means of detecting material carrying self-markers and deflecting it from the possibility of immune response"; (ii)"To account for the persistence of antibody-producing capacity it was postulated that a 'genocopy' of the antigenic determinant was incorporated in the genome of the Stem cell concerned, so allowing the indefinite production of descendant antibody-producing cells"; (iii)"This incorporation of pattern determinants into the genetic structure of antibody-producing cells provided some basis for the changes in antibody character that may result from secondary antigenic stimuli or simple lapse of time" (Burnet, F.M & Fenner, F. The Production of Antibodies. Monograph of the Walter and Eliza Hall Institute, Melbourne, 2nd Edition, 1953).

In 1984, N.K. Jerne received another Nobel Prize for a theory of antibody formation that postulated that: (v)"The spontaneous presence, in the blood of an animal, of small numbers of antibody molecules against all antigens to which the animal can respond, delegates to the antigen the sole role of carrying such specific globulin molecules from the circulation into cells in which these molecules can induce the production of more of their kind" (Jerne, N.K., Proc Nat Acad Sci USA 41:849, 1955).

Yet, as attractive as some of these ideas seemed to be, which became the topic of discussion among vaccinologists and immunologists alike during the launch of vaccine mandates going back Centuries, including the infantile paralysis and then the polio vaccine crusades that caused paralysis as soon as they were introduced (see the chronicles regarding poliomyelitis later in this book), each of these mandates were undermined to a large extent by the introduction of the cellular selection theory, as best articulated by David W. Talmage in 1957 in the context of allergens: "The process of natural selection requires the selective multiplication of a few species out of a diverse population. As a working hypothesis it is tempting to consider that one of the multiplying units in the antibody response is the cell itself. According to this hypothesis, only those cells are selected for multiplication whose synthesized product has affinity for the antigen injected" (Talmage, D.W., Annu Rev Med 8: 239-256, 1957).

As one might guess, this idea led to many refinements of theorizing, such as the clonal selection theory, advocated in revised form by F.M. Burnet, in 1957: "It is postulated that when antigen-natural antibody contact takes place on the surface of a lymphocyte the cell is activated to settle in an appropriate tissue, spleen, lymph node or local inflammatory accumulation, and there undergo proliferation to produce a variety of descendants. In this way preferential proliferation will be initiated by all those clones whose reactive sites correspond to the antigenic determinants on the antigen used. The descendants will include plasmacytoid forms capable of active liberation of soluble antibody and lymphocytes which can fulfill the same functions as the parental forms. The net result will be a change in the composition of the globulin molecule population to give an excess of molecules capable of reacting with the antigen, in other words the serum will now take on the qualities of specific antibody. The increase in the number of circulating lymphocytes of the clones concerned will also ensure that the response to a subsequent entry of the same antigen will be extensive and rapid, i.e., a secondary type of immunological response will occur."

In 1959, Barnett clarified this concept further by stating that: "... in the animal there exist clones of mesenchymal cells, each carrying immunologically reactive sites corresponding in appropriate complementary fashion to one (or possibly a small number of) potential antigenic determinants. This provides a population of cells which, when an appropriate stage of development has been reached, are capable of producing the population of globulin molecules which collectively provide the normal antibodies. When an antigen is introduced, it will contact a cell of the corresponding clone, presumably a lymphocyte, and by so doing stimulate it to produce in one way or another more globulin molecules of the cell's characteristic type" (Burnet, F.M. The Clonal Selection Theory of Acquired Immunity. Vanderbilt University Press. Pp 54-55, 1959). At the end of the 1950's, Joshua Lederberg "blamed" the immune response on mutation(s). (Mutation as a mechanism involved in vaccine resistance will be discussed at some length later on), a phenomenon cited that always can account for anything complex that happens in living systems that is not even remotely understood, similar to a reference to cartoon Super-heroes that acquire supernatural abilities to defeat the forces of evil.

Lederberg received the Nobel Prize in 1958 for arguing that: 1. The stereospecific segment of each antibody globulin is determined by a unique sequence of amino acids. 2. The cell making a given antibody has a correspondingly unique sequence of nucleotides in a segment of its chromosomal DNA: its "gene for globulin synthesis." 3. The genic diversity of the precursors of antibody-forming cells arises from a high rate of spontaneous mutation during their lifelong proliferation. 4. This hypermutability consists of the random assembly of the DNA of globulin gene during certain stages of cellular proliferation. 5. Each cell, as it begins to mature, spontaneously produces small amounts of the antibody corresponding to its own genotype. 6. The immature antibody-forming cell is hypersensitive to an antigen-antibody combination: it will be suppressed if it encounters the homologous antigen at this time. 7. The mature antibody-forming cell is reactive to an antigen-antibody combination: it will be stimulated if it first encounters the homologous antigen at this time. The stimulation comprises the acceleration of protein synthesis and the cytological maturation which mark a "plasma cell". 8. Mature cells proliferate extensively under antigenic stimulation but are genetically stable and therefore generate large clones genotypically preadapted to produce the homologous antibody. 9. These clones tend to persist after the disappearance of the antigen, retaining their capacity to react promptly to its later reintroduction." Lederberg, J., Science 129: 1649-1653, 1959).

None of these concepts elaborated so far, however, could explain some simple long-time known biological facts, such as how any of these postulated mechanisms can allow or explain the life perpetuating process of pregnancy, when a radically dissimilar and genotypically different entire organism(s) (the embryo and then the fetus) develop and persist in a womb harboring a different genotype than the mother without being lethally attacked immunologically as foreign entities are tolerated, or how gut bacteria that are critically important for digestion and which sustain all living systems can live and persist symbiotically to break down nutrients amid a firestorm of self-non-self-directed mechanisms designed to attack and destroy non-self.

One attempt toward a rational explanation for these commonplace facts of the existence of bacterial and fungal symbiosis in the guts of living mammals were set forth by Polly Matzinger in 1994 in a theory she called "The Danger Hypothesis," or more accurately, "The Damage Theory." Consequently, The Danger Hypothesis/ Damage Theory became perhaps the most provocative, and potentially useful immunological idea explaining the nature of immunity and tolerance. In retrospect, however, even these ideas did not even begin to approach anything resembling a coherent hypothesis or explanation for how vaccines may (or may not) protect a living system from future infections, epidemics, or "pandemics."

In all fairness, Dr. Matzinger never pretended or claimed that her hypotheses addressed or explained the issues associated with vaccines and vaccinology in the context of her Damage Theory or Danger hypothesis. Therefore, as a consequence of Matzinger's open honesty and testable model of immunity, her ideas are worth a careful review. In a review of Matzinger's work by Thomas Pradeu and Edwin L. Cooper in Frontiers in Immunology that was published in September, 2012, Mazinger's ideas are reviewed and compared against other noted modern immunologists of her generation, such as C.A. Janeway. In this review, Pradeu and Copper contrast Matzinger's ideas with Janeway's and other noted immunologists notions about the immune system evolving to discriminate between infectious non-self, and non-infectious self (Immunology. Today 19, 11-16. 1992).

Pradeu and Cooper correctly point out, and as Matzinger argued, that immune responses appear to respond to cellular damage in a variety of contexts with the following description, regardless of whether or not the antigen generating the response is foreign or 50 not: "The danger theory [of Matzinger] was explicitly a critique of how immunologists have been trained, namely, within the self-non-self-theory (Matzinger, 1994, 2002). According to the self-non-self-theory, an immune response is triggered against all foreign ("non-self") entities, whereas no immune response is triggered against the organism's own constituents ("self") (Burnet, 1962,1969). For Matzinger, despite the evolution of the self-non-self-theory, between the 1960's and the 1990's, today's immunologists still think of the immune system within this framework, even though this theory may be interpreted as fundamentally flawed."

"Against the self-non-self-theory, the danger theory claims that self-constituents can trigger an immune response, if they are dangerous (e.g., cellular stress, some autografts, etc.; and non-self-constituents can be tolerated, if they are not dangerous (e.g., the fetus or commensal bacteria) (Matzinger) 1984, 2002). According to Matzinger and colleagues, the proper opposition to determine why an immune response is triggered is the presence or absence of danger, not exogenous vs. endogenous characters of any entity under consideration." "Janeway proposed that antigen-presenting cells (APC's) evolved to interact with widespread natural microbial patterns or "pathogen-associated molecular patterns" (PAMP's), e.g., lipopolysaccharide (LPS). APC's do not recognize "non-self"; instead, they recognize foreign patterns that are highly conserved throughout evolution. These legacies from Janeway to Matzinger seemed plausible, but Matzinger emphasized differences between Janeway's view and hers (Matzinger, 2001, 2002). Janeway crucially references to the exogenous nature of rejected entities, whereas Matzinger claims the necessity to fully abandon this perspective. Manzinger asserts that immune responses are not triggered by non-self, but by "endogenous" cellular alarm signals from distressed or injured cells (Matzinger, 2002; 302; see also Matzinger 2001). Even more explicitly, Matzinger wrote: "the 'foreigness of a pathogen is not the important feature that triggers a response, and 'self-ness' is no guarantee of tolerance (Matzinger, 2002; 302)."

Yet despite decades of discussions, ideas, theories, and critiques from the historians of immunology, the Damage theory is rarely if ever discussed in the context of vaccines, to explain how vaccines might theoretically work. Instead, the Jennerian paradigm as it was erroneously proposed by Jenner (1749- 1823) is still in place and implemented as the theoretical basis of most of the vaccinologists justification for mandated vaccinations and used to support the delusional realities to justify booster vaccine schedules.

Adjuvants that non-specifically "boost" the host immune response were designed with a similar motive in mind, except nothing about adjuvants need be facsimiles to induce a ramping up of the immune system. They simply act is generalized immunostimulants, and they greatly "rev-up" the sentinels of the immunity-generating arsenal of the recipient.

Coulter's other principle medical path during medicine's history he termed the "law of contraries," is when and where the therapeutic remedy administered directly "attacks" the microbe or pathogen (like penicillin is believed to disrupt cell membranes of bacteria), and which is a hallmark of allopathic medicine.

Anti-vaxxers (persons who believe vaccines do not confer immunity and are harmful) can list endless side effects to try to convince that vaccines are bad, evil things, and much time has been spent accumulating these data for many years. Pro-vaxxers (persons who believe vaccines work and can immunize) can provide endless arguments about how they believe vaccines do not harm people and how they have helped populations avoid epidemics and disease. I will let the reader judge. But please ask yourself the question why the death rate in the US in 2020 was lower than in 2019 (CDC stats-more about this later)? The RT-PCR tests do not even work so those who are healthy carriers, or false-positives, cannot be determined.

When weighing the relative influences of these various perceptions and the institutions within which they have emerged, the complexity of influences behind vaccine crusades and public health policies become more complex. It is clear from the start, however, that assumptions or any arrogance of knowledge regarding vaccines or vaccine history, epidemics, or endemic illnesses, need serious revisions. Many uncertainties instead of certainties remain the rule. If and when this history can be adequately investigated, finally the ultimate question the philosophers might be in a position to ask is why? **"Why do we vaccinate?"**

430 B.C Athens. The disease, suspected to have been typhoid fever, weakened the Athenians significantly and was a significant factor in their defeat by the Spartans. Inoculations or vaccines played no role in this "disease," nor can it be certain that it was due to typhoid, as other diseases present with these same symptoms. *"The earliest recorded pandemic happened during the Peloponnesian War. After the disease passed through Libya, Ethiopia, and Egypt, it crossed the Athenian walls as the Spartans laid siege. As much as two-thirds of the population died. The symptoms included fever, thirst, bloody throat and tongue, red skin and lesions."*

165 A.D.-185 A.D. Antonine or "Plague of Galen," If it were bubonic plague and not smallpox as written by some historians that afflicted the Roman Empire of this era of Markus Aurelius Antonius, it is certain that no plague preventative or therapeutic measure in the form of inoculations or vaccines could have played a role in the 165-185 epidemic or later in the epidemic of 251-256 AD. The occurrence of the first plague epidemic was described in depth by Galen in during the period of 169-216 A.D as being characterized by victims having *"fevers, diarrhea, vomiting, thirstiness, swollen throats, and coughing. More specifically, Galen noted that the diarrhea appeared blackish which suggested gastrointestinal bleeding, and the coughing of plague victims produced a foul odor on the breath and an exanthema, skin eruptions or rash, over the entirety of the body distinguished by red and black papules or eruptions: Of some of theses which had become ulcerated, that part of the surface called the scab fell away and then the remaining p*art nearby was he*althy and after one or two days became scarred over. In those places where it was not ulcerated, the exanthem was rough and scabby and fell away like some husk and hence all became healthy. (Littman & Littman, p. 246). Those infected suffered from the illness for roughly two weeks. Not all who caught the disease died, and those who survived developed immunity from further outbreaks.*

Based on Galen's description, some modern epidemiology researchers have concluded that the disease affecting the Roman Empire of this period was most likely smallpox (Littman R.J. Littman M.L. "Galen and the Antonine Plague." The American Journal of Pathology 3, 94, pp. 243-255, 1973).Although bubonic plague has its easily visible "buboes" or swollen lymph nodes of the groin and arm pit that are characteristic of this form of plague is known to be spread either by air through the breath or by flea bites that originate from rats that tend to populate times of extreme social disruptions, and although plague has inspired one of the richest mythologies and foremost examples of what primitive religion in the West envisioned a punishment from God for bad behavior, social conflicts, and any kind of "discord," some historians claim, however, that the Antonine "plague" was possibly an early appearance of smallpox that began with the Huns who then infected the Germans, who passed it to the Romans and then returning Roman troops spread it throughout the Roman empire. Described symptoms included fever, sore throat, diarrhea, and pus-filled sores. This plague continued until about 180 A.D. and is said to have killed Marcus Aurelius.

250 A.D. Cyprian Plague In no description of this 250 A.D. 250-occurring plague is dehydration-inductive persistent vomiting described as a symptom as it was described in the Antonine plague occurrence, yet other features of plague were described. But important for this history, again, is the fact that there could have been no preventative or therapeutic inoculation or vaccine intervention in place for any of this series of plague-attributed epidemics during the 195 years between 250 A.D. and 444 A.D.

It is believed to be the first significant appearance of the bubonic plague that clearly featured enlarged lymphatic glands and was thought to be carried by rats and transmitted to man by fleas, yet as previously mentioned, there are other known ways of plague's spread, such as food-transmission, or inhalation of air next to an infected person. *The Cyprian Plague was named after the first known victim, the Christian bishop of Carthage, the Cyprian plague entailed diarrhea, vomiting, throat ulcers, fever and gangrenous hands and feet. There were recurring outbreaks over the next three centuries. In 444 A.D., it hit Britain and obstructed defense efforts against the Picts and the Scots, causing the British to seek help from the Saxons, who would soon control the island.*

541 A.D. Justinian Plague It is uncertain how the census takers have made estimates of population sizes as large as ¼ of the world's human population as long ago as 541 A.D., but we can be fairly confident that inoculations or vaccinations played no role in the occurrence or abatement or severity of this "apocalyptic" epidemic.

"First appearing in Egypt, the Justinian plague spread through Palestine and the Byzantine Empire, and then throughout the Mediterranean. The plague changed the course of the empire, squelching Emperor Justinian's plans to bring the Roman Empire back together and causing massive economic struggle. It is also credited with creating an apocalyptic atmosphere

that spurred the rapid spread of Christianity. Recurrences over the next two centuries eventually killed about 50 million people, 26 percent of the world population.

11th Century: Leprosy is described as first appearing in pandemic proportions in 1100, presumably manifesting physically with clearly visible "skin rot" or gangrenous flesh, loss of certain facial features "*Though it had been around for ages, leprosy grew into a pandemic in Europe in the Middle Ages, resulting in the building of numerous leprosy-focused hospitals to accommodate the vast number of victims. A slow-developing bacterial disease that causes sores and deformities, leprosy was believed to be a punishment from God that ran in families. This belief led to moral judgments and ostracization of victims. Now known as Hansen's disease, it still afflicts tens of thousands of people a year and can be fatal if not treated with antibiotics.*

1349-1350 Black Death. It has been written that this second *large* outbreak of the bubonic plague possibly started in Asia and moved west in caravans. Entering through Sicily in 1347 A.D. when plague sufferers arrived in the port of Messina, it spread throughout Europe rapidly. Dead bodies became so prevalent that many remained rotting on the ground and created a constant stench in cities. England and France were so incapacitated by the plague that the countries called a truce to their war. The British feudal system collapsed when the plague changed economic circumstances and demographics. Ravaging populations in Greenland, Vikings lost the strength to wage battle against native populations, and their exploration of North America halted. Historians often conclude that *"this plague was the "big one and was responsible for the death of one-third of the world population,"* but as mentioned already, as with other "pandemics," the claim should be subjected to modern criteria of pathology instead of dogmatic and dire historical fact.

1492: The Columbian Exchange. Following the arrival of the Spanish in the Caribbean, diseases such as smallpox, measles and bubonic plague were passed along to the native populations by the Europeans. With no previous exposure, these diseases devastated indigenous people, with as many as 90 percent dying throughout the north and south continents. Upon arrival on the island of Hispaniola, Christopher Columbus encountered the Taino people, population 60,000. By 1548, the population stood at less than 500. This scenario repeated itself throughout the Americas.

In 1520, the Aztec Empire was destroyed by a smallpox infection. The disease killed many of its victims and incapacitated others. It weakened the population, so they were unable to resist Spanish colonizers and left farmers unable to produce needed crops. Research in 2019 even concluded that the deaths of some 56 million Native Americans in the 16th and 17th centuries, largely through disease, may have altered Earth's climate as vegetation growth on previously tilled land drew more CO2 from the atmosphere and caused a cooling event.

1665 The Great Plague of London. A graph showing the huge increase in deaths during the Great Plague of London in 1665 and 1666. The solid line shows all deaths and the broken line deaths attributed to plague. In another devastating appearance, the bubonic plague led to the deaths of 20 percent of London's population. As human death tolls mounted and mass graves appeared, hundreds of thousands of cats and dogs were slaughtered as the possible cause and the disease spread through ports along the Thames. The worst of the outbreak tapered off in the fall of 1666, around the same time as another destructive event—the Great Fire of London.

1817 Cholera Pandemic Although many historians claim that the first of seven cholera pandemics over the next 150 years, this wave of the small intestine infection originated in Russia, where one million people died. Spreading through feces-contaminated water and food, the bacterium was passed along to British soldiers who brought it to India where millions more died. The reach of the British Empire and it's Navy spread cholera to Spain, Africa, Indonesia, China, Japan, Italy, Germany, and America, where it killed 150,000 people. A vaccine was created in 1885, but pandemics continued.

1855 The Third Plague Pandemic. Starting in China and moving to India and Hong Kong, the bubonic plague claimed 15 million victims. Initially spread by fleas during a mining boom in Yunnan, the plague is considered a factor in the Parthay rebellion and the Taiping rebellion. India faced the most substantial casualties, and the epidemic was used as an excuse for repressive policies that sparked some revolt against the British. The pandemic was considered active until 1960 when cases dropped below a couple hundred.

1875: Fiji Measles Pandemic. It is widely believed that *"after Fiji ceded to the British Empire, a royal party visited Australia as a gift from Queen Victoria. Arriving during a measles outbreak, the royal party brought the disease back to their island, and it was spread further by the tribal heads and police who met with them upon their return. Spreading quickly, the island was littered with corpses that were scavenged by wild animals, and entire villages died and were burned down, sometimes with the sick trapped inside the fires. One-third of Fiji's population, a total of 40,000 people, died."*

1889: Russian Flu. The official textbook descriptions of the Russian flu continue to claim that it was *"the first significant flu pandemic started in Siberia and Kazakhstan, traveled to Moscow, and made its way into Finland and then Poland, where it moved into the rest of Europe, and by the following year, this flu had crossed the ocean into North America and Africa, and by the end of 1890, 360,000 had died."*

1918: Spanish Flu. Official propaganda still claims that *the avian-borne flu that resulted in 50 million deaths worldwide, the 1918 flu was first observed in Europe, the United States, and parts of Asia before swiftly spreading around the world. At the time, there were no effective drugs or vaccines to treat this killer flu strain. Wire service reports of a flu outbreak in Madrid in the spring of 1918 led to the pandemic being called the "Spanish Flu." By October, hundreds of thousands of Americans died and body storage scarcity hit crisis level. But the flu threat disappeared in the summer of 1919 when most of the infected had either developed immunities or died.* The primary sources of agent isolation by Rosenow and then more definitively by Rosenau (no relation) shows however, that the causative microbe thought to be responsible for this "Great Spanish Flu," which was a misnomer in the first place was not in fact due to Pfeffer's bacillus, which was believed to have been the causative agent for some 36 or more years leading up to this catastrophe. Much more about this will be discussed later.

1957: Asian flu. Starting in Hong Kong and spreading throughout China and then into the United States, the Asian flu became widespread in England where, over six months, 14,000 people died. A second wave followed in early 1958, causing an estimated total of about 1.1 million deaths globally, with 116,000 deaths in the United States alone. A vaccine was developed, effectively containing the pandemic.

1981: HIV/AIDS. First identified in 1981, the cause of AIDS was announced as being a Cytomegalovirus rather than an "HIV" viral infection, but the scientific community after intense analysis had figured it out approximately 8 years later but were ignored, vilified, their careers destroyed, and the knowledge was suppressed by the interests of the United States Government and to be fair, a love of the mental illness known as biological reductionism. Briefly reviewed, here are the facts regarding the connection of "HIV" and the anergy attributed to the collection of some 50+ diseases subsumed under the AIDS disease definition: Cytomegalovirus causes AIDS because Dr. Michael Gottlieb found CMV (cytomegalovirus) in 100% of his first 5 patients at UCLA. (The CDC's Monthly Mortality Weekly Report, and, in the journal Nature, December **1981** issue).

1983 "Black slaves" according to Robert Gallo caused cancer because he saw artwork evidence which proved to him as the head of the laboratory of Tumor Virology of the NIH that the themes of certain artworks depicted slaves who had caught **a cancer virus in the 16th Century from monkeys during the slave trade**. This logic was first used by Gallo to explain the historical reasons as to how RNA viruses (like "HIV") can cause human cancers, and to illustrate this universally discredited notion that viruses cause human cancers. Gallo painted a picture in his writings about how Japanese civilians in and near Nagasaki developed the high rate of leukemias after the atomic bombs were dropped on them because of the retrovirus, "HTLV-I" which was one of his first of 3 precursor mistakes before he claimed "HIV" caused AIDS. This hypothesis was advanced to explain the origins of the lentiviruses culminating with "HIV" as being a "human cancer virus variant" turned human immune suppressive virus, despite the fact that the virus cancer hypothesis had been completely smashed and discredited by Payton Rous in his 1966 Nobel Prize acceptance speech and by many other working biologists of that era (which is a theme that will later be analyzed in some depth in this analysis). Yet Gallo persisted for some years even after he first tried to convince the scientific community that he had discovered **"HTLV-1"** in 1979-81 to explain Japanese leukemias, and then "HTLV-II was named as "the perp" by Gallo, but even after this idea was rapidly dismissed by the scientific community, and abandoned by Gallo, after a brief period, Gallo then again claimed that another cancer virus, "HTLV-III" was the true "perp" and was "the true "first human cancer virus" in order to explain why 339 out of more than 600,000 Japanese acquired cancers in Southern Japan near Nagasaki. This is also why in 1984 when the televised announcement was made for the first time to the American public regarding "the probable cause of AIDS" had been found" by Dr. Gallo in his sunglasses and with Health and Human Services Margaret Heckler standing at his side, the Health and Human Services government official was instructed by Gallo and the US government to use the phrase, "the probable cause of AIDS has been found...to be "HTLV-III...[which is] a known ***variant*** of a "cancer virus." "HTLV-III" was later renamed "HIV" by oncogene Nobelist Varmus's committee. (National Institute of Health: Gallo R.C., Sliski A., Wong-Staal F: Origin of T-cell leukemia-lymphoma virus. Lancet (ii): 962-963, **1983**.

1983 The virus "LAV" (Lymphadenopathy-Associated Virus was associated with AIDS because Luc Montagnier's "Patient 1" had many diseases and was said to have pre-AIDS. Montagnier's so-called "LAV-BRU" or "LAV-LAI" "isolate's" association with pre-AIDS conditions was advanced despite the fact that Montagnier's "Patient One" had been treated for syphilis, gonorrhea, cytomegalovirus, Epstein-Barr virus, and herpes viruses. Yet, even though "Patient One's" lymphocytes were believed to harbor "LAV," (later also named "HIV" by Varmus's committee, Montagnier later admitted they **couldn't** purify "HIV" despite "a Roman effort," a required technical step in proving the association of any virus with disease (Pasteur Institute: Barre-Sinoussi, F,J.C. Chermann J.C., Rey F., Nugeyre MT., Chamaret, S., Gruest J., Dauguet C., Axler-Blin C., Vezinet-Brn F., Rouzioux, C., Rozenbaum R., & Montagnier L. Isolation of a T-lymphotropic retrovirus from a patient at risk for Acquired Immune Deficiency Syndrome. Science 230: 868-871, **1983**).

1984 Gallo's claim with Heckler in 1984 then claimed that "HIV" was actually not a cancer virus but a cancer virus variant, and his claim that "HIV" causes AIDS, was based on the finding that 36% of 72 of his AIDS patients tested "HIV-positive," even though many were not sick. This claim was the basis of the first Abbott Lab "HIV-test kits," which were patented by Gallo and the French that same day (which is also the same enterprise that is said to be the most promising for the patenting of a kit to detect SARS-CoV-2). And it should not escape attention that this claim of virus association was also 64% less of an association that Gottlieb reported for CMV's association with his original AIDS patients he believed harbored cytomegalovirus. These are the four papers, published in the same issue of science that launched the AIDS era: From the National Institutes of Health- Popovic M, Sarngadharan MG, Read E, et al. Detection, Isolation,and Continuous Production of Cytopathic Retroviruses (HTLV-III) from Patients with AIDS and Pre-AIDS. Science, 224:497-500, **1984**; Gallo RC, Salahuddin SZ, Popovic M, et al. Frequent Detection and Isolation of Cytopathic Retroviruses (HTLV-III) from Patients with AIDS and at Risk for AIDS. Science 224:500-502, **1984**; Schupbach J, Popovic M, Gilden RV, et al. Serological analysis of a Subgroup of Human T-Lymphotropic Retroviruses (HTLV-III) Associated with AIDS. Science, 224:503-505, **1984**; Sarngadharan MG, Popovic M,Bruch L, et al. Antibodies Reactive to Human TLymphotrophic Retroviruses (HTLV-III) in the Serum of Patients with AIDS. Science, 224:506-508, **1984**.

1985 "HIV" emerged from barbaric African sexual practices to stimulate a man or a woman and induce them to intense sexual activity, monkey blood [for a man] or she-monkey blood [for a woman] was directly incubated in the pubic area and also the thighs and back. These magic practices would therefore unequivocally constitute an efficient experimental transmission model and could be responsible for the emergence of AIDS in man, as was published in The Lancet. (Noireau F. HIV transmission from monkey to man-Lancet (i):1498-1499, **1987**).

1987 "HIV" is a harmless passenger virus: "HIV" exists but does no harm and does not cause AIDS. (University of California, Berkeley: Peter H. Duesberg, "Retroviruses as Carcinogens and Pathogens: Expectations and Reality Cancer Research 47, 1199-1220, March 1, **1987**).

1987 Smallpox vaccine campaigns in Africa caused AIDS as they woke up latent "HIV" harbored by blacks who were vaccinated. (The World Health Organization, published in Letters to The Lancet, and NEJM, London Times Edition 1 MON 11 MAY **1987**).

1987 AIDS is actually a form of cryptic syphilis, "the great imitator," which presents with identical T—cell disturbances, profound immune suppression, and dementia (Washington's National Library of Medicine. HL. AIDS and Syphilis-The Hidden Link, CA, pps. 20, 21, **1987**).

1988 AIDS is caused by Redox imbalances and by proteins and behaviors that oxidize cells and tissues (Royal Perth Hospital, Perth Australia, Papadopulos-Eleopulos E. Medical Hypotheses. 25: 151-162, **1988**).

1989 Malnutrition, recreational and prescription drugs, and foreign proteins cause AIDS (University of California, Berkeley: Peter H. Duesberg, Proc. Natl. Acad. Sci. USA Vol.86, pp. 755-764, February **1989**).

Yet despite this history that unfolded in 5 years between 1981- and 1989, according to modern textbooks and popular wisdom, AIDS is still caused by "HIV" which over time destroys a person's immune system, resulting in eventual death by diseases that the body would usually fight off. Those infected by the HIV virus encounter fever, headache, and enlarged lymph nodes upon infection. When symptoms subside, carriers become highly infectious through blood and genital fluid, and the disease destroys t-cells. AIDS was first observed in American gay communities but is believed to have developed from a chimpanzee virus from West Africa in the 1920s. The disease, which spreads through certain body fluids, moved to Haiti in the 1960s, and then New York and San Francisco in the 1970s. Treatments have been developed to slow the progress of the disease, but 35 million people worldwide have died of AIDS since its discovery, and a cure is yet to be found.

This addition of "HIV/AIDS" to this "expert's" list of epidemics is not only unjustified, unwarranted, and irrational, and does not belong on this list for more than 100 reasons that will be elaborated at length later, one can argue also that the mode of suspected transmission of plague has never been, or ever will be argued to occur through an infected person breathing "HIV-"-laced air onto a non-infected person. In addition most if not all plague statistics have been gained via the imagined transmission through insect vectors like fleas yet it also has been reportedly in rare instance been transmitted through breathing "very close" to infected persons, and while the statistics regarding cholera is a syndrome spread through contaminated food and again is not transmissible through the air like flus are thought to be (but not proven as will be elaborated at great length later), the non-existence of "HIV" itself discredits its belonging on this list of epidemics). **This topic will be covered at some length later in the text.**

SARS BEGINS IN 2003 AND VACCINES ROLL-OUT IN FEBRUARY 2021

2003 SARS. First identified in 2003 after several months of cases, Severe Acute Respiratory Syndrome is believed to have possibly started with bats, spread to cats and then to humans in China, followed by

26 other countries, infecting 8,096 people, with 774 deaths. SARS is characterized by respiratory problems, dry cough, fever and head and body aches and is spread through respiratory droplets from coughs and sneezes. Quarantine efforts proved effective and by July, the virus was contained and has not reappeared since. China was criticized for trying to suppress information about the virus at the beginning of the outbreak. SARS was seen by global health professionals as a wake-up call to improve outbreak responses, and lessons from the pandemic were used to keep diseases like H1N1, Ebola and Zika under control.

2019: COVID-19. On March 11, 2020, the World Health Organization announced that the COVID-19 virus was officially a pandemic after barreling through 114 countries in three months and infecting over 118,000 people. And the spread was not anywhere near finished. COVID-19 is caused by a novel coronavirus—a new coronavirus strain that has not been previously found in people. Symptoms include respiratory problems, fever, and cough, and can lead to pneumonia and death. Like SARS, it is spread through droplets from sneezes. The first reported case in China appeared November 17, 2019, in the Hubei Province, but went unrecognized. Eight more cases appeared in December with researchers pointing to an unknown virus. Many learned about SARS-CoV-19 when ophthalmologist Dr. Li Wenliang defied government orders and released safety information to other doctors. The following day, China informed WHO and charged Li with a crime. Li died from COVID-19 just over a month later. The virus spread beyond Chinese borders and by mid-March, it had spread globally to more than 163 countries. On February 11, the infection was officially christened COVID-19.There are only two take home messages that we arrive at regarding this morass of confusion, misplaced altruism, and medically justified terrorism.

The first is the concept that will be advanced is our ridiculous car wax analogy of vaccine protection of individuals, and the other concept to be advanced is best described with the term, herd immunity, which is also ridiculous from the standpoint of biological fitness and resistance.

To briefly remind about the concept of car wax or vaccine protection: If citizens believe a vaccine is like car wax that protects a car in the winter from the ice and snow and rain (imagine the ice, snow, rain, hail, as different viruses, bacteria, or other pathogens), if you believe in the efficacy and safety of the vaccines that will protect you acts analogously to the way wax protects a car (and your children), then by all means, wax (vax) your car (and your children) to protect it (them), but my NOT waxing (vaxing) my car (or mandating that I should wax it by coercion by mandate or by law or penalty) should have no bearing on what happens to your car if you "vaccinated it" or "waxxed it" to protect it from winter "rust" (or germs floating everywhere about in the case of COVID-19). Why should we continue to mandate vaccines in the future to attend schools, to obtain honest work as a health care provider, to travel abroad, etc.?

THE EVOLUTION OF THE EARLY VACCINATION PARADIGM AND THE REAL STORY OF POLIO – *SINCE THE DAWN OF VACCINATION THERE HAS BEEN A WAR OF DISINFORMATION AND FALSE NARRATIVES*

The Jennerian paradigm of vaccination proposed by Edward Jenner's vaccination doctrine was based on milk maid cases of cow pox being analogous to human smallpox and was spread all over the world like a mind-virus, and Benjamin Waterhouse of Harvard brought it to the United States while Jenner's medical credentials are deemed fraudulent.

At about this time in 1868, smallpox then emerged in San Francisco.

As a Professor of Hygiene, Robert Koch introduced a remedy for tuberculosis, which caused thousands of deaths in 1899.

At about this time, a paralysis outbreak began to occur in Vermont, and it was non-contagious in families and associated with cotton, apple farming, and arsenate pesticide residues.

As a result of these events, vaccine mandates began to be formulated by "the experts," and for example the baffling nature of tuberculosis ignited the Public Health and Safety eugenicists to begin the coordinated efforts to control citizens and parents via medical terrorism. This was an incredibly important chapter in vaccine history.

In response to this terrorism, the Supreme Court of the United States handed down its ruling in the famous Jacobson case, wherein the Jacobson father refused to have his son vaccinated (Jacobson vs. Commonwealth of Massachusetts, Docket 197 US 11 IN, 1905).

In New England, calcium arsenate came into widespread use primarily on cotton crops and orchards in 1907, and it was noticed for the first time that polio was not apparently transmissible in families.

A few years later, a World prepared to go to war, and mandatory induction vaccination of soldiers began, followed by the greatest influenza epidemic of all time, which spread to the civilian population from military bases. This launched the Great Influenza Era in 1911. Supported by the eugenicists, the concept of "The Healthy Carrier

State" begins to take its full expression as a result of paralysis (polio's) non-contagious modes of acquisition, while at the same time, the Department of the Navy, according to records found in The Naval Historical Center claims that "The Great Spanish Flu" attacked young people in the prime of their lives unlike any other epidemics ever recorded previously.

By **1918**, and although the cause of the greatest disease in human history remaining unknown, 20,000,000 were estimated to have died from flu, but the "Spanish Flu" was not from Spain and is now believed to have been due to vaccination, war, and bacteria.

However, at the time, despite Supreme Court decisions and emphasis on "protecting the greater good," North Dakota enacted laws expressly forbidding the passage of any mandatory vaccination laws, and Wisconsin established personal exemptions from vaccinations.

In **1921**, the events that comprise the story we are all told as children occurred when Franklin D. Roosevelt developed paralysis after he swam in the icy Bay of Fundy in New Brunswick.

Meanwhile, during these years spanning the early 1900's and across the globe in the Pacific, and according to the Congressional Record, The Philippines experienced the worst smallpox epidemic ever after a vaccination rate recorded as being administered to 95% of the Philippine population via a mandated vaccine crusade.

Similarly, West Nile Virus is said to originate from a black woman before electron microscopes could have confirmed the West Nile syndrome was due to a virus, ushering in the beginnings of institutionalized racism.

Viruses are imaged for the first time in 1939, when the tobacco mosaic virus, which was below the wave-lengths of visible light, and which decimated tobacco crops and the tobacco industry, was visualized for the first time by the resolution of the first functional electron microscopes.

During the 1940's, advertisements appeared in American magazines showing cartoons of huge house flies attacking babies as they slept in their cribs, and that flies were the most likely source of paralysis.

Of course, it was ignored that the pesticide, DDT was developed to spray everything, including the household kitchen and the food supply.

At about this time in 1942, a report of the US Secretary of War, Henry L. Simpson regarding the deaths from yellow fever shots state that "recent army experience with the yellow fever vaccine resulted in 28,505 cases of hepatitis with 62 deaths."

1944 was a particularly important year in vaccine history. For instance, early in 1944, pertussis-diphtheria-tetanus tri-valent vaccine was recommended for universal use in infants by the American Academy of Pediatrics for routine use, and across the pond later in 1944, a British authority on immunology, M. Meadow Bayly, M.R.C.S., and author of the book The Shick inoculation against diphtheria wrote:

"Perhaps the greatest evil of immunization lies in its diversion of public attention from true methods of disease prevention…and encourages public authorities to permit all kinds of sanitary defects and social problems to remain unaddressed, particularly in schools." Before the year's end, the NIH claimed that DDT damaged the same anterior horn cells that are damaged in the infantile paralysis syndrome.

It became more and more apparent to inquiring physicians that epidemics corresponded quite closely to pesticides. In 1946, Dr. Gebhaedt showed that polio seasonality, for example, correlated with the fruit harvest each year.

In 1948, the Vaccination Inquirer Newsletter reported that the English and Scotish Health Ministers had acknowledged that more than 25,000 cases of diphtheria had been reported from 1941 to 1945 in immunized children, with nearly 200 deaths.

A few year later, however, the polio era was launched because one "round" particle was found in a human turd, which, in 1948 was supported by the laboratory work of Daldorf and Sickles because they took excrement from a paralysis victim and prepared a 20% suspension with ether and centrifugations and injected it into the brains of suckling 7-day-old mice, which caused the mice to become paralyzed (due to the foreign protein toxicity they administered intracranially). In an epidemiological context, and in **1949**, DDT was linked to similar nervous system paralysis, but the pesticide was ignored, and Enders at Harvard claimed that he could make this "virus" from human embryonic cells, making it far easier to make a vaccine. These events transpired, in addition, at the same time endocrinologist Dr. Morton Biskind who was a practitioner and medical researcher found that DDT causes "lesions in the spinal cord similar to human polio."

In 1950, the US Public Health Industrial Hygiene Medical Director, J.G. Townsend noted the similarity between parathion poisoning and polio and believed that some polio might be caused by eating fruits or vegetables with parathion residues.

Also, in **1950,** and with more science having been accumulated using the electron microscope, a small nanometer-sized ball-like particle that was 24-30 nM in size was isolated from human excrement and further fueled the launch of the polio era. This single ball was made visible for the first time with these new improvements to electron microscope technology, and it was named, "The Polio Virus."

Over the next 30 years, between the 1950's and 1980's, 12 million vaccines were shown to have caused yaws, schistosomiasis, "HIV," and hepatitis C.

During the **1950's**, and with a growing appreciation that animal models of vaccines are of limited interpretational value, in 1972, mentally disabled children at Willowbrook School (NY) were deliberately infected with hepatitis in an attempt to find a vaccine. Participation in the study was a condition for admission to the institution, and the routine and widespread human experimentation on vulnerable populations by the vaccinologists began in full force.

Such human experimentation was questioned, however, when Ralph R. Scobey**, also in 1950,** who was a noted M.D. of his day because he was president of the poliomyelitis Research Institute INC.

in New York listed 170 diseases that exhibit polio-like symptoms and effects but with different names such as epidemic cholera, cholera morbus, spinal meningitis, spinal apoplexy, inhibitory palsy, and others.

The political and social forces of the world again conspired to change medical history during the beginnings of The Cold War, and the days of innocence were over. Cervical cancer cells were obtained from an African American "slave girl" and used without her or her family's consent by a Dr. Gey who used them to test if Henrietta's cancer cells, when injected into more than 600 patients without their consent, into 80 prisoners without their informed consent, and into a number of orthodox Jews, without their informed consent either. Dr, Gey wanted to know if Doctors self injected themselves by accident with a patient's cancer cells, whether they would develop cancer (or not). No cancers were produced, however, in any of these groups Dr. Gey injected with Henrietta's live cancer cells, but Dr. Gey's insanity did usher into the world the first human experimentation laws. Henrietta Lacks cervical cancer cells changed the world and helped win the biological arms race because her cells were also given to a Communist (at that time) Russian delegation to join forces with the Americans and Europeans in the world's pursuit to find the first human cancer virus. Accompanying these unspeakable tragedies and insanity, during the 1950's polio era, hopes and beliefs took shape that there must be human cancer viruses in order to lay the conceptual foundation to launch an extremely lucrative although futile "war on cancer" beginning in the 1960's and into the 1970's. This war waged on during the 1970's when Gallo took up the charge to find the first cancer viruses he first fraudulently passed off as "HTLV-I, HTLV-II, HTLV-III, which became "HIV." This initiative was begun by Mary Lasker, Mathilde Krim, and others. These women had close personal ties to the most powerful circles inside of Washington, and also to Hollywood and the Hollywood stars.

Yet in 1950-1951 at the beginning of the decade, all these politics began to be set into motion at the same time scientists were reporting that they could not find the designated polio virus in many polio paralysis victims, and despite the fact that Dr. Biskind presenting evidence to the US Congress that pesticides were the major cause of polio epidemics, and Dr. Ralph Scobey reporting that he found clear evidence of poisoning when analyzing chemical traces in the blood of polio victims.

But a Dr. Kumm is then appointed as Director of Research of the National Foundation for Infantile Paralysis (NFIP). The NFIP was funded by its "March of Dimes" program, and it sponsored the hasty development of the Salk vaccine in the early 1950's. At the height of the DDT/polio controversy, Dr. Kumm also "served" as a civilian consultant to the Surgeon General…directing field studies of the use of DDT….(American Journal of Digestive Diseases, 20,330, (1953).

And by **1955,** there was still a great deal of social pressure in America to moth-proof clothes by washing them in EQ-53, a formula containing DDT, while legislation recognizing the dangers of persistent pesticides is enacted, and a phase of DDT in the US accelerated along with a shift of sales of DDT to third world countries. Thus, DDT was being phased out as widespread polio vaccinations are about to begin.

While these deliberations transpire, Dr. Jonas Salk develops the first commercial polio vaccine with a virus found "in the pooled feces of three healthy children" in Cleveland (who were not paralysis victims), and the first commercial pooled "polio virus" extract is administered to 400,000 US children. The official safety report stated that it protected 30-90% of recipients…however, manufacturers could make a 300% markup on the vaccine.

On April 16, 1955, an infant with paralysis was admitted to Michael Reese Hospital in Chicago, IL. The patient had been inoculated in the buttock with "Cutter's" polio vaccine and a week later, on April 24, had developed flaccid paralysis of both legs. A month later, in May, ninety-nine cases of polio became eventually attributed to Cutter vaccine in California, with the incidence of polio among other cutter vaccinees exceeding the textbook definition of a wild polio epidemic by nearly 3-fold in Idaho, with eighty-eight cases attributed to Cutter vaccine, the rate was fifteen times greater. Before it was over, the "Cutter incident," as it was called in scientific circles resulted in 260 people contracting polio and almost 200 cases of paralysis, with eleven deaths.

This prompted Canada to suspend the distribution of Salk's vaccine. By November, all European countries had suspended distribution plans, apart from Denmark. By January, 1957, 17 US states had stopped distributing the vaccine. The same year the New York Times reported that nearly 50 percent of cases of infantile paralysis in children between the ages of five and fourteen had occurred after vaccination.

This prompted the CDC to change the rules for defining polio again, and cases of inflammation of the brain that protects the brain and spinal neuron cells, which causes muscular weakness and pain but not paralysis, were no longer classified as polio. The call such collections of symptoms in cases thereafter, "viral or aseptic meningitis." Non-paralytic cases are to be renamed "meningitis" even if the polio virus is present. The reported figures for polio were officially to exclude cases of aseptic meningitis and other enteroviruses. "Reported" cases dropped the same extent following the introduction and widespread use of polio vaccines.

In **1963**, the measles vaccine is licensed: to implement the vaccination strategy a mixture of cooperative appeals and coercive school mandates were set into motion.

Baruck Blumberg at the NIH claims that he is able to isolate some funny-looking "hepatitis B" particles that have 3 different sizes and shapes from a healthy, black, Aboriginal male's blood, and is believed without inquiry.

Similarly, birds are imagined having begun swapping their diseases through genes to humans in Asia after about more than 100 million years of separate evolution, and the Hong Kong flu pandemic is claimed to kill 700,000 people due to "H3N2" virus.

While all this bird business is happening in the early 1970's, the HEW reported that as much as 26 percent of children receiving rubella vaccinations were developing arthralgia or arthritis, and in 1971, the MMR (tri-valent measles/mumps/rubella vaccine is licensed. TRI-VALENT MEASLES/MUMPS/ RUBELLA) LICENSED (1971). In 1975, it is reported that crib death and infantile convulsions virtually disappeared when Japan moved the vaccination age to two years old.

Thus, the era of "hepatitis B, the "slow" virus-like particle, and the origins of most if not all of humanity's epidemics and pandemic afflictions began with institutionalized racist thinking, and perversions of human sexuality.

One of the noted Fathers of "slow virus" theories who influenced an entire generation of biomedical researchers was the 1976 Nobelist, C. Carlton Gajducek, discoverer of Creutzfeldt-Jakob disease (kuru), and bovine spongiform encephalopathies, known as mad cow disease, was the top official in the Brain Studies Laboratory at the National Institute of Neurological Disease and Stroke, which is part of the National Institutes of Health. Although this hypothesis does not make sense because all viruses are made by cells, and because all biologically-made pathogens are formed from common organic biomolecules, to postulate that are "slow in nature," is to suggest they are miraculously not metabolized or degraded, or activated once they enter the organism, as are all other known biological molecules of living systems. This defies both biological and chemical experience. Yet several Nobel prizes have been awarded for work relating to these postulated "slow viruses" by "slow virologists, mostly, including those Nobel Prizes given to Gajducek, Gajdusek's successor, Stanley Pruisner, and Baruck Blumberg for their unsubstantiated and irrational beliefs that slow viruses or other pathogens can cause sudden illness years or decades after infection.

Many scientists, and other Human Beings believe a person's character should matter in life, and especially in the realms where the responsibility of protecting or promoting public health policies and science is bestowed on them. In this context, C. Carlton

Gajdusek with his "prions" or protein-replicating-particles or PrP's was a man who plead guilty and then was convicted of molesting many young boys from New Guinea and Micronesia where his NIH-bestowed grants took him to discover and then study kuru among the Fore Tribesmen of New Guinea. On his way home to the NIH, he brought the boys to Maryland to molest them in a home given him as an Official Head of Neuroscience at the NIH, and then he defended his actions by stating that as a student of Anthropology and different cultures, American values are "prudish," and he should be allowed to molest the children as it was normal, according to him. He plead guilty and spent a year in prison, before fleeing the country to Europe, rather than being brought to the justice he deserved here in the U.S. This says something about a man's world view, including his scientific beliefs. Gajdusek's Nobel was followed up by another one given to Stanley Prusiner, whom everybody liked because he was clever enough to come up with different names for Gajdusek's Prions: PrP, which represented Proteinaceous Replicating Particles which came in 2 kinds, one that always is in our bodies designated as the normal protein, and the disease-associated particle (or rod) that caused the host's normal PrR protein to begin to polymerize, to create brain problems, such as plaques. Although car-accident victims, and anoxic patients also develop similar plaques, there seems to be nothing special about the accumulation of amyloid to form tangles or plaques as a generalized response to any severe neural assault or injury.

For his findings regarding aboriginals and hepatitis B "virus," Baruch Blumberg is credited with the discovery of the AU antigen, HbSAg, that he believed was caused by a virus that could cause liver cancer after decades of incubation of the hepatitis B virus. He found the HbSAg marker in the stored blood sample of a healthy, black, Australian Aboriginal male, for which he is co-awarded The Nobel Prize with NIH's Former Neurobiology Program Director, D. Carlton Gajdusek, for his belief in other so-called "slow virus-like entity" that he believed were responsible for neurological Parkinsonian-like syndrome called kuru. In a bovine context, Gajducek's "prion" diseases were known by such names such as bovine spongiform encephalopathy or mad cow disease, and among small human populations in Europe, it was thought to cause Creutzfeldt Jacob Syndrome. All of these neurological fatal syndromes were attributed to the presence of a new, indestructible, yet infectious "slow-acting" agent that broke all rules of infectious diseases.

Meanwhile, the English begin to notice that there is a marked change in the severity of whooping cough that they are seeing that coincides with before and after administration of the pertussis vaccine, stating that "since the decline of the pertussis vaccine's use, hospital admissions and death rates from whooping cough have fallen unexpectedly."

In **1979**, the consciousness-raising American physician, Dr. Robert Mendelsohn (Author: Confessions of a Medical Heretic, who was the Medical Director of the "Head Start" program, Chairman of the Medical Licensure Committee for the State of Illinois, who was an Associate Professor at the University of Chicago, Illinois, and "The People's Doctor") was quoted as saying: "My suspicion, which is shared by others in my profession, is that the nearly 10,000 SIDS deaths that are routinely given children, the pertussis vaccine, is the most likely villain, but it could also be one or more of the others."

A few years later, Dr. Robert Gallo, MD, Chief Virologist of the NIH's "tumor virology lab" tries to alarm that a cancer virus precursor of "HIV" was endemic in certain Japanese populations who acquire leukemias, and he tried to convince the scientific community that his "cancer viruses," not nuclear weapons, are the cause. He advanced the argument that HIV's precursor "virus variant" probably reached the Americas along with the slave trade and may well have arrived in Japan the same way, carrying on the racial construct as far as it will go.

Luc Montagnier reported that "LAV" (Lymphadenopathy-associated virus) is "isolated" from a young male homosexual with a previous history of two treatments for gonorrhea, one treatment the year before for syphilis, and with antibodies against Herpes I and Herpes II, Epstein-Barr virus, and cytomegalovirus...but Montagnier's "LAV" paper is rejected but then was "shepherded" through by Robert Gallo into the glossy, prestigious Science magazine the next year in 1983. Although Gallo believed Montagnier's LAV could not be a cancer virus like the cancer viruses he had been looking for during the decade before when he first named HTLV-I, and then HTLV-II as cancer viruses in the late 1970's, which were proven not to exist and constituted the basis of ridicule by The Establishment,he then opportunistically took advantage of the establishment's confusion and in the early 1980's convinced them that his latest "cancer virus" HTLV-III was the probable cause of AIDS.

And in 1984, and despite the uncertainties and criminally culpable mayhem Dr. Gallo and Health and Human Services Secretary Margaret Heckler created because of their 1984 science by press release made on International TV in which they stated that "HIV is the probable cause of AIDS," an uncritical world, due to viral terrorism accepted that "HIV" was a lethal and 100% fatal disease that could infect anybody (depending on their sexual partners) when in fact, "AIDS" never has left its original risk groups: IV drug addicts, and iatrogenically damaged people, and those given the toxic AZT and other so-called "anti-HIV" medications.

A few months ago, Robert Gallo at NIH was telling us that an oral polio vaccine might buy us a few months of life as a civilization if we used the oral polio vaccine to combat SARS-COVID-19 until the Pfizer and Moderna, J&J, AstraZenica vaccines were rolled out!

In addition, Gallo envisioned and claimed that "HIV" "jumped" off monkeys to African men during the slave trade that certain art works of old sea travels had revealed to him.

By **1985**, vaccines were mandatorily required for admittance into elementary schools. These vaccines were diphtheria, polio, tetanus (DPT), and pertussis, as well as measles, mumps, and rubella (MMR)

Also, in 1985, "it was concluded that in children living in Britain, the risk of pertussis vaccine during the period of 1970-1983, exceeded those of whooping cough," according to Development of Biological Standards, Vol. 61, 1985, pp 395-405, and the varicella vaccine (for the harmless lesions of childhood chicken pox) is licensed in the US.

Importantly, vaccine injuries were finally acknowledged by the government and they agree on the 1986 Vaccine Injury compensation Act passed and the VAERS (Vaccine Adverse Events Reporting System) was launched at the same time the recombinant hepatitis B vaccine is licensed.

That same year, it was reported that 90% of 1,300 pertussis cases in Kansas were "adequately vaccinated", and in Chicago, 72% of pertussis cases were up-to-date with their vaccinations.

The next year in **1987**, the HiB vaccine is licensed, as the claim is being advanced the smallpox vaccine triggered AIDS in Africa.

More reports begin being published that vaccines do nothing to protect the vaccinated from the diseases they are designed to prevent. For example, it was reported that "17 subjects had been vaccinated for measles and all 17 subjects experienced measles again, showing IgM antibodies indicating acute infection," which concluded by stating that "a history of prior vaccination is not always associated with immunity nor with the presence of specific antibodies." (Journal of Clinical Investigative Medicine, Vol. 11, No 4, Aug. 1988 Pp 304-9).

In **1988**, a serological survey was performed on 573 subjects aged 3-80 years or older to evaluate the presence of neutralizing antibodies for Types 1,2,3, Sabin vaccine strains as well as a wild strain of poliovirus Type I isolated in France, claiming that: "The highest immunity antibody levels were found in Group D, which were children with a recorded history of complete polio vaccination, and in Group A, which were unvaccinated persons but who were contemporary with the past polio epidemics."(Virologie, 1988, Oct. 39 (4): 241-245).

Autism spectrum disorders begin to explode in the United States, and in 1989 the country of Oman experienced a widespread polio outbreak six months after achieving a complete vaccination rate.

In **1990**, the FDA granted the Department of Defense a waiver from The Nuremberg code for use of unapproved drugs and vaccines in Desert Shield.

Although it is known that hepatitis B is a disease of IV drug addicts and alcoholics, and iatrogenically induced cases of hepatitis, the anti-hepatitis B vaccine is recommended for all newborn infants and children, and the predictions of vaccine-induced diseases and syndromes begin to be fully realized, but it is believed these infants will be protected from hepatitis B when some of them grow up and acquire the fatal illnesses of addiction to IV drugs or chronic alcoholism, or haplessly visit their local hospital and receive a transfusion with hepatitis-tainted blood. Following these mandates, and despite a lack of any animal model for hepatitis B (chimps injected with hep-B tainted blood acquire the antibodies but never exhibit hepatitis B syndrome and liver damage), in 1978, experimental hepatitis B trials were conducted by the CDC in New York, Los Angeles, and San Francisco. Ads for research subjects specifically asked for promiscuous homosexual men, and there also is evidence that the first hepatitis B vaccines were also tested on blacks in Central Africa without informed consent, and as mentioned in children with intellectual disabilities.

In 1998, the result of these hysterical vaccine trials eventually came to light by the French when the hepatitis B vaccine was formally linked to autoimmune rheumatoid diseases in 1998, and when 15,000 French citizens filed a lawsuit against the French Government for understating the risks and overstating the benefits associated with the hepatitis B vaccine, after hundreds of people were reported to have suffered from autoimmune and neurological disorders, including multiple sclerosis following hepatitis B vaccinations. As a result of this enlightened progress by the French, the French Health Minister ended the mandatory hepatitis B vaccination program for all school children, as the target population was acknowledged to be prostitutes and drug addicts, and not children, and despite France repealing its mandate for school-aged children and despite the fact that the CDC admitted that the vaccine might not be effective after 7 years in 30%-50% of the vaccinated (titer negative following vaccination), the hepatitis B vaccine is still mandated anyway in the US for school-age children in 48 states.

Hepatitis C diseases are then invented using the smoke and mirrors of serology and molecular markers, because the virus cannot be isolated and photographed and shown to cause anything like hepatitis in an experimental animal, then isolated again and shown to cause disease in a second animal (Koch's postulates for proving the pathogenicity of a microbe).

Coincident with the hepatitis C scare, in 1991, fish farmers become angry when Nature publishes the claim that fish farming causes influenza pandemics.

In **1992** and now well into the AIDS era, the hepatitis B vaccine is said to cause a positive "HIV" test result (Lee D., Eby W., Molinaro G. Lancet 339: 1060). ICL or idiopathic CD4 Lymphocytopenia associated with IV drug use and transfusions becomes the 40th disease subsumed under the AIDS umbrella when no antibodies are detected and victims exhibit any sign of AIDS-indicator symptoms, and America's Centers for Disease Control (CDC) in Atlanta admits polio live-virus vaccine had become the main cause of polio in the United States, while the Lancet publishes claims in 1994 that "the incidence of asthma has been found to be five times more common in vaccinated children."

By **1994**, the failure to reach the goal of measles elimination creates an apparent paradox of measles infections in immunized persons..." The apparent paradox is that as measles rates rise to high levels in a population, measles becomes a disease of immunized persons," and in 1995, the Congress of the United States, Office of Technology Assessment releases its report regarding the failure of the first 33 "HIV" vaccine trials in a brief article entitled:

"Office of Technology Assessment of the failure of the first 33 HIV vaccine trials: adverse reactions to HIV vaccines, medical, ethical and legal issues."

This is the same year it is published that "more companies are engaged in HIV vaccine research than in research for any other type of vaccine, and when reports were being released that experts were now claiming the hepatitis B vaccine actually caused more illness than the disease by a 20 to 1 ratio."

While all the positive developments are happening in the world of human beings, it is claimed that birds are catching a cold flu also, but it is not passed from person to person, and it is decided to slaughter the entire chicken population of Hong Kong, further ushering in the bird flu era, as Donald Rumsfeld reports profits between 5 and 25 million dollars due to his investments.

Really bad news is finally released by the Federal agency known as DIADS: The Division of AIDS (DAIDS) says everybody has got "HIV's" capsid protein in their cells, but they only will convict those persons who harbor more than 30 pg/ml (picograms per milliliter) P24 protein. These proclamations by DAIDS are coming in 1997 at the American public at the same time claims that it is admitted by the CDC that the polio virus has not been eradicated by vaccination, but likely lurks behind a disease redefinition and new diagnostic names like viral or aseptic meningitis, and during a propagandistic campaign for the Lymerix (the Lyme disease vaccine) which was licensed without any isolation of a Lyme disease pathogen, and when a recommendation was promulgated by the CDC that Paul Offit's "rotavirus" vaccine be administered universally in infants.

In **1998** in the arena of pathogen testing, The Cambridge Biotech "HIV-1" Western Blot kit insert was written to state that "the implications of antibodies to HIV-1 in an asymptomatic person are not known."

THE ROTOVIRUS VACCINE ROLL-OUT OF PAUL OFFIT

Although it was "a recommendation" that was promulgated by the CDC that Paul Offit's rotavirus vaccine be administered universally in infants, in 1998 the vaccine is licensed as children begin to develop intestinal intussusception following the rotavirus vaccination. According the MCT law firm who has handled many cases of rotavirus vaccine damage, intussusception is defined as "a type of intestinal blockage. It happens when part of the intestine folds into itself like a telescope causing a blockage that prevents food from passing down through the rest of the intestines. When the walls of the folded intestines become swollen, eventually blood flow is cut off to that part of the intestinal tract, causing the tissue to die. But to receive damage compensation, a patient must experience intussusception symptoms between 1 and 21 days from when they first got the rotavirus vaccine to receive compensation.

The US Department of Health and Human Services defines intussusception as:

> "the invagination of a segment of intestine into the next segment of intestine, resulting in bowel obstruction, diminished arterial blood supply, and blockage of the venous blood flow. This is characterized by a sudden onset of abdominal pain that may be manifested by anguished crying, irritability, vomiting, abdominal swelling, and/or passing of stools mixed with blood and mucus." Several years later, in 2011, the New England Journal of Medicine ran an article in 2011 that minimized the risk of rotavirus vaccine and claimed that: "Recent preliminary studies from Australia also suggest a link between RV5 and intussusception. Hence, we can infer from these studies that any orally administered live rotavirus vaccines will probably carry some detectable risk of intussusception, that the risks associated with RV4 were not unique, and that the risk of intussusception seems to be small." (N. Engl J Med 2011; 364-2354-2355).

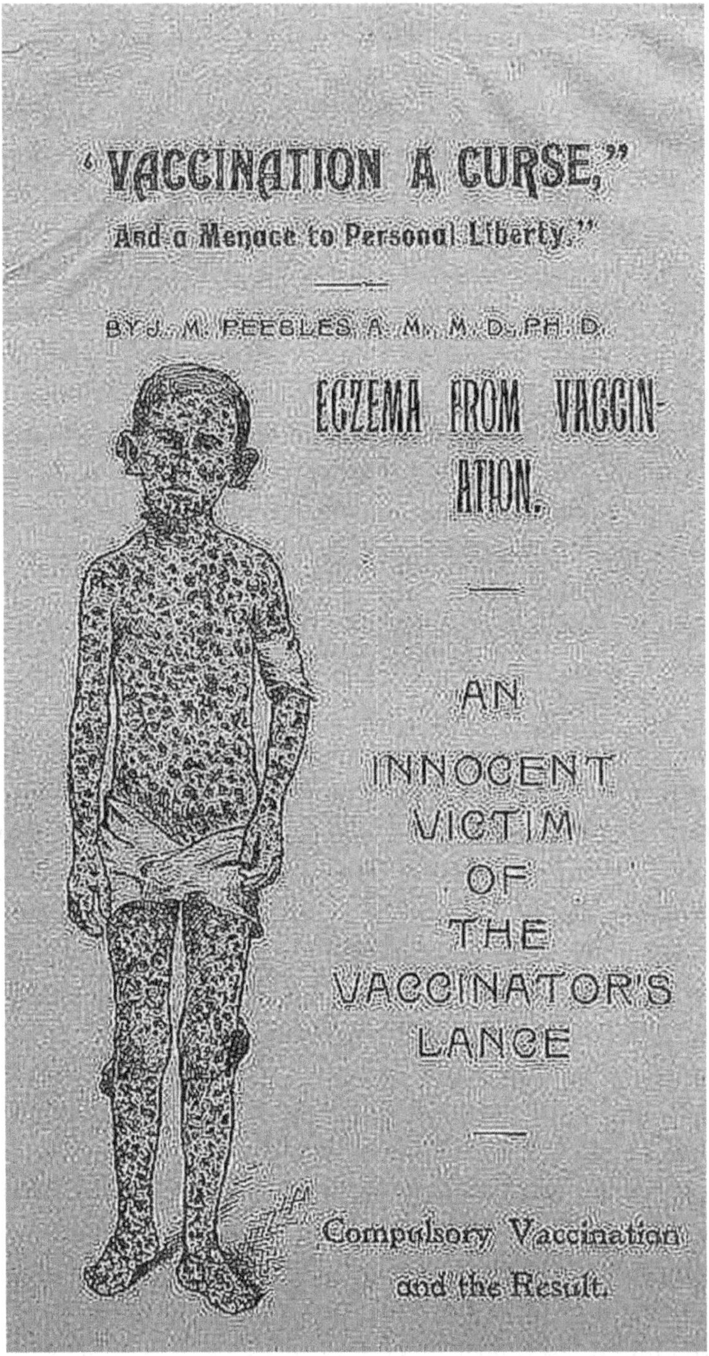
"VACCINATION A CURSE,"
And a Menace to Personal Liberty."
BY J. M. PEEBLES A. M., M. D., PH. D.
ECZEMA FROM VACCIN-
ATION.
AN
INNOCENT
VICTIM
OF
THE
VACCINATOR'S
LANCE
Compulsory Vaccination
and the Result.

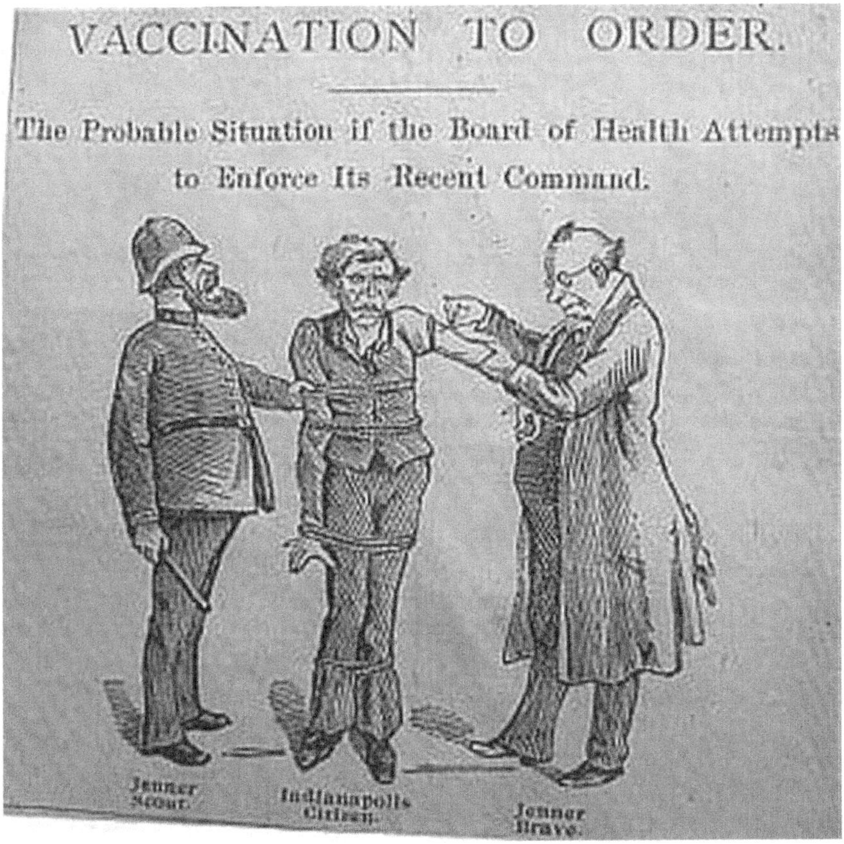
VACCINATION TO ORDER.
The Probable Situation if the Board of Health Attempts to Enforce Its Recent Command.
Jenner Scout.
Indianapolis Citizen.
Jenner Brave.

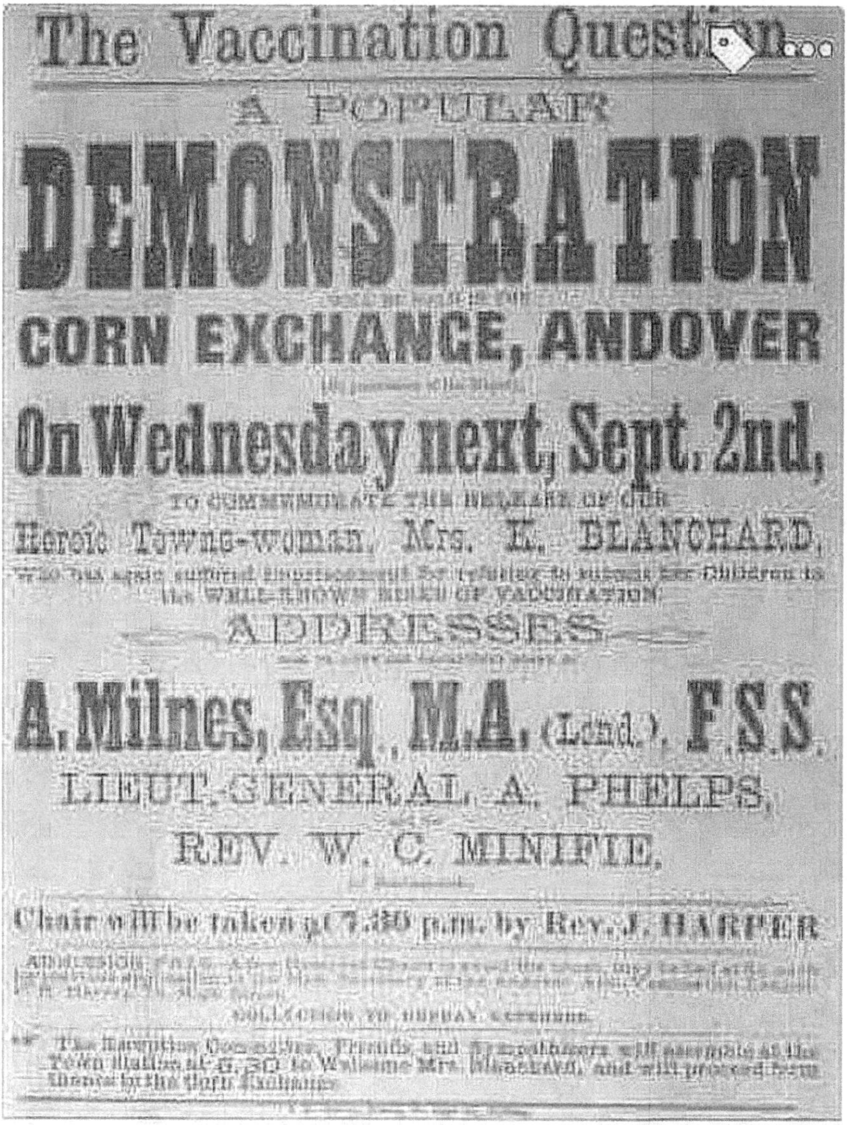
The Vaccination Quest
A POPULAR
DEMONSTRATION
CORN EXCHANGE, ANDOVER
On Wednesday next, Sept. 2nd,
TO COMMEMORATE THE RELEASE OF OUR
Heroic Towns-woman, Mrs. E. BLANCHARD,
ADDRESSES
A. Milnes, Esq., M.A. (Lond.), F.S.S.
LIEUT.-GENERAL A. PHELPS,
REV. W. C. MINIFIE,
Chair will be taken at 7.30 p.m. by Rev. J. HARPER

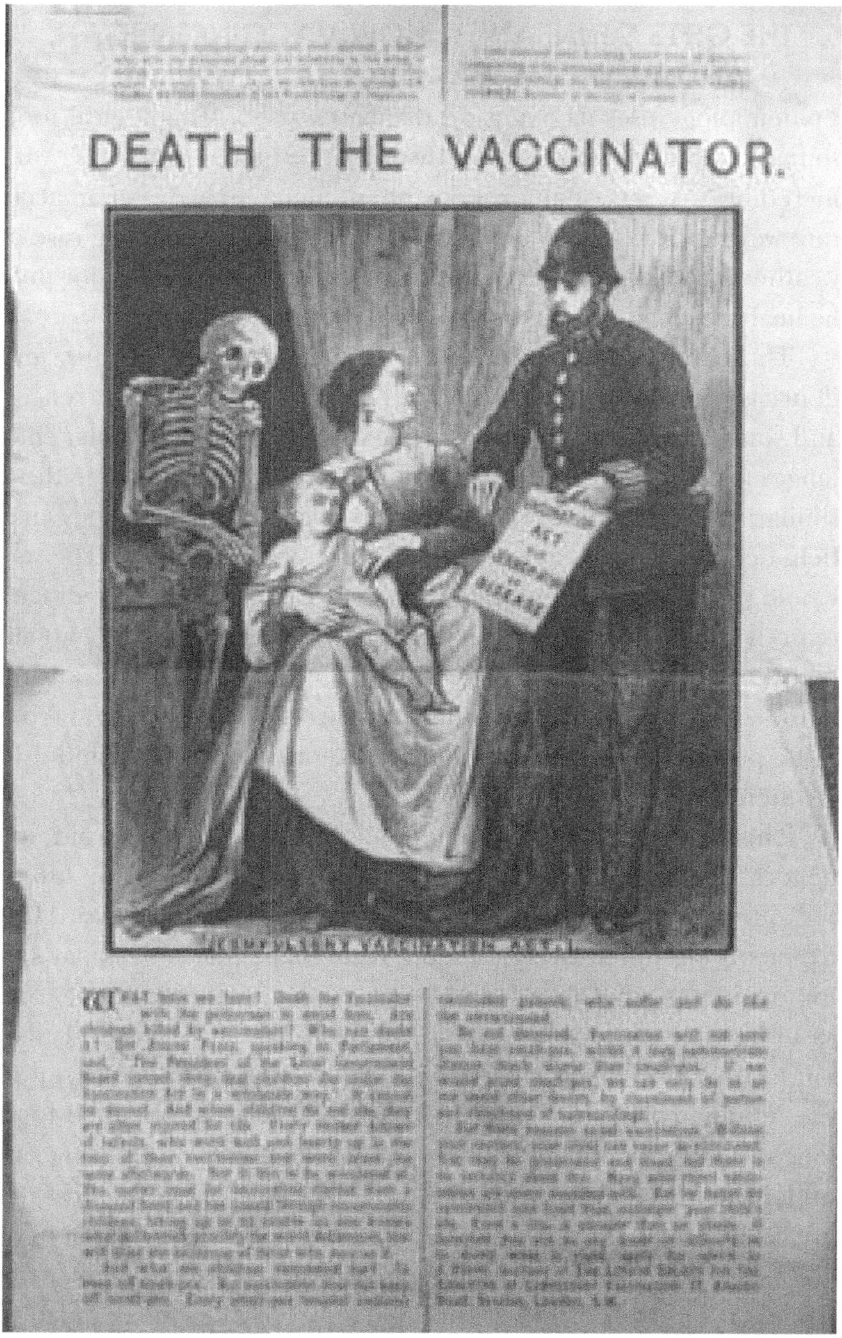
DEATH THE VACCINATOR.

THE GIFTS OF INSANITY, HOW VACCINES BEGAN, AND HOW CAR WAX CAN SAVE YOUR LIFE

Epidemiology uses its extensive databases as epidemiological tools somewhat akin to weather forecasting, in an attempt to cope with incredibly vast sets of amorphous phenomena, to arrive at an accurate weather forecast or prediction of future weather in the case of weather forecasting, and the appropriate recommendation for public health in the future in the case of epidemiology.

Those that come to imagine and then believe their scientific evidence is good enough to predict the future of epidemic occurrences, and your morning local weather woman (or man) have similar challenges to face, and indeed, share similar obstacles. Identifying these similarities in vaccinology and epidemiology, and meteorology, may help define the limits of what is knowable, and what is not. The vaccinologist and the meteorologist both forecast huge phenomena entirely out of human control and try to forecast what will happen and then implement the correct response to the forecast with full knowledge that the object of their focus is constantly changing, has more possible states that can be modeled or even counted, and thus is inherently unpredictable.

The vaccinologist's recommendations about how to avoid epidemics, or non-epidemic diseases that might happen in the future are appreciated, if they are right. In a sense, the vaccinologist is like a meteorologist that tries to discern from maps and radar today's or tomorrow's weather forecast. If sunny picnic weather is in the forecast is coming our way, we can prepare a lunch, and get our blanket out of the closet. Or if Hurricane Mathew is offshore closing in on the Atlantic coast, then perhaps blankets should be obtained for a long-term power outage with no water, electricity, or sleeping out under the stars if evacuation is required. Real epidemics such as the great Philadelphia yellow fever epidemic (spread by mosquitoes as are most modern endemic and epidemic afflictions spread by parasitic life cycles of one kind or another) took out 2/5's the population of Philadelphia as records show, whereas "pandemic flu's" such as the H1N1 or Swine Flu hoaxes and many others are simply propaganda invented to motivate, as records also clearly show, and are invented to serve some other purpose than "the greater good. All forecasts of epidemic emergencies or future predicted illnesses can be life-threatening psychologically, or at a minimum delusional, and those who make such blunders should be held accountable, but also, those who believe them also have to be held accountable for their actions based on that information.

Our timeline begins with sanity because insanity only can begin from there. Epidemic and endemic disease syndromes caused by vaccines in populations have been and are predictable to the extent that vaccine campaigns, epidemics, and chronic endemic maladies have been frequently associated, as carefully kept military records have shown repeatedly. Evidence from the 1800's in the Lancet and from elsewhere shows that the medical profession of that Century was clearly aware of the alarming relationship between inoculation, vaccination, and morbidity, which is why they vigorously attempted and succeeded for a while to end the practice of compulsory vaccinations. In fact, the British Parliament outlawed the practice, for a while. In the 1900's, much evidence demonstrates that through proper nutrition, sanitation, adequate care of the sick, or lack of war or mandated vaccination, that epidemics may be avoided. Examples in which common chronic illnesses were managed without vaccination during and after the FDR era are numerous (De Kruif, 1949), and invite sanity and prudence.

1. The insanity of inoculation and then vaccination began with a history of the inoculations of lymph puss (cells), cellular materials, associated microbes, toxins, and other substances into the human body that are foreign or constitute degrading decaying waste products of one kind or another. From a soluble tissue grafting point of view, inoculation was practiced in Persia and elsewhere as an operation where the surface of the body was injured with needles or lancets, and foreign

puss from "pox" or perhaps other putrid eruptions similar to pox was placed in direct contact with the bloodstream of the inoculated persons (or mucus membranes of the nose-as the case of the Chinese method of smallpox inoculation 1000 years earlier).

This practice suggested in addition, that the smallpox of that era was not particularly frightening with respect to its virulence, although there are reports that natural epidemics carried off 50% of the population during small outbreaks (Crookshank, History and Pathology of Vaccination Vol 1, p 7). These individuals were enlightened, and strongly argued that hygiene, quarantine, and not vaccinations during epidemics "knocked the bottom out of a grotesque superstition" (i.e., vaccination-Charles Creighton, History of Epidemics and Alfred M. Crookshank, The New England Magazine P. pps 14-17, Sept. 1908; in The Great Jennerian Blunder), yet it has been vaccination that has received the credit. In these historical documents, Professor Crookshank emphasized that during epidemics, "isolation has been instrumental in saving lives.

In this context among the proponents of vaccines, there was intense discussion regarding whether to use year-old puss (dried out from a previous bout of illness, versus obtaining material directly from an ill person. The application of aged versus fresh lymph from a pock probably made quite a difference in the severity of the inoculated disease, as Pasteur would later confirm with his first preparations of anthrax vaccines and rabies vaccines).

2. In a real sense, inoculations, as well as vaccinations were and are complex and dangerous medical procedures, not unlike blood transfusions or liver transplants, and should be regarded as such by the scientific and medical communities, as well as the general public. To exclude even more people from medical insurance and save our astronomical

health care debt, on medical questionnaires, next to the box that asks if you have ever had a blood transfusion, organ transplant, or cancer, there should also be a box asking about what vaccines you have had. The infusion of foreign cells such as lymph early during the vaccine era is not unlike the early experiments that revealed graft versus host disease at the beginning of the 1900's. In graft versus host disease, foreign lymphocytes were infused into mice, and these foreign lymphocytes rejected the host's lymph nodes first. The Peyer's patches of the intestines were affected soon after the infusion, as were the cervical, axillary, and inguinal lymph nodes of the neck, arm-pit, and groin, followed by massive rejection of the recipient's tissues, followed by extreme morbidity and death in >50% of the recipients, depending upon their genetic background. In the context of vaccination, history suggests that it should never be forgotten that one is attempting to alter the entire immune system and its future responses to the universe of antigens. Although intact and living eukaryotic cells are no longer infused, their components are, and some of these components can evoke massive responses of the immune system.

3. Vaccines wear off. The "chicken pox vaccine" aimed to avoid a harmless childhood syndrome is a good example of many others mandated for a syndrome such as measles that is also a harmless and normal childhood illness whose virus does not exist. A few examples of this insanity will suffice:

   "Varicella Vaccine Waning -Waning Immunity with the Varicella Vaccine. A population-based study shows declining immunity over time in individuals who receive only a single dose of varicella vaccine."

   "Although varicella incidence has decreased dramatically in the U.S. since the introduction of universal varicella immunization in 1995, disease outbreaks have continued to occur in highly vaccinated populations. Might vaccine-induced immunity diminish with time? To find out, researchers from the CDC and the Los Angeles County Department of Health Services examined varicella surveillance data from Antelope Valley, California (population, 350,000)."

"From 1995 through 2004, 11,356 cases of varicella were reported in this population, including 1080 cases (9.5%) with onset >42 days after vaccination. During the decade of observation, annual varicella incidence decreased by 85%, and the proportion of cases in immunized children increased from 1% to 60%. Among vaccinated children, the incidence of moderate-to-severe disease increased from 18% in 1995–1998 to 31% in 2001–2004. Moderate-to-severe disease was significantly more likely in 8- to 12-year-olds who had been vaccinated 5 years previously than in those vaccinated within the previous 5 years (odds ratio, 2.6; 95% confidence interval, 1.2–5.8). The rate of varicella disease following vaccination increased significantly each year after vaccination, ranging from 1.6 per 1000 person-years in year 1 to 58.2 per 1000 person-years in year 9 which isn't bad because it is only increased 36 times in the disease frequency among the vaccinated compared to the non-vaccinated!"

"These findings were part of the evidence underlying the June 2006 recommendation from the Advisory Committee on Immunization Practices to provide a second dose of varicella vaccine to children aged 4 to 6 years."

"Exogenous re-exposure to varicella virus has probably helped in maintaining immunity to this pathogen. Given the ongoing decline in varicella incidence, and thus in opportunities for community exposure to the virus, a second dose of vaccine may also be needed in the future for high-risk populations such as healthcare workers."

4. If it is not enough to introduce vile poisons into our infants and children: doctors also want to inject premature infants who possess no immune system. (March) MMR, Chicken Pox

Vaccines Work for Preemies. Main Category: Pediatrics News Article Date: 08 Mar 2007 – 11:00 PDT.

"Vaccines for measles-mumps-rubella and varicella, or chicken pox, are effective in extremely preterm infants, even though preemies' immune systems are not as developed as full-term babies. This confirms a long-held assumption by pediatricians and neonatologists across the country."

"The assumption has always been that it would be OK, that very early babies would have enough immunity, but no one had formally researched the subject," said Carl D'Angio, M.D., associate professor of Pediatrics at the University of Rochester Medical Center, and author of a paper on the subject in Pediatrics this month. "I'm happy be able to reassure my colleagues and parents that it is OK." The study, which included 16 term and 16 extremely preterm (born before about 6 1/2 months of pregnancy) infants born between May 2002 and May 2005, is the first of its kind to examine the antibody levels of measles, mumps, rubella, and varicella in this population before and after vaccination. It was published in this month's Pediatrics."

"The same number of preterm infants and full-term infants in the study reached a level of immunity considered protective against the diseases. This positive outcome, however, was not guaranteed because preemies' immune systems do not always react the same way as full-term infants [probably because they are in a sterile environment known as the womb and are protected by maternal antibodies post-partum for 9-18 months-my comment]. "For instance, a change in the types of vaccine used in the UK apparently resulted in an increase in Haemophilus influenzae type b infections, like bloodstream infection or meningitis, in children. Children born prematurely appeared to be particularly at risk for this, alluding to potential problems this population may have with responding to vaccines. That isn't the case for the MMR and chicken pox vaccines."

"Now we can all breathe a sigh of relief. We were right," D'Angio said. Although not generally life-threatening, measles, mumps, rubella, and chicken pox can all have serious complications. While many adults contracted chicken pox as a childhood rite of passage, the varicella "virus" killed 100 and hospitalized 11,000 people every year before the vaccine became available. (How many are currently hospitalized or killed/year in hospitals from non-defined entities)? Generally, the virus causes a rash, itching, fever, and fatigue, but it can also cause severe skin infections, scars, pneumonia, and brain damage. And a person who has had chicken pox can get a painful rash called shingles years later, according to the Centers for Disease Control and Prevention. The measles virus causes a rash, cough, runny nose, eye irritation and fever, but it can also lead to ear infections, pneumonia, seizures, brain damage, and rarely, death." The mumps virus causes fever, headache, and swollen glands, but it may also cause deafness, meningitis, painful swelling of the testicles or ovaries, and rarely, death. The rubella virus causes a rash, mild fever, and arthritis, but in pregnant women, it can lead to a miscarriage or birth defects, according to the CDC. D'Angio's study was funded by the National Institute of Allergy and Infectious Diseases and the National Center for Research Resources, both part of the National Institutes of Health. D'Angio is finishing a similar study on the pneumococcal conjugate vaccine, which helps prevent meningitis and blood and ear infections, and is in the process of studying the influenza vaccine."

5. Soldiers (young adults) have always been the best victims for vaccine experimentation, and war efforts have always been associated with epidemic disease, and with mandatory vaccination and revaccination. Thus, the negotiating tongue, rather than the poisoned needle, might go far in preventing epidemics such as the 1918 "Spanish Flu," or "Gulf-War Syndrome." Next in the hierarchy of human guinea pigs have

been unsuspecting new parents, who would do anything authorities told them to do to protect their cherubs. Blacks, gay persons, and those groups deemed to be impoverished, inferior, prisoners, or handicapped, have also been extensively used as victims of vaccinology.

6. Vaccine contamination has always been a central issue regarding their danger and capacity to cause diseases unrelated to the disease vaccinated against. **Early vaccinologists in the middle 1800's were afraid that diseases such as leprosy were transmitted through cuts caused by the vaccinator's lancet in regions of the world such as Hawaii, where lymph was derived from potentially leprosy-bearing peoples, and there is some evidence from the middle to late 1800's to support the idea that in some instances, smallpox vaccination caused outbreaks of both leprosy and syphilis, as well as outbreaks of other diseases**.

   Similarly, vaccinologists in the middle of the 1900's, were afraid that the Salk and Sabin vaccines were contaminated with SV40, the so-called simian virus that was shown to be capable of causing mesotheliomas, lymphomas, brain tumors, and other cancers in animals (hamsters), and feared that it would cause cancers in humans. During the "polio era" this fear accounted for published statements suggesting that "The Soviets would lose the 1964 Olympics because their athletes would all have tumors thanks to SV40" (Bookchin and Schumacker, 2004). Even in the 35-year post-polio vaccine mortality studies, initiated because a so called potent cancer-causing virus, SV-40 was inoculated into millions of people, along with the polio virus, has not been long enough to determine if SV-40 is contributing to escalating cancer rates. Indeed, the thirty-five year mortality study on people now in middle age or who are now seniors following receipt of SV40-simian-(cancer) virus-contaminated polio vaccine in the 1960's showed that out of 1073 newborns that were vaccinated and carefully followed for 35 years, between 1959 and 1963, there was no apparent increase in cancer above the expected background incidences in this carefully followed subgroup (Carroll-Pankhurst et al., British Journal of Cancer 85 (9) 1295-1297, 2001), although others would contest this claim and argue that the polio vaccine has contributed greatly to certain cancer rates.

7. Among the acellular or molecular vaccines, the fear is finally beginning to register in the ears of the eugenicists that the effects of contaminants such as adjuvants like squalene used by vaccinologists to bolster the non-specific immune response can cause massive inflammatory responses and cause autoimmune diseases with high frequency. Yet, these adjuvants still are thought to be necessary in modern vaccinology because it is clear that the "molecular "vaccines with their highly purified components of antigens seldom can be shown to evoke an adequate, or any, immune response on their own, probably because the antigens are too pure, too fragmentary, or they are non-immunogenic. This state of affairs has been largely due also to faulty isolation.
8. Also, the injected molecular components of modern vaccines often have proven to be chemically denatured because of harsh reagents used to isolate or purify the various pathogens or their parts, or because the immune system does not really work the way the textbooks say it does (or the way Jenner hypothesized that it does). The Jennerian idea that a single or even multiple exposures of a foreign substance, organism, or molecular epitope will protect for life has long been shown to be an absolutely worthless assumption. The frequent tetanus vaccines foisted on us at hospitals every few years, despite the fact we constantly are cutting ourselves, despite the well-publicized success of the hepatitis B vaccine **to promote** rather **than prevent** hepatitis B in Gambian teenagers, and the despite the increase in polio and smallpox

rather than their abatement following near universal vaccination campaigns each are good examples of this eugenic insanity because Mr. Jenner's hypothesis is not applicable in practice.

9. So-called epidemic diseases have historically been, and continue to be, a hodge-podge of various syndromes and symptoms lumped together under a single name or disease entity. This is a complex topic and more about this will be elaborated later.
10. Vaccinology has always been fraught with politics and financial interests. Despite the fact that inoculation was outlawed by the British Parliament in 1840, in 1853, The Compulsory Vaccination Act in England was passed by Parliament and every parent was required to have their baby vaccinated within 3 months of birth or face a fine of 20 shillings. In modern times, we face similar threats that our children will not be admitted to school unless they are jabbed with the hepatitis B vaccine (a rare syndrome), or now the SARS-COVID-19 arsenal of highly damaging and frequently lethal vaccines, and whose safety or efficacy data are truly causes of grave concern. Yet the school nurse and Public Health Department, or school admittance policies can threaten you into believing that you cannot enroll your kid in school without proof of a hepatitis B vaccine or many others, based on the madness surrounding the possibility in the case of hepatitis B, that your 5-year-old will transmit a sexual, or needle-borne, or blood-product-transmitted "syndrome" that has a 99% or greater spontaneous resolution rate in otherwise healthy individuals, to someone else's 5 year old, (when they have sex or shoot heroin in the gym locker-room in elementary school or Junior High School, or if they share razor blades in High Schools-are the reasons typically given to support mandatory vaccination). This is how the pharmaceutical company, Public Health Service logic, and The Church of Modern Medicine's

logic goes. Currently, parents are being threatened that their daughters have a 70% chance of acquiring cervical cancer if they test "HPV" positive, unless they fork over $300.00 dollars for a series of 3 HPV shots. More frightening and more egregious, and as the co-founder of the National Vaccine Information Center recently wrote after 9/11:

"There is no question that, right now, the fear and hysteria that is being whipped up by politicians and public health officials about bioterrorism in the aftermath of September 11 is paving the way for a serious threat to informed consent to vaccination. The passage of oppressive Emergency Health Powers Acts in the states will allow public health officials to use the state militia to arrest, quarantine and forcibly medicate and vaccinate citizens without their consent. It gives unprecedented power to public health officials who, in some states, will not even have to have a state of emergency declared by the Governor in order to detain and forcibly vaccinate whole families without a court order if they so choose. It is the most serious threat to civil liberties since the Constitution was written..." (Barbara Loe Fisher, co-founder of the National Vaccine Information Center (NVIC)

11. With all the modern propaganda concerning bioterrorism, and regarding conflicts of interests and fear-mongering, is it ethical or for the good, that VaxGen, and similar Challenger-sized disasters, be awarded an $877.5 million contract from our tax money to produce and manufacture a new Anthrax vaccine (potentially loaded with squalene or other adjuvants) as a reward for failing to provide any protection with a previous AIDS vaccine for an invented virus such as "HIV?"

Where is there any sanity in this life? In this regard, since 9/11, there has been much discussion and even Hollywood movies made regarding the destructive potential of technological achievements such as a few "box-cutters" that changed the world, and which launched us into the longest war profiteering in US history, but by contrast, very little discussion for some reason regarding the source and destructive potential of the weaponized Iowa Strain of weaponized anthrax derived from Utah's Dugway Proving Ground "found" in the mail of Tom Brokaw and Senator Tom Daschle shortly before the Homeland security vote in the Senate. This could have been a new chapter in the History of Vaccine timeline but wasn't. No doubt the terrorists parked their camels outside the perimeter of Dugway proving ground where supposedly the weaponized anthrax was kept, as it is the Nation's most guarded military installation.

CAN A POLIO VACCINE HELP STOP THE CORONAVIRUS, OR WOULD IT BE MORE EFFECTIVE TO STOP COVID-19's REIGN OF TERROR SIMPLY BY REMOVING LEADING PUBLIC HEALTH OFFICIALS WHO HAVE BEEN GIVEN LEADERSHIP ROLES AND HAVE INVENTED OTHER PAST HOAXES?

In response to the current COVID-19 madness, Robert C. Gallo, who heads the NIH's Institute of Human Virology was quoted here as offering his wisdom again and is now on record advocating that these people with or without the flu receive the failed and dangerous, oral polio vaccine of Albert Sabin.

Dr. Robert Gallo, who helped identify HIV in the 1980's, is leading an initiative to use the oral polio vaccine for short-term coronavirus treatment. He believes it could provide a couple of months of immunity, buying time for anyone infected to develop the antibodies to fight it. It still awaits FDA approval, but Dr. Gallo believes there is cause for hope — as he explained:

"https://www.pbs.org/wnet/amanpour-and-company/video/can-an-oral-polio-vaccine-help-stop-the-coronavirus/ Can an Oral Polio Vaccine Help Stop the Coronavirus? 04.13.2020

Yet let us never forget how Gallo and the other thought police became the assassins and jailers of academic freedom, who then forced people with failing populations of T-cells to take shelved cancer chemotherapy drugs such as AZT (azidothymidine). Not to use AZT like cancer patients who cycle the drugs so they will not die in a year or so, but brow beat physicians to "become compliant" with the regimen of continued administration of cancer drugs to AIDS victims. The higher doses given in the 1980's and early to mid-1990's, wiped out a generation of newly liberated men, and hundreds of thousands of children and even entire families. Unless something is done, it is clear now more than ever that still today, these Gallo and other sociopathic forces will expand their reign of terror and fear and will succeed as never before to propagandize legions of all hapless victims of COVID-19, and through citation of the same erroneous facts and devious tactics that succeeded to implement vaccine mandates in the past, and which was directly responsible for the iatrogenic gifts euphemistically called The AIDS era. More disturbingly, Fauci has now in the last several months been joined by a notorious criminal who still heads the Laboratory of Human Virology at the NIH: Dr. Robert C. Gallo.

As far as how the mechanism of immunity is achieved, which theory of immunity should be employed and what safety tests can justify the vaccination of 4.9 billion people that The WHO recently said it wants to vaccinate during a recent International Meeting. The long-term potential cancer effects of vaccines have never been tested on any human F2 generation. Will the WHO's zeal to jab 4.9 billion people be a replay on a massive human scale of Herbst and Bern's DES study? During this study it was revealed that a drug, DES, given to a generation of women to ease their pregnancies during the 1960's, induced ovarian cancers in the female children of the mothers given this untested, "anxiety-relieving" drug known as DES. Does the word "eugenicists" even come close to the criminal behavior and insanity the WHO proposes to foist on the world now with the SARS-COVID-19 hot shots?

HEALTHY CARRIERS/ASYMPTOMATICS

Are fear-mongering campaigns, and other initiatives and infrastructure that accompany vaccinology anything more than government-promulgated propaganda and implements of disease and death? Why isn't accurate factual information regarding the risks of vaccine campaigns perhaps the most important issue of our times? Is it because of our almost instinctive fear of contagion and epidemics and "healthy carriers"? Healthy carriers are those individuals or groups of individuals who exhibit some serological or molecular marker of a disease process, that do not show or display any symptoms of that malady. This "state" of "healthy carriers" is what vaccine proponents apparently fear the most, and this fear of contagion and a "healthy carrier state" has become one of the most powerful forces that shape our collective behavior and laws that compel and coerce about 55% of Americans currently to decide to expose the children or themselves to superstitious practices like vaccination.

However, like a prosecuting attorney might present arguments against the accused, there is scant if any evidence in the history of vaccinology or epidemics to support the claim either that inoculations or vaccinations have had any impact whatsoever on avoiding illnesses or epidemics, but there is considerable evidence that can be presented to show how inoculations and vaccinations have ignited epidemics and fueled endemic diseases following nearly universally mandated medical vaccine experiments.

If, for example, it was widely known that the "polio" era was founded on a single, submicroscopic, round piece of cellular garbage initially discovered in feces extracts which looked like a submicroscopic ball, would proponents be so rabid about defending the implementation, and then the almost immediate recall of the first polio vaccines?

This piece of cellular junk was deemed "the polio virus" and was so Christened to justify the infusion of it into millions of arms and buttocks.

What fears compel us to jab our infants with hepatitis B vaccines before their immune systems are even developed, a decade and a half before we are told we should prepare for the possibility that our children, when grown, might become IV drug addicts, health care workers, or prostitutes? Is the vaccine more risky to the infants than the potential future problem it is alleged to address? Although it is written on the package inserts that the hepatis B vaccine causes a plethora of life-time chronic disabilities in about 10% of its recipients, these warnings are ignored, and claims are made that the hep B vaccine will protect them from serum hepatitis and liver cancer decades later.

And as perhaps one of the worst offenders of logic of all, how can we come to believe that an HPV vaccine could ever protect our daughters from developing cervical cancer 50 years hence, if only our daughters are virgins before they get the HPV vaccine? Similar arguments were made about the suspected etiological agent of kuru and other "slow unconventional" long latency syndromes. "Slow virologists" thought these long neurodegenerative syndromes were caused by virus-like entities they called prions, which had no genes, and whose latency periods were postulated to be on the order of decades, like the "slow cancer viruses," (e.g. HPV, HBV, and "HIV").

These hypothesized contagious entities, and nobody can explain how, are postulated to sit dormant for years or decades without participating in any of the normal chemical processes inside an organism, to cause disease at some imagined time in the future. One of the noted Fathers of these "slow virus" theories, the 1976 Nobelist, C. Carlton Gajducek, discoverer of Creutzfeldt-Jakob disease (kuru), and bovine spongiform encephalopathies, known as mad cow disease, and he led the research of the brain studies laboratory at the National Institute of Neurological Disease and Stroke, which is part of the National Institutes of Health. Although this hypothesis regarding a proteinaceous replicating agent always has been controversial, several Nobel prizes have been awarded for work relating to it.

There indeed appears to be certain principles surrounding vaccines that seem to emerge repeatedly, through an examination of vaccination history, other than they do not work and they do much harm, as more than 4 Billion dollars/year in this country is given out as partial financial compensation for a fraction of individuals damaged by them. How they may affect entire populations will be a topic speculated about in the second part of this book.

In this direction, if and when scientifically valid associations between vaccines and epidemics are more fully understood and as a consequence when harm is avoided, hopefully the conceptual advances this chronology delivers might serve to improve human health and well-being, and ward off tragedy due to misplaced eugenic ideas, practices, and thinking. Most importantly perhaps, the following information should raise the critical question: what is the evidence that widespread or universal vaccination of a population will generate immunity, or are there perhaps better preventative measures that are yet to be discovered in the context of communicable pathogens and epidemics?

A more precise way to consider these questions perhaps is to ask them in the following way:

Is our ongoing superstitions and fear of a healthy carrier state derived from the biological basis of human behavior, from our culture and our learned behavior, from any solid science, or from some mixture of these phenomena? What compels some parents who belong to day care centers or groups, to shun other children and their parents from those day care centers, if those parents refuse vaccinations, and who, as religiously faithful pro-vaccinators, seemingly believe with all of their hearts, that not to vaccinate everybody is to recklessly endanger the life of their own child?

A process of discarding hypotheses along the path toward one, good, solid, testable hypothesis, is what science is all about: a method of asking questions so one can disprove one's hypothesis and go on to formulate a better one, and then test it. There are no truths, or assumptions that are exempt from the scientific method: these are the domains of mathematics, where assumptions are required to begin a process of steps that are in routine usage, "formulaic." Through running experiments, or by excluding the experience and data already obtained by many others, the question will come to focus on a key issue that will be tested, and results obtained, which then leads to a decision and yet another hypothesis, followed by more experiments, that must be repeatable by other investigators.

This rigorous process is especially important to feel comfortable with before any recommendation is tested on human beings. In essence, science is simply a tool to ask questions, not find The Truth. Epidemiology uses its extensive databases as epidemiological tools that are somewhat akin to weather forecasting, in an attempt to cope with incredibly vast sets of amorphous phenomena, to arrive at an accurate weather forecast or prediction of future weather, and the appropriate recommendation for public health in the future, instead of whether it will rain or be sunny.

The study of vaccine history and its relationship to epidemics, endemic diseases, vaccine hesitance, natural immunity, acquired immunity, adverse reactions, autism spectrum disorders, seizures, epidemiology, pathology, and indeed every aspect of our lives, have in some way been influenced by the history of vaccines, epidemics, endemic disease burdens, and the politics, biases, and economic motives that drive these things. Historically, it has been a common theme that disease definitions change, they are classified as other syndromes and diseases, or certain exhibited symptoms are "outliers." It is common knowledge among those who have wrestled with diagnostics, that to arrive at an unequivocal diagnosis, the deeper pathologists look into the nature of pathological syndromes to diagnose them, the more most if not all illnesses have at times in the past been subsumed under other existing diseases.

For example, here is one example from a President of an institute devoted to a single malady, polio: "Here is a [partial] list of 170 diseases of polio-like symptoms and effects but with different names such as: epidemic cholera, cholera morbus, spinal meningitis, spinal apoplexy, inhibitory palsy, intermittent fever, famine fever, worm fever, bilious remittent fever, ergotism, and others.... There are also such common nutritional deficiency diseases as beriberi, scurvy, Asiatic plague, pellagra, prison edema, acidosis, and others." "No drugs, medicines or medical treatments have ever been able to cure any of these diseases and no germs have been isolated as the cause. But they all respond to fasting, cleansing, proper diet and improved circulation. And the history of vaccines is no exception." (Ralph R. Scobey, M.D., president of the Poliomyelitis Research Institute, Inc). Syracuse, New York; Archives of Pediatrics, Sept. 1950).

The question to ask then becomes – If diagnostics remain at best, like any science, a process of elimination, then how is it possible to make conclusions that vaccines are Mankind's greatest medical achievement, or the most damaging invention of all time? And let's address the elephant in the room- Can an epidemiological or pathological approach with such constraints even conclude anything without taking into account the phenomenon of disease resistance? Yet it is a fact that for any malady, a majority of those exposed to it resist it, overcome it, or avoid it completely. How do we classify diseases when in some victims they are "latent," and never express recognizable symptoms?

How did the human populations of our past survive without "immunizations"? If we concede as a starting assumption that vaccines and inoculations were not yet used, invented, or a thought on somebody's blackboard? Well, here come those with certainty to tell us: Mankind is living longer today than in our past. Methuselah was a myth. Aristotle was a statistical "outlier" at 70 when he died way back when. Survive as a population and pass along their genes, however, the ancients somehow managed. They must have survived and reproduced because we are here asking why we are here. Maybe we have it all wrong about epidemics and our growing endemic disease-afflicted population(s)? Perhaps there is an easier way to come at this important question that affects all of us to some extent?

Those that come to imagine and then believe their scientific evidence is good enough to predict the future of epidemic occurrences, and your morning local weather person have similar challenges to face, and indeed, share similar obstacles. Identifying these similarities in vaccinology and epidemiology, and meteorology, may help define the limits of what is knowable, and what is not. The vaccinologist and the meteorologist both forecast huge phenomena entirely out of human control and try to forecast what will happen and then implement the correct response to the forecast with full knowledge that the object of their focus is constantly changing, has more possible states that can be modeled or even counted, and thus is inherently unpredictable.

The vaccinologist's recommendations about how to avoid epidemics, or non-epidemic diseases that might happen in the future are appreciated, if they are right. In a sense, the vaccinologist is like a meteorologist that tries to discern from maps and radar today's or tomorrow's weather forecast. If sunny picnic weather is in the forecast and coming our way, we can prepare a lunch, and get our blanket out of the closet. Or if Hurricane Mathew is offshore closing in on the Atlantic coast, then perhaps blankets should be obtained for a long-term power outage with no water, electricity, or sleeping out under the stars if evacuation is required. If real epidemics such as the great Philadelphia yellow fever epidemic (spread by mosquitoes as are most modern endemic and epidemic afflictions spread by parasitic life cycles of one kind or another) took out 2/5's the population of Philadelphia as records show, whereas "invented influenzas" such as the 1976 swine flu influenza are simply propaganda tactics invented to motivate and frighten, as records also clearly show (**and as it was documented on Mike Wallace's interview about Swine Flu vaccine fraud in 1976 on 60 minutes https://www.youtube.com/watch?v=g5jx243DHyg** with a woman school teacher named Judy Roberts, who acquired Guillain Barre Syndrome after receiving the swine flu vaccine, and who never recovered from her immune system attacking her peripheral nerves, part of her central nervous system, and leaving her semi-paralyzed and in need of leg braces for the rest of her life. Guillian Barre Syndrome (GBS) also causes a partial loss of sensation as well as loss of movement, and even changes in cognitive ability and personality, which she also experienced because she could no longer smile, blow out birthday candles, or drink through a straw on one side of her face.

It was discovered that the CDC had lied about testing the vaccine given to 46 million Americans, which, like the 1918 Spanish Influenza began on the Fort Dix Army base, where it attacked four soldiers killing one of them. The CDC lied by concealing the fact that the prototype swine flu vaccine was tested in mice, but its second version that was derived from it and jabbed into some 46 million plus innocents was never tested for safety of efficacy. A safety monitoring agency headed by a Dr. Michael Hatwig warned the CDC about the severe neurological effects of the revised swine flu vaccine, but they ignored his warnings and then lied about the fact that they had been informed by Dr. Hatwig. In their media campaign to get Americans to accept the vaccine, the CDC also lied about famous people having had the shot without adverse effects: names were mentioned such as then President, Gerald Ford, Rudolph Nereyev, Walter Cronkite, Edward Kennedy, Ralph Nader, Mary Tyler Moore and others.

Mary Tyler Moore admitted on 60 Minutes that she never had given her consent to use her name in association with having taken the swine flu shot, and she emphasized that she never even received the vaccine. Incidentally, Judy Roberts was never compensated for her paralysis even years later following her GBS paralysis, and despite years of litigation. She didn't even receive an apology from the government. [In 1976] the swine flu "pandemic" claimed a mere 429 lives WORLDWIDE (as of July 15), while the regular flu (not the swine flu) allegedly killed 13,000 in the United States alone since January of that year (although there is strong support that even these types of figures are grossly exaggerated to increase vaccine sales). However, in the aftermath of the 1976 swine flu, claims totaling $1.3

billion had been filed by victims who had suffered GBS paralysis from the vaccine.

The 1976 swine flu vaccine was also blamed for 25 deaths in the US. Several hundred people also developed crippling Guillain-Barré Syndrome after they were injected with the swine flu vaccine. Even healthy 20-year-olds ended up as paraplegics. And the swine flu pandemic itself? It never materialized. So the fact remains that the regular flu at this point in time was FAR more dangerous than the swine flu. Just like in 1976, today there is clearly a lot of fear-mongering going on, fear-mongering that has a noticeable subplot preparing you for draconian measures to combat a future pandemic as well as forcing you to accept the idea of mandatory vaccinations. "Pandemics" are invented to serve some other purpose other than "the greater good."

In this particular 1976 "pandemic," more than 40 million Americans were the targets of an aggressive CDC propaganda campaign. Forecasts of epidemic or pandemic emergencies or future predicted illnesses can be life-threatening psychologically, or at a minimum delusional, and the vaccines conjured up to prevent them proved toxic and paralytic or lethal for some victims.

When people continue to question what they are told about vaccines, however, they become mandated or forced by incarceration and fines if you do not act, or with the banning of your child from school so they cannot learn to read or do arithmetic.

As emphasized several times in this indictment's evidence presented in this book: that the charge or indictment that virologists went "off the rails" some time ago (and took the biomedical sciences with them off a cliff), doesn't require much more evidence provided in the pages ahead to understand how and why this perversion of science and medicine has occurred, and this topic will be elaborated on and justified at length and in great detail in this indictment later, as it has consumed me for many years. This is because the viral hoax "iatrogenocide" was accompanied during the 2000-2012 years by threatening phone calls threatening dire consequences if I did not shut up.

During this period of time, extreme pressure was applied by NIH's Robert Gallo to President White of the entire University of Illinois system where I worked as an Associate Professor, my Executive and other Deans, my department Chairman, Dr. Robert Folberg, and to me and my family personally...to fire me if I did not shut up.

I, however, have survived my heresies (so far) against the AID$ establishment despite Robert Gallo from NIH, a close colleague and confidante of Tony Fauci, calling me by phone in my office on a frequent basis to try to compel me to retract everything I said about him and the AIDS agenda, "or else" there would be "dire consequences." Some of these letters are also included in this "indictment."

These threatening letters and phone calls during this period began during the middle of my academic research and teaching career at the University of Illinois at Chicago Medical School, and I rapidly became aware that many basic observations and medical protocols that appeared to violate common sense, such as the idea of toxic cancer therapies, herd immunity through the use of toxic medications, were being used on human beings, sometimes deadly, and which were associated with the appearance of imbalances of certain tissue-building processes, such as laminin or fibronectin, as shown in the vaccine induced cancer observations of the veterinarians presented earlier.

The "HIV-AIDS" era was justified and forms the basis our current COVID-19 crisis because a high-ranking appointee named Robert Gallo still runs the National Institute of Health's Institute for Human Virology, supported by Anthony Fauci, and with the highest biomedical budget of them all, brokered by our current executor of the Global coronavirus "pandemic," Debora Birx, and admitted thief and former appointed head of the CDC, Robert Redfield. Robert Gallo, Anthony Fauci, Barbara Birx, Robert Redfield, the CDC, the

NIH, and many others foisted the "HIV" hoax upon a generation of gay men, and later their viral-phobia restricted the freedom of the heterosexual community as well, when it was pronounced that these folks who practice "normal sex" are "equally susceptible" and at "equal risk" of acquiring "HIV" and developing "AIDS," because after all "AIDS" ("HIV") [does not] discriminate we were lectured, which has become the buzz phrase of two generations of human beings.

Of course, nobody wants to discuss the elephant in the room... that those who "test positive" are typically IV drug injectors, as the drugs, not the virus is leading to collapse, and also starvation because the T-cell diagnostic reverses when starvation conditions, as they are prevalent in places such as Africa, occurs. In a non-addicted individual that does not have a past of IV drug use or who has become positive by some other means but still is healthy and "HIV-positive" should according to all theories of the principle of vaccination, be immune for life, or as long as they have titres present to measure in their sera. This same conundrum now plagues the testing proposals of COVID-19. The nucleic acid tests, which are the PCR tests, measure a non-specific gamish from a lung aspirate, that was assumed to possess a novel CoV-2 virus because some sequences did not line up as they did before, and they instead resembled a sequence derived from a bat, or was it a camel? (Chinese have camels too).

One issue that needs to be carefully addressed is vaccine safety. The question most urgent to ask the proposed pre-clinical testing of the proposed COVID-19 vaccines, and the past track record(s) regarding CoV-2 vaccines that have been deployed already in a number of contexts and analyzed with varying degrees of rigor.

And similarly like the coronavirus tests have not been validated in asymptomatic positive testing individuals, beginning in the early 1980's, it was known that "HIV" tests were not based on reality as we know it in this universe, and that AIDS had little if anything to do with sexual preferences, or race, but that isn't how the AIDS era played out at all. Yet despite these diagnostic uncertainties, the first of the more than 200 failed "HIV" vaccine trials began only 2 years after the press announcement with HSS Margaret Heckler standing at Gallo's side proclaiming the "the probable cause of AIDS has been found....to be a variant of a known cancer virus." This gross violation of science and medicine clearly illustrated how the molecular reductionism of virology was able to usher in the destruction of millions of lives deemed to be "HIV" positive via phony, non-validated, fraudulent, "HIV" tests.

By allowing AZT to be consumed at a dose of 1.6g/kg after a lousy, fraudulent drug trial that was terminated in only 4 months, a toxic chemotherapeutic agent was fed to millions (and in places it still is), although that drug was shelved in the 1960 because it was too toxic for rats. The drug, AZT, was made by the same folks who are involved with COVID-19 proposals for therapeutics. Until they lowered the dosages of this "life-ending" drug, they had succeeded in nearly wiping out a generation. The AIDS era currently is the model and politics upon which this so-called pandemic is being based-its phony non-validated testing, with its insistence on not isolating COVID-19 although Co-2 was properly isolated in 1996 by Tyrrell and Bycoe, with the currently proposed "vaccine" that was already patented by Gates with 2 pharma companies in 2016 before anyone heard about COVID-19, the toxic drug treatments, and most egregiously, with the proposal of a universal vaccine "passport" being proposed as the answer.

The lies and distortions of these folks would of and could have never occurred, if Gallo initially did not want so much to have his face appear next to a cancer virus in some medical dictionary. Besides, "HIV" wasn't sexually transmissible between 175 condom-using and condom avoiding serodiscordant sexual partners (where one sexual partner tests "HIV-positive" and the other sexual partner tests "HIV-negative) if folks receive expert counseling. Therefore, lack of expert counseling causes AIDS because transmission rate was reported in this experiment to have been 0% in victims who had received "expert counseling:" Padian, et al. Heterosexual Transmission of HIV in Northern California: Results from a Ten-Year Study." American Journal of Epidemiology. August, **1997**.

SARS COV-2 COVID-19 RHETORIC IS BASED ON "HIV" TESTING RHETORIC AND TREATMENT CATASTROPHES AND OTHER "CHALLENGER-SIZED DISASTERS"

The following letter I wrote to President Obama when he was my Illinois US Senator (2005-2008) conveys this idea perhaps better than any long-winded explanation.

We can substitute "HIV testing" for Covid-19 testing to get the general idea of how foolish it is to engage in mass testing of populations for viruses using PCR and antibody tests as it guarantees a wide net to generate hundreds of thousands of false positive test results.

It is NO COINCIDENCE that the same exact scientists and personalities (Dr. Fauci, Dr. Birx, Dr. Redfield) who hyped AIDS and HIV unproven and inaccurate lab tests, as confirmed by the very scientists who developed these virus testing technologies such as Dr. Rodney Richards and Dr. Kary Mullis, are today hyping Covid-19 lab tests using the same testing technology used for HIV decades ago today to determine Covid-19 infectious status and following the same corrupt, unscientific playbook.

The public health officials pushing mass Covid-19 testing using either PCR or antibody tests without any shred of scientific evidence or justification for their use for people with no symptoms are all criminals and guilty of crimes against humanity.

You are a wonderful Senator, and I will vote for you again. But you should be aware that Representative Mary Flowers promotion of the CDC and IDPH recommendation for universal "HIV" screening of all Illinois citizens and indeed all Americans is a faith-based recommendation, and not a scientific one. Due to your recent media-projected "HIV" testing, you could be in grave if not mortal danger. I would hate to see your life ruined, and the potential good you will do for Illinois and the nation thwarted, because of medical and scientific ignorance, and because of institutionalized racism regarding "HIV" among many of my peers in the scientific/medical establishment.

I am aware that your wife, as well, has pioneered outreach programs at the University of Chicago. These are the programs that are most needed, not for "HIV" testing, or drugging, but for high blood pressure, diabetes, and other programs. I hope that she knows about the testing issue as I have tried to convey here to you. Below I have brought some facts including their references for your consideration.

The U.S. medical establishment and Public Health Service agencies are currently pressing for legislation requiring mandatory "HIV" testing for Americans between the ages of 3 and 80. This is the biggest mistake that the U.S. could make and the most costly mistake and the most damaging mistake for the largest amount of people possible because when you test populations of people that are considered what the promoters of AIDS say are "low risk," you are going to get a huge number of false positive test results, which is essentially going to ruin the lives of tens of thousands or perhaps as many as hundreds of thousands of people. All who test "HIV-positive" in a "low risk" population are false positives, ***by definition****. All who test "HIV-positive," or whose T-cells are deemed "too low" are selectively biased by these tests,* ***by definition.***

Why?

You are going to get a number of people who really are not sick in any way, shape, or form, to test positive. And they will not be able to get health insurance. They may be fired from their jobs. The stigma of having AIDS causes suicide, as it did with David Acer, the dentist whom the CDC later exonerated (after his suicide), because the CDC could find no evidence after he committed suicide that the dentist's 5 "HIV-positive" patients contracted their "HIV" signatures from him. There is evidence, however, that countless others who have been given the diagnosis of an "HIV infection," in addition to Dr. Acer, have chosen to end their lives upon getting an "HIV-positive" test result. "HIV" terrorizes both parents and children that are split apart by The State when children are placed into foster care, and people are forcibly drugged. I am not understating these facts and egregious violations of human rights.

On February 10th, 2005, three articles appeared in the New England Journal of Medicine advocating that it would be timely and cost effective to test every man, woman, and child for "HIV" at least once in their lifetime.

"In all but the ***lowest-risk*** *populations, routine, voluntary screening for*

HIV ***once every three to five years*** *is justified on both clinical and cost-effectiveness grounds. One-time screening in the general population may also be cost-effective" [****1-3****].*

The authors of these articles do not define with precision who should be selectively targeted "in all but the lowest risk populations," but they now recommend testing for children, and monogamous adults, in addition to "high risk" people who are African Americans, Hispanics, alcoholics and drug addicts, pregnant women, and men who have sex with men. Some have suggested, in addition, routinely testing persons during every emergency room visit.

Other "HIV" "experts" more recently have claimed screening for AIDS would be cost-effective based on parallels with results obtained through screening for cancer (emboldened words or underlined words are my emphasis and are highlighted to point out baseless or non-scientifically validated assumptions):

"In the United States, approximately 1 million persons are living with HIV ***infection*** *or AIDS, and 164,000 to 312,000 of them remain unaware of their* ***infection****. Experts* ***hypothesize*** *that most of the 40,000 new* ***infections*** *that occur annually in this country arise from contact with these undiagnosed persons. Given this* ***likelihood****, investigators have examined the* ***potential*** *benefit of routine screening, rather than testing of* ***only those perceived*** *to be at increased risk. This strategy* ***appears*** *to be as cost-effective as screening for colon, breast, or prostate cancer, and the availability of* ***a rapid oral test*** *has simplified broad scale testing" [****4****].*

One problem with these proposals, Mr. Obama, is that "HIV" has no unique and isolatable identity or proven molecular signature as an exogenous retrovirus (a virus that comes from outside of a cell or organism) that is the cause of AIDS. "HIV" gene sequences can be detected in ***non-infected*** *humans, chimps, and monkeys:*

"HIV-like sequences" exist in ***normal*** *human, chimpanzee, and rhesus monkey DNAs...Herein we describe the first report of the presence of nucleotide sequences related to HIV-1 in human, chimpanzee, and rhesus monkey DNAs from* ***normal uninfected*** *individuals." [****5****].*

Because the primate test subjects in this study were normal and healthy (no low lymphocyte counts or detectable illness), yet "HIV" sequences were detected, the molecular signature attributed to an assumed exogenous retrovirus, "HIV," may represent an inducible HERV (Human Endogenous Retroviral Sequence) molecular sequence or inducible genetic polymorphism, which has not in itself been adequately demonstrated to be causal of immune suppression, or illness, but has been merely associated with less than 1/3 of human subjects who may be immune suppressed, according to the original studies of Robert Gallo's group that claimed a causal connection between "HIV's" molecular signature, and AIDS.

The unproven exogenous retroviral identity of so-called specific "HIV" derived proteins also can be appreciated, for instance, by considering what Nobelists Howard Temin and David Baltimore once proposed, who discovered reverse transcriptase (RT), and what Nobelist and former NIH head Harold Varmus wrote regarding reverse transcriptase, an enzyme once thought to be solely specific to retroviruses:

"[Reverse transcriptase] is a normal protein found in the uninfected cells of ***yeasts, insects, and mammals****"[6].*

More recently, other investigators have claimed RT is an endogenous cellular enzyme that can assume various forms and it is important for telomere replication at the tips of normal chromosomes ***[7]*** *and may have nothing to do with exogenous retroviruses. Once claimed by AIDS scientists to be a specific molecular component required for "HIV" replication, RT is now seen in market magazines concerning biotechnology stocks* ***[8, 9]****, in the context of normal, non-pathological situations, despite what AIDS proponents continue to claim about the specificity of RT to exogenous retroviruses.*

*p24, another protein once thought to be unique to "HIV" is known to be expressed in the thymus glands of "****HIV-negative*** *children* ***[10]****." Other studies show that goat and cow milk that is unpasteurized induce positive "HIV" tests for proteins once thought to be derived from exogenous "retroviral HIV." Fifty percent of dogs in one study also exhibited "HIV" structural proteins but did not develop "AIDS" either* ***[12]****. Experiments testing the hypothesized ability of "HIV" integrase to interact with normal chromosomes revealed that the enzyme has no activity when compared side by side with histone H1 or polyamines, or the topoisomerases, and thus* *constituted a negative control for the minor groove-binding of the topoisomerases [**13**].*

Although the template for the molecular signatures of "HIV" may derive from common endogenous DNA sequences whose proteins are expressed by normal uninfected yeast, insects, dogs, rhesus monkeys, chimps, humans, and even in allo-immunized mice (non-"HIV-infected" mice given sera from other "non-infected" mice), as has been known by scientists since this experiment was published in 1991, neither "HIV's proposed 9,150 base pair molecular sequence, or its proteins have been isolated or identified without contaminating cellular components. For instance, it has been repeatedly shown more than 64-100 times in "HIV" vaccine trials that antibodies against "HIV" proteins aren't evoked even when the so-called unique and diagnostic "HIV"" antigens are injected directly into the bloodstream of healthy humans. According to "experts," no molecular entity associated with "HIV" sequences, proteins, or glycoproteins such as GP120, has been shown to be immunogenic in humans, perhaps because it is a case of self being challenged by molecules derived from self? The Merck "HIV" vaccine was just announced in September of 2007 as a complete and disappointing failure, not only in preventing acquisition of "HIV," but in the failure to evoke anti-"HIV" antibodies in the 741 volunteers:

"In a major setback, one of the leading experimental AIDS vaccines not only failed to prevent test subjects from becoming infected with HIV, but it didn't offer any indication it might delay the onset of full-blown AIDS, which had been a key hope."

"24 of 741 volunteers who got the vaccine in one segment of the experiment later became infected with HIV, the virus that causes AIDS. In a comparison group of volunteers who got dummy shots, 21 of 762 participants also became infected."

"The ultimate fear among researchers is that the whole theory underlying the Merck vaccine might be flawed, which, if true, could doom an entire class of experimental vaccines."

As mentioned before, it may be more appropriate to say that the whole theory of "HIV=AIDS" is flawed, because there is no evidence that an exogenous "AIDS virus" has been isolated and shown to evoke an antibody response in vaccine recipients or cause disease in either an animal model or a human being.

Unless one would like to make unfounded assumptions that the 24 of the 741 volunteers that "became infected" in this last of more than 60 failed "HIV" trials actually represents an extremely low rate of seroconversion due to exposure of isolated "HIV" components to the human immune system (24/741), and that these 24 individuals are now immunized against "HIV" instead of having acquired an "HIV" infection, the similar rate of seroconversion in the control group (21/762) suggests that this cannot be the case, and it is more likely, that seroconversion in both groups represents mere testing artifacts.

In support of this seemingly radical idea, "AIDS experts" themselves like Anthony Fauci have just canceled the new PAVE vaccine trial, and Robert Gallo wrote in the pages of science several years ago that:

*"A sound rationale (is) needed for Phase III HIV vaccine trials" [**14**].*

"In 2006, Barre-Sinoussi (of the Luc Montagnier team) has "come out of the closet," so to speak on this issue at the Toronto International AIDS conference, where she said:

"It is not clear if therapeutic vaccines might be useful, since 15 trials to date have not demonstrated definitive evidence of improved outcomes."

Perhaps more importantly, even after the 120-million-dollar failure called AIDSVAX was announced in 2004 that prompted Dr. Gallo to state: "a sound rationale is needed for Phase III HIV vaccine trials," no re-evaluation of the basic premises of AIDS science has taken place. Instead, following that failure, Donald Francis's 120-million-dollar AIDSVAX program and his company VaxGen has now been rescued with our tax dollars by the military to produce a new anthrax vaccine that also failed-but that is a different $857 million dollar story.

Other "HIV" vaccine enthusiasts claim that although "HIV" vaccines do not work because they are not immunogenic, it is asserted tacitly that certain vaccine adjuvants will do the job (because the so-called proteins of "HIV" repeatedly fail to evoke humoral immunity, mucosal immunity, cellular immunity, or even T-cell activation). Vaccine adjuvants like squalene (MF-59), however, when they have been added to certain lots of anthrax (and "HIV") *vaccines given to soldiers and other "volunteers" on threat of court martial if they don't roll up their shirt on command (in contrast to Walter Reed's voluntary experiment with yellow fever), It is now established that some of these vaccine adjuvants have been responsible for autoimmune syndromes in most of the sick Gulf-War I veterans tested, as evidenced by the fact that sick veterans invariably generate antibodies to vaccine adjuvant, squalene, in their blood [**15, 16**]. This type of "promising vaccine experimentation" on our young soldiers is particularly disturbing in light of the fact that squalene and other similar vaccine adjuvants have been traditionally used by scientists who study rheumatoid arthritis, lupus, or demyelinating syndromes, because experimental rodents will reliably develop experimental arthritis, macrophagic myofasciitis, multiple-sclerosis (demyelinating syndromes), and lupus-like syndromes upon intravenous exposure to squalene [**17, 18, 19**].*

*The proposal for universal "HIV" testing raises other issues about "HIV-testing" itself. In 1985, at the beginning of HIV testing among sperm donors, it was known that "68% to 89% of all repeatedly reactive ELISA (HIV antibody) tests [were] likely to represent false positive results" [**20**]. This and many other similar false-testing trials all support the hypothesis was suggested above regarding testing artifact to explain the 24/741 and 21/762 numbers obtained in the context of the failed Merck STEP vaccine trial mentioned above.*

*The modern "HIV" screening tests, especially the rapid ones, are contradictory from test result to test result, they are inconsistent across national boundaries, and no consensus about their validity exists. An "HIV" positive test result obtained with an ELISA, Western Blot, or PCR, may not even mean that a person who tests positive is infected with a virus, or is expressing evoked "HIV"-endogenous sequences or molecular markers [**5**]. Cross reactivity has also again and again been shown to exist regarding "HIV" sequences and proteins, and normal endogenous cellular components are expressed or shed under certain conditions of immunological or other types of physiological stress [**10**]. In this regard, a principal issue to reconcile before universal testing is implemented is that the makers of the test kits used to measure "HIV" or progression to "AIDS" are themselves aware of these issues, because they all claim their ELISA, Western Blot, and PCR-based kits cannot really detect "HIV" virus in their package inserts:*

"ELISA testing alone ***cannot*** *be used to diagnose AIDS" [**21**].*

*"**Do not** use this kit as the sole basis for HIV infection," [**22**].*

"The Amplicor HIV-1 monitor test ***is not*** *intended to be used as a screening test for HIV,* ***nor as a diagnostic test*** *to confirm the presence of HIV infection" [**23**].*

"The NucliSens(R) HIV-1 QT assay ***is not*** *intended to be used as a screening test for HIV-1 nor is it to be used as a diagnostic test to confirm the presence of HIV-1 infection" [**24**].*

"COBAS AmpliScreen HIV-1 Test ***is not*** *intended for use as an aid in diagnosis" [**25**].*

*The Cambridge Biotech HIV-1 Western Blot Kit insert: "The clinical implications of antibodies to HIV-1 in an asymptomatic person are not known"[**26**].*

*"The OraSure HIV-l Western Blot Kit is not intended for use with blood, serum/plasma or urine specimens, or for screening or reinstating potential blood donors" [**27**].*

*The Red Cross recently reported in the New England Journal of Medicine that even after repeated testing using different test kits, low-risk populations, such as blood donors (or military recruits) will typically yield 12 (PCR-positive) or 2 (ELISA positive) out of 37,000,000 samples, leaving potentially 10 out of 12 false positives, depending on which test kit you believe accurately detects "HIV's" molecular signatures [**28**]. While it has been pointed out that of the 2 of the 12 who initially tested positive on ELISA seroconverted in subsequent months to the molecular signature of "HIV" detected on PCR, and thus may warrant an investigation as to what the meaning of these molecular markers represent among persons who exhibit clinical symptoms, it could be argued that 2 or 8 out of 37,000,000 does not constitute a national health crisis, or communicable illness of the proportions of other STD's, and certainly doesn't warrant research budgets in the billions or trillions, or universal testing of "low risk" individuals, or anybody else.*

The value of the rapid "HIV" test kits is even more problematic, and some of them have been banned from the US:

"A District Court in Seattle has granted a request from the Federal Trade Commission and issued a temporary restraining order to prevent the sale and

distribution of "defective" home HIV test kits. According to FTC, the kits' maker, Seville Marketing of British Columbia, Canada, on two Web sites had advertised the "Discreet" home HIV test kits as producing 99.4% accurate results based on three independent studies. However, CDC studied the test kits and found they were not as accurate as the company claimed on its Web site."

*"FTC will seek a permanent ban on sales and advertising of the kits in the United States and a permanent order to seize any kits that are imported. Consumers who have used the kits are advised to see a health professional for another test to determine their HIV status, according to the release"[**29**].*

None of these tests have been validated against the isolation of pure "HIV" itself. They have been validated instead against other test kits that were assumed to detect "HIV."

Moreover, it has been recently proposed that viral load does not correlate with T-cell numbers, and the **rate** *of progression (when an individual will exhibit symptoms of AIDS) can only be predicted in 4%-6% of HIV-positives studied (out of 2,800):*

*"A nationwide team of orthodox AIDS researchers led by doctors Benigno Rodriguez and Michael Lederman of Case Western Reserve University in Cleveland are disputing the value of viral load tests-a standard used since 1996 to assess health, predict progression to disease, and grant approval to new AIDS drugs after their study of 2,800 HIV positives concluded viral load measures failed in more than **90%** of cases to predict or explain immune status..."“Viral load is only able to predict progression to disease in 4% to 6% of HIV-positives studied, challenging much of the basis for current AIDS science and treatment policy"[**30, 31**].*

*In 1992, the Lancet reported that for 66 true positives, there were 30,000 false positives. And in pregnant women, "**there were 8,000 false positives for 6 confirmations.**" [32].*

*In 1995, the CDC recommended offering HIV testing to all pregnant women, but according to official AIDS websites like the CDC's and on package inserts of "HIV" test kits, false positives due to pregnancy occur frequently [**33**]. There are some 70 factors or conditions that are known to generate false positive test results including flu vaccination [**34**] and hepatitis B vaccination [**35**], although it still is not clear that these conclusions were not due to* *vaccination cross-reactivity, or attributable to problems with the "HIV" test kits themselves. Different testing standards in different countries makes it possible that if you test "HIV" positive in the US in the morning, one can fly the same day to Canada, the UK, or Australia, where different standards are considered diagnostic, and you will be considered negative the same day and thereby retain your insurance, job, relationships, pregnancy, or life. Many countries such as England do not use a confirmatory WESTERN BLOT.*

By 18 months after birth, in 1993, Parekh et al. reported:

"a 60% rate of seroreversion in infants born of "HIV-positive" mothers ***[36, 37]****.*

Seroreversion means, that the infants may test positive at birth, but that 60% of them will generate a negative test if tested at 12 or 18 months. Thus, under the new mandate to universally test infants, 60% of infants who initially test positive will serorevert by 18 months post-partum, and if 60% of infants who initially test positive serorevert (change from a positive to a negative "HIV" test result) are forced to imbibe "anti-retrovirals," then 60% of infants will be needlessly exposed to toxic chemo (either in utero, post-partum, or through surgically inserted gastric feeding tubes placed there by doctors to force compliance of these deadly medications).

PCR results in infant testing are not diagnostic in infants either, because the inventor of PCR, the Nobel Laureate Kary Mullis, has repeatedly claimed that PCR can only amplify the assumed nucleic acid signature of "HIV," which again, has not been validated against the isolation of "HIV" itself (Kary Mullis in numerous writings and statements that are typically ignored, belittled, and derided by "AIDS experts" and the promoters of AIDS). ***<u>If junk goes into the PCR cycles of amplification, then junk will be amplified. One must begin with a purified isolate.</u>***

"If "HIV/AIDS" is chemotherapeutically hit hard and early as a consequence of an impassioned crusade to provide what amounts to toxic chemotherapy (see any Antiretroviral-ARV- package insert) to millions of those who test positive (even those who live in Kenya who only have a cup of diluted gruel paste/day as food-liquid to wash down their medications-see Christine Amanpour's July 19, 2006 documentary on CNN-http://www.cnn.com/2006/WORLD/africa/07/17/amanpour.africa.btsc/index.html),

universal testing for "HIV" "infection" would increase morbidity and death amongst those designated as "HIV/AIDS" patients, rather than decrease morbidity and death.

For example, de Martino et al. concluded that children born to ZDV-treated mothers (ZVD is AZT, or the AIDS drug, Azidothymidine):

*"are **more likely** to have a rapid course of HIV-1 infection compared with children born to **untreated mothers**, as disease progression and immunological deterioration are significantly more rapid, **and the risk of death is actually increased during the first 3 years of life**"[38].*

In the journal Pediatrics, Antoni Noguera et al reported that:

*"Almost **half** of the children (63 of 127) who were exposed to nucleoside analogues developed benign and self-limited hyperlactatemia when symptomatic, nucleoside analogue–induced toxicity affected **neurologic development** " [39].*

*In 1992, The Veterans Affairs Co-operative Study Group reported that AZT disproportionately harmed Blacks and Hispanics and provided no benefit to the quelling of advancing immune suppression in Caucasians and harmed healthier subjects (early treated) more than persons considered to exhibit clinical symptoms of AIDS [**40**].*

*The Concorde trial, which was published without endorsement by Burroughs Wellcome's Coordinating Committee who declined to endorse the final report, and which was the largest, longest, and best controlled adult AZT trial concluded: "The results of Concorde do not encourage the early use of zidovudine in symptom-free HIV-infected adults. They also call into question the uncritical use of CD4 cell counts as a surrogate endpoint for assessment of benefit from long-term antiretroviral therapy" [**41**].*

When considering "HIV" testing all infants and all subjects who visit their doctor or emergency rooms, faith-based science and medicine currently dominate ideas and therapies that address the imagined "mutability" of the "HIV" virus, and the failure of ARV-therapy is always based on mutation, rather than toxicity caused by the drugs. Individuals who fail ARV therapy are told their virus has mutated and is no longer sensitive to the drugs. The impact of this hypothesis on persons living with "HIV" or "AIDS" is unfair, uninformed, and cruel. For example, Mark Harrington, a member of The

*Treatment Action Group (TAG) summoned "the power of prayer" over "HIV" mutability, and discussed "The Chinese Menu Approach" in a description of a meeting he attended on developments regarding anti-retrovirals that included AIDS leaders such as Marc Wainberg, Director, McGill AIDS Centre, and the 2006 Chair of The Toronto International AIDS Conference-who possesses several "HIV" drug patents such as lamivudine (3TC), and grants from GlaxoSmithKlein, Bristol-Myers Squibb and Boehringer-Ingelheim. Also present at the meeting was Emilio Emini, Tufts University's John Coffin, Roche's Noel Roberts, the CDC's Harold Jaffe, Chiron's David Chernoff, the ACTG's Robert ("Chip") Schooley and John Mellors (developer and champion of the viral load tests now known to be invalid [**30**]), as well as treatment activist Dawn Averitt-Doherty of Atlanta-based Woman's Information Service and Exchange (WISE):*

"During the coffee break, I (Harrington) joined three activists outside to share nicotine and despair. What was the point of quitting smoking if we were still all passengers on the speeding train heading for the cliff? The Birmingham resistance data were wrenching. Our fears of multiple cross-resistance, from November 1995's 3TC and saquinavir FDA approval hearings, reared their ugly heads. Several months of post-Vancouver euphoria crumbled in a moment as it became clear that many of those who developed resistance to ritonavir and indirovine-as thousands clearly would-might have no protease inhibiting options ahead of them. Today's resistance news made for a toxic cocktail. As I left the auditorium I bumped into Emilio Emini."

"Harrington: So, what do you do if you fail Crixivan?"

"Emini: [sighs] We don't know what to do."

"Harrington: Take two new nucleosides and nevirapine?"

"Emini: Yeah. And pray."

"No one had yet assessed the healing effects of prayer on viral load. This was what we had come to. I rushed into the lobby of the Interior Department and ran into a colleague, who was wild with fear and disappointment."

"Sometimes the gap between how the researchers felt and how we felt became an abyss. They were excited about the endless possibilities opened up by the research advances of 1996; we were terrified about the limited treatment options facing people who had exhausted most of the current arsenal

of antiretroviral therapy. What to do with those whose viral load refused to go undetectable? What to do with those who added a protease inhibitor to a failing two-drug regimen and appeared doomed to develop resistance, most of it-especially with ritonavir and indinovir-cross-resistant to all other protease inhibitors? What to do with those who jumped aboard last year's bandwagon, AZT+3TC, and now appeared likely to have developed 3TC resistance and, with it, cross-resistance to ddI, ddC and possibly 1592? ***The Chinese menu approach to antiretroviral treatment suddenly looked much less appetizing, and much less nourishing****"[42].*

These same results also have been advanced in frequent warnings on MedWatch:

"Early virologic ***nonresponse*** *(91%) and nucleoside reverse transcriptase inhibitor (NRTI)* ***resistance*** *(50-95%) has been observed at a high rate in a Gilead Sciences-sponsored clinical study. Participants in the study were treatment-naive (i.e, no previous treatment for HIV) took a once-daily, 3-drug NRTI regimen. The NRTI regimen contained didanosine enteric coated beadlets (Videx EC), lamivudine (Epivir), and tenofovir (Viread)."*

"The new information is consistent with several recent clinical studies evaluating the use of 3 NRTIs simultaneously. Suboptimal virology response has also been reported with abacavir, didanosine, and stavudine, as well as another regimen containing abacavir, didanosine, and zidovudine. Similarly, early virologic failure and high resistance rates have been reported with abacavir, lamivudine, and tenofovir (see eMedicine Recalls and Alerts 8/1/03, Nonresponse Reported in HIV Infection Treated with 3-Drug Regimen Including Lamivudine, Abacavir, and Tenofovir."

Other warnings on FDAMedWatch support Mr. Harrington's sentiments regarding liver toxicity, and also warn about neural tube defects in fetuses from woman who test positive and who are treated with "the lifesaving" AIDS medicines:

"Increased Liver Toxicity with Nevirapine (Viramune) and Higher CD4 Counts...Revised prescribing information for nevirapine (Viramune) includes a new recommendation against starting nevirapine treatment in women with CD4 cell counts above 250 cells/mL and males with CD4 counts above 400 cells/mL unless benefits clearly outweigh risks. The new recommendation is

based on an increased risk of serious liver toxicity with higher CD4 cell counts prior to starting therapy. with nevirapine."

"Females and patients with higher CD4 cell counts are at increased risk of liver toxicity. Females have a three-fold higher risk of symptomatic nevirapine liver toxicity than males, and females with CD4 cell counts above 250 cells/mL have a 12-fold higher risk of symptomatic liver toxicity than females with CD4 cell counts below 250 (11% vs. 0.9%). Males with CD4 cell counts above 400 cells/mL have a five-fold higher risk of symptomatic liver toxicity than males with CD4 cell counts below 400 (6.3% vs. 1.2%)."

New Drug Interaction Warning with Rifampin and Combination of Ritonavir and Saquinavir. 'Drug-induced liver toxicity with highly elevated liver enzymes (greater than 20 times the upper limit of normal) has been observed in 39% of ***healthy volunteers*** *receiving rifampin 600 mg once daily in combination with ritonavir 100 mg/saquinavir 1000 mg twice daily (ritonavir boosted saquinavir).*

Neural Tube Defects with First Trimester Efavirenz (Sustiva) Use. "The prescribing information for efavirenz (Sustiva) has been changed to include new information. The revision result of four reports linking neural tube defects in infants born to women with first trimester exposure to efavirenz. The four cases of neural tube defects include three cases of meningomyelocele and one Dandy Walker Syndrome. Pregnancy should be avoided in women receiving efavirenz...Efavirenz is an antiretroviral drug indicated for acquired immune deficiency syndrome (AIDS, HIV-1 infection). ***A registry has been established to monitor fetal outcomes born to women exposed to efavirenz.***

Perhaps from the standpoint of imagining genetic mutation abilities or inventing viral characteristics that defy all biological evidence, a Century of genetics, and all common sense, there is no bigger tragedy than what was reported several years ago with nevirapine. Virological failure or drug resistance are technical terms among "HIV-AIDS" proponents that have come to mean that an anti-retroviral drug does not work (fails to suppress virus), or that disease progression is more rapid in those that take a particular drug. In the New England Journal of Medicine, it was reported (and despite its known toxicity and withdrawal from the U.S. several years ago):

"Well over ***875,000*** *women and infants have received a single dose of*

nevirapine. A single dose of nevirapine is the cornerstone of the regimen recommended by the World Health Organization (WHO) to prevent mother-to-child transmission among women without access to antiretroviral treatment and among those not meeting treatment criteria. However, nevirapine ***resistance*** *is detected (with the use of standard genotyping techniques) in* ***20 to 69%*** *of women and* ***33 to 87%*** *of infants after exposure to a single, peripartum dose of nevirapine. Among 60 women starting antiretroviral treatment within 6 months after receiving placebo or a single dose of nevirapine,* ***no women in the placebo group and 41.7% in the nevirapine group had virologic failure (P<0.001).*** *Women who had received a single dose of nevirapine had significantly higher rates of virologic failure on subsequent nevirapine-based antiretroviral treatment than did women who had received placebo. This apparently deleterious effect of a single dose of nevirapine was concentrated in women who initiated antiretroviral treatment within 6 months after receiving a single dose of nevirapine. We did not find that a previous single dose of nevirapine compromised the efficacy of subsequent nevirapine-based antiretroviral treatment in women who started antiretroviral treatment 6 months or more after delivery. Among the 30 HIV-infected infants, a single dose of nevirapine (one each to mother and infant) as compared with placebo was associated with significantly higher rates of virologic failure and smaller CD4+percentage increases in response to subsequent nevirapine-based antiretroviral treatment".*

Universal "HIV" screening of certain groups is nothing new, and it hasn't improved the health or reduced "infection rates" of those populations for which routine screening is already in place: military recruits, medical students, "disease ridden foreigners" (immigrants who apply for permanent residence, and any participant in the Gay Games in Chicago, despite "some conservative groups who oppose(d) the federal government's decision to waive the ban on HIV-positive travelers to the U.S., saying it threatens public health)", and, universal screening of pregnant women. The reason why none of these groups have benefited by universal testing is because of the false positive rate of the test results, especially among those "low risk" groups that will now be tested routinely at their doctor's office, or perhaps in emergency room visits.

If you test positive because you recently had a flu vaccine or are pregnant, grave psychological consequences can result. Has universal "HIV" screening within mandatory medical resident training programs ever prompted a letter of apology by the CDC to the family of Dr. David Acer, for his committing suicide on the basis of their mistaken charges that he spread "HIV" to his patients, which the CDC later exonerated him of doing (after his suicide), because the CDC could "find no evidence the dentist's HIV-positive patients contracted their infections from him because their virus' DNA did not match his, and also concluded the dentist's patients did not contract the virus from one another — in effect, that unclean dental implements did not act as conduits." Other studies and thousands of anecdotal reports that have followed exposure of health care workers have also reported no transmission of an "HIV-positive" test result, or AIDS.

Not only does transmission of AIDS not occur between 60% of positive mother-infant pairs because infants serorevert, but it also has not occurred in health care settings such as dentist's offices, hospitals, or sperm banks, or between sexually active serodiscordant couples, such as hemophiliacs. It has not even been scientifically shown to be transmitted between persons who have frequent unprotected sex in any context. From the study called "Heterosexual Transmission of HIV in Northern California: Results from a Ten-Year Study:"

*"We followed up 175 HIV-discordant couples [one partner tests positive, one negative] over time, for a total of approximately 282 couple-years of follow up… No transmission [of HIV] occurred among the 25% of couples who did not use their condoms consistently, nor among the 47 couples who intermittently practiced unsafe sex during the entire duration of follow-up…" "**We observed no seroconversions** after entry into the study [nobody became HIV positive]…This evidence argues for low infectivity in the absence of either needle sharing and/or other cofactors."*

No scientific evidence has shown that the "HIV" "retrovirus" causes the immunodeficiency illness symptoms called AIDS. We have requested the scientific paper(s) that prove that "HIV" is the causative agent. "HIV" sequences and proteins are found in a variety of non-disease-associated contexts, and "HIV" vaccines do not evoke antibodies and are provided with dangerous adjuvants like squalene. The "HIV" screening tests are contradictory, inconsistent across national boundaries, and no consensus exists regarding their validity. ARVS induce immune suppression according to their manufacturer's package inserts, and fears of HIV's mutability provide excuses for drug makers claims to conceal the fact that ARV's do not work. Seropositivity reverts to seronegative in infants and in single patients and vice versa even when compared on the same test. Transmission studies show no transmission. Universal screening has not protected groups where universal testing is already in place, and the stigma associated with testing positive has caused many to commit suicide, has prevented them from getting health insurance, has caused uncounted abortions, and has ruined and ended countless lives.

Because of these considerations, the assumptions underlying universal testing are flawed. It is an idea predicated on faith rather than scientific evidence. Moreover, the numbers of "infected individuals" provided in references, by the CDC, by the WHO, or others, are fictitious.

"Estimates on HIV called too high. New data cut rates for many nations."

"Statisticians traditionally have had a difficult time estimating the size of the pandemic. In 1986, Jim Chin, then a state epidemiologist in California who later developed models for the World Health Organization to calculate HIV prevalence, and several other US officials met in a West Virginia hotel room to figure out how many Americans had HIV."

"Chin recollected that the group arrived at a range of 1 million to 1.5 million people; 18 years later, the number is at about 1 million Americans. "A lot of it was guesswork, based on limited studies," Chin said. "It was the best we could do".

Regarding the imagined similarities between universal "HIV" testing and early detection of cancer with routine screening, unlike cancer, early screening does not matter with profound immune suppressive states: the symptoms considered diagnostic for "AIDS" cannot simply be removed with a surgeon's knife, with radiation, or with a "chemical knife" once it is detected, like a non-invasive melanoma. When considering assays in human patients which diagnose "AIDS" by quantifying the number of lymphocytes/ml, patients are not considered to have an AIDS-defining illness if they have suffered from chronic starvation, as these individuals are known to possess a helper T-cell ratio in the AIDS-defining range or even lower (< 250 cells/ml), and can present with as much as a 90% reduction in their normal T-cell number which is reversible *upon nutritional supplementation and a normal diet. In this regard, it has been several years since the announcement in the New England Journal of Medicine that vitamin supplements can ward off progression to AIDS in the absence of HAART (Highly Active Anti-Retroviral Therapy).*

The recommendation handed down from CDC for universal "HIV" screening, universal screening of pregnant woman, universal screening in routine doctor office visits, and routine testing in emergency room visits are reminiscent of the hepatitis B vaccine era. Twenty years later, the evidence shows that the current hepatitis B mandate in place not only threatens our children's health, but also serves in the future to threaten our children's education and admission to all kinds of institutions (day care and school admission).

So, Mr. Obama, please do not think about science at a time like this: either allow your people to refuse or obtain a religious or philosophical exemption from undergoing an "HIV" test. Faith-based exemption means that God told you not to get tested, and who can argue with that?

Sincerely,
Andrew Maniotis, Ph.D.
Program Director in the Cell and Developmental Biology of Cancer
Departments of Pathology, and Bioengineering,
University of Illinois at Chicago, Chicago, IL 60607

REFERENCES

1. Sanders et al., Cost-Effectiveness of Screening for HIV in the Era of Highly Active Antiretroviral Therapy; NEJM, Volume 352:570-585, February 10, Number 6, 2005.
2. Paltiel et al. Expanded Screening for HIV in the United States – An Analysis of Cost-Effectiveness. Volume 352:586-595, February 10, Number 6, 2005.
3. Samuel A. Bozzette, M.D., Ph.D. Routine Screening for HIV Infection – Timely and Cost-Effective. Volume 352:620-621, February 10, Number 6, 2005.
4. Kent A. Sepkowitz. N. England Journal of Medicine 354:23, June, 2006.
5. Horwitz MS, Boyce-Jacino MT, Faras AJ. Novel human endogenous sequences related to human immunodeficiency virus type 1. J Virol. Apr;66 (4):2170-9, 1992.
6. Varmus H, Reverse transcription Sci. Am. 257:48-54, 1987.
7. Ghori A. 1; Usselmann B. 2; Odogwu S. 1; Fraser I. 1; Morris A. 2 Colorectal Disease, vol. 2, no. 2, pp. 106-112, 2000.
8. Pachez M. No need to be phased. Shares, 28-32, 2001.
9. Papadopulos-Eleopulos E, Turner VF, Papadimitriou J, Page B, Causer D, Alfonso H, Mhlongo S, Miller T, Maniotis A, Fiala C. A critique of the Montagnier evidence for the HIV/AIDS hypothesis. Med Hypotheses 63(4):597-601, 2004.
10. Dura WT, Wozniewicz BM. Expression of antigens homologous to human retrovirus molecules in normal and severely atrophic thymus. Thymus 22 (4):245-54, 1994.
11. Willman et al., Heterophile Antibodies to Bovine and Caprine Proteins Causing False-Positive Human Immunodeficiency Virus Type 1 and Other. Enzyme-Linked Immunosorbent Assay Results. Clinical and Diagnostic Laboratory Immunology, p. 615-616, Vol. 6, No. 4, July 1999.
12. Strandstrom et al., Studies with canine sera that contain antibodies which recognize human immunodeficiency virus

structural proteins Cancer Res 1990 Sep 1;50 17 Suppl: 5628S-5630S.

13. Bojanowski, K., Maniotis, A., Ingber, D. DNA toposiomerase ll can control chromatin topology and drive chromosome condensation without enzymatically modifying DNA. J. Cellular Biochem. Vol. 69:127-142, 1998.
14. Gallo and others, Science, Vol 303 16 January, 2004.
15. P. B. Asa et al., Exp. Mol. Pathol 68, 196-197, 2000.
16. Asa PB, Wilson RB, Garry RF. Antibodies to squalene in recipients of anthrax vaccine. Exp Mol Pathol. Aug;73(1):19-27, 2002.
17. Gary Matsumoto. Vaccine A, Basic Books Publisher, 2005.
18. Holmdahl et al. Arthritis induced in rats with nonimmunogenic adjuvants as models for rheumatoid arthritis Immunol Rev. Dec;184:184-202, 2001.
19. Gherardi NK. Lessons from macrophagic myofasciitis: towards definition of a vaccine adjuvant-related syndrome. Rev Neurol (Paris). Feb;159(2):162-4), 2003.
20. Schiff I, Correia B, Ravnikar VA, Schur PH. HTLV-III antibody testing in sperm donors.N Engl J Med. Jun 20;312(25):1638, 1985.
21. Abbott Package HIV-I ELISA Test Kit insert, 1997.
22. Epitope Package HIV-I Western Blot Test Kit insert, 1997.
23. Roche's amplicor HIV-1 monitor test, 1996.
24. NucliSens HIV-1 package insert, Nov. 13, 2001. http://www.fda.gov/cber/pmalabel/P0100010LB.pdf
25. COBAS AmpliScreen HIV-1 Test, version 1.5 Approval Date: 12/19/2003 (www.fda.gov/cber/label/hiv1roc121903LB.pdf).
26. The Cambridge Biotech HIV-1 Western Blot Kit. www.fda.gov/cber/label/hiv1cam052898Lb.pdf)
27. OraSure(R) HIV-1 Western Blot Kit (www.fda.gov/cber/pmalabel/P950004Lb.pdf)
28. Stramer et al. "Detection of HIV-1 and HCV Infections

among Antibody-Negative Blood Donors by Nucleic Acid–Amplification Testing. New England Journal of Medicine, Volume 351:760-768, August 19, Number 8, 2004.

29. John Bulloch, Wall Street Journal, June 9th, 2004.
30. Rodriquez B, Sethi AK, Cheruvu VK, et al. Predictive value of plasma HIV RNA level on rate of CD4 T-cell decline in untreated HIV infection. JAMA 296(12):1498-506, 2006.
31. Cohen J. Study says HIV blood levels do not predict immune decline. Science 313(5795):1868, 2006.
32. Lancet 339; 1992.
33. Doran TI et al. False-Positive and Indeterminate Human Immunodeficiency Virus Test Results in Pregnant Women. Arch Fam Med. Sep/Oct; 9: 924-9, 2000.
34. Simonsen L, Buffington J, Shapiro CN, et al. Multiple false reactions in viral antibody screening assays after influenza vaccination. Am J Epidemiol 141:1089 1096,1995. http://content.nejm.org/cgi/content/extract/354/13/1422.
35. Lee, D, Eby W, Molinaro, G. HIV false positivity after Hepatitis B vaccination. Lancet 339: 1060, 1992.
36. Parekh BS, Shaffer N, Coughlin R, et al. Dynamics of maternal IgG antibody decay and HIV-specific antibody synthesis in infants born to seropositive mothers. The NYC Perinatal HIV Transmission Study Group. AIDS Res Hum Retroviruses 9:907-12, 1993.
37. Chantry CJ, Cooper ER, Pelton SI, Zorilla C, Hillyer GV, Diaz C. Seroreversion in human immunodeficiency virus-exposed but uninfected infants. Pediatr Infect Dis J 14:382-7, 1995.
38. de Martino et al., Rapid disease progression in HIV-1 perinatally infected children born to mothers receiving zidovudine monotherapy during pregnancy. AIDS. 13(8):927-933, May 28, 1999. The Italian Register for HIV Infection in Children AIDS, 13:927-933, 1999.
39. Antoni Noguera et al. Pediatrics, Vol. 114 No. 5 November, pp 598-603, 2004.

40. JD Hamilton et. al. and the Veterans Affairs Cooperative Study Group. A controlled trial of early versus late treatment with zidovudine in symptomatic human immunodeficiency virus infection." New England Journal of Medicine, 326: 437-434, 1992.
41. Seligmann et al., Concorde: MRC/ANRS randomised double-blind controlled trial of immediate and deferred zidovudine in symptom-free HIV infection. Concorde Coordinating Committee. Lancet, Apr 9;343(8902):871-81, 1994.
42. TAGline/Volume 4 Issue 2 February 1997.
43. FDAMedWatch *1/19/2005.*
44. FDAMedWatch *2/9/2005.*
45. FDAMedWatch *6/10/2005.*
46. Lockman S. et al., Response to Antiretroviral Therapy after a Single, Peripartum Dose of Nevirapine. The New England Journal of Medicine 356 January 11, 2007.
47. DS Burke et al. Human immunodeficiency virus infections among civilian applicants for United States military service, October 1985 to March 1986. Demographic factors associated with seropositivity. Volume 317:131-136, July 16, Number 3, 1987.
48. Sateren et al., HIV-1 Infection Among Civilian Applicants for US Military Service, 1985 to 2000: Epidemiology and Geography. Epidemiology and Social Science Journal of Acquired Immune Deficiency Syndromes. 32(2):215-222, February 1, 2003.
49. Awash in controversy. Is city ready for Gay Games? By Alexia Elejalde-Ruiz RedEye. Chicago Tribune, June 14, 2006. http://www.chicagotribune.com/news/custom/redeye/red-061406-gay1,1,170181.story?coll=chi-news-hed
50. Ted Anthony. STUDY: HIV not contracted from dentist. Associated Press, Thursday, December 1, 1994. ww2.aegis.org/news/ap/1994/AP941233.html
51. Hirsch MS, Wormser GP, Schooley RT, Ho DD, Felsenstein

D, Hopkins CC, Joline C, Duncanson F, Sarngadharan MG, Saxinger C et al. Risk of nosocomial infection with human T-cell lymphotropic virus III (HTLV-III). N Engl J Med. Jan 3;312(1):1-4, 1985.

52. Padian, et al. Heterosexual Transmission of HIV in Northern California: Results from a Ten-Year Study." American Journal of Epidemiology. August, 1997.
53. John Donnelly, The Boston Globe June 20, 2004.
54. Parent et al. In vitro lymphocyte-differentiating effects of thymulin (Zn-FTS) on lymphocyte subpopulation of severely malnourished children. Am. J. Clin. Nutr. 60(2):274-8, 1994
55. Chevalier et al. Immune recovery of malnourished children takes longer than nutritional recovery: implications for treatment and discharge. J. Trop Pediatr 44(5):304-7, 1998.
56. Wafaie W. Fawzi, et al. A Randomized Trial of Multivitamin Supplements and HIV Disease Progression and Mortality Volume 351:23-32, July 1, Number 1, 2004.
57. Maniotis Andrew, Maniotis Rita, Espat N. Joseph; Chen Xue, Lycos Peter. Why is the Hepatitis B vaccine still mandated? Medical Veritas, Nov; 3(2):1206-1210, 2006.

VACCINES AND BRAIN DAMAGE

When our young children do not want to pay attention and want to play well with others in elementary school, a healthy course of Ritalin, or Adderall will fix them we are told, which sets many of them up for the disease of methamphetamine addiction to everyone's surprise, and which has been left to be managed by the criminal justice system instead of being managed as a disease (McCauley, "Is addiction really a disease?" https://www.youtube.com/watch?v=b2emgrRoT2c).

Dr Robert Mendelsohn, who was Professor of Pediatrics at Northwestern University Medical School, also the United States federal government's first National Medical Director for Project Head Start, also Professor at the University of Illinois at Chicago Medical School where I taught, and finally who was Chairman of the State of Illinois medical licensing board appointed by the Illinois Governor to oversee licensing of MDs in Illinois, said repeatedly that every vaccine causes brain damage.

In California special education rates increased from 1 in 50 in the year 2000 to 1 in 8 kids needing special education in the year 2017. This is a 600% increase in children requiring special education in 17 years.

See https://edsource.org/2019/california-governor-and-lawmakers-at-odds-over-new-special-education-funding/612935

Also read this article from EdSource about skyrocketing special education costs and rates https://edsource.org/2019/california-spending-over-13-billion-annually-on-special-education/619542

Dr. Mendelsohn was tireless in his efforts to warn how vaccines were causing pediatric brain injuries, auto-immune diseases, and cancers http://whale.to/vaccines/mendelsohn.html.

Another perspective of how vaccines cause brain damage can be read here in this interview with Dr Andrew Moulden, an MD and neuropsychologist who taught at several Canadian universities, and who has done some of the most elegant SPECT imaging of ischemic zones that he claims are present in a wide array of morbid syndromes that all involve ischemia.

(http://vactruth.com/2009/07/21/dr-andrew-moulden-interview-what-you-were-never-told-about-vaccines/).

In an online article (http://vactruth.com/2009/08/03/vaccinations-are-causing-impaired-blood-flow-ischemia-chronic-illness-disease-and-death-for-us-all-hp/), Dr. Moulden concludes that

> *"ALL vaccines are causing immediate and delayed, acute and chronic, waxing and waning, impairments to blood flow, throughout the brain and body. This IS causing us all to become chronically ill, sick, and causing brain damages along a continuum of clinically silent to death. This is causing ischemic "strokes". In some respects, this is also "aging." Since the damages are microscopic, we cannot see them as they occur. However, we can now see the neurological aftermath of these damages – within hours and days of vaccination – all vaccinations."*
>
> *"Remarkably, it is not so much the specific "germs and toxins" that are causing death and disease. It is the response of the body and blood to foreign substances entering the blood and tissues that causes pathology. The state of the blood, the nature of the triggers, the state of the immune system relative to repeat antigenic challenges, conspires to effect damages along a continuum of harm – all organ systems can be affected."*
>
> *"The cellular and tissue damages are additive with each exposure. Direct vaccination is no longer necessary to be vaccine injured. Vaccinations are not the only trigger to pathology. Serial (repeat) vaccinations aggravate the core problems. Once the blood vessels are damaged, to a critical point, the pathological process can take on a self-perpetuating life of its own accord from infants to teenagers to adults, to companion pets alike."*
>
> *"The ischemic brain damages, after vaccination, from infants to adults, cut across all symptom based medical diagnostic end points."*

We require vaccination throughout our lives during our "yearly wellness checkups," and indeed, we need a flu vaccine every year for the rest of our medicalized lives, and other vaccines for international travel. Finally, we arrive at our dying moments in a hospital and are drug-managed to death. However, when it comes to addressing an intention to deliver a pharmaceutical drug to 4.9 billion healthy people, isn't it time for a moment of reflection and perhaps have a small talk?

Although these pharmaceuticals are supposed to have been "scientifically-proven" and extensively safety tested in at least 3 levels of clinical trials and preferably also during a period of post-marketing experience before the FDA permits their wide release to the public, they are not. Now we are instructed that EUA (Emergency Use Authorization) for proclaimed epidemics and pandemics is needed, and that the "maladies" these medical interventions given to healthy populations will "treat but not cure." We also are told that without them, a plethora of pathogens out there will likely later do us in, if we are not compliant with the prescribed pharmaceuticals coursing through our veins. For example, we should receive a hepatitis B vaccine within minutes to months of our births, to protect us from acquiring hepatitis B when we become IV drug addicts in our teens, and also, to protect us from developing hepatitis B-induced liver cancers when we are 60, although the vaccine "wears off" in 7 years, "according to the data."

"Go ask your doctor if this drug is right for you"...is the responsible thing "the educated thing to do," and now we are even told that, even your neighborhood pharmacist has been given license to give you vaccines upon the asking. What is especially egregious, is that they will provide you with this or that new vaccine for the asking, and without accountability or monitored registration for possible long-term vaccine side effects either to VAERS (Vaccine Adverse Events Reporting System), datalink's database, or now the new one made just for the expected toxic adverse events of the most dangerous vaccines of them all, the SARS-CoV-2 vaccines, and they should be approached with a significant measure of caution, according to Baylor College researchers during the 2012

SARS-COVID "epidemic," according to vaccine scientists who attended the WHO's Global Vaccine Safety Summit who confirmed major problems with coronavirus vaccine safety around the world on December 2-3, 2020, according to Paul Offit, the inventor of the rotavirus vaccine that was immediately recalled because it caused intestinal intussusception, and many other usually pro-vaccine advocates. Because there has been concern about the new Moderna and Pfizer-BioNTech vaccines, a new adverse events database has been established called the V-safe database and another injury database is being planned.

In the context of SARS-COVID-19, and from the tone and demeaning assumptions that characterize these pharmaceutical litanies, it seems as if a premeditated marketing strategy was set into place years ago to currently convince a "heathy-sick audience," that they are doomed, unless they comply with "the vaccine," "the mask," the social distance," and to be OK with the joblessness.

Another dimension to the madness asks weather health in the context of individuals or populations should be biologically defined as the ability of an individual or a population to avoid illnesses, or overcome illnesses if and when it occurs? A familiarity with the life cycles of living systems favors the interpretation that health is best defined as an ability to overcome, not to avoid diseases and illnesses, which begs the question about the purpose of vaccines given to hundreds of millions or 4.9 billion healthy folks, as proposed by the WHO.

What do our policy decision makers that we elect and believe say about this question? In this context, the wisdom of living systems, with their natural variation in populations, and their natural mechanisms of resistance is ignored…the human manufactured artifact and technology of vaccination along with its witchcraft and sorcery rule! But shouldn't policy decisions "toward the good" that affect our children's and future's health and well-being be the product of reason, historical facts, science, and compassion, and not the prognostications of witchcraft and sorcery?

INDICTMENTS

Scientifically speaking, we know so little about vaccines and their relationship to epidemics. Biologically speaking, we know so little about human variation, specifically of the immune system, and its relationship to epidemics. There are certain principles that seem to emerge though. One fact that becomes evident, however, is that inoculations and vaccines and vaccination campaigns, or epidemics, seldom appear to behave the way we have been told they have behaved. Questions far outnumber any certainties, regarding inoculations, vaccines, or epidemics.

Natural epidemics, or "pandemics" have been hypothesized by some to have severely culled the populations of our ancestors. It has even been suggested on the basis of no evidence that perhaps the Neanderthals were carried off by a virus or some other pathogen. Climate changes could have led to their disappearance (if indeed Neanderthals constituted a different species from modern man as some believe because their heads were larger, their skeletal frames more robust than ours, and some would even say, that the artwork they left behind was more inspired than some of ours as shown by some of their cave paintings).

New conceptual problems have emerged because of modern molecular testing which is increasingly used and trusted to inform and then to guide critical therapeutic decisions. A more informed awareness needs to be in place that does not exist yet in current standards of care, to better assure the safety and effectiveness of therapeutic interventions that have been shown to do no harm under any circumstances.

Although during desperate health crisis and chronic illness, there sometimes is an acute urgency to abandon standards of care and medical intervention successfully used in the past in the hopes that some panacea will emerge to somehow cheat death itself, direct pathogen testing by Electron Microscopy (EM) can make a positive difference in weeding out the false positive lab test results from indirect testing from the legitimate cases that may want to stay in bed for a few days.

Many have advanced the idea that vaccination and antibiotics are perhaps Mankind's greatest medical achievements because therapeutic decision-making often is based on the **findings of indirect tests**, imagined fears, and well-orchestrated propaganda. Particularly worrisome are therapeutics applied to diagnoses of illnesses that have been shrouded in social stigmas, in which especially those syndromes that have been associated with certain racial groups, classes, genders, or occupations.

This fear mongering has dramatically gained credence during our own lifetimes, especially during certain critical periods in the human life cycle, such as during normal human pregnancy, normal infancy, and indeed during the entire duration of the era we have chosen to live in best described as humanity's historical era of "healthy sickness," which is mandated by the urgency of yearly "wellness checks".

This era and thinking have ushered us through the revolving doors of cardiology practices, hypertension diagnoses, pain clinics, and the like. The most heinous example of this unforgivable and unspeakable delusion are mandated vaccines, yet other iatrogenic practices also claim as many victims as possible. Fierce objections have been forcefully and articulately advanced toward policy changes regarding over-vaccination and re-vaccination schedules and antibiotic over-prescription during infancy, childhood, adolescence, middle age, and old age. An entire spectrum of what amounts to even costlier and problematic and highly adverse event-inducing lifelong maladies and endemic illnesses are increasing exponentially, and when drugs are given to treat the side effects of previous drugs, these arguments have been ignored and censored. Too much profit is made by the medical system treating their own mistakes and treating endemic iatrogenic diseases caused by the medical system itself.

Consider the invitations, advertising, and even legally enforced mandates to herd our children and seniors into the slaughter-house of ever more drugs and vaccines that continues to this day. Almost each month there are new so-called "preventive" vaccines and drugs that are being aggressively advertised and marketed for new ailments you have never heard of or never known that you or your children are suffering from, without your awareness.

When obedience is not willingly provided to the agenda of Big Pharma, even by the asking of a simple question about seeing the safety data for such "staples" as the hepatitis B vaccine, some parents have been threatened with incarceration by governmental agencies at the insistence of certain factions of the medical establishment. Children in fact have been illegally prevented from attending school, and in other situations, parents have been incarcerated until they "listen" to doctor's orders and force their adult children to follow "standards of care" rather than try alternative therapeutics they want to explore that involve no toxicity and can do no harm.

Yet we are forced to accept that these medicines do no harm and are beneficial. We are counseled that we should blindly accept them without a discussion, or without harboring any concerns for the long-term effects they may have and which they could potentially unleash on entire populations because of an "impassioned crusade" to vaccinate and medicate the entire human race to establish "herd immunity" and to accomplish disease "eradications" through vaccines.

But are these projections really true, or are they simply cruel violations of human potential and the common good? Vaccine makers in some cases have admitted or include on the package inserts page-long lists of adverse reactions associated with many vaccines prescribed to children, teens, adults, and seniors.

A common but by no means exhaustive list of these maladies in humans include arthritis, asthma, seizures, ADD, shingles, AIDS and other ill-definable autoimmune syndromes, diabetes, meningitis, pneumococcal illnesses, hypertension, and a plethora of "pulmonary hypertensive disorders," and cancers.

Vaccines and drugs are even given anyway at the expense of the taxpayer. Yet healthy children, adolescents, and young adults in fact appear in many statistical surveys to becoming "sicker" without any concerns raised about the long-term effects on health of preventative interventions such as the so-called "hepatitis B" and "HPV" vaccines that supposedly protect against cancers that will occur 50 years later, with their > 10% severe and often life-long adverse event profiles. Vaccines and drugs are even given anyway at the expense of the tax-payer. It doesn't even ring any alarms among most people, such as parents,that we are being subjected to increasingly promoted programs of seasonal influenza vaccinations, and experiencing drug-associated liver diseases, and immunosuppression-associated diseases, and ever increasing complex vaccine schedules

(see: https://www.netce.com/coursecontent.php?courseid=1754;scrollTo=chap.4

https://www.cdc.gov/vaccines/schedules/hcp/imz/child-adolescent.html

https://www.cdc.gov/vaccines/vpd/vaccines-list.html

Yet despite package inserts accompanying these products, and which the doctor's never disclose to their healthy-sick "patients," even when the vaccines or drugs include the putrid and often proprietary molecules in vaccines and immunizations designed to prime the non-immunologically mature normal soil bacteria such as tetanus and tetanus "spores" and bacteriophage particles, and non-specific immunoglobulins, people are either coerced or forced to comply, by allowing these experimental potions to be injected into their bodies or their children.

As all the media pundits and Anthony Fauci who is now the de facto ruler of the United States wants to jab all of us with vaccines and not let us leave our house or get jobs bagging groceries without first showing a "vaccine passport". Yet other well established scientists are telling the truth regarding these new vaccines, although they are censored. One such article was published in Reuters on March 9, 2020 entitled: "As pressure for coronavirus vaccine mounts, scientists debate risks of accelerated testing." One such article was published in ***Reuters*** on March 9, 2020 entitled: ***"As pressure for coronavirus vaccine mounts, scientists debate risks of accelerated testing."***

The abstract claims the following:

> *"Behind the scenes, scientists and medical experts are concerned that rushing a vaccine could end up worsening the infection in some patients rather than preventing it.*
>
> *"Studies have suggested that coronavirus vaccines carry the risk of what is known as vaccine enhancement, where instead of protecting against infection, the vaccine can actually make the disease worse when a vaccinated person is infected with the virus.* ***The mechanism that causes that risk is not fully understood and is one of the stumbling blocks that has prevented the successful development of a coronavirus vaccine. Normally, researchers would take months to test for the possibility of vaccine enhancement in animals. Given the urgency to stem the spread of the new coronavirus, some drug makers are moving straight into small-scale human tests, without waiting for the completion of such animal tests."***
>
> ***"There is a risk of immune enhancement,"*** *said Hotez. "The way you reduce that risk is first you show it does not occur in laboratory animals." "Hotez testified before the U.S. House Committee on Science, Space and Technology about the need for sustained funding for vaccine research"...that "There remains no vaccine for any of the new coronaviruses that have caused outbreaks in the past 20 years."*

In more recent times, experiments using monkeys have shown some clinical indicators of a lung condition known as a "ground-glass" MRI, but these experiments also yielded some rather unexpected results also. Because of the **legacy** of ethical laws that came into effect following the reign of terror perpetrated by a Doctor Chester Southam who during the 1950's injected cervical cancer cells into more than 600 of his uninformed gynecology **patients** (should be pluralized... patients not patient), into 40 extremely ill Jewish citizens without their informed consent, and 80 prison volunteers, the same standard imposed after Southam's iagrogenocide should be applied to the approval of the SARS-COVID-19 arsenal of vaccines.

HeLa cells are commonly used cancer cells used in most cancer research laboratories. During the early 1950's they were used without success to generate yet another failed "polio vaccine". But perhaps most significantly, HeLa cells were injected into some 80 or more Ohio prisoners' forearms by a Dr. Chester Southam following the first hepatitis B vaccine trials on those same prisoners that were conducted by Nobelist Dr. Baruch Blumberg and Saul Krugman and others (who would launch the hepatitis B era and its associated iatrogenic carnage that will be discussed later). Before Chester Southam would admit later that he failed in his live cancer cell injections to induce cancer in those prisoners, 3 Jewish student doctors refused to follow Southam's orders, and they alerted the hospital's top administrator. Southam had and wanted to continue to perform the same experiment on 40 old sick Jewish folks at this Jewish Chronic Disease Hospital in Brooklyn, who only spoke Yiddish, and could not understand the purpose of Southam's experiment if they wanted to. It also would become revealed later that Southam also had already subjected more than 600 gynecological surgery patients to his inoculations of live HeLa cancer cells and other cells at Sloan-Kettering, without their consent either.

Why were Henrietta Lack's cervical cancer cells injected into the arms of 40 non-informed and aged and quite ill Yiddish-speaking Jews at the Jewish Chronic Disease Hospital in Brooklyn, and also, without their knowledge, into more than 600 women in New York who had undergone gynecological surgeries of various kinds under his knife? Because Dr. Southam wanted to know that if such cells as HeLa were accidently needle-stuck into doctors or researchers, if they might acquire cancer, since doctors and scientists were special soldiers on the front lines to rid the world of that disease.

The work was published. It made little impression on those doctors or scientists that an African American woman's living malignant cervical cancer cells did not cause cancer even when directly injected into a human being's skin by a tuberculin syringe and repeatedly into some 80 healthy white prisoners, into 40 morbidly sick and aged old persons some of whom already had cancer, or into 600+ unsuspecting females. All that happened was a small lesion formed at the inoculation site, and the lesions became rejected, and the injection site healed in every human case that he followed.

After the student doctors refused to aide in Southam's experiment at the Jewish Chronic Disease Hospital, the ethical conundrum Dr. Chester Southam's "human experiments" created became the focus of the world's attention, that led to many our modern experimentation rules and informed consent laws that are currently in place when human beings are ever used in medical research (see Sacrifice of the Virgins, and **Another First Anti-cancer Vaccine, Andrew Maniotis, 2010-free on my website** andrewmaniotis.wordpress.com; Also see: **"The Virus and The Vaccine-The True Story Of A Cancer-Causing Monkey Virus-Contaminated Polio Vaccine, And the Millions Of Americans Exposed**, by Debbie Bookchin and Jim Schumacher, St. Martin's Press, 2004).

EPIDEMIC, ENDEMIC, AND HERD IMMUNITY

The original definitions of the words epidemic and endemic were derived from the Greek words "demos," which means people, and epidemic which combined means: *excessively prevalent "upon" the people affecting many people at the same time,* whereas endemic means "in" the people at a low but constant frequency. Do these terms apply to all declared epidemics even though the symptoms of the "disease" of seasonal flues are accompanied by fever, chills, and respiratory distress, whereas the symptoms of addiction are manifested in unwanted behaviors?

Over the past several thousand years, inoculations and then vaccinations became a global phenomenon. Yet vaccines and the inoculations preceding them have not accomplished the "immunization" and "herd immunity" that the vaccinologists and epidemiologists in theory hoped they could achieve. Pandemic, epidemic, and endemic diseases, syndromes, and maladies, and Humanity's unique degree of forethought among all mammals as far as we know, has evolved the concept, and practice of immunizing against future harms. The "harms" perceived are both physical harms, and material harms, financial harms, behavioral harms, and future times of hardship. What have been the historical tendencies and trends associated first with inoculations and then vaccinations, and are there any new and useful insights about this centuries-old human activity that can be revealed by History itself? How have epidemics, now pandemics, and vaccines influenced every conceivable dimension of our past, present, and future lives, and the lives of our offspring?

Are there elements about vaccination mandates that are based upon social pressures we might not be aware of, that emerge from some of humanity's deeper, more distant to emerge characteristics that may be an anathema to the essence of science as a specific way of asking questions to disprove hypotheses-characteristics that aren't necessarily uniquely human characteristics, such as fear, altruism, other instincts, or perhaps other "capacities", which began their expression among human beings even before our species was considered as being in the taxonomic group of Homo sapiens, or even members of the primate order?

What is sought in public discussion is to decipher an incredibly complex and ancient practice, that touches all aspects of our modern lives, and through an historical approach, and with a little deduction and luck, illuminate the "how's," "what's," "when's," "where's," and then try to ask the most important question, why have we inoculated and vaccinated for centuries, even before any germ theory was in place, and why do we vaccinate today? Why should we continue to mandate vaccines in the future to attend schools, to obtain honest work as a health care provider, to travel abroad, etc.?

Natural Selection is important to address regarding the topic of pandemics, epidemics, and endemic disease, and also in the context of inoculations and the heavily publicized promoted "miracle cure" or dampening effect of Co-2 SARS vaccines in particular.

A fundamental question raised is do we know or can we know if vaccine acquired "herd immunity," if it were even something vaccines could achieve, is something that is desirable in the first place for a species, or might it be something to fear and avoid because it may immunologically accomplish a loss or lack of Natural immunological diversity or "species-wide homogeneity", which has been a fundamental tenet that has insured our survival.

What information should be believed and what should we teach our children to be true, and on what evidence should we then decide is solid enough to take some decisive and measured action?

In this same general context, and as the immunity myth goes, if humans believe that vaccines protect them, then why should they insist on others being vaccinated if they believe they themselves are protected by the vaccine they received? This would be akin to two next door neighbors living with their driveways adjacently positioned, and neighbor A waxes his car to protect it, he has been taught, from rust. If he believes the wax (vaccine) will protect his car from rusting in the rain and bad weather, then why should he or she insist that neighbor B who lives next door, and whose car is parked only 6 feet away, refuses to wax his car parked only feet away? Is it logical that neighbor A be imprisoned for 30-60 days, or fined $ 1000.00 or both, as NYC Mayor De Blasio threatened the Orthodox Jewish people in Brooklyn who refused vaccines if they did not submit to a measles vaccine within 48 hours, and that somehow, if neighbor B's unwaxed car rusts, then A's rust will somehow rust neighbor B's waxed car?

EVOLUTION DOES NOT ANTICIPATE FUTURE EVENTS

Evolution does not anticipate future events, yet many believe that vaccination is perhaps Mankind's greatest medical achievement. Nobody predicted The Black Death which happened at the time of Greece's Golden Age, or the plague of 1347- 1353. As far as we know, there were no plague vaccines or plague treatments in existence then that worked.

In 1889, Alfred Russel Wallace, who was Darwin's collaborator and the co-discoverer of Natural Selection perhaps more than anyone else, changed the practice of forced vaccine compliance to the centuries-old superstition of inoculations and the vaccinations that were ushered in a century before by The Jennerian paradigm of vaccination, by publishing two extensive volumes in 1889 that he first submitted to The British Parliament entitled: **"VACCINATION-PROVED USELESS AND DANGEROUS FROM FORTY-FIVE YEARS OF REGISTRATION STATISTICS"** (The Reese Collection, 1957), and in another that followed, entitled, **"THE ARMY AND NAVY: A DEMONSTRATION OF THE USELESSNESS OF VACCINE."**

Scientifically speaking, we know so little about vaccines and their relationship to epidemics. Biologically speaking, we know so little about human variation, specifically of the immune system of populations, and its relationship to epidemics. Certain principles that seem to emerge though, by examining a chronological history of epidemics and vaccines. One fact that becomes evident from the beginning, however, is from examination of historical records from many sources, vaccines and vaccination campaigns, or epidemics seldom appear to behave the way we have been told they have behaved. Questions far outnumber any certainties, regarding vaccines or epidemics.

Natural resistance to disease and epidemics is a fundamental part of our biology. Natural biological diversity at the immunological level more than any other biological factor kept our kind alive before the advent of any human intervention. Inoculations and vaccinations are superimposed upon this natural resistance, and arguably confound the already complex problem of resistance. Human attempts to "homogenize" the immune response of populations through mass vaccination programs have complicated the problem of background incidence and resistance of infectious disease occurrence even more.

VAERS (the **V**accine **A**dverse **E**vents **R**eporting **S**ystem that is maintained by the CDC and FDA) is a system in place where by many estimates 1-10% of vaccine injuries are recorded by many estimates. If and when scientifically valid associations between vaccines and epidemics, and more importantly, between natural resistance and variation are more fully understood, perhaps the 4+ billion dollar (VAERS) budget can be spent elsewhere? If examined scientifically, can an argument be made in favor of an older and much improved new emerging technology known as hyperbaric medicine? Hopefully, the conceptual advances this chronology delivers might serve to improve human health and well-being, and ward off tragedy due to misplaced eugenic ideas, practices, and thinking.

As absence of evidence is not evidence of absence, and a lack of epidemics between two points in time does not imply that that human forethought in the form of a technology such as inoculation or vaccination immunized populations protecting them from an epidemic. Most importantly perhaps, the following information should raise the critical question: what is the evidence that widespread or universal vaccination of a population will generate immunity? And is there reason to hope that perhaps better preventative measures or strategies that are already widely available simply need to be repurposed in the context of communicable pathogens and epidemics to accomplish the "immunization" that vaccines have not so far delivered?

It appears that nutrition and hygiene have worked historically as preventatives against many diseases and syndromes, whereas the assertion that inoculations or vaccinations have prevented any diseases or epidemics is less certain. Hippocrates famous statement: "Let the food be the medicine and the medicine be the food" is still true today. Recent evidence suggests that this wisdom should be more of a primary concern for maintaining good health and overcoming even the most severe known human afflictions. What is immunity, what does immunity mean, and is it obtainable?

Historically, it has been documented that the inoculation of dried pox-pus was practiced in Persia and India as an operation where the surface of the body was injured with needles or lancets, and foreign puss from "pox," or perhaps from other disease effusions were placed into direct contact with the bloody wound or bloodstream of the inoculation recipient. It is uncertain whether or not this practice "immunized" against smallpox or spread the illness throughout the inoculated.

In China, it is claimed that dried material from pox and other disease-derived effusions were introduced in the nostrils of both children and adults. There is evidence that controversy raged regarding the use of fresh disease-derived material versus dried, old material, which could have made a substantial difference in the virulence of an inoculum. It is unclear also whether or not this practice immunized against smallpox or served to spread the illness.

Among the Arabs, there are accounts that citizens would "purchase the pox," by exchanging raisins and other fruits with an infected person who would serve as the donor of the lymph (Pylarini, Phil Trans., 1716 Vol XXIV., p, 393). We do not know the effective outcome of this practice.

Nobody predicted The Great Plague that killed a fifth of London's population in 1665-1666. There was no universally mandated plague vaccine back then. Nor were there plague vaccines during the 313 years (between 1353 and 1665) to prevent a plague epidemic during those years. Therefore, we may assume a plague vaccine played no role whatsoever in the occurrence, prevention, or recurrence of these two plague epidemics, and nobody could have predicted that the two great epidemics would be separated by 313 years. Plague is spread by rats, and fleas, but other "forms" are thought to exist. The great yellow fever outbreak said by medical historians to have killed 2/5 of the Philadelphia population in 1793 was not prevented by a universally-implemented vaccine program because one did not exist ("Bring Out Your Dead," Powell, Time Reading Program Special Edition Books, 1949). In this disease context, historical accounts claim that the famous Dr. Benjamin Rush (the revered signer of The Declaration of Independence) thought yellow fever to be caused by rotting coffee on the Philadelphia docks! Dr. Rush also thought the best therapeutic approach for yellow fever consisted of near lethal doses of mercury, combined with exsanguinations (bloodletting) to the extent that many of his patients were poisoned or bled to death until French physicians pointed out to him the blood to body weight ratio. No mention of vaccination regarding yellow fever can be found in any historical reference from this era. This is to be expected, because it was not until Christmas morning in the year 1900, when Walter Reed conducted his yellow fever transmission experiment, which showed that yellow fever was transferred via the mosquito. The relationship between epidemics, prevention of epidemics, vaccine campaigns, other types of interventions, and recurring epidemics must be clearly defined with respect to causality or lack of causality in modern epidemic occurrences. These relationships shall be examined in this analysis, including SARS-COVID-19 and the prospect of the impending vaccination campaign that some claim "will save us."

Paul De Kruif convincingly emphasized that nutritional additives to foods, as well as improvements in the realization of civil hygienic programs (like the Roman aqueducts), have most likely reduced the spread of pathogens and, prevented epidemics historically, and have improved the quality of life for that portion of humanity that has instituted these habits and technologies in a not well-known book entitled, "*Life Among Doctors*" (Harcourt, Brace, New York, 1949).

There is no evidence or proof that any primate pathogen had led to the extinction of any non-human primate species, or group(s) of early humans, except for a mythology that arose in the 1980's: that "HIV" is 100% fatal without "life-extending" toxic and life-ending treatments with the nucleoside analog, AZT or other rank poisons. But at the same time, we were told we are in the capable hands of physicians and scientists, backed by political and financial mandates about their ability to conquer all obstacles by "practicing scientifically-based medicine" and through drug discovery using "scientifically-designed clinical trials." For instance, in 1984 Margaret

Heckler, the U.S. Government, and Dr. Robert C. Gallo promised in a press conference that an "HIV" vaccine would be forthcoming in 2 years (by 1986), and now he wants to give an oral polio vaccine to SARS-CoV-2-positives. This is particularly relevant to the subject of SARS-COVID-19 because again, Dr. Gallo is behind the curtains of the SARS-CoV-2 global lockdown, and he has been pushing for a COVID-19 vaccine without any remorse or apology for the carnage he, Dr. Fauci, and the other "virologists" have wrought during the past 35 years during the AIDS era (Can an Oral Polio Vaccine Help Stop the Coronavirus? | Video | Amanpour & Company | PBS https://www.pbs.org/wnet/amanpour-and-company/video/can-an-oral-polio-vaccine-help-stop-the-coronavirus/ Can an Oral Polio Vaccine Help Stop the Coronavirus)?Perhaps the most "vicious criminal" of them all, who has not only driven the current SARS-COVID-19 madness with his "economically-inspired" models, is Neil Fergusson who has brought us once again (incorrectly) with his "weather forecasts" involving global pandemic shutdowns, as he has before without any whimper of protest from the virologists or from those in the biological or medical communities. In the words of Jon Rappoport:

> *Claiming a new "mutant strain" of SARS-CoV-2 is 70% more deadly than the original, computer modelers in the UK have advised Prime Minister, Boris Johnson, to lockdown the country at a much stricter level. The computer model was concocted at the Imperial College of London. The accompanying text actually admits it is too early to tell whether the mutant strain is a major threat. Nevertheless, Boris Johnson has issued the new vast lockdown order.*
>
> *Who is on television promoting the need for the lockdown? None other than Neil Ferguson, the disgraced and failed computer modeler. He did not author the new model/study at the Imperial College, but he is now the face of the "science." Ferguson's prior model predicted 500,000 COVID deaths in the UK and 2 million in the US would occur by last summer. This absurd and criminal estimate directly influenced Boris Johnson and Donald Trump to declare states*

> *of emergency, and abandon plans to keep their national economies open. And now he is back, on television, warning citizens about the new "mutant strain" of the virus and the need for a higher level of lockdown.*
>
> *Other scientists are outraged at the latest computer model; they are demanding to see the actual evidence of the increased threat. They are saying they do not even understand what "70% more deadly than the original strain" means. How much more economic devastation can the people of the UK take?*

In hindsight, and as presented to the 1995 Congress of the United States by their Office of Technology assessment, we know that none of these or many other modeling prophesies have been realized, nor are they likely to ever materialize. Despite the fact that (as admitted in that 1995 Technology Assessment presented to Congress following 30 then failed "HIV" vaccines:

"More companies are engaged in HIV vaccine research than in research for any other type of vaccine. Potential liability may have discouraged some companies, but liability has not stopped HIV vaccine development."

The "experts" have said that vaccines are both safe and they are effective. To better understand the point, and the importance of a chronology of the harms vaccines have caused as documented by some of the most reputable medical men in recorded history, a brief look at some well documented history as to these assertions is presented below, yet the same type of propaganda that Fergusson invented took place even during the polio and their incredibly damaging propaganda campaigns that minimized the now known calcium arsenate poisoning of orchards back at the end of the 1800's, and the paralysis and the concomitant DDT poisonings that happened during the polio era of the 1950's.

In 1860 The following is part of a letter which appeared in the Lancet on July 7th, 1860, signed a "Military Surgeon:" *"VACCINATION AT SHORNCLIFFE.— SIR,— Having seen in the Lancet of last week an* *article commenting on a return moved for by Mr. DUNCOMBE, respecting those who have died from Vaccination, the number of amputations required to save life at the camp at Shorncliffe, I can only say that it would be advisable to extend this return, and ask for the number of those who have died or had their arms amputated since the promulgation of an order from the late Director-General ALEXANDER...*

The military always has kept the best records of the carnage caused by vaccination, and the Navy in particular because entire crews of ships were mandated to be vaccinated:

1864 A US Department of Navy record was found stating: *"Upon the U.S. steamship Jamestown, serving in Japanese waters, there occurred, in 1864, among a ship's company of 212 persons, 31 cases of small-pox, with four deaths. The entire crew had been vaccinated after leaving the United States."*

1868 JOSEPH JONES, M.D., Professor of Physiology and Pathology, University, Nashville, U.S.,1868, wrote: *"The Federal prisoners confined in Camp Sumpter, Andersonville, Georgia, were vaccinated, and, in a number of cases, large gangrenous ulcers appeared at the points where the vaccine lymph had been inserted, causing extensive destruction of tissues, exposing arteries, nerves and bones, and necessitating amputation in more than one instance. From the establishment of the prison, on February 24th, 1864, to October 1st, over 10,000 Federal prisoners died, i.e., near one-third of the entire number perished in less than seven months. These accidents led to the belief among some of the prisoners that the surgeons had intentionally introduced poisonous matter into their arms during vaccination. No wonder they had such a persuasion, seeing that about 100 of them lost the use of their arms, and about 200 were so injured that they soon afterwards died. Though some medical officers were tried before a special military commission, convened in accordance with orders from the War Office at Washington, on the charge of having willfully poisoned the Federal prisoners with vaccine lymph, it was shown that the unhappy consequences of vaccination at Andersonville were paralleled in the Northern prisons. 'After careful inquiries,' says Dr. JONES, 'among returned Confederate prisoners, I am convinced that the accidents* *attending Vaccination were quite as numerous and severe in Northern prisons as in Southern."*

What about the experience recorded by other countries during that era?

1871 *"Europeans resolutely object to be vaccinated with lymph from native sources; and, notwithstanding the law, when imported lymph cannot be obtained, they and their children remain unvaccinated. As a consequence, the population of Europeans attacked with leprosy is comparatively small and, indeed, of rare occurrence, except in the case of soldiers who are subject to the military regulation of revaccination. This repugnance to native lymph on the part of Europeans in the West Indies was pointed out by Dr. R. Hall Bakewell, Vaccinator – General, Trinidad, in his remarkable evidence before the Select Parliamentary Committee of 1871, and has been referred to by Dr. Castor, of British Guiana, and other authorities."*

The famous London physician, medical journal editor, author, and harsh critic of vaccines, Dr. Charles Creighton worked in London as a hospital registrar until his appointment in 1876 as demonstrator of anatomy at the University of Cambridge. Over the next five years he wrote his first book, *Bovine Tuberculosis in Man* (1881), and published several articles on anatomy in the *Journal of Anatomy and Physiology*. He became co-editor of the journal in 1879. He devoted most of his later career to exposing vaccines as dangerous and useless as an active member of the London Society of the Abolition of Compulsory Vaccination.

1879 Mr. P. A. TAYLOR reveals his intention to introduce a Bill during the next Session for the Repeal of the Compulsory Clauses of the Vaccination Acts, and told the House of Commons, in April, 1879, that he had *"seen dozens and scores of persons who had stated to him that they honestly believed that their children had died from vaccination. They took perfectly healthy children to be vaccinated, an incision was made in the arm, in a few days a sore appeared on the arm, from thence it spread all over the body, and finally the children died in agony"* (Lancet, August 21st, 1881).

In the 20th Century, perhaps the best documented examples that were not able to be censored or "cleansed" by the powerful vaccine interests (The Rockefeller Foundation for one) comes from the polio era because paralysis greatly ***increased*** following the Salk polio vaccine era in the 1950's, which was one reason why the Sabin vaccine was quickly developed and then adopted. In 1972, for example, Jonas Salk, who became a bitter critic of Sabin (the inventor of the IPV-inactivated polio vaccine), testified before a Senate subcommittee said that:

CDC ADMITS THAT "NEARLY ALL POLIO OUTBREAKS SINCE 1961 WERE CAUSED BY THE ORAL POLIO VACCINE"

And by 1992, America's Centers for Disease Control (CDC) in Atlanta admitted that the polio live-virus vaccine had become the main cause of polio in the United States. Specifically, the CDC asserted that:

"From 1973 to 1983, **87%** of all (non-imported) cases of polio resulted directly **from vaccine administration**. Even more amazingly, it was asserted that **every** non-imported case of polio in the United States from 1980 to 1989 was vaccine-induced." (Strebel, P. M., et al., Epidemiology of Poliomyelitis in the U.S., One Decade after the Last Reported Case of Indigenous Wild Virus Associated Disease, *Clinical Infectious Diseases, CDC, February, pp. 568-579, 1992*).

By 1997 it was admitted that:

> ***"Polio is not eradicated by vaccination, but likely lurks behind a disease redefinition and new diagnostic names like viral or aseptic meningitis.......According to one of the 1997 CDC issue of the MMWR, there are some 30,000 to 50,000 cases of viral meningitis per year in the United States alone. That is where it is thought that 30,000 – 50,000 cases of polio disappeared after the introduction of mass vaccination."..."Today, various other forms of the word "polio" are still used to describe the effects of poisoning, though usually with regard to paralysis in animals. A search of Medline ("polio" and "poison") finds about 45 contemporary articles where poisoning causality is attributed to polio."***

The various terms used to describe "polio-like symptoms were compiled from, The Health and Research Publications of Jim West:

"polioencephalomalacia","poliomyelomalacia","polyradiculoneu ritis","neurological picture similar to that of poliomyelitis", "polio-encephalo-myelomalacia", "lumbal poliomyelomalacia", "cerebro-cortical necrosis (polioencephalomalacia)", "Lead poisoning in grey-headed fruit bats (Pteropus poliocephalus)", "multifocal-polio-myelomalacia", "spinal poliomalacia", "Polio and high-sulfate diets", "atypical porcine enterovirus encephalomyelitis: possible interaction between enteroviruses and arsenicals", "polioencephalomalacia and photosensitization associated with kochia scoparia consumption in range cattle", "bovine polioencephalomalacia." Viral or aseptic meningitis, Guillaine Barre Syndrome (GBS), Chinese paralytic syndrome, chronic fatigue syndrome, epidemic cholera, cholera morbus, spinal meningitis, spinal apoplexy, inhibitory palsy, intermittent fever, famine fever, worm fever, bilious remittent fever, ergotism, ME, post-polio syndrome, acute flaccid paralysis.

By the several examples given so far, it should begin to become confusing that vaccine injuries are not simply a damage issue. Disease definitions are changed-vaccines cause diseases they were not designed to prevent, in a majority of a population, they seem to be as if a syringe were filled only with water, and absent some epidemic vaccines are assumed to protect the majority, and so forth. In fact, there are 7 distinct categories, including the category which clearly shows that vaccines do no harm at all-as if the syringe were filled with water, and absent an epidemic, assumed to protect the masses.

The hepatitis B era of Baruch Blumberg during 1990's brought us not only rising rates of allergies, and brain damage among children jabbed with the hepatitis B vaccines. Hepatitis B vaccine is not only mandated for most modern children who enter schools or daycare, but also it many contexts is delivered within hours or even minutes of birth, as they tried to do to one of my children (but I intervened). How does an immune system that is minutes to hours old know how to "process" an attenuated antigen? Now some virology "experts" are urging us to vaccinate "preemies." Does this make any sense?

The long-awaited AIDS vaccines that were promised to us in 2 years following Robert Gallo's and Margaret Heckler's famous **1984** Springtime TV announcement that "the probable cause of AIDS has been found"…to be a "cancer virus variant" have not "arrived"?

2003 "*Weeks after the announcement that the HIV vaccine, AIDSVAX, had failed, VaxGen (the makers of AIDSVAX) was hit with a shareholder lawsuit that accused the company's officials of continuing to make positive statements about their vaccine to artificially pump up the company's stock price, despite mounting evidence that it was not effective. The suit was dismissed last year and VaxGen, under new management, remade itself into a biodefense company, and is now supported with 887 million of our tax dollars.*"

2005 (November) Chinese scientists reported H5N1 avian flu infection in pigs, *raising concerns that the virus could exchange genes with human flu strains in this 'mixing vessel'. None of these pigs was ill, according to National Geographic article. By November 2005, H5N1 virus had spread throughout most of SE Asia, resulting in the culling of over 100 million chickens. In Vietnam and Thailand, the pandemic infected at least 37 people, with 26 deaths.*

2006 "*One of the chief dissenters of AIDSVAX, the failed program now funded to make an anthrax vaccine for 887 million of taxpayer money following announcement of that failure of AIDSVAX, Robert C. Gallo, who helped discover "the human immunodeficiency virus" not only in artwork, but in the black slaves he imagined coming to America after the AIDS virus had jumped onto them from monkeys during the slave trade, scoffed at the notion that the trial would be successful.*"

2007 September. "*AIDS Effort Suffers Big Blow as Merck Vaccine Fails to evoke seroconversion or protection from "HIV,*" by Marilyn Chase and Mark Schoofs:

> *"In a major setback, one of the leading experimental AIDS vaccines not only failed to prevent test subjects from becoming infected with*

> *HIV, but it didn't offer any indication it might delay the onset of full-blown AIDS, which had been a key hope."*
>
> *"The collapse of the trial leaves Merck & Co., which had spent a decade developing the vaccine, with no remaining prospects in the global hunt for an AIDS immunization. The vaccine was tested in a network funded by the National Institutes of Health."*

"*We've been kicked in the teeth,*" said Bruce Walker, a veteran AIDS researcher at Harvard University who was not involved in the study. Lawrence Corey, a leader of the NIH-funded HIV Vaccine Trials Network, said he was in 'mourning." The vaccine's failure to protect recipients from acquiring "HIV" was also a big disappointment to the recipients of the anti-HIV vaccine.

> *"The "HIV" vaccine recipients tested positive for "HIV" slightly more frequently than the non-HIV-vaccinated, but the differences between the groups* ***were not significant*** *in any arms of the STEP trial, or in any other "HIV" vaccine trial. All of these men who now test "HIV-positive" will be regarded and treated now as AIDS patients."*

NO VACCINE EVER HAS BEEN RIGOROUSLY SAFETY TESTED FOR CARCINOGENIC POTENTIAL IN HUMANS HOWEVER AMPLE ANIMAL STUDIES INDICATE VACCINES CAUSE CANCERS IN MAMMALS

Despite the constant clamor from pharma and the Public Health Agencies that vaccines first are tested for safety before they are administered to tens to hundreds of millions of human arms (and into most of our companion animal dogs and cats), this clearly has not occurred to the standards of other pharmaceuticals that have been FDA evaluated in the past. For example, a tranquilizer given to women during the 1950's for a variety of reasons was found to damage the ovaries of those women and were linked to high levels of ovarian cancers in the daughters of those women in the next generation. Eventually the drug was banned. What vaccines have been held up to this simple though rational strategy to test their effects on the next generation of children? Answer: 0.0%:

(Modified from DES action of Australia https://www.desaction.org.au/):

"Synthesized in 1938, laboratory studies showed animals administered DES developed mammary cancer, with high rates of fetal death, sterility and cancer in the offspring. Despite this, DES was approved for use in humans in 1940. Initially used to treat late pregnancy complications, by the mid-1940s the use was widened to include the prevention of miscarriage, i.e., for prophylactic use by women who had a history of miscarriage."

"However, by 1949, DES was seen as making "a normal gestation more normal". By the early 1950s DES was being prescribed and marketed as a general pregnancy "tonic", mixed with vitamins, and recommended for all pregnant women to ensure healthier pregnancies with "bigger and stronger" babies. A 1953 study showed, to the surprise of the researchers, that the DES-treated group experienced higher rates of miscarriage, premature labor, and neonatal death than the control group, and the 1953 Dieckmann study was ignored.

DES was already entrenched as standard obstetric clinical practice. Also, by this stage, DES was being aggressively promoted by the drug companies for use in all pregnancies."

"In 1971 it was discovered that DES caused clear cell cancer of the vagina/cervix in DES daughters. DES was thus proven to be carcinogenic in humans. Regardless of these findings, it was continued to be used as a treatment for acne, to dry up breast milk, as a contraceptive like a morning after pill, as hormone replacement therapy during menopause, as a treatment for "tall girls" to stunt their adult height, and to fatten up livestock to increase profits. In 1981 a landmark publication, Arthur L Herbst and Howard A. Bern edited a book which brought together leading experimental researchers and expert clinicians on DES, and with an experiment on mice, Herbst and Bern showed that in later life, the immune system of DES exposed mice was suddenly compromised. Preliminary studies of DES daughters in the early 1980s indicated that DES exposure is linked with immune system problems, including a higher incidence of autoimmune disease, such as asthma, arthritis, diabetes, systemic lupus, and thyroid dysfunction in addition to cancers (Herbst AL, Bern, HA. (eds) Developmental effects of Diethylstilbestrol (DES) in pregnancy." New York. Stratton).

Despite this knowledge has been around for 40 years, no vaccine ever has been rigorously tested for cancer inductions like DES was.

VACCINE INDUCTION OF CANCER AND THE SCIENCE OF VACCINE DAMAGE: VACCINE INJECTION SITE SPACIAL AND TEMPORAL ASSOCIATIONS WITH MALIGNANT CANCERS AND OTHER MALADIES

If a person decided to receive a vaccine after the insanity of testing then they should know about the lengthy evidence of spatial and temporal associations between vaccination site locations and cancers. Records kept by military medics and surgeons have been among the best objective records chronicled documenting vaccination injuries in such journals as The Lancet, with reports dated as far back as the 1860's. Yet the best evidence that is readily available regarding vaccine injuries are being filed by veterinarians regarding how our pets are acquiring a range of endemic illnesses associated with vaccines, including cancers, nervous system disorders, degenerative diseases, drug-toxicity effects, abnormal sclera, plaques, or fibrotic tissue all have been characterized in the advancing deconditioned states and disease processes.

A new revolution in the biological sciences began with the discovery and many confirmations that factors outside of cells control diverse essential functions of living systems. It is now realized also that the biofilms produced by microbes play important roles in resisting any and all environmentally harsh or pharmaceutical interventions, and the matrix scaffolds produced by multicellular organisms function as critical master regulators of many critically important cellular processes. Single-celled and multi-celled organisms even share some the same extracellular matrix molecules such as fibronectin and laminin.

There is accumulating evidence that vaccines have been known to initiate cancers at or near the vaccine site, and cancers remain as one of the best and most studied examples and insights as to the baffling nature of cancer initiation and resistance of cancers. Inoculations and vaccinations also have been causally linked to "mini-strokes," or more accurately described, to ischemic episodes and life-long autoimmune diseases by exhaustive use of new technologies such as CT scans, PET scans, and other technologies now routinely used by physicians and scientists such as Andrew Moulden and countless other investigators.

It seems to be true that both naturally occurring severe syndromes such as cancers and a host of neurological and long-term immunological issues as well as these same injuries caused by vaccines all appear to be due to a lack of oxygen available to tissues of varying degrees (collectively called ischemia). These vaccine injuries are also mechanistically believed to be the result of a phenomenon known as molecular mimicry (when the body detects a foreign molecule and doesn't fully recognize it as foreign, but instead, undergoes the mysterious process of tolerance, yet reacts against some of the organism's own molecules in tissues, as if they were foreign and the immune response rejects them by attacking those molecules and tissues of the body which the immune system senses structurally mimic to some extent the foreign antigen).

This phenomenon of vaccine-induced cancer induction has been appreciated since early during the first decades of the 1900's when tissue grafting experiments in mice revealed "graft versus host disease"-a pathological and potentially fatal process wherein the body's immune system "rejects" the foreign tissue and sometimes its own tissues also. In a real sense, inoculations, as well as vaccinations were and are complex and dangerous medical grafting procedures, not unlike blood transfusions or liver transplants, and should be regarded as such by the scientific and medical communities, as well as the general public. Next to the box on the medical form you fill out when you go to the doctor's office that asks if you have ever had a blood transfusion, organ transplant, or cancer, there is a box to check that asks about what vaccines you have had for this reason.

The infusion of foreign cells such as lymph early during the vaccine era revealed that when graft versus host disease occurs, and when foreign lymphocytes were infused into mice, these foreign lymphocytes rejected the host's lymph nodes. Peyer's patches (lymph nodes along the intestines to guard against food-borne pathogens that enter the body through eating) were often affected soon after the foreign molecules were infused, as were the cervical, axillary, and inguinal lymph nodes of the neck, arm-pit, and groin, followed in some cases by a massive immune rejection of the recipient's tissues, followed by extreme morbidity and death in >50% of the recipients, depending upon the vaccine or inoculum, and depending on the recipient's genetic background. In the context of vaccination, history suggests that it should never be forgotten that one is attempting to alter the entire immune system and its future responses to the universe of antigens. Although intact and living eukaryotic cells are no longer infused in most vaccines, their molecular sub-components are, and some of these components can evoke massive responses of the immune system.

An understanding and review of the cancer extracellular matrix phenomenon known as vasculogenic mimicry and its likely biological significance in malignant tumor progression may provide important insights about the processes known as induration (hardening), fibrosis and perhaps even hemorrhaging in SARS-COVID-19 lung and kidney pathogenesis, as well as vaccine injuries. Many laboratories working on basic and clinical research on cancer and vasculogenic mimicry (**VM**) during the last 20 years, and especially in China, have suggested that vasculogenic mimicry channels 1) are important regulators of genomic function, 2) are regulators of differentiation, regulate the mechanical properties of tumor cells, and notably, 3) serve as a resistance mechanism of cancer cells and colonies (tumors). It is possible that perhaps matrix formation not only contributes to the inflexibility of lung tissue as it does to the hardening of malignant tumors, but also serves as a primary resistance mechanism and irreversible pathogenic change in atypical pneumonias. This similarity between the vasculogenic tumor matrix of malignant tumors and the induration in SARS-COVID-19 atpyical pneumonia victims' lungs suggest that certain therapeutic strategies that can penetrate through these matrices may be more effective than others. Fibrosis and fibrotic reactions may in fact be common features of pathogenic processes of many kinds?

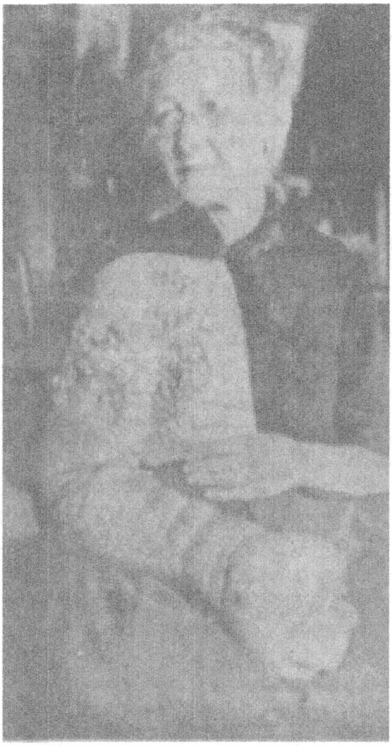

Photograph by permission of Harbison Printers, Oceano, Calif.

Mrs. Helen Goates of Bolivar, Missouri was a strong, healthy woman with no skin trouble or chronic disease when she was persuaded, during a vaccination drive, to submit to vaccination. Almost immediately, after the injection, an inflamed swelling started to develop around the vaccination. It continued to increase in size and intensity until it covered her entire arm and hand. After a period of time, it spread over her back and breast as is shown in the photograph.

She was treated by more than a dozen doctors and cancer specialists, but the condition grew steadily worse until death relieved her of her agony. Before her death she requested that a photograph be taken of the cancer in order that others might see the results of vaccination and be warned, in time against this ever-present danger of vaccine poisoning.

The cancer does not always start immediately. It usually takes months or years for the poisons to degenerate enough tissue for a cancer to form.

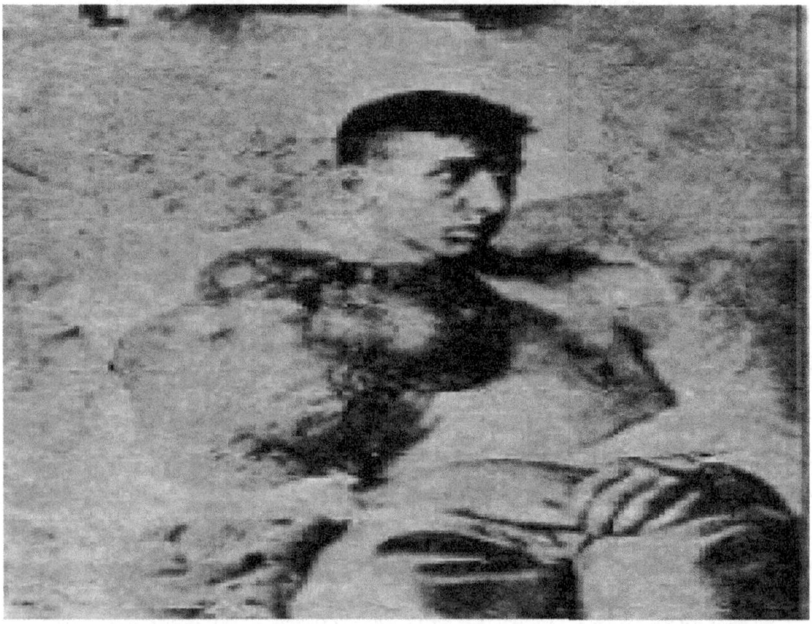

Giant tumor growing from the site of vaccination. Courtesy of Eleanor McBean

More specifically, there appears to be several specific molecules that are known to be deregulated due to vaccines when vaccines induce cancers systemically, and at the site of injection, and several of these same tissue-controlling molecules have been found to be present in fatal atypical pneumonias. Perhaps this is nowhere more clearly evident than in the field of veterinary medicine, because of the yearly vaccine mandates directed at our companion animals. The phenomenon regarding tumors appearing at or near the vaccination site(s) has been known for more than a Century, and was discussed in depth by Eleanor McBean, in her book, "The Poisoned Needle." Also, she quotes some of most celebrated physicians of past eras, regarding their surmise of vaccines and cancers.

"The chief, if not the sole cause of the monstrous increase in cancer has been vaccination."—Dr. Robert Bell, the famous cancer specialist of the British Cancer Hospital.

"We do not claim that vaccination is the only cause of cancer although Dr. Bell (quoted above) observed so many cases of cancers at the site of the vaccination and elsewhere, but directly traced to this cause that he affirmed that vaccination was the cause of the great increase in the cancer rate."

Many highly regarded physicians of the past decried the linkage between vaccines and the occurrence of cancers following the widespread use of vaccines. Many of these physicians were initially vaccine advocates until they experienced first-hand the carnage of vaccination site-linked cancers.

Dr. E. J. Post, a prominent physician of Berlmont, Michigan, said: **"I HAVE REMOVED CANCERS FROM VACCINATED ARMS EXACTLY WHERE THE POISON WAS INJECTED."**

In the New York Press, January 26, 1909, W. B. Clark stated:

> "Cancer was practically unknown until cowpox vaccination began to be introduced. I have had to do with 200 cases of cancer and I NEVER SAW A CASE OF CANCER IN AN UNVACCINATED PERSON."

Dr. Herbert Snow, Surgeon of the London Cancer Hospital, had this to say:

> "I am convinced that some 80 per cent of these cancer deaths are caused by the inoculations or vaccinations they have undergone. These are well-known to cause grave and permanent disease of the heart also."

Dr. Dennis Turnbull, who had studied cancer for 30 years declared:

> "I have no hesitation in stating that in my judgment the most frequent disposing condition for cancerous development is infused into the blood by vaccination and re-vaccination."

Dr. Forbes Laurie, late Medical Director of the Metropolitan Cancer Hospital, (London) said:

> "I am thoroughly convinced that the increase of cancer is due to vaccination."

Over-responses of immune cells have repeatedly been linked for many decades to vaccines and vaccine adjuvants which is no surprise because adjuvants were designed to non-specifically ramp-up the immune response. Adjuvants also have been linked to various tissue ischemias and various deregulations that occur in many disease syndromes. Some of these syndromes that have been triggered by aluminum-adjuvated vaccines include Parkinson's and Parkinson's-like syndromes, multiple sclerosis, Alzheimer's, arthritis, demyelination syndromes, autism spectrum disorders, and Gulf War syndrome.

In the case of Gulf War Syndrome, the debilitating malady was linked to the administration of squalene in anthrax vaccines during the First Gulf War, and which is an adjuvant that has been indicted by many studies to constitute its direct cause. An excruciatingly painful syndrome called myofacciitis also has been linked to seasonal flu vaccines, as well as gulf war syndrome of veterans to the anthrax vaccine.

Squalene, a hydrocarbon chain made from shark oil was experimentally used to reliably cause arthritis models in rats to find drugs to interfere with the development of arthritis, as it has been shown to repeatedly occur in certain lots of vaccines and not in other lots of the same vaccines not containing squalene. These adjuvants indeed do "ramp-up" the non-specific immune response-and at the same time they reliably accomplish these unwanted adverse events and side effects. Again, the vaccination records kept by the armed forces are instructive:

Pamela B Asa, Russell B Wilson, Robert F Garry. Clinical Trial Exp Mol Pathol **73(1):19-27, Aug, 2002.**

Abstract

"We previously reported that antibodies to squalene, an experimental vaccine adjuvant, are present in persons with symptoms consistent with Gulf War Syndrome (GWS) (P. B. Asa et al., Exp. Mol. Pathol 68, 196-197, 2000). The United States Department of Defense initiated the Anthrax Vaccine Immunization Program (AVIP) in 1997 to immunize 2.4 million military personnel. Because adverse reactions in vaccinated personnel were similar to symptoms of GWS, we tested AVIP participants for anti-squalene antibodies (ASA). In a pilot study, 6 of 6 vaccine recipients with GWS-like symptoms were positive for ASA. In a larger blinded study, only 32% (8/25) of AVIP personnel compared to 15.7% (3/19) of controls were positive (P > 0.05). Further analysis revealed that ASA were associated with specific lots of vaccine."

...These results suggest that the production of ASA in GWS patients is linked to the presence of squalene in certain lots of anthrax vaccine."

This isn't the only group claiming that squalene causes this "new disease" called "Gulf War syndrome". It turns out that the World Health Organization agrees with this claim:

Macrophagic myofasciitis and aluminum-containing vaccines

https://www.who.int/vaccine_safety/committee/reports/october_1999/en/

"The emergence of a new type of histopathological lesion of unknown origin called macrophagic myofasciitis (MMF), characterized by a unique myopathological pattern, has been reported by the Groupe d'études et recherche sur les maladies musculaires acquises et dysimmunitaires (GERMMAD) of the Association française contre les myopathies."

From the WHO's 2021 Newsletter they now claim the following regarding myofaciitis:

> "MMF is characterized by centripetal infiltration of the epimysium, perimysium and perifascicular endomysium by non-periodic-acid-shiff (PAS) positive cells of macrophage lineage with osmiophilic crystal inclusions. MMF has been mainly detected by deltoid muscle biopsy in adult patients, although it has also been detected by quadriceps muscle biopsy in 3 young children. The histopathological lesion is localized at these sites. There is absence of necrosis (of both epithelioid and giant cells) and of mitotic figures, and inconspicuous muscle fiber damage."

> "MMF can only be associated with vaccines containing aluminum hydroxide or also with those containing aluminum phosphate;

- a vaccine antigen can be detected in the affected muscle;

- deltoid biopsies were performed at the site of the injection (it is likely however that this was done in the majority of cases since the recommended practice is to give vaccinations and take biopsies from the nondominant arm).

> "From an epidemiological perspective, MMF has with few exceptions—only been observed in France. MMF was first seen in 1993 and has been recognized with increased frequency since then."

Adjuvants or preservatives such as aluminum that contaminate many vaccines also have been linked to many kinds of autoimmune disorders including cancers (Katarzyna Zabielska-Koczywąs, Anna Wojtalewicz and Roman Lechowski. Current knowledge on feline injection-site sarcoma treatment. Acta Vet Scand (2017) 59:47. DOI 10.1186/s13028-017-0315-y).

IRREFUTABLE SCIENTIFIC EVIDENCE OF VACCINE-INDUCED CANCERS IN DOGS AND CATS AT THEIR VACCINE INJECTION SITES

"Tail vaccination in cats: a pilot study ..." Abstract from University of Florida College of Veterinary Medicine Report

https://sheltermedicine.vetmed.ufl.edu/files/2013/10/Tail-vaccination-cats-jfms-hendrix-levy.pdf

"Feline injection site sarcomas affect 1–10 cats per every 10,000 vaccinated and are associated with high mortality. *Radical resection may be curative, but is often associated with prolonged recovery, disfigurement, and loss of function when tumors occur at currently recommended injection sites.* ***The objective of this study was to assess alternatives to currently recommended vaccination sites in terms of preference by oncology practitioners,*** *ease of injection and serological responses.* ***Surgical, radiation and medical oncology practitioners were surveyed regarding their preference for vaccination sites based on the ease of tumor resection.***

Original Article

Journal of Feline Medicine and Surgery
0(0) 1–6
© ISFM and AAFP 2013
Reprints and permissions:
sagepub.co.uk/journalsPermissions.nav
DOI: 10.1177/1098612X13505579
jfms.com
SAGE

Tail vaccination in cats: a pilot study

Cleon G Hendricks[1], Julie K Levy[1], Sylvia J Tucker[1], Shaye M Olmstead[2], P Cynda Crawford[1], Edward J Dubovi[3] and Cathleen A Hanlon[4]

Abstract

Feline injection site sarcomas affect 1–10 cats per every 10,000 vaccinated and are associated with high mortality. Radical resection may be curative, but is often associated with prolonged recovery, disfigurement and loss of function when tumors occur at currently recommended injection sites. The objective of this study was to assess alternatives to currently recommended vaccination sites in terms of preference by oncology practitioners, ease of injection and serological responses. Surgical, radiation and medical oncology practitioners were surveyed regarding their preference for vaccination sites based on the ease of tumor resection. A six-point Likert scale was used to measure each cat's behavioral reaction to vaccination when injected subcutaneously in the distal hind limb or the distal tail. Serum collected before and 1–2 months after vaccination was tested for antibody titers against feline panleukopenia virus (FPV) and rabies virus (RV). The preferred sites for vaccination by 94 oncology practitioners were below the stifle (41%) and the tail (30%). There were no significant differences in the cats' behavioral reaction to vaccination below the stifle (n = 31) and in the distal tail (n = 29). Of the cats seronegative for FPV at the time of vaccination, 100% developed protective antibody titers (≥40) against FPV 1–2 months following vaccination. For cats seronegative for RV, all but one cat (tail vaccine) developed acceptable antibody titers (≥0.5 IU/ml) against RV. Tail vaccination was well-tolerated and elicited similar serological responses to vaccination in the distal limbs.

Accepted: 22 August 2013

Introduction

Vaccines have been associated with life-threatening sarcomas in 1–10 of every 10,000 cats vaccinated.[1] Although the proportion of affected cats is low, vaccination is such a common procedure that several thousand new cases occur each year in the USA. Feline injection-site sarcoma (FISS) is poorly controlled with conservative surgery, chemotherapy and radiation therapy, and most cats die of local recurrence or distant metastasis. Recently, radical excision by surgical specialists incorporating surgical margins of at least 5 cm laterally and resection of two muscle planes deep resulted in long-term survival of a majority of cats.[2]

Historically, cats were commonly vaccinated in the interscapular region owing to ease of administration. Following the recognition that vaccination was associated with malignant tumor development and that wide and deep surgical excision was difficult to achieve at that site, international guidelines were developed that recommended vaccination in sites more amenable to radical excision. Currently, the American Association of Feline Practitioners recommends that vaccines containing feline panleukopenia virus (FPV), feline herpesvirus-1 and feline calicivirus antigens be injected subcutaneously below the elbow joint of the right forelimb, and vaccines containing feline leukemia virus (FeLV) or feline immunodeficiency virus (FIV) antigen or rabies virus (RV) antigen be injected below the stifle joint on the left and right hind limb, respectively.[3] The World Small Animal

[1]Maddie's Shelter Medicine Program, Department of Small Animal Clinical Sciences, College of Veterinary Medicine, University of Florida, Gainesville, FL USA
[2]Operation Catnip, Gainesville, FL, USA
[3]Animal Health Diagnostic Center, College of Veterinary Medicine Cornell University, Ithaca, NY, USA
[4]Kansas State University Rabies Laboratory (Hanlon), Manhattan, KS, USA

Corresponding author:
Julie Levy DVM, PhD, DACVIM, Maddie's Shelter Medicine Program, Department of Small Animal Clinical Sciences, College of Veterinary Medicine, University of Florida, Gainesville, FL 32610, USA
Email: levyjk@ufl.edu

A six-point Likert scale was used to measure each cat's behavioral reaction to vaccination when injected subcutaneously in the distal hind limb or the distal tail. Serum collected before and 1–2 months after vaccination was tested for antibody titers against feline panleukopenia virus (FPV) and rabies virus (RV). The preferred sites for vaccination by 94 oncology practitioners were below the stifle (41%) and the tail (30%). There were no significant differences in the cats' behavioral reaction to vaccination below the stifle (n = 31) and in the distal tail (n = 29). Of the cats seronegative for FPV at the time of vaccination, 100% developed protective antibody titers against FPV 1–2 months following vaccination. For cats seronegative for RV, all but one cat (tail vaccine) developed acceptable antibody titers (0.5 IU/ml) against RV. Tail vaccination was well-tolerated and elicited similar serological responses to vaccination in the distal limbs."

"The vaccinated Purdue dogs also developed autoantibodies to laminin, which is involved in many cellular activities including the adhesion, spreading, differentiation, proliferation and movement of cells. Vaccines thus appear to be capable of removing the natural intelligence of cells....Autoantibodies to cardiolipin are frequently found in patients with the serious disease systemic lupus erythematosus and also in individuals with other autoimmune diseases. The presence of elevated anti-cardiolipin antibodies is significantly associated with clots within the heart or blood vessels, in poor blood clotting, hemorrhage, bleeding into the skin, fetal loss and neurologic conditions."

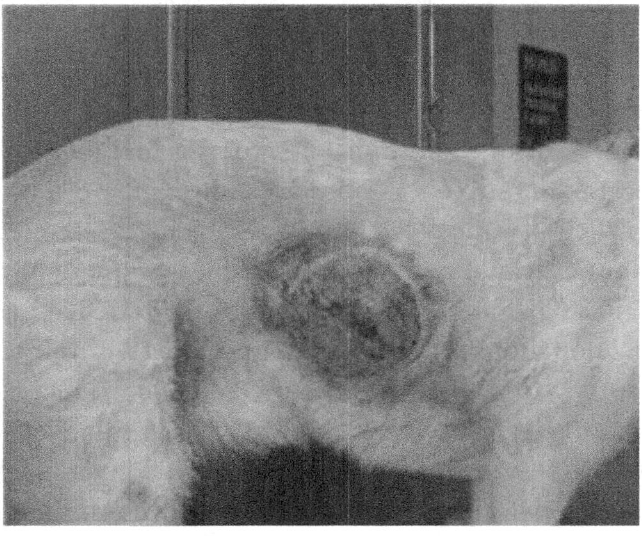

A vaccine-linked tumor lesion following vaccination.

http://www.thedogplace.org/VACCINES/vaccine-reaction-tumors-photos-Jordan-DVM.asp

"The Purdue studies also found that vaccinated dogs were developing autoantibodies to their own collagen. About one quarter of all the protein in the body is collagen…it is no wonder that Canine Health Concern's 1997 study of 4,000 dogs showed a high number of dogs developing mobility problems shortly after they were vaccinated (noted in my 1997 book, What Vets Don't Tell You About Vaccines)."

"It is also widely acknowledged that vaccines can cause a fast-acting, usually fatal, disease called autoimmune hemolytic anemia (AIHA). Without treatment, and frequently with treatment, individuals can die in agony within a matter of days. Merck, itself a multinational vaccine manufacturer, states in The Merck Manual of Diagnosis and Therapy that autoimmune hemolytic anemia may be caused by modified live-virus vaccines, as do Tizard's Veterinary Immunology (4th edition) and the Journal of Veterinary Internal Medicine (Duval, D. and Giger,U., 1996). "Vaccine-Associated Immune-Mediated Hemolytic Anemia in the Dog." Journal of Veterinary Internal Medicine 10:290-295). The British Government's Working Group, despite being staffed by vaccine-industry consultants who say they are independent, also acknowledged this fact."

"However, no one warns the pet owners before their animals are subjected to an unnecessary booster, and very few owners are told why after their pets die of AIHA."

The owners could not pay again for the surgical removal of this cancer and so had to have their pet destroyed by lethal injection. It has been known for decades that vaccine-induced cancers often first appear at the vaccination site on our companion animals and then proceed more aggressively than typical cancers (some 60,000 cats/year develop these more than normally-aggressive tumors that originate from the injection site). Patricia Jordan, DVM, CVA, CTCVH, and Doctor of Veterinary Naturopathic Medicine. Dr. Driscoll wrote an article about some of our conversations:

"Having seen an article in which I quote the Purdue study, Andrew Maniotis, Ph.D., Visiting Associate Professor of Bioengineering: Program of tumor mechanics and tissue regeneration, University of Illinois at Chicago, contacted me."

He wrote: **"I don't think it is coincidental that two of the molecules that the vets find (especially the tissue-controlling two molecules laminin and fibronectin) that are deregulated in vaccine-induced, cancer-harboring animals, are the same ones we have found reverse, kill, or promote tumors. It is logical that these two tissues constructing molecules in the correct or incorrect amounts induce tumor dormancy or killing as we have found, and at different amounts (as when a vaccine disturbs a tissue and fibronectin is produced in abundance while laminin is suppressed) they can, when not in proper amounts, induce tumor growth and metastasis."**

Canine Health Concern was formed in 1994 by Catherine O'Driscoll, after two of her beautiful young Golden Retrievers – Oliver and Prudence – tragically died. She asked, why? Catherine was sent scientific papers which told her that commercial pet food was nutritionally inadequate, and that many deficiency diseases are the direct result of poor feeding. She also learnt that the annual shots we give to our pets each year, in the belief that we are protecting them from disease, are actually the largest cause of ill health in our pets today.

This proposal to monitor these 160,000 cats/year that develop tumors at their injection sites and dogs experiencing cancers and other maladies associated with vaccines, is ethical, in addition, as long as vaccine mandates and laws are in place to vaccinate our pets, and there is no legal recourse not to comply with the law to subject our pets to a rabies or distemper vaccine except to go to jail or pay stiff fines. In fact, because our pets that develop cancers spontaneously, or as a result of vaccines with such frequency, and immune-system manipulated rodent models typically used in cancer research are so inadequate as their immune systems aren't "robust" as they are in our companion animals prior to vaccination, a new horizon in cancer therapeutics has been available and as a huge resource (as long as these laws are in place) to explore cancer induction due to vaccines in the context of an immune suppressive drug free, large bodied, relatively long lived mammalian living system (that also with some owners, eat similar diets as humans, so that most if not all of the environmental controls can be identified).

When vaccination site tumors occur, and because the primary tumor inducer can be controlled with respect to where the vaccine is given, many questions about the nature of cancer inducers can finally be answered. This spatial relationship between vaccines and vaccine-site tumor occurrence, prompted international meetings of veterinarians to propose to come to an agreement to change the location of vaccination sites away from more centrally located anatomical sites, toward more distal locations on limbs (although many vaccines still are given behind the nape of the neck).This change in the preferred amputation location was proposed because veterinarians made aware of the vaccination site-tumor relationship reasoned that it therefore is within their power to save a pet's life from its metastasizing vaccine-induced cancer simply by sacrificing the necrotic or cancer-bearing limb where the vaccine was given and where the primary tumor starts growing.

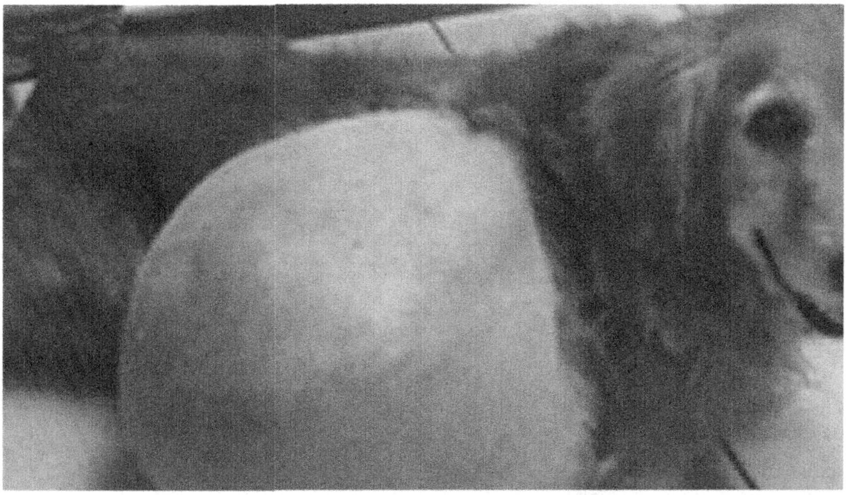

Vaccine-associated tumor of the shoulder

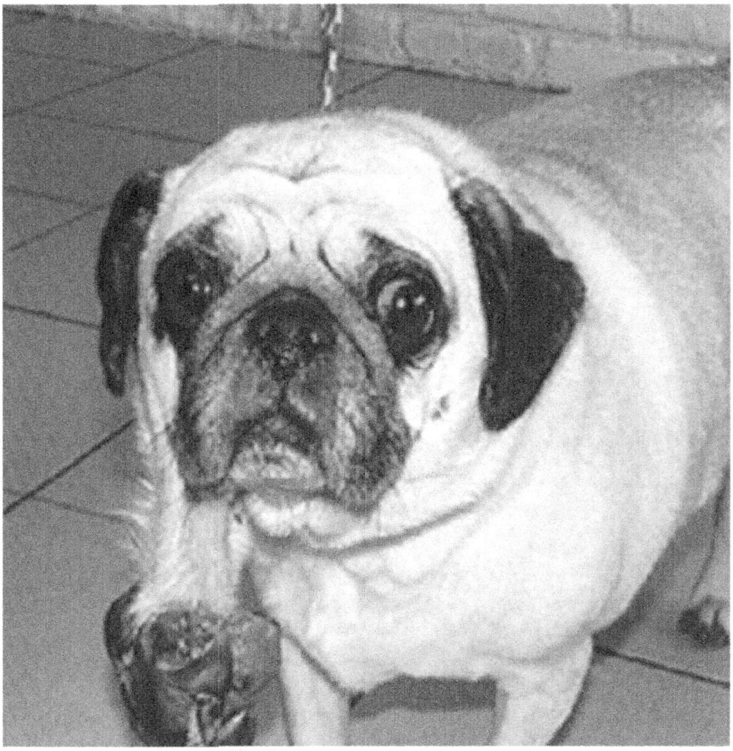

Vaccine associated tumor of the head.

From: www.thedogplace.org/VACCINES/vaccine-reaction-tumors-photos-Jordan-DVM.asp

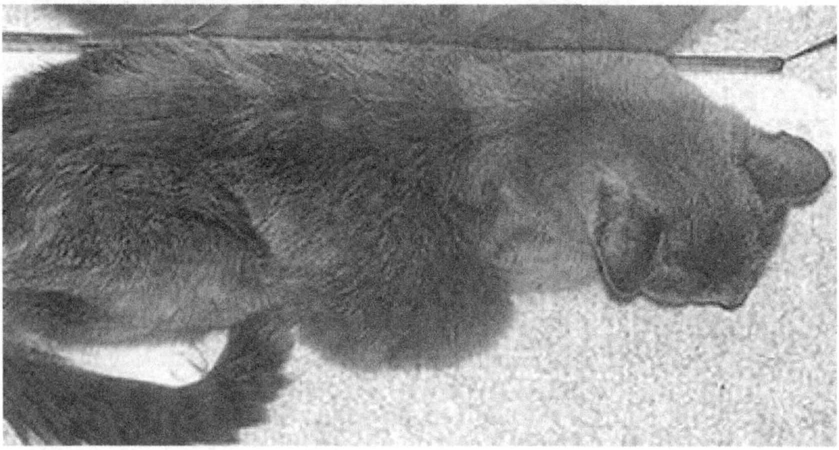

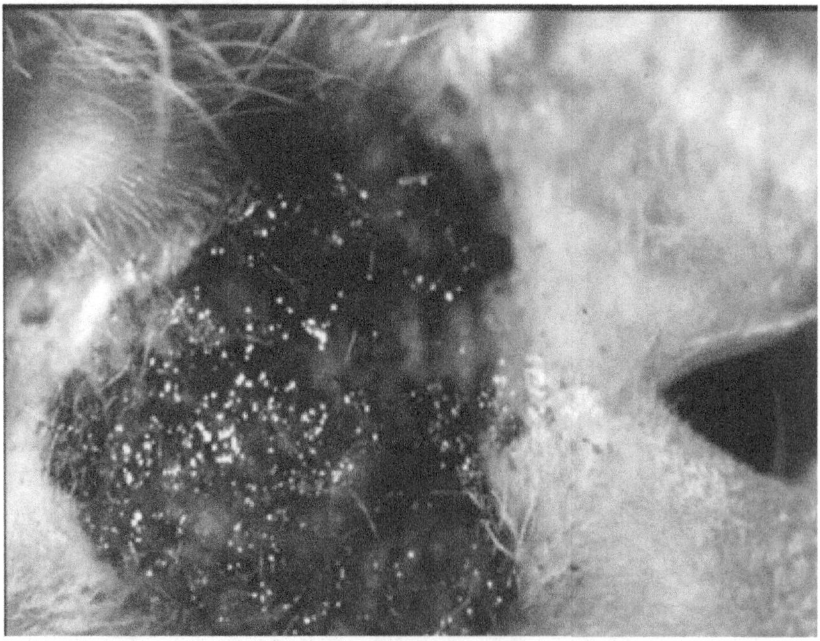

VACCINE-ASSOCIATED CANCERS IN CATS. Left: Tumor in a cat's side after a flea vaccine (lufenuron). Right: Squamous cell tumor on the face of a cat after shortly following vaccination

This potential ability to prevent metastatic spread depends on the assumption that if the primary tumor associated with the vaccine site were placed distally enough from the animal's trunk, that complete removal would be possible. As the reasoning in this regard went, the veterinarians took solace in the fact that the pet owner would be left with a three-legged dog (or cat), but that pet could still live if the limb were amputated but would invariably die if it were not removed. **The veterinarians also noticed that it did not appear to matter what vaccine is given: all of them can induces cancers.**

The passage of time, vigilance, and research have made it increasingly clear that feline injection-site sarcomas (FISS) are malignant skin tumors of mesenchymal origin that develop in 1–10 of every 10,000 vaccinated cats, and significantly, these same cancers do also occur when non-absorbable surgical stitches are used, or microchips, or injections of antibiotics or cortisone, or anti-flee injections as with the cat shown in these above pictures. These are important observations because they lend more support to the hypothesis that carcinogenesis is a process often initiated by foreign bodies or proteins that cause an "irritation," or from an irritation generally caused by the organism's exposures to immunological "non-self."

Our US National Cancer Institute (NCI) has also claimed that there is evidence that most enforced vaccines of one kind or another have been linked to childhood cancers (in humans) which has been increasing during the last several decades.

An article entitled, "**Temporal Trends in The Population Structure of Bordetella pertussis During 1949-1996 In A Highly Vaccinated Population**" in the journal Health: Immune and Brain Disorders, written by Rishma Parpia was published asking the question: "Is there a link between vaccines and the rise of human pediatric cancer?" The conclusion of this study was startling:

"The National Cancer Institute (NCI) at the National Institutes of Health (NIH) estimated that 10,270 new cases of pediatric cancers would be diagnosed in 2017 in children from birth to the age of 14. Approximately 1,190 of these children were expected to die as a result of cancer."

"According to the American Cancer Society, after accidents, **cancer is the second leading cause of death in children between the ages of one**

and four. Although pediatric cancers account for less than one percent of all cancers diagnosed each year, the number of children diagnosed with cancer has **been rising steadily over the last few decades."** These studies also concluded that:

> **"Pediatric cancer has been increasing over the last few decades,"**

and

> **"The causes of most pediatric cancers are not known. The possible link between vaccines and pediatric cancer has not been fully investigated...."**

The escalating cancer rates in older humans are also cause for alarm, which according to the CDC, have sky-rocketed, especially during this era of an accelerated and more complex vaccination schedule.

IF, as it is with our companion animals, there also is growing evidence that the most enforced vaccines have been linked for more than a decade to childhood cancers in humans whose rates have exploded during the last several decades and if the "The National Cancer Institute (NCI) at the National Institutes of Health (NIH) estimated that **10,270 new cases** of pediatric cancers would be diagnosed in 2017 in children from birth to the age of 14; And **IF** approximately 1,190 of these children were expected to die as a result of cancer."

And **IF** "According to the American Cancer Society, after accidents, cancer is the second leading cause of death in children between the ages of one and four. And **IF** the number of children diagnosed with cancer has been rising steadily over the last few decades." The analysis highlighted the observations that human pediatric cancers have been increasing over the last few decades, and the causes of most human pediatric cancers are not known."

THEN, DO THESE KINDS OF NUMBERS SUGGEST THAT WE SHOULD MANDATE INFANT OR SCHOOL-AGE VACCINATIONS FOR ANY CHILD?

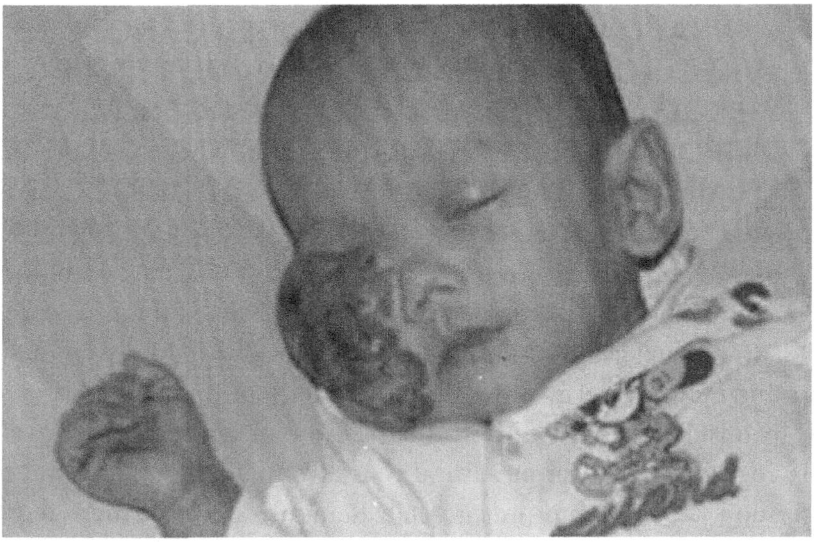

A vaccinated child exhibiting a tumorous growth on his face – possibly caused by over-vaccination. Most pediatric cancers occur between ages 1 and 4, the same years children receive the vast majority of childhood vaccinations

The link between vaccines and cancer induction is especially difficult to prove occurs in humans because of our long lifespans compared to laboratory rodents or our own cats and dogs, where the induction(s) of cancers is quite clear because they often occur first at the injection site of a vaccine, and then metastasize (spread) to kill the animal (cats, dogs, livestock).

These observations of induction of tumors both temporally and spatially with respect to vaccine administration along with the production of antibodies to laminin and fibronectin mechanistically had been shown previously under organ culture conditions with human breast cells where every variable can be controlled. In these studies (See Sandal et al., cited above) extracellular matrix, and specifically laminin and fibronectin have been implicated as being the master control molecules that regulate, direct, and halt growing tissues, especially breast cancers (and melanomas).

WHAT CAUSES VACCINE INDUCED CANCER: VASCULOGENIC MIMICRY AS A TUMOR TISSUE-PRODUCED BIOFILM AND AN "APOGENETIC" CONTROLLING ELEMENT SUGGESTS A MECHANISM TO EXPLAIN HOW DAMAGE BY VACCINATION OCCURS VIA DYSREGULATION OF FIBRONECTIN AND LAMININ

What is Vasculogenic Mimicry? A consensus became established that anti-angiogenesis would succeed against cancer. It was reasoned that, as normal cells, endothelium could not or would not "mutate" around blood vessel growth inhibitors, like "highly mutable," "genetically unstable" tumor cells. In this as in other contexts, tumor cells are regarded still as supernatural cells. Eventually, the important realization was born and pre-clinically demonstrated that there might be both positive and negative regulators of tumor angiogenesis, or by default, molecularly definable positive and negative regulators of tumor growth, dormancy, and metastasis. Vasculogenic mimicry (VM) as a tumor derived extracellular matrix (ECM) phenomenon appears to almost always signal accelerated or enhanced malignancy. From research surveying dozens of human tumor types, the association has been established that cancers harboring VM are refractory to therapeutic intervention.

Reasons that have been advanced to account for the general failure of cancer therapeutics, it could be argued, include the use of immune modified animal models implanted with foreign tumor cells, and the widespread belief that irritants, toxins, viruses, or growth factors are specific cancer inducers. While these systems and observations have been modestly informative as to some basic mechanisms of tumor growth and rejection phenomenon, the nearly universal use and study of animal models lacking a complete or functional immune system, or animal models that are genetically weakened or modified to be susceptible to cancers has failed us in the context of therapeutics.

According to what is now known, these immune compromised systems are like studying knee-replacement surgery using a snake as an animal model.

Vaccine-induced tumors in both animals and man could provide better therapeutic models of cancer, or better non-toxic methods for cancer reversal, dormancy, and rejection. Vaccine-induced tumors that arise at vaccine sites and then spread to kill the animal (or human) are immunologically derived from "self," circumventing the need for weakened hosts that are made to harbor foreign tumor cells. In light of these data and conceptual advances, a number of recently published primary reports and reviews regarding malignant cancers support the idea by noted cancer immunologists that the plasticity inherent in tumor vasculogenic mimicry is now being considered as a likely reason that the war on cancer via "proven" and often life-ending cytotoxic and immunotoxic drug remedies and radiation have not succeeded. Anti-tumor angiogenesis approaches are now believed even to accelerate certain brain malignancies.

TISSUE MIMICRY IS CONROLLED BY FIBRONECTIN AND LAMININ-A CLUE AS TO HOW BOTH VIRUSES AND VACCINE INJURIES OR VACCINE INDUCTIONS OF CANCERS LEAD TO FIBROSIS

It appears as though not only molecular mimicry is operational in vaccine-associated injuries, but also tissue-level mimicry also may be playing an important role. One manifestation of tissue mimicry is "vasculogenic mimicry," where in two dimensions, tumor cells appear to form barriers between nests of malignant tumor cells that appear in 2-dimensional sections as "channels" because they splay open in various regions, and trap leaked red blood cells as the malignant tumor burrows its way through normal tissues.

Recent studies show that these patterns of matrix probably are tumor biofilms secreted by the malignant tumor cell nests, making these tumor nests impervious to soluble anti-cancer drugs or anti-cancer antibodies. In 3-dimensional tissue reconstructions, we documented over a 20 year period, that these vasculogenic mimicry patterns constitute tightly packed spheres of tumor cells surrounded by semi-hollow extracellular matrix coatings (in places) that trap red blood cells.

Vasculogenic mimicry in melanomas constituted a challenge at first to a 4 Billion dollar new industry that sought to disrupt blood vessels to tumors in an attempt to starve them of nutrients, blood flow, oxygen, and clearance of wastes non-toxically, yet it was not considered that these malignancies didn't require oxygen as they may be anaerobic (not need O2 to grow) according to Warburg, and the ideas that malignant tumors switch to glycolysis and neither require oxygen or the blood vessels to deliver it as they run on glucose.

The tumor anti-angiogenesis research initiative collapsed shortly thereafter and the world then pursued vasculogenic mimicry to try to block these channels from forming in tumors and again tried to starve them, ignoring the fact, once more, that 100% of malignant tumors are known to be anaerobic and not require O2 (see Warburg).

And what evidence had ever been obtained in the past, that MALIGNANT cancer cells need oxygen, and nutrients, clearance, and waste removal like normal cells in the first place and why was the work of Otto Warburg and the anaerobic nature of all cancers he described so thoroughly not investigated with respect to fermentation measurements. He discussed these experiments and received a Nobel Prize in the 1960's, and if he was correct, there is a possibility that tumors do not require blood or nutrients or oxygen, but grow as anaerobes?

It was on the eve of the first Human clinical trials of endostatin, when two blood-vessel inhibitory molecules found in mouse urine entered human clinical trials, following previous attempts using compounds using compounds derived from from fungal sources (TNP—470 fumagillin, and TNP-1470, a less toxic but still toxic fumagillin derivative) that had both been proven to be unacceptably toxic, when the observation of vasculogenic mimicry (VM) was reported in 1999.

VM was first described as a tumor-specific extracellular matrix (ECM)-dominated phenomenon that harbored what looked to some critics like tumor-made vascular channels made by the tumor cells themselves, circumventing the need for any host-formed neovasculature made out of endothelial cells that are part of us.

From research surveying dozens of human tumor types harboring VM, the association also has been established by numerous pathological studies and different groups that cancers harboring VM are typically aggressive and malignant. By August, 2021, and 20 years after the discovery of vasculogenic mimicry, The National Library of Medicine's (PUBMED) NCBI's website listed 3801 PUBMED Central (PMC) journal articles, 14 books, and 19 protein databases that have archived the developing science of vasculogenic mimicry. Top tier journals that have featured work on VM are listed on the National Library of Medicine's website: (https://www.ncbi.nlm.nih.gov/pmc/?term=vasculogenic+mimicry).

Not all of these reports are focused on defining and trying to kill these tumors, but a majority of them probably have this goal in mind. If they all fail because the strategy is flawed, then will it signal a green light for other alternative approaches that do not employ toxic targeted strategies to be funded? The veterinary community may provide a clue, and the tumors of our pets have not been systematically studied for VM, although VM has been found in other mammals upon autopsy, even whales. Vasculogenic mimicry patterns have also been called "the fluid conducting meshwork" by other scientists who have validated their existence and their functions in different contexts.

This tumor biofilm may be the prime reason mutation is not required to form resistance to radiation, heat, drugs, or any type of medical intervention currently used. Yet, the patterned VM matrix, as shown above is largely composed of molecules such as fibronectin, laminin (not shown), and other molecules that are used in normal tissue building and differentiation.

And immunotherapeutic methods against cancer have and are still being tried on dying cancer victims, failed many times, and continue to fail. It is perhaps even safe to say that these "immunotherapeutic" approaches will continue to be supported and will continue to fail, because the obvious sameness of molecular participants in VM to those found in normal matrix is ignored with the hope that somehow, the immune system will "know" and will selectively attack the tumors surrounded by the patterns. The VM patterns appear to be an essential structural control apparatus to understand how rational and non-toxic therapeutics can circumvent these above defined factors of resistance to new promising non-toxic therapeutic interventions, and help cancer victims recover from critical and fatal illnesses or deconditioned states of health.

This database lists both the scientifically peer-reviewed published research and therapeutic programs underway under the heading of Vasculogenic mimicry, and there are hundreds of labs full of critically-minded researchers who have found evidence that VM may hold some clues.

With such examination of both current and past approaches to the topic of **VM** that have transpired since 1999 when **VM** was first described, the peer-reviewed record suggests that cancer centers and researchers throughout the world also have engaged in an allopathically directed yet failing effort, as they are almost exclusively developing therapeutics on the basis of the same target-directed thinking, hypotheses, and approaches of the past, and ignoring what has been learned about the nature of the VM patterns.

The following work and excerpts were compassionately penned by a concerned and compassionate veterinarian named Catherine O'Driscoll in 2009, and evidence has been presented by Dr. Jordan, DVM.

"A team at Purdue University School of Veterinary Medicine conducted several studies to determine if vaccines can cause changes in the immune system of dogs that might lead to life-threatening immune-mediated diseases...The vaccinated, but not the non-vaccinated, dogs in the Purdue studies developed autoantibodies to many of their own biochemicals, including **fibronectin, laminin,** DNA, albumin, cytochrome C, cardiolipin and collagen. This means that the vaccinated dogs —but not the non-vaccinated dogs– were attacking their own fibronectin, which is involved in tissue repair, cell multiplication and growth, and differentiation between tissues and organs in a living organism."

In a 1999 study from a study at Purdue University in Indiana by members of its veterinary college, which is a nationally praised veterinary college, an article was published on November 1st, 1999 entitled:

"Effects of Vaccination on the Endocrine and Immune Systems of Dogs, Phase II" (https://www.homestead.com/vonhapsburg/haywardstudyonvaccines.html).

Also see: https://www.vet.purdue.edu/epi/gdhstudy.htm

This article should have changed the world but has not. In an effort to avoid the lethal cancers that are induced by vaccines, the Feline Sarcoma Society held a conference about strategies to keep their "patients" alive following vaccine administration in 2013 and decided to amend their current medical procedure of front or hind limb administered vaccines, or administrations behind the neck, and decided to begin to administer vaccines in their tails.

These dedicated vets simply want to avoid the horrendous limb or torso amputations caused by vaccine "tissue rot," and because vaccine morbidity could be more easily coped with if tails were vaccinated because tail amputations were far less traumatic to their cat patients than were cancers that would form and spread from injection sites, or which formed close to them. Cat owners were also more likely to detect tumors that were forming on the tail than they were to see tumors beginning under the fur of the limbs or trunk.

The new directive was discussed by Cleon G Hendricks, Julie K Levy, Sylvia J Tucker, Shaye M Olmstead, P Cynda Crawford, Edward J Dubovi, and Cathleen A Hanlon and published in The Journal of Feline Medicine and Surgery (0(0) 1 -6 © ISFM and AAFP 201, Accepted: 22 August 2013).

A WIDE RANGE OF VACCINE-INDUCED DISEASES BESIDES CANCERS IN DOGS AND CATS

In the practice of veterinary medicine, vaccine injuries are more readily noticed because of the animal's lifespans compared to humans. In a discussion among certain of the most highly regarded veterinarians, other syndromes other than cancers are frequently discussed, as the dialog below indicates:

"We also found some worrying correlations between vaccine events and the onset of arthritis in our 1997 survey. Our concerns were compounded by research in the human field."

"The New England Journal of Medicine, for example, reported that it is possible to isolate the rubella virus from affected joints in children vaccinated against rubella. It also told of the isolation of viruses from the peripheral blood of women with prolonged arthritis following vaccination (New England Journal of Medicine, vol. 313,1985)."

"Then, in 2000, CHC's findings were confirmed by research which showed that polyarthritis and other diseases like amyloidosis, which affects organs in dogs, were linked to the combined vaccine given to dogs.(8) There is a huge body of research, despite the paucity of funding from the vaccine industry, to confirm that vaccines can cause a wide range of brain and central nervous system damage. Merck itself states in its Manual that vaccines (i.e., its own products) can cause encephalitis: brain inflammation/damage. In some cases, encephalitis involves lesions in the brain and throughout the central nervous system. Merck states that "examples are the encephalapathies following measles, chickenpox, rubella, smallpox vaccination, vaccinia, and many other less well-defined viral infections".

The dog owners were given a CHC survey, and they reported that their dogs developed short attention spans, and that 73.1% of the dogs did so within three months of a vaccine event. The same percentage of dogs was diagnosed with epilepsy within three months of a vaccine (but usually within days and it did not appear to matter which vaccine was received). The veterinarians also found that 72.5% of dogs that were considered by their owners to be nervous and of a worrying disposition, first exhibited these traits within the three-month post-vaccination period.

"I would like to add for the sake of Oliver, my friend who suffered from paralyzed rear legs and death shortly after a vaccine shot, that "paresis" is listed in Merck's Manual as a symptom of encephalitis. This is defined as muscular weakness of a neural (brain) origin which involves partial or incomplete paralysis, resulting from lesions at any level of the descending pathway from the brain. Hind limb paralysis is one of the potential consequences. Encephalitis, incidentally, is a disease that can manifest across the scale from mild to severe and can also cause sudden death. Organ failure was also suspected to have occurred when it happened shortly after a vaccine event. Dr Larry Glickman, who spearheaded the Purdue research into post-vaccination biochemical changes in dogs, wrote in a letter to Cavalier Spaniel breeder Bet Hargreaves:

"Our ongoing studies of dogs show that following routine vaccination, there is a significant rise in the level of antibodies dogs produce against their own tissues. Some of these antibodies have been shown to target the thyroid gland, connective tissue such as that found in the valves of the heart, red blood cells, DNA, etc. I do believe that the heart conditions in Cavalier King Charles Spaniels could be the end result of repeated immunizations by vaccines containing tissue culture contaminants that cause a progressive immune response directed at connective tissue in the heart valves. The clinical manifestations would be more pronounced in dogs that have a genetic predisposition [although] the findings should be generally applicable to all dogs regardless of their breed. Some specific commentaries of veterinarians who attended this forum are worth noting. In addressing the topic of cancers, the following information was presented:

"Modified live-virus (MLV) vaccines replicate in the patient until an immune response is provoked. If a defense is not stimulated, then the vaccine continues to replicate until it gives the patient the very disease it was intending to prevent. Alternatively, a deranged immune response will lead to inflammatory conditions such as arthritis, pancreatitis, colitis, encephalitis, and any number of autoimmune diseases such as cancer and leukemia, where the body attacks its own cells. A new theory, stumbled upon by Open University student Gary Smith, explains what holistic practitioners have been saying for an exceptionally long time. Here is what a few of the holistic vets have said in relation to their patients:

Dr Jean Dodds: "Many veterinarians trace the present problems with allergic and immunologic diseases to the introduction of MLV vaccines..." (Dodds, Jean W.,DVM, "**Immune System and Disease Resistance**" (https://www.dogsnaturallymagazine.com/purdue-vaccination-studies/).

Christina Chambreau, DVM: "Routine vaccinations are probably the worst thing that we do for our animals. They cause all types of illnesses, but not directly to where we would relate them definitely to be caused by the vaccine." (Wolf Clan magazine, April/May 1995).

Martin Goldstein, DVM: "I think that vaccines...are leading killers of dogs and cats in America today."

Dr Charles E. Loops, DVM: "Homoeopathic veterinarians and other holistic practitioners have maintained for some time that vaccinations do more harm than they provide benefits." (Wolf Clan magazine, April/May 1995).

Mike Kohn, DVM: "In response to this [vaccine] violation, there have been increased autoimmune diseases (allergies being one component), epilepsy, neoplasia [tumors], as well as behavioral problems in small animals)."

By some of these statements, it becomes increasingly clear that we are currently living in a crisis of our perceptions about causality. Cause and effect have become confused, and along with this confusion, sanity has been temporarily misplaced or lost. Many of the biological and medical issues have been solved regarding the best way to prevent or reverse cancers, influenzas, traumatic and other brain injuries, infections, and a plethora of other human maladies, yet the philosophical and psychological dimensions of insanity are currently in a state of crisis in the realms of vaccinology and virology. Therefore, it becomes essential that assumptions need to be critically examined, by many, and often. For instance, it is becoming increasingly certain that the "classic" clonal selection models of how the immune system works, and other models are too simplistic.

WITH ANTHONY FAUCI AND OTHERS LEADING THE CHARGE, PERHAPS THE LARGEST FAILURE OF THE AIDS ERA WAS PUBLISHED IN 2009 IN THE NEJM: A 3% RATE OF PROTECTION (OVER BACKGROUND LEVELS WITHOUT THE VACCINE)

If you look at the numbers published regarding the "HIV" vaccine trial involving 16,000 recipients and 8,000 controls injected with aluminum, and 8,000 injected with aluminum and gp120, a difference in "true seroconversion" between the two groups was reported as 0.6% (of 8,000) aluminum "HIV": versus 0.8% with aluminum.

However, the CIA website (of all places) you will find that the rate of seroconversion in Thailand at background levels is 1.3 percent without any vaccination. From these numbers, one only can conclude that the cheapest way to "immunize" those promiscuous _________ is to inject them with aluminum (it's cheap)! (you will see later how Bill Clinton and these agencies deemed "HIV" a National Security Issue in the information presented about A History of AIDS on this website).

Here are the numbers more visibly:

Aluminum boosted Aluminum without Background "HIV" detection:

-gp120 "background"-	-gp120 Military-	-Thailand trial aluminum-
1.3%	0.6%	0.8%

The numbers would make it appear that it is a good idea to inject everybody with aluminum only because it is cheap-and will reduce the levels of "HIV" detection by 0.5% in the absence of co-injected and expensive to acquire and manufacture gp120 (1.3 is the background levels) -0.8=0.5%).

This trial cost 101 + million? But that is not all we got for that expenditure combined with the 500 million a year spent for the 172 vaccines currently in "the pipeline?" What a corrupt racket!

RELIGIOUS TERMINOLOGY, FOOTBALL STRATEGIES, AIDS RESEARCH, AND ORIGINAL ANTIGENIC SIN

The term, "Hail Mary," has been used after numerous failures of the "HIV equals AIDS hypothesis" to describe the 100-billion-dollar failures of AIDS research (HIV vaccine may never be found, warns leading scientist Mark Henderson, Science Editor, in Boston. From Times Online, February 14, 2008):

> *"Professor David Baltimore, a Nobel laureate who is President of the American Association for the Advancement of Science, told its annual conference in Boston that the failure of every promising approach to an HIV vaccine had led many scientists to wonder whether it would ever be possible to create one."*
>
> *"While Professor Baltimore has a major grant from the Bill and Melinda Gates Foundation to research a new approach to HIV therapy and treatment, he said it was a last-ditch effort with only a slim hope of success. He compared it to a "Hail Mary" play in American football – a desperate attempt at a long pass, in which the quarterback throws the ball up and prays it will be caught by a teammate."*

Specialized proteins that are not found in nature that can attack "HIV?" Yikes!

Hail Mary indeed!

These kinds of strategies based upon football, and faith-based science and medicine have been employed since the first decade of "HIV" vaccine research. As shown a book obtained from The Office of Technology Assessment of "HIV" vaccine development, up until 1995, the recommendations of The Office of Technology presented to the 1995 Congress by the AIDS Research Advisory Committee (ARAC) of the National Institute of Allergy and Infectious Diseases (NIAID) were no more promising than those statements about the failed STEP trial we hear about from Dr. Baltimore and others today (1995 Congress of the United States:

Office of Technology assessment. Adverse Reactions to HIV Vaccines: Medical, Ethical, and Legal Issues. Roger C. Herdman, Director).

The conclusions of this 1995 assessment recommended that Phase III clinical trials with enveloped vaccines should not proceed in the United States because of scientific, political, and ethical issues, and because of the significant level of scientific uncertainty about the wisdom of immediate trials. Not only were warnings presented about the danger of giving an "HIV" vaccine to already immuno-compromised individuals (such as ARC or AIDS patients), but many "HIV" vaccine recipients were harmed.

This push and flurry of activity and funding to test, inoculate, and vaccinate every moving creature on the planet continued unabated until about the year 2000, when the projected 225 "HIV" vaccines that were on the NIH's website were removed because every single one of them failed. And when the SARS-COVID-19 panic began, there is Fauci again before the American public and the world again, sheepishly claiming that the largest "HIV" vaccine trial in history, the Thai-Military Trial finally had been "a success" which is far from truth as we will examine in some depth later on. By January, 2012, there had been 64 smaller yet failed "HIV" vaccine trials and at that time there were 172 "candidate" "HIV" vaccines in the U.S. "HIV" pipeline that were supported by a $500 million/year price tag (at that time). Such easily available facts should make it clear that the AIDS era itself has played a relatively small, if any role in either scientific or medical progress in the context of human health, and perhaps has played a late and significant role at best in the history of vaccines and vaccination due to the massive, often prematurely halted failures of any and all "HIV" vaccine components to evoke immunity, or in many cases even evoke seroconversion. So, in effect, the AIDS era confirms vaccination results from approximately the past 150 years-worthless at best even going back to small-pox inoculations during the Civil war days, where soldiers lost their arms due to "the rot."

RUMOR BIOLOGY

The term "rumor biology" was coined during the AIDS era to broadcast the idea that since the time of Payton Rous who was said to discover a tumor virus against his protests that he had indeed discovered a tumor virus, the same applies to a vast array of other viruses, as they have been shown to be particles associated with, but not causal of many syndromes repeatedly.

> *"While smallpox vaccine is no longer kept for public health purposes, new recruits to the American armed services are immunized as a precaution against possible biological warfare. Routine vaccination of a 19-year-old recruit was the trigger for stimulation of dormant HIV virus into Aids. This discovery of how people with subclinical HIV infection are at risk of rapid development of Aids as a vaccine-induced disease was made by a medical team working with Dr Robert Redfield at Walter Reed. The recruit who developed Aids after vaccination had been healthy throughout high school. He was given multiple immunizations, followed by his first smallpox vaccination. Two and a half weeks later he developed fever, headaches, neck stiffness and night sweats. Three weeks later he was admitted to Walter Reed suffering from meningitis and rapidly developed further symptoms of Aids and died after responding for a short time to treatment..."*

In the US, and Europe, the ***claimed*** spread of "HIV infection" in the 1980's coincided with the IV drug epidemic almost exclusively, whereas the explosion of AIDS in Africa and elsewhere coincided with poverty, starvation, and the most intense immunization programs, with the number of people immunized being as follows: Zaire 36,878,000; Zambia 19,060,000; Tanzania 14,972,000; Uganda 11,616,000; Malawai 8,118,000; Ruanda 3,382,000 and Burundi 3,274,000. Brazil, the only South American country covered in the eradication campaign, has the highest incidence of AIDS in that region. About 14,000 Haitians,second to Central Africa, were covered in the campaign. They began to return home at a time when Haiti had become a popular playground for San Francisco homosexuals and illicit IV drug usage.

Although the National Childhood Vaccine Injury Act created the VAERS system (Vaccine Adverse Events Reporting System) in 1990, which is a mechanism whereby anyone-doctors, nurses, and any member of the general public can submit a report to VAERS, and the Armed Forces have historically and up to the present day remained a more reliable source of information for reporting adverse events about vaccine injuries, and have kept accurate records because soldiers have to be in top shape to execute actions against other nations, whereas, children and their developing minds and bodies aren't as immediately critical for carrying out aggressive policies of our government or corporate economic interests and conquests in foreign countries.

It is important to know, in addition, that with the VAERS system of reporting and tabulating vaccine injuries, although anyone who receives a **licensed** vaccine in the US is encouraged to report any significant health problem that occurs after vaccination, the **Reportable Events Table** (known as **RET**) only lists conditions and provides entry spaces to report injuries that are believed to be caused by vaccines, and in drawing up the form space entries in this manner, excludes possible adverse events which are not on this approved list. Another way of describing this system is that the Vaccine Injury Compensation Program (VCIP) administered by the **Health Resources and Services Administration** compensates only those people whose injuries may have been caused by certain vaccines (but not others). The VCIP is separate from VAERS, and reporting an event to VAERS does not file a claim for compensation to the VICP.

(cdc.gov/vaccinesafety/ensuringsafety/monitoringvaers).

In 2019, VAERS received over 48,000 reports. VAERS reports include such items as **death, permanent disability, hospitalization, life-threatening illness, or temporary acute symptoms including injection-site injury or inflammation. VAERS does a poor job at capturing long-term impacts of vaccines such as autoimmune diseases that**

develop months later or cancers that develop months or years later due to vaccination.

On November 8, 2002, the Pentagon's mandatory anthrax shots caused adverse reactions in most recipients and helped prompt many Air Force Reserve and National Guard to transfer to other units or leave the military between 1998 and 2000, according to a survey by Congress's General Accounting Office (GAO). The survey indicated that 85% of the troops who received an anthrax shot had an adverse reaction, a rate far higher than the 30% claimed by the manufacturer in 2000.

What about childhood vaccines and adverse events reporting? In 2004, Pilar Carrsco-Garrid, Carmen Gallardo-Pino, and Rodrigo Jimenez-Garcia et al., published a report entitled, "Incidence of Adverse Reactions to Vaccines in a Pediatric Populations" (Journal Clinical Drug Investigation 24, 8, 264-263. 2004) that concluded that:

> Of 946 children reported who exhibited adverse reactions to vaccinations, 191 of them were non-serious or suspected reactions that represented 19% of the vaccinated children, but that "a more intensive search for suspected adverse reactions revealed adverse reactions that are not usually reported," and that "primary care physicians and nurses must be vigilant for information on adverse reactions to vaccines in pediatric populations".

Do pharmacists or pharmacist's assistants giving out vaccines at Walgreens or CVS stores ever report vaccine adverse side effects from yearly Flu vaccines to VAERS (the US Government's **V**accine **A**dverse **E**vent **R**eporting **S**ystem) if vaccine injuries and adverse events occur? Only less than about 1% of licensed physicians ever report adverse vaccine reactions, so who is it at Walgreens or Walmart that will be reporting adverse reactions following this year's seasonal flu shots? The cashier? Are USA hospitals reporting vaccine injuries to VAERS?

Are deaths from COVID-19 in New York State nursing homes partly the result of so many senior citizens having been vaccinated this year against flu? These questions all need to be carefully looked into.

It is not likely that the Walgreens cashier will advise you on the risks of a flu vaccine that might increase your likelihood of having lung complications. This well-known reaction to seasonal flu vaccines is anticipated. With the unleashing of new RNA vaccines and other vaccine designs against SARS-CoV-2, some small fraction of the vaccinated population will almost certainly experience these and other reactions as is expected with all vaccines. It is believed these reactions are due to the placing foreign proteins, adjuvants, and other irritants in the vaccines into the bloodstream which bypasses mucosal immunity which normally processes foreign entities that enter the body.

FOUR AXIOMS REGARDING VACCINES, GENETICS, AND EPIDEMICS

These concerns can be stated as axioms that will emerge throughout this analysis of vaccines and epidemics. These axioms include:

Axiom A) No inoculation or vaccine has ever been tested for safety in a scientific manner, especially in the context of influenza vaccines such as those now being developed for SARS-CoV-2, but many others if not all of them also have not been tested to the standards of other pharmaceuticals;

Axiom B) No vaccine in history has ever shown anything resembling "efficacy" except in a few well-documented experiments on animals which have many caveats that never are mentioned, and as time has passed, uncertainties appear to increase and accumulate rather than decrease and diminish regarding both the modes of transmission of agents that are assumed to be infectious agents (as has recently been called to attention again in the case of HPV-more about this later), and especially, uncertainties have increased rather than decreased regarding any and all remedies for any endemic or epidemic (or pandemic) human malady.

For instance, the polio vaccine is often cited as a great example of a successful effective vaccine campaign in the manner that any catechism of a religion is promulgated, but this surmise is incorrect and not scientifically (or historically) justified. Polio decreased at the same time and at same rate in Europe which had no widespread use of a polio vaccine as in the USA which widely vaccinated against polio during that same time period, until it was abruptly halted due to all the increasing cases of paralysis concomitant with the polio vaccine crusade of the 1950's-60's. This fact is one of many that will be revealed in this book with many references given, and an historic timeline will be presented that raise questions about myths we have been told about eradication of various historic plagues by vaccination.

Axiom C) Vaccines and inoculations have been and continue to be the most efficient disease-spreading or causing devices and endemic syndrome-inducing pharmaceuticals that ever-victimized large groups of innocent individuals and entire societies. **For example, the leading cause of polio over the last few decades has been polio vaccination itself. Another example was the rotavirus vaccine that also was quickly withdrawn after its first roll-out (but then replaced by something else that may not even be a rotavirus vaccine at all but something like a "shot filled with water.") More about this phenomenon will be discussed at length.**

AXIOM D) Genes are important and function as a necessary information storage system but are not sufficient to cause normal or physiological processes without extensive interactions with epigenetic and as I will argue, **"apogenetic" (the matrix outside the cell that controls the genotype)** environmental systems/ interactions. In other words, genes are necessary but not sufficient to predict normal physiological processes or pathological disease syndromes without understanding what Dr. Mina Bissell first described as "dynamic reciprocity" between the extracellular environment and the genes, and between the genes and the environment.

In effect, both inoculations of past Centuries, and the vaccines of today, are a kind of "operation" that introduces a foreign substance to a healthy organism's bloodstream or tissue, and thereby that foreign material circumvents the body's mucosal front-line immune mechanisms which are the sentinels and gate-keepers of the body's immune defense.

Vaccines therefore should be considered along with the history of all drugs immunologically foreign substances. In this current SARS CoV-2 atypical pneumonia crisis, this information is of grave and immediate concern.

The history of vaccines, and their relationship to the wellness or illness of populations is a complex issue that demands careful, scientific consideration. In some way vaccines have and will continue to touch all of our lives. The history of vaccines physically affects us as individuals, as families, and as a society. Millions of people are vaccinated, and they aren't harmed. Vaccines also have been associated with severe cognitive, developmental, and emotional impairments. They have been linked to countless autoimmune maladies, and cancers. In this context, observations of routine vaccinations of our pet dogs and cats suggest that vaccines are directly-linked to cancer initiation at the sites of vaccination, and other studies show initiations of cancers that erupt in close timing to vaccinations.

Regarding their influence on society as a whole, vaccines have caused spiritual and financial devastation. The evidence is indisputable that inoculations and vaccinations have had major impacts both on our physical health, as well as on our thinking and world views regarding disease resistance. It is precisely for these reasons, the vaccine topic must be subjected to intense scientific investigation, instead of past and current appraisals which have been rooted in fear, religion, uncertainty, and political and financial gain. Many of these past assessments of vaccination can be likened to assessing auguries of bird migration in relationship to predicting omens in Ancient Roman religions or likened to assessing the predictability of weather forecasting based on cloud formations. An attempt at a **true scientific appraisal** cannot afford to be avoided any longer. But how is it best to proceed?

Auguries are a sign of what may happen in the future, which cannot be known. Millions are vaccinated around the world without immediate visible harm. Yet there still is a $4 Billion-dollar vaccine injury compensation court system in place in the US alone compensating vaccine-damaged individuals and families every year (credible estimates exist that this represents only 1% of the actual vaccine injuries). Millions become infected with feared lethal strains of microbes including viruses, yet they do not become ill and remain asymptomatic, which serves to emphasize the importance of how genetic sequences dynamically interact with their extracellular environments, and vice versa.

How will current vaccines affect the future of populations of humans? How do they affect our overall resistance to disease as a population?

What are supposed to be "scientifically-proven" vaccines and other pharmaceuticals are in fact not scientifically proven at all. They have not been scientifically tested for either safety to the extent that other pharmaceuticals have been tested, or for efficacy over sufficiently long periods of time. Yet vaccines still are marketed as if they were "proven medicines." With this assurance, these potions are given to millions of "healthy sick folks" (asymptomatics and pathogen naive individuals alike). These rituals occur during the yearly confessionals of wellness checks, military inductions, travel, pregnancy, early infancy, childhood, and indeed every aspect of their lives, including some are suggesting, a condition of employment in industries other than the medical industry.

Many who were not yet aware they are inherently sick must be taught that they are sick or are "healthy carriers" by public health officials. Yet these new rituals are accompanied also by a constant clamor of unrelenting lawsuits and warnings about each vaccine's side-effects and contra-indications. Yet the Pharma funded TV commercials increasingly present hopeful pictures of what are supposedly potentially vulnerable people climbing mountains or playing sports with children with smiles on their vaccinated and drug managed faces. We are shown images of young virginal girls smiling saying, "just one less," in the context of a so-called anti-HPV and anti-cervical cancer vaccines.

It is also in this context that the modern virologists and others offer their prophesies about the emergence of new epidemics, and over time, the prescription for any illness, infirmity, and aging itself, typically is "pharmaceutical" in nature.

As we now sit in a global "pandemic" lockdown the likes of which has never been seen in human history and which has currently exploded globally, we are all assured that our salvation is around the corner, and that "the calvary is coming" in the form of yet more untested EUA-sanctioned vaccines (Emergency Use Authorization) act, which is not FDA-approved for a year or at least 9 months.

Perhaps this failure to demonstrate safety or efficacy or benefit with any and all vaccines is due to the religious belief that vaccines ward off epidemics, they are needed to cope with normal childhood illnesses, and they are absolutely required to avoid illness in the future-they are "insurance" against something vague in the future that one in principle would rationally want to avoid...vaccines bestow some kind of magical protection against something that does not yet exist, but when it will exist and come to strike us down-vaccinations will be there to save us somehow.

In the minds of many, vaccinations and inoculations are sort of like a magical car wax applied in the summer that protects a car in the winter from the ice and snow and rain (imagine the ice, snow, rain, hail, as different viruses, bacteria, or other pathogens). The wax is so durable, that it can miraculously protect from rust for decades.

In fact, it is believed so tacitly that it is absolutely inconceivable for many *not* to give one's infant or child a hepatitis B vaccine so that when their child grows up to become an IV drug addict or is exposed to infected blood products later in life (the two major hepatitis B risk groups), they will be "protected" not only from the hepatitis B, but also to prevent it from causing liver cancer decades later! In a similar mythology, another "preventative "cancer" vaccine known as the HPV vaccine protects girls from acquiring the virus, if given the shot before they lose their virginity, according to Merck, and miraculously, the HPV vaccine will protect them from developing cervical cancers decades later (See my book "Sacrifice of the Virgins" free on my website andrewmaniotis.wordpress.com).

And when vaccines are administered to millions, and millions do not get ill when the seasonal flu comes around, it must be of course because they were vaccinated. We do not see paralysis anymore, of course because of the OPV (oral polio vaccine) or its predecessor which caused paralysis only weeks after its first release, the Salk type vaccine injection. And vaccines of course are responsible for ridding the world of smallpox, we are told. Mankind, once again, has outsmarted nature's evils, because with our relatively highly developed degree of forethought, unlike the relatively short-ranged degree of forethought chimps that termite prepare in advance to fashion their twigs in shapes to facilitate their termite-fishing behavior in advance of doing it, or even Betty the crow's apparent displays of pre-thought, we can read the future-we have become smarter than Nature and have become God-like. The reason the millions do not get sick could not possibly be because most populations of living organisms on earth, as long as they are alive, are not sick but are in this "vague" state called- "health" or homeostasis.

But are the real reasons they are well or stay well is because they listen to their doctors, or would they be healthy anyway because they take responsibility for their own health? Is the real reason modern epidemics do not happen is because of vaccines can protect populations, and is the most likely reason why these diseases like smallpox or acute infantile paralysis (polio) no longer plague us because of vaccination? Do immunologists really understand the human immune system?

Are epidemics sporadic and unpredictable throughout history (predictable only as a result of preparation or execution of wars and other massive social upheavals, or is it possible that vaccines cause epidemics, and can epidemics be predicted by being aware of when and where the next vaccine roll-out will occur (or has occurred)?

Are we now seeing a classic demonstration of this possibility in countries like India and in Africa, where polio, once thought to be eradicated in the world, has emerged again seemingly out of nowhere, after the vaccine crusades of Bill Gates and the WHO assaulted these countries with their polio vaccines?

Does it make sense that a child not be allowed to enter a school to learn to read or write without first getting jabbed with all manner of some now more than 26 "protective" vaccinations and more than 100 foreign antigens? Will my kid possibly "catch it," even though I have had my kid vaccinated many times with all their jabs if you do not make sure to have your kid vaccinated or inoculated? Do the pro-vaxxers really have it all figured out regarding how human immunity works, and are anti-vaxxers fighting the "good" fight against vaccination and inoculation for the right reasons?

Is the Mayor of a large city (New York) justified in threatening Jews and parents with incarceration and $1000.00 fines or both if they do not get themselves and their kids vaccinated and are able to prove that they have obtained a measles vaccine. This phenomenon is now happening in many places, and world-wide.

These are among only a few of the catechisms we are promulgated to learn from the time we were small, and indeed today in these troubled apocalyptic times. But what do "the infectious disease experts" say, who hold high ranking positions in public health decision making to direct much of current biomedical policy and who dictate mandates and call them laws?

What do trusted gatekeepers of the most highly regarded

biomedical journals say about the science underlying these public health mandates and strongly held beliefs?

"It is simply no longer possible to believe much of the clinical research that is published, or to rely on the judgment of trusted physicians or authoritative medical guidelines. I take no pleasure in this conclusion, which I reached slowly and reluctantly over my two decades as an editor of The New England Journal of Medicine." (Marcia Angell, MD ("Drug Companies and Doctors: A story of Corruption." NY Review of Books, Jan. 15, 2009).

In 2008, Dr. K.P. Stoller wrote a resignation letter and published it in the journal Medical Veritas entitled: Les Incompétents: My open letter to the American Academy of Pediatrics. K. Paul Stoller, MD. President, International Hyperbaric Medical Assoc Medical Director, Hyperbaric Medical Center of New Mexico (Stoller K.P. Medical Veritas 5, Pps. 1699-1700, 2008).

Abstract

A protest resignation from the American Academy of Pediatrics (AAP), by a pediatrician with two decades of membership, is precipitated by the organization's sellout of the world's children by a policy that arrogantly and blindly ignored basic toxicology and safety limits when it involved vaccine and enabled a dangerous immunization mandate by the compromised Centers for Disease Control (CDC) via publication of CDC sponsored low quality epidemiology studies showing no connection between vaccines with Thimerosal written by individuals involved in producing Thimerosal-containing vaccines without disclosure (the conclusion of the studies showed Thimerosal removal caused autism). The AAP is fully aware of the untainted CDC analysis presented at the secret Simpsonwood conference and has known for almost a decade that Thimerosal causes neurodevelopmental disorders. Perpetuating the myth that affected children have come to the fore only because of better diagnosing, or because of a genetic epidemic (there are no genetic epidemics), the AAP has helped to subject the world's children to environmental triggers that effect both mitochondrial function and brain activity.

Driven by hubris and the largesse of vaccine manufacturers, the AAP has helped cause the loss of valuable time to rectify the crisis, the loss of a generation of children and perpetuated untold suffering worldwide. As a pediatrician, who has been a fellow of the American Academy of Pediatrics (AAP) for two decades, I find the AAP's approach to the autism epidemic to be deeply disturbing. Not only have they allowed the myth of better diagnosing (as the reason for all the notice given to affected children) to be perpetuated, but when they were put on notice at the Center for Disease Control and Prevention's (CDC's) Simpsonwood meeting in 2000, that the mercury in the preservative Thimerosal was causing speech delays and learning disabilities, they obfuscated and hid that information. They never made good on their 1999 pledge to have Thimerosal eliminated from vaccines and almost a decade later joined in the protest against a fictitious TV show (Eli Stone) because it was critical of mercury being in vaccines. Out of about 120 million doses of the worthless [1] flu vaccine shipped for the 2007-08 flu season, no more than about 15 million doses, including the less than 4 million live-virus doses, were no-Thimerosal doses. That means that about 87% contained some level of Thimerosal and at least 42% contained the maximum level (0.01%) of Thimerosal.

If a pregnant woman got a flu shot in 2001 and her child followed the flu shot recommendations, the baby/fetus would have received six flu shots with the full amount of Thimerosal by the year 2005. Today, in some states, the flu vaccine given to those under 3 year of age are supposed to contain no more than a trace level of Thimerosal, but with no government agency testing vaccines for mercury, the only ones who know whether a preservative-free vaccine (flu or otherwise) actually mercury is free are the manufacturers themselves. Vaccines with "trace" amounts of Thimerosal are supposed to contain less than 1 microgram of mercury (Hg) per 0.5 ml dose (1 microgram of Hg per 0.5 mL is the same as 2 micrograms of Hg per mL which is the same as 2000 liter; micrograms per liter is parts per billion [ppb].

–0.5 parts per billion (ppb) mercury = Kills human neuroblastoma cells (Parran et al., Toxicol Sci 2005; 86: 132-140).

–2.0 ppb mercury = U.S. EPA limit for drinking water. Http.

–20 ppb mercury = Neurite membrane structure destroyed (Leong et al., Neuroreport 2001; 12: 733-37).

–200 ppb mercury = level in liquid the EPA classifies as hazardous waste http://www.epa.gov/epaoswer/hazwaste/mercury/ regs.htm#hazwaste

–25,000 ppb mercury = Concentration of mercury in multi-dose, Hepatitis B vaccine vials, administered at birth from 1991-2001 in the U.S.

—–50,000 ppb mercury = Concentration of mercury in multi-dose DTP and Haemophilus B vaccine vials, administered 8 times in the 1990's to children at 2, 4, 6, 12 and 18 months of age and currently "preservative" level mercury in multi-dose flu, meningococcal and tetanus (7 and older) vaccines.

For years, the Infectious Disease division at the CDC (and others) have said the reason for the dramatic increase in autism is due to "better diagnosing" and "greater awareness." They have encouraged those like the AAP to manufacture uncertainty by publishing articles that were less than truthful. The AAP shame-fully played along, perhaps encouraged by the largesse of vaccine manufacturers who significantly contribute to the AAP's yearly budget. To publish studies that showed the removal of a known neurotoxin (mercury) from vaccine caused the incidence of autism to increase was shameful pseudo-science. There is another budget to consider for eighty percent of autistic Americans under the age of 18, and we will soon begin to see a dramatic impact on Social Security in coming years as these children become dependent adults. There are no studies that have found the previously undiagnosed or misdiagnosed autistic individuals among older Americans. They simply are not there. So, what is coming will significantly impact on society. As there are no genetic epidemics, which leaves an epidemic linked to some sort of exposure. Now, the increase of autism has been linked to the increase in mercury exposure through fish and industrial sources, amalgam and additionally, through increased parenteral exposure to Thimerosal – no controlled, randomized study regarding the safety of amalgam or Thimerosal exists.

A recently released Scientific Consensus Statement on Environmental Agents Associated with Neurodevelopmental Disorders (by the Collaborative on Health and the Environment's Learning and Developmental Disabilities Initiative) concludes that environmental contaminants are an important cause of learning and developmental disabilities. Delayed detoxification of mercury severely impairs methylation reactions (required for the correct expression of DNA, RNA, and neurotransmitters), which further adversely affects growth factor derived development of the brain and attention abilities. Phospholipid methylation, which is crucial for attention, is impaired in autistic and attention deficit hyperactivity disorders.

In a first analysis of the VSD datasets, Verstraeten et al. had described a 7.6-to-11.4-fold increase of autism risk in children at one month, with the highest mercury exposure levels compared to children with no exposure. In four subsequent separate generations of the analysis, which involve the exclusion of children with no Thimerosal exposure and less than two polio vaccines, the statistical significance disappeared. This is what was published by the AAP even though they knew the truth. How did they know the truth?

Again, they were presented at the Simpsonwood meeting in June 2000, a meeting that was illegal to hold. No Federal agency is allowed to call a meeting together with representatives of private industry (all the vaccine manufacturers were represented at this meeting) without opening the meeting to the public. Thimerosal was tested only once, by Eli Lilly on 22 adult patients suffering from meningitis. There was no chance for follow- up to observe long-term effects, as all of the patients in this "study" died. Even if follow-up had been possible, damage to the developing brains of incredibly young children would have remained an unknown. Eli Lilly said it was safe and the medical community accepted it. After the creation of the FDA, its use was simply continued. The federal government has never tested the type of mercury in vaccines for toxicity. This is an unconscionable oversight failure at best, at worse it is an example that we have left consensus reality to be created by the liars, thieves, cheats, killers, and the junk scientists they employ. How it came to pass the AAP joined these rogues and became an active participant in this skullduggery is beyond reason even beyond greed. They have remained silent as mercury-laden vaccine continues to be exported and used in all third world and second world countries.

We are living in a time where an incredible overplay and lies, self-aggrandizing behavior and non-science are the norm. We have tolerated the junk science that has covered up the true cause of this epidemic at a considerable cost to science, the public, and our very way of life in this country. Is it a stretch to realize that by putting our collective heads in the sand about the autism epidemic we have made it possible for the destruction of our very civilization? Not something easy to contemplate.

Then ask why haven't pediatricians come forward to demand the end of the use of Thimerosal once and for all, and to advocate for the treatment of these children before it is too late? Why are they not at the front of the line protesting the amounts of mercury allowed to come out of coal-fired power plants? Why aren't they leading the charge to stop the use of mercury amalgam dental fillings that are placed in the mouths of young children and pregnant women? The very Federal agencies that should have been sounding the alarm bell about environmental pollution creating future generations of mentally disabled citizens did less than remain silent because they have become arms of the very corporations that profit from selling and distributing poisons. Just look who sits on the FDA's Scientific Advisory Boards the conflicts of interest are so glaring as to suggest that the FDA has become a trade arm of Big Pharma. Nevertheless, the handwriting is on the wall as the US government has quietly conceded a vaccine-autism case in the Court of Federal Claims [3]. Pediatricians will no longer be able to hide behind the skirts of "Standard of Care" if they are giving autistic children heavy-metal laden vaccines, or children with mitochondrial dysfunction vaccine, or when it is established most "autistic" children have mitochondrial dysfunction.

The AAP should proactively be bringing in risk management specialists to determine how this could affect pediatricians in civil litigation for following the CDC recommendations on vaccinations after a diagnosis of any type of neurodevelopmental delay in a child. Of course, this is what they are afraid of and this is what the law of attraction will bring in upon the AAP and their minions who just followed the recommendations and drank the Kool-Aid that Big Pharma wanted them to drink. For all the above reasons, I will no longer enable the AAP to be party to the damage that is being done to the world's children by sending in my dues for a third decade. It is a token protest, but it has to begin with someone.

References cited in Dr. Stoller's letter:

1. a. Jefferson T. Influenza vaccination: Policy versus evidence. BMJ 2006; 333: 912-915 (28 October), doi: 10.1136/bmj.38995.531701.80b.
2. Geier DA, King PG, Geier MR. Influenza Vaccine: Review of

effectiveness of the U.S. immunization program, and policy considerations. JAPS (Journal of American Physicians and Surgeons) 2006 Fall; 11(3):69-74[2].

3. http://www.ajph.org/cgi/eletters/AJPH.2007.113159v1[3] http://www.huffingtonpost.com/david-kirby/government-concedes-vacci_b_88323.html

In 1999, Dr. Jane Orient, MD, President of the American Association of Physicians and Surgeons (AAPS) testified before the U.S. House of Representatives on the Hepatitis B Vaccine. It was a meeting held by the Criminal Justice, Drug Policy & Human Resources Subcommittee of the Committee on Government Reform. Here is what she had to say:

> *"Mr. Chairman and Members of the Subcommittee: My name is Jane Orient, M.D. I am a practicing internist from Tucson, Arizona, and serve as the Executive Director of the Association of American Physicians & Surgeons ("AAPS"). "For most children, the risk of a serious vaccine reaction may be 100 times greater than the risk of hepatitis B. Overall, the incidence of hepatitis B in the U.S. is currently about 4 per 100,000. The risk for most young children is far less; hepatitis B is heavily concentrated in groups at high risk due to occupation, sexual promiscuity, or drug abuse. VAERS contains 25,000 reports related to hepatitis B vaccine (in 1999-it is about 40,000 as of 2003), about 1/3 of which were serious enough to lead to an emergency room visit, hospitalization, or death. It is often assumed that only 10% of reactions are reported."*
>
> *"Striking increases in chronic illnesses have occurred in temporal association with an increase in vaccination rates. Asthma and insulin-dependent diabetes mellitus, causes of lifelong morbidity and frequent premature death, have nearly doubled in incidence since the introduction of many new, mandatory vaccines. There is no explanation for this increase. The temporal association (with universal*

hepatitis B vaccination), although not probative, is suggestive and demands intense investigation. Instead of following up on earlier, foreign studies suggesting a greater-than-chance association, the CDC, through vaccine mandates, is obliterating the control group (unvaccinated children)."

"Nonetheless, the implications are so grave that immediate investigation is needed. Measles, mumps, rubella, hepatitis B, and the whole panoply of childhood diseases are a far less serious threat than having a large fraction (say 10%) of a generation afflicted with learning disability and/or uncontrollable aggressive behavior because of an impassioned crusade for universal vaccination. There are plausible mechanisms such as molecular mimicry whereby vaccines could have such effects. Basic research, as well as epidemiologic studies (starting with a long-term follow-up of reactions reported to VAERS), is urgent."

Dr. Orient concludes her assessment and condemnation of the mandated hepatitis B vaccine thus to the Criminal Justice, Drug Policy & Human Resources Subcommittee:

"AAPS opposes federal mandates for vaccines, on principle, on the grounds that they are:

An unconstitutional expansion of the power of the federal government.

An unconstitutional delegation of power to a public–private partnership.

An unconstitutional and destructive intrusion into the patient-physician and parent-child relationships.

A violation of the Nuremberg Code in that they force individuals to have medical treatment against their will, or to participate in the functional equivalent of a vast experiment without fully informed consent.

A violation of rights to free speech and to the practice of one's religion (which may require one to keep oaths)."

Just as it is widely accepted nowadays, even from all disparate political persuasions, that there is “fake news,” many have become to believe there too is fake medical science. Fake medical science has destroyed the medical profession over the last 200 years because of faulty medical paradigms about pandemics and vaccines adopted as gospel centuries ago, that are based on faith and religion instead of rigorous scientific evidence.

About Covid-19 testing: A principal problem all along (and in the past during other epidemics) is testing, and the deontology surrounding testing. Deontology is defined legally as the rightness of action as a function of whether the action is required, prohibited, or permitted by a moral duty, as in the case with wearing a mask or socially distancing, or submitting to a “test” in the first place, especially among asymptomatics. This is important because the CDC in August 2020 released a report to the NY Times suggesting that asymptomatics need not get tested (Katherine J. Wu, *New York Times*, 8/27/2020).

A recent study out of Johns Hopkins looking at medical errors stated that modern medicine is the 3rd leading cause of death in the United States, with modern medicine & pharmaceuticals causing over 250,000 deaths in the USA alone annually.

(https://hub.jhu.edu/2016/05/03/medical-errors-thirdleading-cause-of-death/) When it comes to SARS COVID-19, we are living through the fruit of over 200 years of fables told to the public about the causes and solutions to pandemics, epidemics, and endemic diseases. We are living through a SARS COVID-19 era of delusional public health paradigms based on sloppy and at times outright fake SARS CoV-2 medical science. What we are witnessing is the complete collapse and reset of the entire epidemic disease and vaccine paradigms as public confidence has plummeted in public health and government authorities and the healthcare system generally. We reached a tipping point prior to SARS COVID-19 but SARS COVID-19 is the final nail in the coffin of our diseased and corrupted public health establishment. For example, prior to SARS COVID-19 a recent Gallup poll showed that the pharmaceutical industry was the least trusted industry in the United States and even less respected than government itself, with less than 30% of the American public having a favorable opinion of pharma and over 58% having a negative view. Additionally other recent polls as described in this Science magazine article show at least 50% of Americans will opt to not get the SARS CoV-2 vaccine(https://www.sciencemag.org/news/2020/06/just-50-americans-plan-get-covid-19-vaccine-here-s-how-win-over-rest)

Another recent Gallup poll showed only 9% of the US public thought a Covid vaccine was necessary to reopen the US from poorly thought-out lockdowns. The foundations for this public health and public relations catastrophe were laid centuries ago. In order to understand where we are today, we need to understand our public health and epidemic history. This book analyzes the historic timeline of epidemics and vaccines going back to the first vaccines and pandemics in recorded modern history that brought us the current SARS COVID-19 pandemic paradigm and SARS COVID-19 media InfoDemic and the push for SARS CoV-2 testing and anti-SARS CoV-2 vaccines. The actual science shows that Sars CoV-2 tests used to scare the public are faulty at best and useless at worst giving off a majority of false positive and false negative test results. Early on in the epidemic in many countries around the world even the very tests being used to diagnose people with SARS CoV-2 infection were found to be contaminated and giving off false positive results. See:

(https://www.cbc.ca/news/canada/new-brunswick/test-kits-contaminated-new-brunswick-1.5534125)

Additionally, over 80% of positive cases are without symptoms and contributing to an "InfoDemic" of fear mongering by the corrupt, bought and paid for pharma controlled mainstream media whose advertising dollars mostly come from the actual pharmaceutical industry.

(https://www.bmj.com/content/369/bmj.m1375)

What we really suffer from is an epidemic of fake COVID-19 science being pushed by the corrupt, bought-and-paid-for pharma-sponsored,

corporate media and corrupt government public health agencies and corrupt "philanthropic foundations" that are funded by plutocrats who are invested in pharmaceutical companies. Here is a small sampling of accurate science on SARS CoV-2 that illustrates that the terror created by the media about SARS CoV-2 – the InfoDemic – is far more dangerous than the virus itself. SARS COVID-19's lethality rate is equivalent to a bad flu season, lower than .1%, and for adults younger than age 70 far lower than this 0.1% death rate. The danger to the general population is equivalent to driving your automobile. See:

(https://www.medrxiv.org/content/10.1101/2020.04.05.20054361v2)

The median age of death from SARS CoV-2 is over 80 years old and the majority of deaths have occurred in people over age 75 with co-morbidities and in nursing homes or similar circumstances and questions remain if most of these patients died from co-morbidities, lockdown side effects, iatrogenic causes (ventilators & other medical interventions), and whether they died with or from SARS CoV-2 as recent medical billing changes incentivized labelling every patient who tested positive on one of these defective SARS CoV-2 tests as "died from SARS CoV02". For 6% of the deaths, SARS CoV-2 was the only cause mentioned. For deaths with conditions or causes in addition to SARS CoV-2, on average, there were 2.6 additional conditions or causes per death. See: (https://www.cdc.gov/nchs/nvss/vsrr/covid_weekly/index.htm 19)

It is worth mentioning also, that before CoV-2 emerged in 2002-3 and received wide attention, coronaviruses were principally a malady known to veterinary science. A canine coronavirus infection (CCV) is a highly contagious intestinal disease that can be found in dogs all around the world. This particular virus is specific to dogs, both wild and domestic. The coronavirus replicates itself inside the small intestine and is limited to the upper two-thirds of the small intestine and local lymph nodes. A CCV infection is generally considered to be a relatively mild disease with sporadic symptoms, or none at all. But if a CCV infection occurs simultaneously with a viral canine parvovirus infection, or an infection caused by other intestinal enteric pathogens, the consequences can be much more serious. There have been some deaths reported in vulnerable puppies.

Symptoms and Types

The symptoms of a CCV infection vary. In adult dogs, the majority of infections will be inapparent, with no symptoms to show. Sometimes, a single instance of vomiting and a few days of explosive diarrhea (liquid, yellow-green or orange) may occur. Fever is typically exceedingly rare, while anorexia and depression are more common. Occasionally, an infected dog may also experience some mild respiratory problems. Puppies may exhibit protracted diarrhea and dehydration and are most at risk of developing serious complications with this virus. Severe enteric inflammation of the small intestine in puppies will occasionally result in death.

Causes

This intestinal disease is believed to be caused by the canine coronavirus, which is closely related to the feline enteric coronavirus (FIP), an intestinal virus that affects cats. The most common source of a CCV infection is exposure to feces from an infected dog. The viral strands can remain in the body and shed into the feces for up to six months. Stress caused by over-intensive training, over-crowding and generally unsanitary conditions increase a dog's susceptibility to a CCV infection. Additionally, places and events where dogs gather are the most likely locations for the virus to spread.

Diagnosis

A CCV infection will usually have some symptoms in common with other bacterial, viral, or protozoic infections, or with general food intoxication or intolerance. Therefore, certain tests may have to be administered to determine the actual cause of the infection. Biochemical analysis and urinalysis will typically show normal physiology, so sometimes specific serologic (serum) tests or antibody titers (measurement of antibody strength) may need to be used.

And finally, the realm of human beings, the reports of large number of deaths in the elderly, increasing evidence is accumulating that these deaths were likely from the side effects, isolation, and harm from the lock-downs themselves.

NOW WE ENTER THE WONDERFUL WORLD OF SARS-COV-19. WHAT DO THE PRELIMINARY STUDIES WITH SARS VACCINES SHOW?

"IMMUNIZATION WITH SARS CORONAVIRUS VACCINES LEADS TO PULMONARY IMMUNOPATHOLOGY ON CHALLENGE WITH A SARS NATURAL INFECTION"

Going back to 2004, we find many titles such as the following printed in prestigious journals:

Marshall E, Enserink *Medicine*. **Caution urged on SARS vaccines.** Science Feb 13, 303 (5660) 994-6, **2004.**

"Immunization with SARS Coronavirus Vaccines Leads to Pulmonary Immunopathology on Challenge with the SARS…"

which was published in PLoS ONE | www.plosone.org, Volume 7, Issue 4, e35421, 1 April 2012 by:

Chien-Te Tseng1,2, Elena Sbrana1, Naoko Iwata-Yoshikawa1,2, Patrick C. Newman1, Tania Garron1, Robert L. Atmar3,4, Clarence J. Peters1,2, Robert B. Couch 3,4* from these research institution collaborations:

1. Department of Microbiology and Immunology, The University of Texas Medical Branch, Galveston, Texas, United States of America,
2. Center for Biodefense and Emerging Disease, The University of Texas Medical Branch, Galveston, Texas, United States of America,
3. Department of Medicine, Baylor College of Medicine, Houston, Texas, United States of America,
4. Department of Molecular Virology and Microbiology, Baylor College of Medicine, Houston, Texas, United States of America

Abstract Background:

Severe acute respiratory syndrome (SARS) emerged in China in 2002 and spread to other countries before brought under control. Because of a concern for reemergence or a deliberate release of the SARS coronavirus, vaccine development was initiated. Evaluations of an inactivated whole virus vaccine in ferrets and nonhuman primates and a **virus-like-particle** vaccine in mice induced protection against infection but challenged animals exhibited an immunopathologic type **lung disease**.

Conclusions: These SARS-CoV vaccines all induced antibody and protection against infection with SARS-CoV. However, challenge of mice given any of the vaccines led to occurrence of Th2-type immunopathology suggesting hypersensitivity to SARS-CoV components was induced. **Caution in proceeding to application of a SARS-CoV vaccine in humans is indicated.**

This "pulmonary immunopathology" finding due to a coronavirus vaccine was published in 2012.

Meanwhile, doctors and vaccine companies are continuing to promote the vaccination of everything that walks or breathes, except perhaps for the ongoing effort to vaccinate premature infants which can neither walk nor "breathe" yet. For instance, in January 25, 2012, an article appeared that suggested that premature babies should be used as subjects of vaccine trials, as reported by the organization SANEVAX (http://sanevax.org/premature-babies-used-as-lab-rats-in-manipulated-vaccine-trials/).

This following title was published in Nature in 2020 regarding SARS-CoV-2 vaccines:

Jiang S. **Do not rush to deploy COVID-19 vaccines and drugs without sufficient safety guarantees.** *Nature* March; 579 (7799):321, 2020.

Why are all these vaccinologists calling for caution regarding SARS-CoV-2 vaccines?

Dr Peter Hotez, dean of the National School of Tropical Medicine at Baylor College of Medicine, told Reuters.

Hotez worked on development of a vaccine for SARS (Severe Acute Respiratory Syndrome), the coronavirus behind a major 2003 outbreak, and found that some vaccinated animals developed more severe disease compared with unvaccinated animals when they were exposed to the virus. Even Paul Offit, the vaccine "guru" has been seen on self-posted Youtube videos decrying the SARS-CoV-2 vaccine roll-out until safety tests are done.

"***There is a risk of immune enhancement,***" said Hotez. "The way you reduce that risk is first you show it does not occur in laboratory animals."

"I understand the importance of accelerating timelines for vaccines in general, but from everything I know, this is not the vaccine to be doing it with..."

As of 1/1021, there are 296 peer-reviewed articles on MEDLINE with the search terms coronavirus, enhancement, 2020, with titles such as:

Molecular Mechanism for Antibody-Dependent Enhancement of Coronavirus Entry, by Yushun Wan, Jian Shang, Shihui Sun, et al., *Journal of Virology*, Feb 14:94 (5):e02015-19, 2020.

Antibody-dependent enhancement and SARS-C0V-2 vaccines and therapies, by Lee WS, Wheatley AK, Kent SJ, DeKosky BJ. *Nature Microbiol.* Oct 5 (10):1185-1191, 2020.

Consensus summary report for CEPI/BC March 12-13, 2020 meeting: Assessment of risk of disease enhancement with COVID-19 vaccines. *Vaccine,* Jun 26:38 (31): 4783-4791, 2020.

These three citations are the first of the 296 citations warning against COVID-19 vaccines for the year of 2020 alone. Yet the risk(s) are not only present for coronavirus vaccines: intensive studies in recent years looking at a phenomenon known as "viral interference" have been published by such agencies as the armed forces when vaccines other that SARS-CoV-2 vaccines have been administered, showing as much as 30% more injury following routine yearly flu vaccinations. In a relatively large study published in 2020 (Vaccine Vol. 38, Issue 2, Pages 350-354, January, 2o2o):

"Influenza vaccination and respiratory virus interference among Department of Defense personnel during the 2017–2018 influenza season," by Greg G. Wolff. The study wanted to assess if: *"Receiving influenza vaccination may increase the risk of other respiratory viruses, a phenomenon known as virus interference."*

Of 9,469 men who met the test criteria, it was concluded that "Vaccine derived virus interference was significantly associated with coronavirus (36% more likely to find coronaviruses following the mandatory flu vaccine upon entering the armed force induction process), and human metapneumovirus.

In other words, yearly flu vaccines can increase the odds of acquiring a coronavirus than if no vaccine is administered. Yet these kinds of data, even coming from the US military do not stop the World Health Organization from promoting any and all vaccines.

The most heinous consequence of this unforgivable and unspeakable testing delusion are mandated vaccines. Fierce objections have been forcefully and articulately advanced toward policy changes regarding over-vaccination and re-vaccination schedules and antibiotic over-prescription during infancy, childhood, adolescence, middle age, and old age. An entire spectrum of what amounts to even costlier and problematic and highly adverse event-inducing life-long maladies and endemic illnesses are increasing exponentially, and when drugs are given to treat the side effects of previous drugs, these arguments have been ignored and censored and veer off toward insanity. Too much profit is made by the medical system treating their own mistakes and treating endemic iatrogenic diseases caused by the medical system itself. Consider the invitations, advertising, and enforced mandates to herd our children and seniors into the slaughter-house of ever more drugs and vaccines that continues to this day.

Although The New York Times on August 27th, 2020 published a report that the CDC had modified its coronavirus testing guidelines to exclude people who do not have symptoms of SARS-CoV-2, international and some national air flight officials are announcing still in January 2021, that people must test negative at least 3 days before being allowed to travel as of 5 months later, and there have been discussions in other news reports of internment camps for folks until they test SARS-CoV-2 negative.

Almost each month there are new so-called "preventive" vaccines and drugs that are being aggressively advertised and marketed for new ailments you have never heard of or have never known that you or your children are suffering from, without your awareness. When obedience is not willingly provided to the agenda of Big Pharma, even by the asking of a simple question about seeing the safety data for such "staples" as the hepatitis B vaccine, some parents have been threatened with incarceration by governmental agencies at the insistence of certain factions of the medical establishment.

Children have been illegally prevented from attending school, and in other situations, parents have been incarcerated until they "listen" to doctor's orders and force their children to follow "standards of care" rather than try alternative therapeutics they want to explore that involve no toxicity and can do no harm. Yet we are forced to accept that these medicines do no harm and are beneficial. We are counseled that we should blindly accept them without a discussion, or without harboring any concerns for the long-term effects they may have and which they could potentially unleash on entire populations because of an "impassioned crusade" to vaccinate and medicate the entire human race to establish "herd immunity" and to accomplish disease "eradications."

But are these projections really true, or are they simply cruel violations of human potential and the common good? Vaccine makers in some cases have admitted or include on the package inserts page-long lists of adverse reactions associated with many vaccines prescribed to children, teens, adults, and seniors. A common but not exhaustive list of these maladies include arthritis, asthma, seizures, ADD, shingles, AIDS and other ill-definable autoimmune syndromes, diabetes, meningitis, pneumococcal illnesses, hypertension, and a plethora of "pulmonary hypertensive disorders," and cancers.

Yet healthy children, adolescents, and young adults in fact appear in many statistical surveys to becoming "sicker" without any concerns raised about the long-term effects on health of preventative interventions such as the so-called "hepatitis B" and "HPV" vaccines that supposedly protect against cancers that will occur 50 years later, with these vaccines'> **10% severe and often life-long adverse event profiles**. It does not even ring any alarms among most people, such as parents, despite package inserts accompanying the products themselves, or which the doctor's never disclose to their "patients," even when the vaccines or drugs include the putrid and often proprietary molecules in vaccines and immunizations designed to prime the non-immunologically immature immune system known as adjuvants. The gateway problem to this kind of insanity always will be the testing and our faith and understanding of the testing for disease. **But again, this psychosis dates back to the AIDS era, Anthony Fauci, and Robert C. Gallo's "vira-topian" delusions, as it is clear by a few reminiscences of the past, and now it is being re-enacted by Christian Drosten's invalidated RT-PCR test and others, which amounted to nothing more than some Internet published sequences that they claimed was "viral isolation."**

GENETIC ENGINEERING, MOLECULAR BIOLOGY, GAIN OF FUNCTION MUTANTS, AND BIO-WARFARE

Aside from the proposed menagerie or zoos full of proposed potential animal sources of pathogenic rumor viruses such as "HIV" from monkeys, or bat origins of real viruses such as the coronaviruses such as SARS CoV-2, or camel origins of MERS virus, many conspiracy theorists speculate the source of SARS CoV-2 was due to intentional or accidental tampering with coronavirus genomes. Ice-minus was a genetically modified bacteria used in the attempt to change the freezing temperature of water on strawberry plant fields unleashed into the environment during the 1980's in California and elsewhere to keep strawberry plants from freezing, can lead to disastrous consequences.

The Gain Of Function research with coronaviruses, advocated and funded by the likes of Fauci and his eugenicists are now tinkering with the genetic structure of viruses in China and elsewhere for use in human beings has been interpreted as a form of bio-warfare, and it is this topic that drives home once again the absurdity of testing, as well as the absurdity of genetic engineering more generally. In other words, if Fauci deliberately sent the Wuhan lab a GOF (gain of function) sequence that could render harmless coronaviruses deadly respiratory pathogens, this in effect would be nothing but bio-weapons development, by America's long-time rival, China, funded by our own government. But this is not the case, nor is it possible. Here is why.

First of all, why would the US give its long-time communist foe a capacity to biologically engineer a lethal pandemic flu virus that could in principle sweep the world and end up infecting Anthony Fauci's mother on this side of the world? If this is indeed what took place hypothetically, the inefficiency of this new influenza "bio-weapon" falls into the same category as other so-called bio-weapons of the past such as weaponized anthrax surrounding the events of 9/11-worthless in terms of actually piling up bodies-any bodies. If it were an intentionally engineered or even accidently engineered flu bio-weapon, then would not the perpetrators enter the deal expecting more than just emergency rooms being busy for a month on the other side of the world, and then having to close because there simply weren't enough victims? The anthrax in the mail killed 5 human beings that had direct contact with the anthrax in extremely high concentrations. Gain of function coronavirus, if we assume that is what SARS CoV-2 is, has caused a flu affecting a small number of people over 70, and by all appearances simply looks like an atypical pneumonia in even the most severe cases, which can be reversed easily now using hyperbaric oxygen therapy (HBOT). Most "cases" remain either mild or asymptomatic (and after the information is absorbed regarding all of the caveats regarding probabilistically being infected and prevalence in populations determining infection, it begs the question whether or not any of these people who do not develop an atypical pneumonia have COVID-19 in the first place). Lousy bioweapon I would say!

This line of thinking speaks to the absurdity of bio-warfare more generally since the days of its first inception decades ago. To think militarily that scientists are cleaver enough to engineer such a weapon in the form that disrupts the enemy biologically, reveals a deep ignorance of how intricately woven Nature's ecosystems are, and how difficult it is to bend the natural forces that maintain them to suit malevolent or even beneficial human purposes.

What is insane, and should be called as such, is the willingness to play with fire in so far as tinkering with Nature's natural genomics. This is because, and this is hypothetical, if you create a strawberry plant that outgrows other plants and crops like a weed, at least with enough shovels and spades you could recruit armies of people to dig up the plants, although it would be more difficult to chase down and kill genetically modified bees, or other insects if they had a genetic modification we created that "turned on us" or the balance of Nature. However, it is beyond imagination to conceive of how armed with a shovel or chemical or any other "weed-out" agent, how human beings could be successful in terminating or controlling in any way the results of an environmental release of either a bacterium, mycoplasma, or, a virus that was genetically modified by humans, released in a biological population or in Nature, and by some quirk of recombination or fecundity, become spread globally and began to cause unforeseen and unwanted harm.

The surmise of species jumping viruses such as "HIV" or SARS CoV-2 is somewhat different than the establishments' view regarding the similarities of the molecular signatures of these viruses. A more likely explanation of the origin of "HIV's" molecular signature comes instead not from racist notions, or from species hopping, but from recent studies in genomic research that suggests that the so-called template for the protein molecular signatures of "HIV" or SARS CoV-2 may derive from endogenous DNA sequences (coming from cellular origin instead of viral origin).

It is known that these cellular proteins are expressed under certain conditions by normal uninfected yeast, insects, dogs, rhesus monkeys, chimps, and humans. "HIV" is said to have 9150 base pairs, but again, this template has not been purified without contaminating cellular nucleic acids. "HIV's" molecular signature could represent a HERV (Human Endogenous Retrovirus) nucleic acid sequence, or what is called a 'retroid' of one kind or another. A retroid is a special kind of mobile gene associated with diseases such as multiple sclerosis, and with normal biological functions involving the placenta. That these endogenous human genetic elements exist and are important has been shown again and again to be likely from studies on HERV's such as "the Phoenix viruses," that can be produced by infecting cells with certain sequences of DNA, which then are replicated and packaged by the cells into virus-like particles.

Are viruses causal of disease and diseased cells, or are they by-products cast off by cells sickened because of some other causes? Are viruses simply cellular "shit?" Tobacco mosaic virus is a true virus with a definitive morphology and has a specific tropism and pathological effect. But are all vesicle-like "endosomes" we see actual viruses, if they are round, endosomal-appearing spheres that contain a dark core, or even if they sport a crown of proteins? I think not. This is why it is so important to identify viremia in a victim.

Cancer cells In Vitro, for instance, can frequently be seen to shed these hundred-nanometer particles, as can normal cells that are grown in media that is not supportive of cellular well-being. Without proper viral isolation and identification using electron microscopy, we cannot be sure, and even then, not sure that object is causing any illness unless other tests are employed following the algorithm of Koch's postulates. Also, any modern analysis of the human genome database will reveal more than 120, 000 full-length retroids containing reverse transcriptase transcripts (See: Marie Dewannieux, Francis Harper Aurelien Richaud, Claire Letzelter, David Ribet, Gerard Pierron, Thierry Heidmann. Identification of infectious progenitor for the multiple-copy HERV-K human endotheous retroelements. Genome Res. Oct 31, 2006; Marcella A. 316 McClure, Hugh S. Richardson, Rochelle A. Clinton, Crystal M. Hepp, Brad A. Crowther, Eric F. Donaldson. Automated characterization of potentially active retroid agents in the human genome. Genomics 512-523, 2005; David J Griffiths. Endogenous retroviruses in the human genome sequence. Genome Biology 2001,2:reviews1017.1- 1017.5).

http://genomebiology.com/2001/2/6/reviews/1017.

Although "HIV=AIDS" proponents are always saying the "HIV virus's" reverse transcriptase sequence is mutating when patients die on "lifesaving" anti-retroviral drugs that supposedly target this enzyme, genomic analyses show that reverse transcriptase is among the most stable transcripts that make up these retroids, and it is the sequence stability rather than the instability or mutability of the reverse transcriptase sequence itself that make these 120,000 retroid sequences possible to classify. What is also remarkable about the data regarding retroids and HERV's is that reverse transcriptase was once thought by all working in AIDS research to be specific to retroviruses, and this is the enzyme they first measured, and indeed some labs continue to measure, as evidence of "HIV infection." As CoV-2 is also a retrovirus, the same issues apply regarding reverse transcription.

We are all made up partly of "retroviral" components, they are part of us, and these components require reverse transcriptase for normal replication. What they call "HIV" and what they have successfully branded as the most dangerous and infectious virus known to man, is (and can be evoked), and what has been mistaken for these "viruses" are artifacts of the technologies for detecting them, without any of the sober analysis of what those tests are actually detecting or what "HIV's" molecular signature means for a human being. Same holds true for SARS CoV-2. The probable "cause of "HIV" could be these retroids and/or endogenous HERV sequences, that can be evoked, under stress conditions, or which may become expressed in healthy persons as part of a relatively rare genetic polymorphism. Without proper viral isolation and verification with electron microscopy, there is no way of knowing. More of this same kind of analysis needs to be done with SARS CoV-2 in victims with atypical pneumonias.

Robert Gallo, Anthony Fauci's side-kick who was credited with being the co-discoverer of "HIV" with Luc Montagnier, and although Gallo did not receive any of the Nobel Prize prizes that Montagnier received, used to call me in my office in the afternoons to threaten me over the phone if I did not shut up. He believed that...black slaves caused cancer because art work evidence proved to a scientifically epidemiologically established and on this basis justified a racist construct, that these slaves that were depicted in works of art caught and contagiously transmitted a cancer virus called "HTLV-I" and then HTLV-II in the 16th Century from monkeys during the slave trade, which caused 0.6 % of approximately 330,000 serologically tested Japanese near Nagasaki to develop a leukemia 40 years or so after the atomic bombs were dropped on them. This hypothesis was advanced for the origins of "HIV's" suspected "cancer virus" relative or precursor(s), "HTLV-I and II" by Robert Gallo in 1979-81, to explain why a few (out of hundreds of thousands of) "HTLV-1" seropositive individuals acquired cancer in Southern Japan near Nagasaki. This is also why, a year later, when the announcement was made to the

American public by Dr. Gallo and Margaret Heckler in 1984, the phrase, "the probable cause of AIDS has been found…to be "HTLV-III," a known "**cancer virus**" was used. As mentioned, "HTLV-III," was later renamed "HIV" by oncogene Nobelist Varmus's committee (please see National Institute of Health: Gallo R.C., Sliski A., Wong-Staal F. Origin of T-cell leukemia-lymphoma virus. Lancet (ii): 962-963, 1983).

Now Gallo is telling us to be open to receiving an oral "polio vaccine" for COVID-19 until we allow ourselves and our children to accept the untested COVID-19 vaccines now being prepared. The AIDS vaccine program has been an absolute catastrophe from its inception. All of this thinking about animal origins of viruses eventually led to the "sexual distancing" we have all come to love and know during the AIDS era…with "safe sex," and a few years ago, this idea was used again with camels with MERS (Middle Eastern Respiratory Syndrome), as it is widely believed by the biomedical establishment that the MERS virus "jumped" from camels to humans. And now with CoV2, we have viruses "jumping off" bats, and pangolins and various small carnivorous mammals as the source of "jumping viruses." As long as we continue to ignore that AIDS never have really left risk groups…starvation is one of the most certain ways of acquiring the helper-T-cell ratios characteristic of AIDS, as is IV drug use, we will be reminded how viruses jump species. Or perhaps in the case of COVID-19, CoV-2 had a little help with Fauci's grants to Wuhan's virology labs to play around with "Gain of Function" sequences (GOF sequences) genetically engineered onto harmless CoV-2 sequences as some conspiracy theories go. But all this amounts to is stupidity, not intentional or accidental bio-warfare or malevolence, and as yet, nobody has reported seeing a leaping virus.

None of this would have happened without the blind faith in molecular reductionism of the DNA or RNA sequence, which worships and pays homage to Watson and Crick's "secret of life." For almost two generations now, this religion has been practiced, and as their God, DNA and RNA sequences are the cause and creator of everything living, and has essentially destroyed the science of biology, physiology, and replaced them with chemistry. The problem of origins has always been problematic in biology as it indeed is in all sciences because we did not see it happen: The origin(s) of The Universe? The origin of life? The origin of vertebrates? The origin of humans? With viruses, which are not living things, but byproducts of healthy and diseased cells, we do know their origins are always and necessarily from the cells they are associated with.

And finally, regarding the results of such delusions about origins, we now instead of only enjoying "sexual distancing" bought to us by our friendly Robert Gallo and Anthony Fauci during the 1980's, now we have "social distancing" with COVID-19 and are living now in Faucitopia. So much more effective than "HIV" being an equal opportunity pathogen, don't you agree? To have an endogenous, ubiquitous gastrointestinal virus, such as CoV2 and many other coronaviruses that all are typically characterized as being normal intestinal subcellular passengers in a variety of mammals including man and man's best friend, the dog, the opportunities seem endless in social engineering based on fear tactics. The little blue masks worn over the face and probably a second one wrapped around the buttocks like a diaper, as it is endogenously an intestinally localized entity in most contexts that have been very well characterized for more than two decades, should become part of an educated and politically correct person's wardrobe for some time, lest they face incarceration or fines or internment camps.

A SOLUTION TO THE 12 HOUR SARS-CoV-2 CRISIS WINDOW THAT HAS SHOWN NEARLY 100% SUCCESS RATES

It should be mentioned that there is a therapeutic device that ensures that most hypoxic victims can acquire enough oxygen under all circumstances during the 12-hour crisis window. Respirators simply cannot provide enough oxygen to these critically ill people- and of this minor population of the most ill, about 60-68% do not make it on respirators. However, preliminary trials with hyperbaric oxygen chambers in China (35/36 victims) of morbidly ill end-stage COVID-19 victims within this 12 hour window show almost 100% cure rate, and trials now ongoing in the US hyperbaric oxygen therapy (for these most desperately ill victims) have among several smaller groups shown 100% cure rates. One trial by Paul Harch showed that 9/9 recovered with HBOT, and several other trials in the ORCCA network in Florida, especially in the clinics of Raymond Cralle, who has reported 19/19 patients pulled through who are in this crisis window (Tel: 561-819-0412; Email: orccahbo@yahoo.com).

ORCCA stands for the Oxygen Rescue Care Centers of America. Hyperbaric chambers are in most major hospitals also, to treat carbon monoxide poisoning, crushing wounds and wounds that do not heal, all manner of drug-resistant infections, and HBOT is especially useful for traumatic brain injuries and other neurological deficits, and it is used for many other indications as well.

HYPERBARIC OXYGEN THERAPY (HBOT)

Most cities possess hyperbaric oxygen chambers that are used in the US for about 16 FDA-approved indications, and principally, they are used for smoke inhalation victims. Yet there are many other uses and benefits of hyperbaric oxygen, and it should be kept in mind that >90% of people who contract full-blown SARS-COVID-19 recover without any medical intervention, so we are talking about those few who are experiencing the most profound effects of this atypical pneumonia. Hyperbaric oxygen or, simply pressurized 21% atmospheric air has been shown to reverse cerebral palsy, and other maladies that are not improved by standard medical procedures.

The list presented below is from William S. Maxfield, M.D. who is Board Certified in radiology and hyperbaric medicine for 16 years and has served as a consultant for Hyperbaric programs and hyperbaric medicine at many locations in the US. In the beginning of his talk, he claims that from the perspective of his medical credentials, that HBOT is "medicines best-kept secret" (http://www.orccahbo.com/). See also; (https://www.lifesupport-usa.com/about-us/) for information about "Life Support Technologies Group"- a company that provides services for a network of clinical hyperbaric centers, NASA, commercial diving, altitude sickness, Department of Defense work, and tunnel, and which provides hyperbaric education and training. They also are leaders in limb salvage and wound care services, training, and HBOT certification.

Below is a partial list of the uses and benefits of hyperbaric oxygen (HBOT):

A. **Cancer chemotherapy-associated brain injuries (Duke University's data)**
B. **Cognitive defects after surgical procedures (Duke University's data)**
C. **Stroke-(See: Conquering Stroke by Valery Green-her book about her experience with HBOT and her stroke) (and see…4 of Maxfield's patient histories with stroke as well). Also See: PLos One. 2013;8(1):e53716. doi: 10.1371/journal.pone.0053716. Epub 2013 Jan 15, for a list of clinical studies regarding treatment of stroke. Also see: "Hyperbaric oxygen induces late neuroplasticity in post stroke patients—randomized, prospective trial. Efrati S1, Fishlev G, Bechor Y, Volkov O, Bergan J, Kliakhandler K, Kamiager I, Gal N, Friedman M, Ben-Jacob E, Golan H.**
D. **Cerebral palsy (See: (http://www.cerebralpalsysource.com/treatment-and-therapy/hbot/) for actual clinical reports of controlled clinical trials of HBOT's improvement effects on CP).**

E. **Asthma-Steroids are typically given in required hospital stays and as prophylaxis (needed hospitalization typically occurs about 3X/year, but with HBOT steroid use can be completely avoided, 2 and the dwarfism it causes in children. Also, steroid side effects can be avoided by HBOT treatments in kidney transplant patients.**
F. **Traumatic brain injury-e.g. Oxygen is fuel of the body and brain is 8% of body weight-and uses 20% of the O2: therefore increasing O2 is an important goal to accomplish this deficit rapidly for any injuries involving cerebral edema (excellent response to HBOT, accept that its use in Maxfield's experience was resisted and then removed as a once recommended approach and various drugs were sought to replace HBOT because HBOT coincided with the garden industry of MRI and CT imaging by the Medical Establishment in favor of allopathic approaches only, or other currently and ineffectively used interventions). Cells in the damaged area regenerate with HBOT. HBOT for traumatic (blast) brain injuries (because of the pressure on the brain bombs create when they detonate) as have been proliferated as the "signature wound of "The War on Terror" in Iraq and elsewhere shows marvelous efficacy in not only physical amelioration but in suicide progression, and even with the airplane transport involved in flying soldiers from these modern George Bush recreated battlefields to Germany for treatment. Traumatic brain injury severity and its long-term sequelae even have been significantly improved with transport in HBOT placed on wounded transport planes, and the immediate supplying of pressurized O2 with HBOT provides this emergency period aide. This benefit is rational because it also fits into the long-time experience of deep sea and deep scuba divers: If you have been deep sea diving without developing divers bends due to too rapid a pressure changes in O2, then this explains (supplying HBOT to TBI-afflicted soldiers)**

why HBOT reduces morbidity and explains why you are not supposed to fly immediately after deep sea or deep scuba diving. Air transport after the pressure created by traumatic injury due to bomb blasts mimic sea diving bends because of the rapid change in O2 bomb blasts generate due to overpressure, so HBOT reverses or diminishes this pathological process when given during soldier transport. Also, neuropsychiatric problems seem ameliorated in returning vets is associated with decreased suicides (using SPEC scans show dramatic improvements)

G. MS (excellent data and Maxfield's experience) (England study-20-year experience of Parent and James 10-year follow-up of their patients in England-but not approved in US).
H. Emphysema- (a patient given less than 6 months with emphysema lived 6 years with HBOT
I. Rheumatoid arthritis
J. Colitis
K. "Infected or vibrating prosthesis" after joint surgery.
L. Cancer and cancer care-E.G. Extravasation of chemo-and radiation-damaged children-Norway's recent study shows HBOT treatment of animals.
M. AIDS
N. Cortical blindness due to a lightning strike
O. Congenital Deficiencies-Mitochondrial C-Disease. (No patients have survived longer than 7 years unless HBOT treated).
P. Ataxia Telangiectasia does not develop because of HBOT's activity.
Q. AIDS patients do not develop malignancies.
R. Horse Pneumocystis carinii does not develop in horses (or in AIDS patients)?
S. Fertility of difficult-birth and miscarrying mares is ameliorated with HBOT.
T. Stem cell take in skin grafts are vastly improved.

U. **A course of HBOT can increase endogenous stem cells to accelerate all wound healing.**
V. **Gas gangrene**
W. **Alzheimer's disease X. Perinatal asphyxia**

It should be emphasized that much of the early work with HBOT, and cancer treatments was aimed at determining if HBOT promoted rather than retarded tumor growth or killed tumors. Many decades were devoted to this question. The consensus among many different teams of skilled and thorough investigation found universally, and unequivocally, that HBOT never has been shown to accelerate or increase tumor growth, in fact, the opposite has been consistently found to be the case.

"The consensus today is that research performed hitherto has failed to demonstrate that HBO has a cancer-promoting effect or that it enhances recurrence. Nevertheless, both recent and older research studies have shown that HBO can be inhibitory and reduce cancer growth in some cancer types, like breast cancer. On the other hand, cervical and bladder cancers appear to be nonresponders to HBO" Ingrid Moen & Linda E. B. Stuhr. Hyperbaric oxygen therapy and cancer—a review. Targ Oncol (2012) 7:233–242).

Originally HBOT was initially used in the context of altitude sickness, and then in the later 1800's, it was used to rescue divers suffering from "the bends" brought on by nitrogen bubbles that form in the blood if a diver should descend or ascend from water that only needs to be 10 feet deep, as the Greek ship maintenance crews have learned during their long-duration shallow dives to clear and repair the bottom of ships, if not enough time is given for "equilibration."

During the past 5 years, hyperbaric oxygen therapy (HBOT) has been shown to hold great promise for treating cancers because pressurized gases penetrate tumor matrices and malignant tumors, or simply "burn cancer cells out" differentially, while nourishing the normal cells of the body:

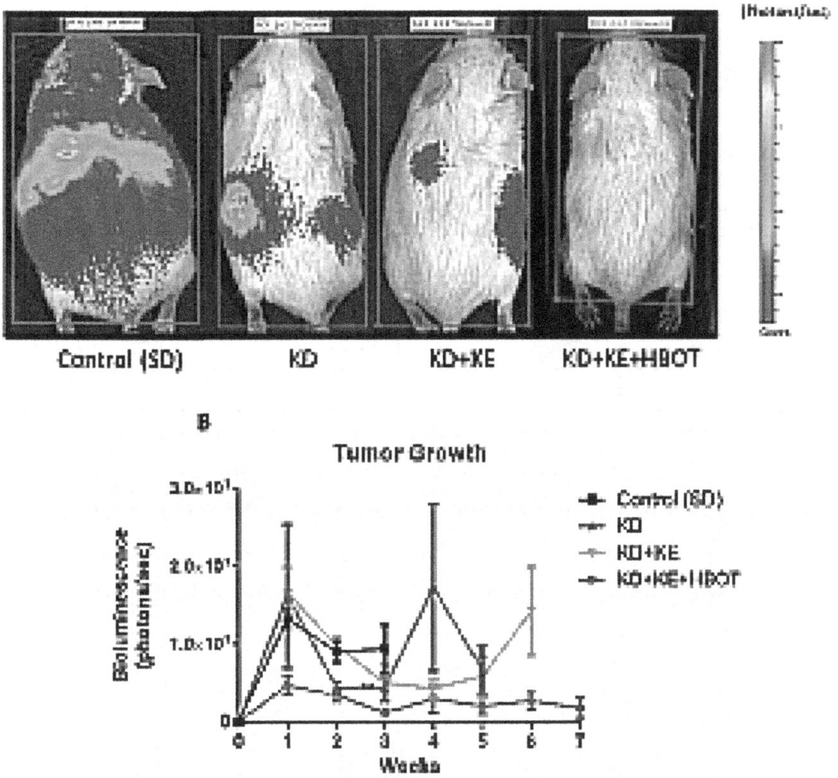

Combination metabolic therapy slows tumor growth. (A) In Vivo bioluminescence imaging of representative animals from each treatment group 3 weeks post tumor cell inoculation. Treated mice exhibited reduced tumor burden and metastatic spread. (B) Whole animal bioluminescence (photons/ sec) was tracked over time as a measure of tumor growth rate. In order to avoid misleading representation of tumor burden, data for treatment groups were 50% of animals had succumbed to diseases progression are no longer shown. Tumor bioluminescence was highly variable, but treated animals demonstrated a notable trend of slower tumor growth compared to controls throughout the study. KD treated mice had less bioluminescence than controls at week 2, while KD=KE+HBOT mice also had less bioluminescence than KD=KE mice at weeks 1,2,3, and 5, and had less

tumor bioluminescence than KD mice at weeks 3 and 5. Error bars represent +-SEM. Results were considered significant when op< 0.05.

The supplemental nutrients used in this amazing experiment were as follows:

Micronutrient Information	Standard Diet (SD)	Ketogenic Diet (KD)	Ketone Ester KE
% Kcal from Fat	18.0%	77.1	NA
% kcal from Protein	24.0%	22.4%	0.5
Coloric Density	3.1 Kcal/g	4.7 Kcal/g	56 Kcal/g

Also, new adjuvants that and are in Phase II human clinical trials and which have shown no toxicity and great efficacy as stand-alone therapies may synergize with HBOT to provide the best solutions discovered so far for the penetration of VM matrices, and treatment of malignancies non-toxically.

What this study above shows is that metabolic therapy (a ketogenic diet devoid of sugars) plus HBOT plus a ketone supplement can completely block the growth of injected tumor cells weeks before. Therefore, as these tumors were metastatic, they undoubtedly harbored VM, signifying that the combination of diet and supplements and HBOT may defeat cancer (at least gliomas) as this study above shows.

What is remarkable about this study is that this group had done a similar experiment 2 years earlier in 2013 and did not have results as significant as shown above. The mouse groups represented by the mouse on the far right that exhibits no bioluminescence and 100% effocacy. The earlier study they published in 2013 was done without the supplement, and there still was visible tumor present. In this study shown above from 2015, along with a ketone diet and with 100% HBOT, it appears that a complete blockage of tumor growth is achieved (in mice).

Certain caveats must remain in place. First the glioblastoma cells were xenographed into these mice, and thus are foreign to the host.

This type of model, rather than a spontaneously arising tumor, may not be representative of the true efficacy of the combination approach they tried. Moreover, we have seen seemingly perfect results like these before in mouse models (for example, endostatin), which was Dr. Folkman's protein that had similar dramatic results in rodents.

HBOT is non-toxic (when appropriately applied), it can penetrate VM matrix "biofilms," as it employs a gas instead of a soluble agent, and of course the ketogenic diet gets into every cell of the body. I feel this approach is exceedingly promising and wish to explore it using companion animals that develop spontaneous tumors. It would be as ethical to try as any other treatment currently in use for pets that develop tumors. This group, situated at The University of Florida in Tampa is part of the Florida ORCCA network I have been working with these past 5 years (ORCCA-Oxygen Rescue Care Centers of America).

ORCCA is a network of HBOT providers dispersed all over Florida, and I am in close contact daily with many of them. They are deeply committed to saving lives non-toxically with the use of HBOT. Currently, the US FDA approves HBOT for 15 conditions that mainstream medicine cannot help or improve. These include traumatic brain injuries, wounds that will not heal, infections that do not respond to any anti-microbial drug, and many other applications. The Russians, on the other hand, have approved HBOT for 73 different maladies that their best mainstream medicine cannot ameliorate.

Many cancers have not been adequately tested for their responses to HBOT combined with various new and promising adjuvants. Most of the studies of HBOT and cancer historically have been devoted toward determining if HBOT enhances tumor growth, but a consensus has emerged over several decades that it does not enhance growth but retards growth, impedes cell division, retards cancer angiogenesis, and is highly effective against several cancers such as human glioblastomas and breast cancers, and with co-administration of various anti-cancer adjuvants, has shown promise in colon cancer, osteosarcomas, and non-small-cell lung cancers.

So far, however, several other cancers do not appear to be responsive to HBOT (head and neck, leukemias, prostate, cervical or bladder). It should be mentioned that the conditions under which some of these "failures" haven't been successful significantly vary in the pressures and protocols used (lengths and frequencies of HBOT "dives"), and types of adjuvants co-administered.

The following recommendations were advanced by The Director of Hyperbaric Oxygen Therapy (HBOT) Authority, Dr. Zhong Xiaoling, of the army HBO Professional Committee, and Deputy Director of the Diving Medicine Laboratory, Chen Ruiyong, that he published on February 17, 2020:

From the pathophysiological characteristics of new coronavirus pneumonia (NCP) and the effect mechanism analysis of hyperbaric oxygen therapy (HBOT), HBOT may have a good effect in the treatment of NCP persistent hypoxemia.

In view of the NCP guidelines (National Health Commission) and various clinical reports, the fact that the oxygen therapy method of NCP patients is continuously upgraded, and the beneficial attempts of the Department of Hyperbaric Oxygen of Changjiang Shipping General Hospital are optimistic, it is recommended to include HBOT in the guidelines as NCP One of the means of clinical treatment, for first-line doctors to choose.

Analysis of the possible effects of HBOT on NCP

1 Pathological characteristics of NCP

The National Health Commission issued a report on the treatment of pneumonia caused by new crown virus infection (fifth edition, here after referred to as the guideline) and interviews with multiple expert treatment teams. The guideline reported that HBOT reverses diffuse, progressive lung tissue inflammation, persistent progressive hypoxemia, multiple organ failure (especially liver and heart function) failure, and inflammatory cytokine waterfall (cytokine storm).

2 Deficiencies in atmospheric oxygen therapy

Various reports show that the oxygen therapy measures in NCP treatment have been continuously upgraded from nasal catheters, non-invasive ventilation to invasive mechanical ventilation, and even ECMO. This indicates that there may be treatment needs that cannot be met by oxygen at atmospheric pressure. The underlying reasons may be:

Severe gas diffusion disorder and ventilation / blood flow ratio caused by interstitial lesions of the lung tissue are important reasons for the inability to correct hypoxemia with the support of ventilation. The systemic metabolic rate continues to increase due to inflammation. The amount of oxygen trioxide transported by hemoglobin transport cannot meet the body's metabolic needs. The body is in a "chronic" hypoxic state of systemic tissues, especially the liver and heart tissues' dependence on oxygen. Therefore, in some patients, ECMO may still be insufficient to correct hypoxia in deep tissues and vital organs. The cumulative effect of "oxygen debt" may be one of the important triggers of the cytokine storm.

ADVANTAGES OF HBOT

HBOT is based on the laws of gas physics related to pressure. The differences and advantages of HBOT from atmospheric oxygen absorption are:

1. Improve the diffusion efficiency of oxygen, overcome the gas diffusion obstacle caused by interstitial lesions, as long as there is a certain amount of ventilation, you can obtain better gas exchange efficiency than normal people when breathing.
2. The physically dissolved oxygen content in the blood is much larger than the combined hemoglobin transport capacity. It does not depend on the oxygen transport function of hemoglobin and can meet the oxygen consumption of the body's metabolic state.

3. The diffusion distance of oxygen is increased, and the aerobic metabolism needs of deep tissues and hypoperfusion tissues are solved.
4. HBOT can complete the repayment of "oxygen debt" in a short period of time, provide aerobic metabolism windows for deep hypoxic tissues and important organs, and play a good role in supporting treatment.

A number of studies have confirmed the effect of HBOT on immune cells and inflammation. The therapeutic effect of hyperbaric oxygen in acute high altitude pulmonary edema as well as diver's bends has been confirmed for at least a century by a lot of literature. Intermittent HBOT can reduce the accumulation of "oxygen debt" load, or it can play a role in delaying and blocking cytokine storms.

LIMITATIONS OF HBOT

1. HBOT requires special large-scale equipment, complex structure, and limited number of one-time treatments.
2. Although there are systematic hygienic management regulations (cabin sterilization, etc.), in view of the high infectivity of the new crown virus, it is necessary to further strengthen the sensory control management. Especially with cabin medical care, there is a possibility of ineffective protective equipment under normal pressure, and the risk of infection increases sharply.

Summary

1. The toxic side effects of conventional HBOT are not obvious, but the theoretical expected effect is good, and the actual effect of the case is significant. It is harmless and likely to be beneficial.

2. HBOT is not a specific medicine, but as a good oxygen therapy method, early intervention can be expected to reduce the incidence of severe and critical illness, thereby reducing medical care pressure, improving treatment efficiency and bed turnover rate. Properly applied, it can play a good role in the treatment of existing large numbers of patients.
3. It is recommended to include hyperbaric oxygen therapy in the Guidelines as a means of choice for the treatment of patients with severe NCP for clinicians to choose.

A clinical trial also was held in New York at NYU Winthrop Hospital in collaboration with New York University and the results were published on-line at 11:15 AM EDT August 4, 2020.

https://www.wusa9.com/article/news/investigations/doctors-say-hyperbaric-oxygen-therapy-as-covid-19-treatment-shows-promise-weve-made-tremendous-strides/65-c797dba0-f609-4e93-9e9c-5bc9e7e9ea74.

Doctors examined whether or not hyperbaric oxygen therapy could help people suffering from coronavirus. Ninety-percent of the patients in this study recovered and were able to go home to their families. The biggest problems with the novel coronavirus are the respiratory issues and subsequent low blood-oxygen levels it can cause.

For more than 80 years, hyperbaric oxygen therapy has been used to treat similar issues in scuba divers who develop decompression sickness.

The treatment works by placing the patient into pressure chamber filled with 100% oxygen. The pressure forces the oxygen into the body, and also increases the blood's capacity to store and transport oxygen to tissues.

In the NYU clinical trial, doctors treated 20 coronavirus-positive patients with hyperbaric oxygen. While two of them died, the remaining 18 patients recovered and were discharged from the hospital – a 90% recovery rate Doctors compared this group to similar patients who did not receive the treatments.

They said they found hyperbaric oxygen decreases the number of deaths and the number of patients that required ventilators.

China is currently leading the world in cancer therapeutics with respect to hyperbaric oxygen treatment of cancers, and also in its use for the treatment of SARS CoV-2 victims because they realized in February that respirators used for Covid-19 simply cannot provide enough oxygen to these critically ill people-and of this minor population of the most ill, about 60-68% do not acquire enough oxygen to make it (live) on respirators. However, China's success rate using HBOT in treating SARS CoV-2 is reported as being a 100% rate of success so far.

Small clinical HBOT trials for SARS CoV-2 atypical pneumonia infections have begun in Florida in its many Oxygen Rescue Care Centers of America network clinics of HBOT providers (HBOT), and in the HBOT clinics in New Orleans headed by Dr. Paul Harch, MD. Harch's New Orleans hyperbaric center and network, is one of the Nation's largest, while Harch himself is one of the world's foremost HBOT exponents because he has the largest HBOT case history in the world. Dr. Harch has authored a book entitled: **Oxygen Revolution** with Virginia McCullough.

Dr. Harch also has won many awards and been honored before US congress 4 times for his contributions that adapted the use of HBOT in wound healing to a host of non-treatable syndromes seen in neurology. Dr. Harch demonstrated that HBOT could be used with amazing success for brain injured divers, boxers, for the reversal of cerebral palsy and autism spectrum disorders, and also, he was the first to document the process of oxygen's curative process and brain regrowth (due to HBOT) in a brain-damaged drowning victim using PET scan technology (Proton Emission Tomography-a way of observing brain activity and regrowth in real time).

During our Bush-launched 21 year-long war in countries that had nothing to do with any buildings or anthrax spores, which is the longest war in American history, Harch and many other HBOT providers all over the nation have been "diving" American servicemen with traumatic brain injuries (TBI's) due to blast concussive injuries and dramatically rescuing severe traumatic brain injury victims, and also, importantly, reducing the appalling suicide rate among these children of war upon returning home ("diving" means putting victims in HBOT chambers).

Dr. William Maxfield in Florida, former Chair of Johns Hopkins School of Medicine's department of radiation oncology, left his position at Johns Hopkins years ago to help establish the ORCCA network here in Florida, and trained the current leadership of the American College of Hyperbaric Medicine in Wisconsin to provide HBOT for a variety of indications.

Jeff Neizgoda is Director of the American College of Hyperbaric Medicine in Milwaulkee, Wisconsin.

Dr. Maxfield has one of the most extensive experience histories anywhere in the context of remediating TBI's and especially obviating suicides of the returning children of war and continues to dive the veterans returning home from Iraq and Afghanistan. A long-accepted and perhaps most successful use of HBO therapy is its use for healing wounds that will not heal using the best-known mainstream medical care.

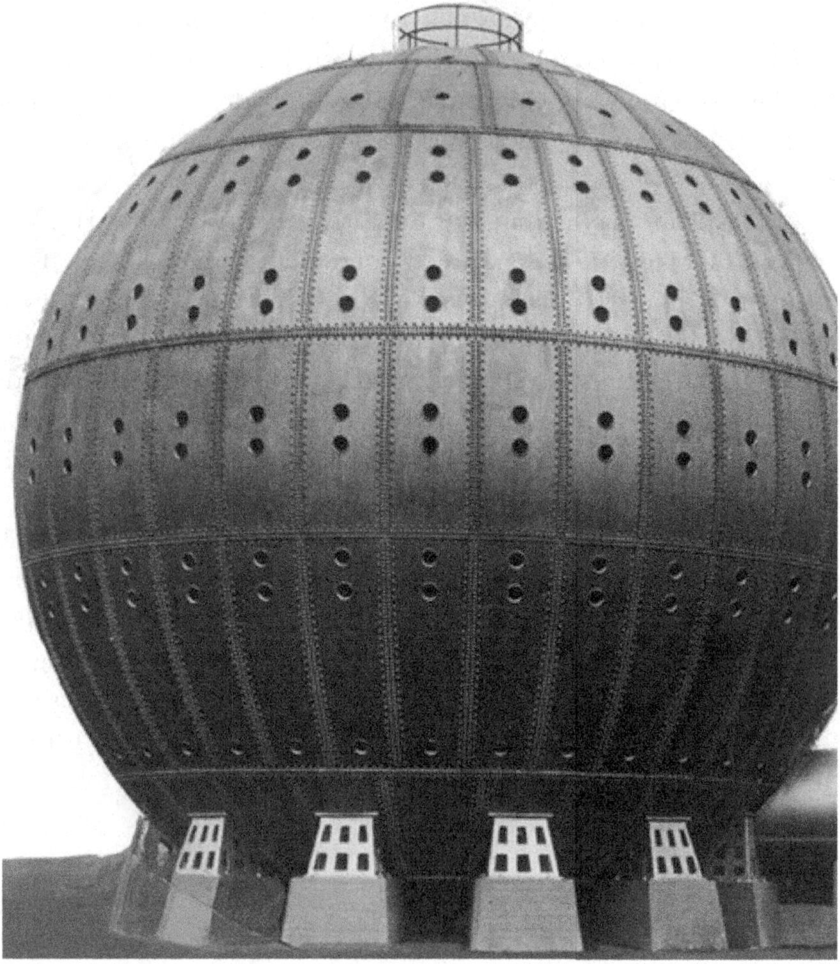

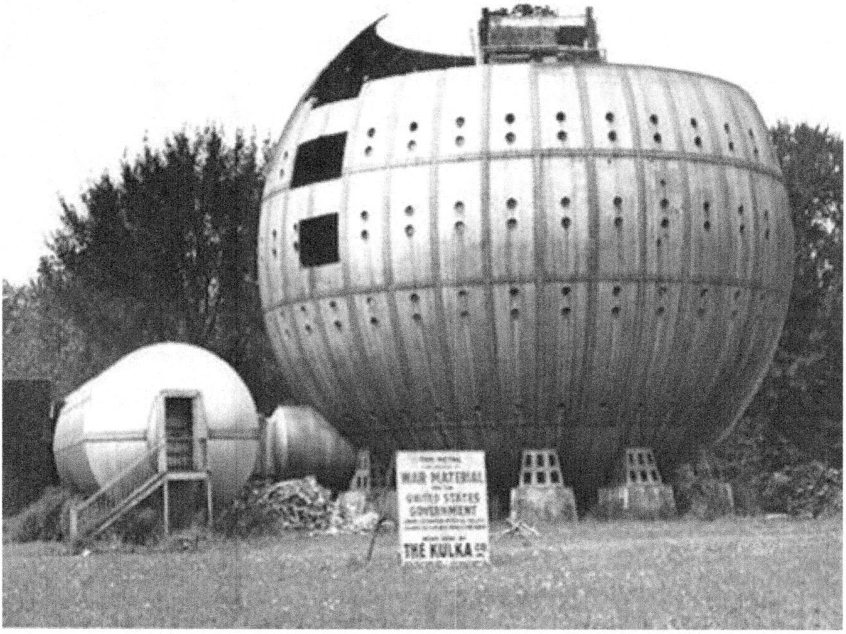

Orval Cunningham's Hyperbaric Sanitarium being torn apart and sold for scrap metal for the upcoming WW II cataclysm, because of FDR's indifference toward this new therapeutic gift.

HBOT chambers are available in most major metropolitan hospitals in the US because it is the only successful device known to reverse smoke inhalation injuries due to fires, and the only recourse known that can "burn out" antibiotic resistant infections, cure wounds that will not heal, and which are used to treat 16 maladies that standard mainstream approaches cannot heal, and which our FDA approves currently. The Russian FDA has approved 73 uses for HBOT, and therefore, they may indeed be more enlightened than our FDA.

The Cunningham Sanitarium was an institution that focused on clean-air breathing treatment. Air was pressurized (probably in the large tube-like apparatus to left of sphere) and pumped into the air-tight sphere, so that occupants inhaled air at 30 pounds per square inch. This is double normal sea level air pressure of 14.7 psi.

The theory was that the pressurized air, by providing double the normal oxygen concentration, would alleviate many diseases (wrongly attributed) to anaerobic bacteria, such as some cancers, diabetes, pernicious anemia, and others. It was built in 1928, only eight miles east of the industrial heart of Cleveland, near East 185th Street at 18485 Lake Shore Boulevard. Named after a Kansas City physician specializing in hyperbaric oxygenation (or "tank treatment,") Doctor Orval J. Cunningham, and funded by Canton-based Timken Roller Bearings Company's owner Henry H. Timken, the Sanitarium's coastal property was chosen because it was aesthetically pleasing.

Dr. Cunningham based his treatment on the belief that diabetes and cancer are caused by living organisms that fail to grow in the presence of oxygen. Therefore, by increasing the oxygen, the organisms fail to multiply and eventually die off. To do this accurately, Cunningham would sequester his patients in highly oxygenated environments for long periods of time cycled with periods of normal atmospheric conditions.

The American Medical Association severely challenged his claims. In May, 1928 (while the tank was under construction), the AMA Journal published a negative assessment of Dr. Cunningham's hyperbaric treatments.

Although not stated in the AMA review, the extra oxygen afforded by the high atmospheric pressure could just as easily — and far more cheaply — have been delivered from a tank of pressurized oxygen delivered to the patient under ambient atmospheric oxygen tension of 21%Oxygen therapy under ambient air oxygen concentrations was certainly available in the 1920s, though not widely used (see Haldane's work from the 1920s). In any case, the Cunningham Steel Ball fell into disrepute among the AMA, and was no longer used after a few short years and sold for scrap metal for the war effort.

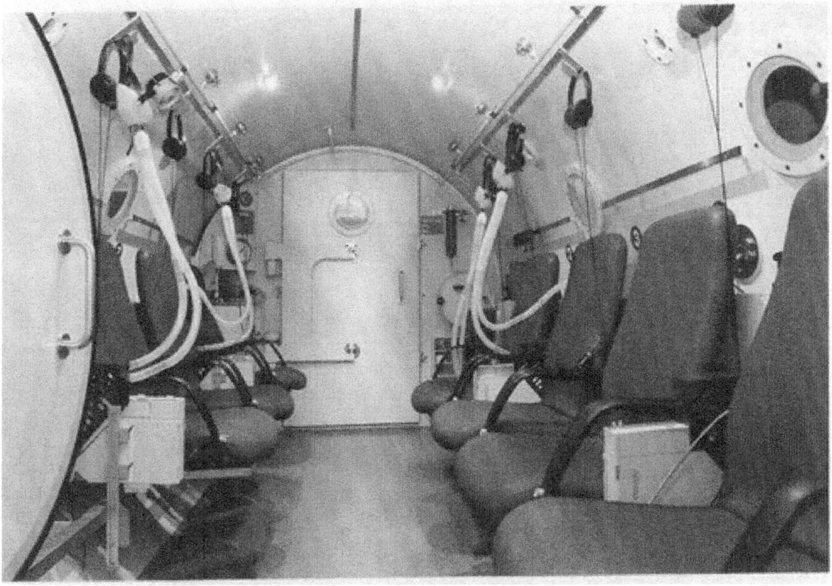

A large modern large hyperbaric chamber in Maroussi, Athens

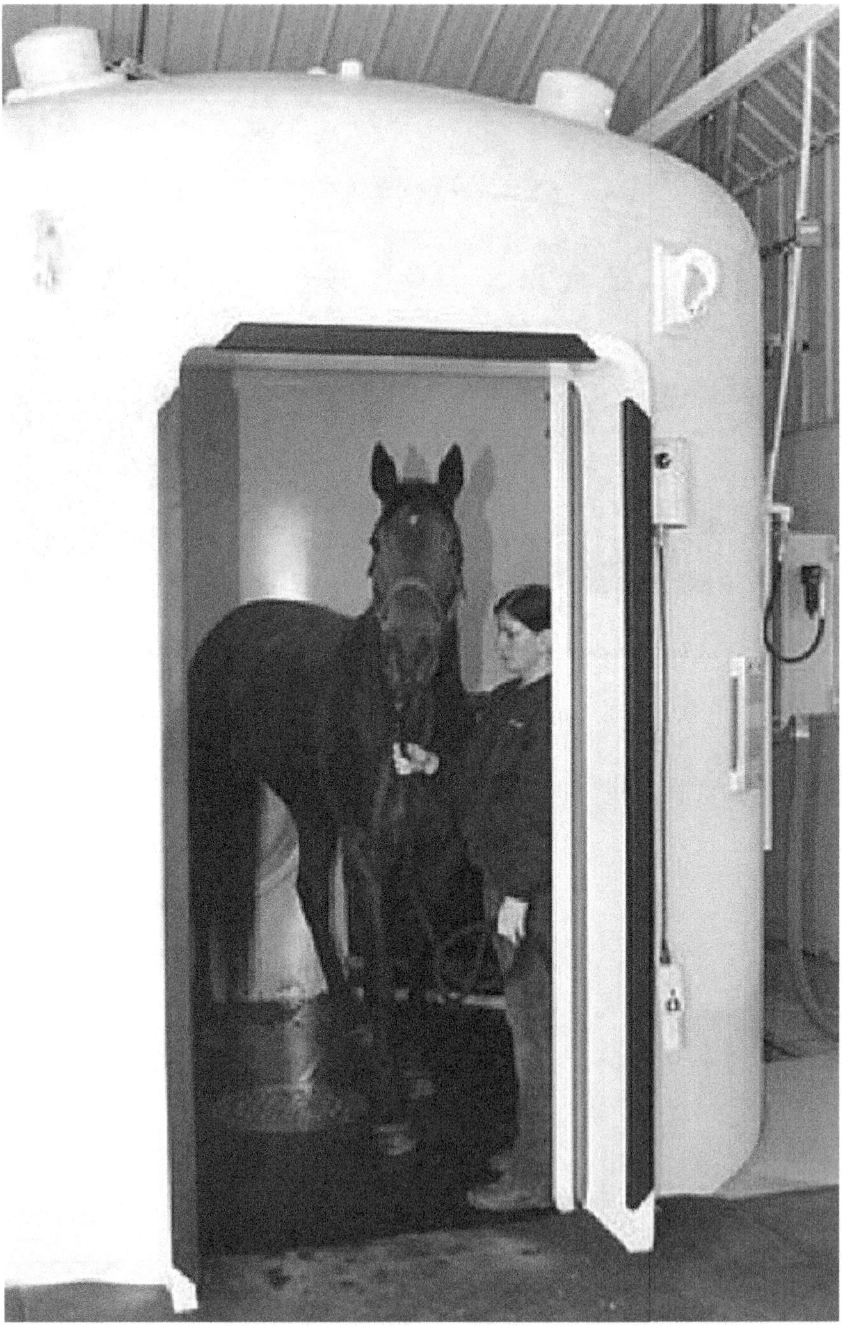

A hyperbaric chamber built for $ 20 million dollar horses that become injured or acquire infections while training for the Kentucky Derby. The horse and the horse's trainer (and friend) are both about to enjoy a hyperbaric "dive" together in this horse-sized hyperbaric chamber. The chambers of the Kentucky Derby primarily treat leg injuries which HBOT can repair in half the time of any other known treatment.

HBOT is currently showing almost 100% cure rates for COVID-9 in current ongoing trials in China, New Orleans, Wisconsin, and elsewhere.

Oxygen was not discovered until the mid-1800's nor was it able to be used or handled until the 1930's effectively. In the past several years, there has been a rebirth of HBT (Hyperbaric Therapy, not Hyperbaric oxygen therapy or HBOT)-only the pressure is used with ambient 21% normal atmospheric oxygen, and in a recent trial in Canada in the context of cerebral palsy, a control group was dived at normox (21%) concentrations, alongside an experimental group that was dived at 2.0 ATA with 60% O2 and both groups exhibited similar degrees of recovery. This is very significant because if this is the case, and only pressure is required using normox levels of oxygen gas, the process eliminates all danger of oxygen use and transport and also eliminates the costs of oxygen storage. Physiologically, the result also suggests that it is not so much the amount of oxygen that is at the basis of all of these ischemic syndromes mentioned in Dr. Maxfield's list, but it is the access of normal atmospheric oxygen into the tissues that is at the basis of avoidance and reversals of all of these syndromes.

New studies have shown, seductively, that 100% O2 may not be needed to reverse cerebral palsy, or any malady currently treated using 100% O2 under pressure, because normox oxygen concentrations (21% O2) were recently used in a cerebral palsy clinical trial as a control for the 100% O2 experimental group, only to find that the long-term outcome for both groups, the 100% 2ATA group, and the

21% O2 2ATA group, did equally well and significantly improved by a number of criteria.

Hyperbaric oxygen has a 300+ year history of safety, with only 2 reported deaths in the US due to an explosion before more stringent precautions were put into place to avoid sparks in the chambers that use 100% O2.

There are currently a number of new articles and clinical trials including several at the NIH for the validation and promotion of HBOT in the context of SARS-CoV-2 and atypical pneumonias which have emerged and which continue to validate the claim that HBOT is medicine's best kept secret. Listed below are several of them:

Ciceri F, Beretta L, Scandroglio AM, Colombo S, Landoni G, Ruggeri A, Peccatori J, D'Angelo A, De Cobelli F, Rovere-Querini P, Tresoldi M, Dagna L, Zangrillo A (2020) Microvascular COVID-19 lung vessels obstructive thromboinflammatory syndrome (MicroCLOTS): an atypical acute respiratory distress syndrome working hypothesis. Crit Care Resusc, April 15. Online ahead of print.

Conti P, Ronconi G, Caraffa A, Gallenga CE, Ross R, Frydas I, Kritas SK (2020) Induction of pro-inflammatory cytokines (IL-1 and IL-6) and lung inflammation by coronavirus-19 (COVI-19 or SARS-CoV.

De Maio A, Hightower LE (2020) COVID-19, acute respiratory distress syndrome (ARDS), and hyperbaric oxygen therapy (HBOT): what is the link? Cell Stress Chaperones 18:1–4. https://doi.org/10.1007/s12192-020-01121-0. Online ahead of print

Moon RE, Weaver LK (2020) Hyperbaric oxygen as a treatment for COVID-19 infection? Undersea Hyperb Med 47(2):177–179.

Milovanova TN, Bhopale VM, Sorokina EM, Moore JS, Hunt TK, Hauer-Jensen M, Velazquez OC, Thom SR (2009) Hyperbaric oxygen stimulates vasculogenic stem cell growth and differentiation in vivo. J Appl Physiol (1985) 106(2):711–728.

Thom SR, Bhopale VM, Velazquez OC, Goldstein LJ, Thom LH, Buerk DG (2006) Stem cell mobilization by hyperbaric oxygen. Am J Physiol Heart Circ Physiol 290(4):H1378–H1386.

Peng Z, Wang S, Huang X, Xiao P (2012) Effect of hyperbaric oxygen therapy on patients with herpes zoster. Undersea Hyperb Med 39(6):1083–1087.

Bosco G, Vezzani G, Mrakic Sposta S, Rizzato A, Enten G, Abou-Samra A, Malacrida S, Quartesan S, Vezzoli A, Camporesi E (2018) Hyperbaric oxygen therapy ameliorates osteonecrosis in patients by modulating inflammation and oxidative stress. J Enzyme Inhib Med Chem 33(1):1501–1505.

ECHM-EUBS (2020) Position statement on the use of HBOT for treatment of COVID-19 patients. http://www.eubs.org/?p=1163. Accessed on 1 May 2020.

Gardin C, Bosco G, Ferroni L, Quartesan S, Rizzato A, Tatullo M, Zavan B (2020) Hyperbaric oxygen therapy improves the osteogenic and vasculogenic properties of mesenchymal stem cells in the presence of inflammation in vitro. Int J Mol Sci 21(4):1452

Gabrilovich DI, Musarov AL, Zmyzgova AV, Shalygina NB (1990) The use of hyperbaric oxygenation in treating viral hepatitis B and the reaction of the blood leukocytes. Ter Arkh 62(1):82–86.

Giamarellos-Bourboulis EJ, Netea MG, Rovina N, Akinosoglou K, et al. (2020) Complex immune dysregulation in COVID-19 patients with severe respiratory failure. Cell Host Microbe S1931–S3128(20):30236–30235.

Guo D, Pan S, Wang MM, Guo Y (2020) Hyperbaric oxygen therapy may be effective to improve hypoxemia in patients with severe COVID-2019 pneumonia: two case reports. Undersea Hyperb Med 47(2):177–183.

Kim KS, Jung H, Shin IK, Choi BR, Kim DH (2015) Induction of interleukin-1 beta (IL-1) is a critical component of lung inflammation during influenza A (H1N1) virus infection. J Med Virol 87(7):1104–1112.

Kowalewski M, Fina D, Słomka A, Raffa GM, Martucci G, Lo Coco V, De Piero ME, Ranucci M, Suwalski P, Lorusso R (2020) COVID-19 and ECMO: the interplay between coagulation and inflammation-a narrative review. Crit Care 24(1):205.

Lodigiani C, Iapichino G, Carenzo L, Cecconi M, Ferrazzi P, Sebastian T, Kucher N, Studt JD, Sacco C, Alexia B, Sandri MT, Barco S, Humanitas COVID-19 Task Force (2020) Venous and arterial thromboembolic complications in COVID-19 patients admitted to an academic hospital in Milan, Italy. Thromb Res 191:9–14.

Mehta P, McAuley DF, Brown M, Sanchez E, Tattersall RS, Manson JJ, HLH Across Speciality Collaboration, UK (2020) COVID-19: consider cytokine storm syndromes and immunosuppression. Lancet 395(10229):1033–1034.

Below are listed 4 HBOT clinical trials that are recruiting or are already in progress world-wide, as well as several ongoing trials with other promising approaches as listed below:

1. **Hyperbaric Oxygen Therapy Effect in COVID-19 RCT (HBOTCOVID19).** Recruiting. Sponsor Assaf-Harofeh Medical Center. April 24, 2020. Interventional study. Randomized. Parallel Assignment intervention model. ClinicalTrials.gov.
2. **A Randomized, Controlled, Open Label, Multicentre Clinical Trial to explore Safety and Efficacy of Hyperbaric Oxygen for preventing ICU admission, Morbidity, and Mortality in Adult Patients with COVID-19.** Deutsches Register Klinischer Stuidien. No. 5.1-2020-36673, Swedish Medical Products Agency. 05.11.2020. Primary Registry ID: NCT04327505 (clinical trials.gov).
3. **Safety and Efficacy of Hyperbaric Oxygen for ARDS in Patients with COVID-19 (COVID-19-HBO).** Sponsor: Karolinska Institutet. University of California, San Diego, Blekinge County Council Hospital, JK Biostatistics AB, The Swedish Research Council. Purpose: To evaluate if HBO reduces the number of ICU admissions compared to best practice for COVID-19. ClinicalTrials.gov.
4. **Management by Hyperbaric Oxygen Therapy of Patients with Hypoxemic Pneumonia With SARS-CoV-2 (COVID-19).**

Sponsor: Direction Centrale du Service de Sante des Armees. Completion date: May, 2021. Purpose: To test HBOT's ability to limit the risk of respiratory decompensation requiring admission to intensive care units for patients with SARS-CoV-2. Clinical trials identifier: NCT04344431. ClinicalTrials.gov.

Another highly successful approach to 19 SARS-CoV-2 has been infusions of high-dose vitamin C. SARS-CoV-2 clinical trials were recently registered on clinicaltrials.gov (Identifier: NCTO 4264533), and which is a new clinical trial to investigate vitamin C **infusion** for the treatment of severe 2019-nCoV infected pneumonia victims.

High-dose C infusions are also being pursued in Wuhan, China and which has been one of the first clinical trials to test the effects of IV vitamin C in patients infected with this virus that first reported successes in the ranges of 100%. High-dose vitamin C with HBOT, and other measures to increase oxygenation also hold promise for a host of reasons as described by the following reports, and vitamin C should be consumed by all humans anyway for too many reasons to list:

Fowler AA, 3rd, Truwit JD, Hite RD, et al. **Effect of vitamin C infusion on organ failure and biomarkers of inflammation and vascular injury in patients with sepsis and severe acute respiratory failure: the CITRIS-ALI randomized clinical trial**. JAMA; 322(13):1261–1270, 2019.

A new clinical trial to test high-dose vitamin C in patients with COVID-19 is being undertaken in China and elsewhere to assess the rectification of apparent vitamin C deficits in critically ill atypical pneumonia patients was described by Anita Carr in the journal, Critical Care (24: 133, 2020) describing the frequent finding of vitamin C hypovitaminosis that is known to affect many critically ill syndromes, and especially those associated with pulmonary distress as is the case with SARS-CoV-2. Moreover, Carr described that despite high dosing with vitamin C have vitamin C deficiency, victims still suffered from a lack of vitamin C, and in the journal, she described the frequent finding of vitamin C hypovitaminosis that is known to affect many critically ill syndromes, and especially those associated with pulmonary distress as is the case with SARS-CoV-2. (Carr AC, Rosengrave PC, Bayer S, Chambers S, Mehrtens J, Shaw GM. Hypovitaminosis C and vitamin C deficiency in critically ill patients despite recommended enteral and parenteral intakes. Crit Care 21:300, 2017; also see: Carr AC. Critical Care (24: 133, 2020).

In this trial, the investigators will treat 140 patients with a placebo control or intravenous vitamin C at a dose of 24 g/day for 7 days. They are assessing the requirements for mechanical ventilation and vasopressor drugs, organ failure scores, ICU length of stay and 28-day mortality. The investigators of the new study hope to complete the trial by the end of September. Although the findings of this trial will be too late for the many thousands of people currently infected with the virus, the study will provide valuable information as to the potential mitigation of symptoms by vitamin C during ongoing and future viral outbreaks.

Another therapeutic that claims to achieve a near 100% success rate for the most compromised atypical pneumonia SARS victims, and which has a rational mechanistic basis has been reported to be an inhaled nebulized steroid, called Budesonide. This approach's reported success underscores the hypothesis that it is the victim's response to the viral antigen rather than the antigen itself that causes the demise of the individual via inflammation. An inhaled nebulized steroid, budesonide, if indeed it has efficacy and is widely verified through empirical experience, would indeed be a rational approach to treating the most compromised of the atypical pneumonia SARS CoV-2 victims.

It has also been claimed that nebulized hydrogen peroxide plus high-dose vitamin C also has shown efficacy, and although not as reliable for the desired result of immediate lung clearance, hydroxychloroquine has been successful in many cases. The principal problem with respirators is that they do not provide enough oxygen to the atypical pneumonia SARS CoV-2 victim, and if no other intervention is applied while a face mask is in place, the victim slowly simply becomes increasingly hypoxic.

Lack of sunlight-driven cutaneous production of about 1000 IU vitamin D3 or a lack of vitamin D supplements in food also has been shown to be associated with epidemics of different syndromes including influenzas, but most visibly with epidemics of rickets which was thought to be due to a communicable pathogen. (Michael F. Holick.The vitamin D epidemic and its health consequences. J Nutr 2005 Nov; 135 (ll): 2739S-48S).

> **"There is mounting scientific evidence that implicates vitamin D deficiency with an increased risk of type I diabetes, multiple sclerosis, rheumatoid arthritis, hypertension, cardiovascular heart disease, and many common deadly cancers."**

Vitamin D deficiency causes poor mineralization of the collagen matrix in young children's bones leading to growth retardation and bone deformities known as rickets. In adults, vitamin D deficiency induces secondary hyperparathyroidism, which causes a loss of matrix and minerals, thus increasing the risk of osteoporosis and fractures. In addition, the poor mineralization of newly laid down bone matrix in adult bone results in the painful bone disease of osteomalacia. Vitamin D deficiency causes muscle weakness, increasing the risk of falling and fractures. Vitamin D deficiency also has other serious consequences on overall health and well-being.

If a population were deficient in vitamin D, it could appear as though a transmissible communicable agent might be responsible, without the science of nutrition guiding decisions to place the vitamin in milk following its discovery and isolation.

In a major 2017 collaborative study, 23 authors concluded that:

"25-hydroxyvitamin D supports induction of antimicrobial peptides in response to both viral and bacterial stimuli, suggesting a potential mechanism by which vitamin D inducible protection against respiratory pathogens might be mediated. Vitamin D metabolites have also been reported to induce other innate antimicrobial effector mechanisms, including induction of autophagy and synthesis of reactive nitrogen intermediates and reactive oxygen intermediates. These epidemiological and in vitro data have prompted numerous randomized controlled trials to determine whether vitamin D supplementation can decrease the risk of acute respiratory tract infection. A total of five aggregate data meta-analyses incorporating data from up to 15 primary trials have been conducted to date, of which two report statistically significant protective effects and three report no statistically significant effects. All but one of these aggregate data meta-analyses reported statistically significant heterogeneity of effect between primary trials.

The study, "Vitamin D supplementation to prevent acute respiratory tract infections: systematic review and meta-analysis of individual participant data", was published in the British Medical Journal on Feb. 5, 2017 (356: i6583) by Adrian R Martineau, professor of respiratory infection and immunity, David A Jolliffe, postdoctoral research fellow, Richard L Hooper, reader in medical statistics, Lauren Greenberg,medical statistician, John F Aloia, professor of medicine, Peter Bergman, associate professor,4 Gal Dubnov-Raz, consultant pediatrician, Susanna Esposito, professor of pediatrics, Davaasambuu Ganmaa, assistant professor, Adit A Ginde, professor of emergency medicine, Emma C Goodall, assistant professor, Cameron C Grant, associate professor, Christopher J Griffiths, professor of primary care, Wim Janssens, professor of pneumonology, Ilkka Laaksi, chief administrative medical officer, Semira Manaseki-Holland, senior clinical lecturer, David Mauger, professor of public health sciences and statistics, David R Murdoch, professor of pathology, Rachel Neale, associate professor, Judy R Rees, assistant professor, Steve Simpson, Jr, postdoctoral research fellow, Iwona Stelmach, professor of pediatric allergy, Geeta Trilok Kumar, associate professor, Mitsuyoshi Urashima, professor of molecular epidemiology, and

Carlos A Camargo, Jr, professor of emergency medicine, medicine, and epidemiology.

More recently, John C. Umhau MD on March 25, 2020 2020, published an article in MEDPAGE TODAY entitled, "Casting Sunlight on an Epidemic— **Is vitamin D a critical host factor to prevent COVID-19?"**

Dr. Umhau emphasized in his article that:

> "As a public health specialist at the National Institutes of Health, I outlined how a lack of sun-induced vitamin D in the winter and early spring leads to epidemic acute respiratory infections (and this probably includes COVID-19)."
>
> "That review, cited almost a thousand times, argued that groups with low vitamin D levels — the obese and the elderly and those with dark skin — may require 5,000 IU of vitamin D each day to obtain the 25-hydroxyvitamin D levels of 50 ng/mL that appear to protect against viral respiratory infection."
>
> "A government-sponsored research strategy to address this issue has not been developed, as officials explained that there was no mandate to explore an alternative to the existing vaccination program. However, other researchers picked up the ball and provided convincing evidence that vitamin D could reduce the incidence of acute respiratory infection."

Dr. Umhau also cited the international 2017 meta study cited above by stating that:

> "In 2017, *The BMJ* released a systematic review and meta-analysis using data from 25 randomized controlled trials. In these studies, the incidence of acute respiratory infection was evaluated in participant-level data from more than 11,000 participants given either vitamin D or placebo. The international team of authors concluded that vitamin D supplementation is safe and that it protects against acute respiratory tract infection."

Importantly, it has been widely broadcast by international media, and in a few prominent scientific journals reports that the first "epicenters" of SARS COVID-19 in Wuhan, China, and in Lambardo, Italy are among the most two polluted places on the continents of Asia and Europe, with air pollution levels increasingly measured at alarming amounts, which has been discussed many times in international reports. Such environmental toxins also could confound the perception of an epidemic or pandemic being the result of a contagious microbial pathogen of the respiratory tract.

SLOW VIROLOGISTS

In 1985, a year after the AIDS hoax was first announced, fears ran like wildfire throughout the biomedical community, especially among those who handled human blood products.

This was the beginning of the era of "slow virologists," and lab personnel who handled human tissues were warned about a deadly new threat to their everyday lives because of an unsubstantiated threat of prion diseases, which we were told could resist gamma radiation sterilization, autoclave sterilization (extreme pressurized steam), and all known pathogen drugs and inhibitors, and cause a fatal, debilitating Parkinsonian-like destruction of the brain in a year, shaking the person violently until they died.

This insanity about these slow virus-like entities, were given two Nobel Prizes as New Infectious Disease agents because they were thought to be transmitted by protein rods that caused polymerization of a normal human cellular protein to form tangles and destruction of large areas of the brains of various ungulates (cows and sheep) and humans. The first of these Nobel Prizes went to D. Carlton Gajducek, who was a National Academy of Science Member, and The Neurobiology Section Chief at the NIH, after he announced his belief that he had found that proteins can behave as infectious agents without harboring any gene(s) or nucleic acid template. His discovery was then recreated experimentally in hamster animal model by UCSF's Stanley Pruisner, who also was later and separately awarded the Nobel Prize for his mechanistic clarification(s) of prions and prion generated neurological demise.

Pruisner had proposed a mechanism to explain Gajducek's findings that involved an interaction between an endogenous normal cellular protein he called PrP C (the "C" signified a normal "cellular protein" that was made by all non-afflicted persons or animals) which was also found in all non-afflicted and afflicted alike. Pruisner had argued that the normal "C" protein somehow was then abnormally polymerized to combine with the foreign, eaten form of PrP Sc of prion protein, and then rapidly form brain tangles resembling

Alzheimer's plaques after the exogenous was eaten by the Papua New Guinea tribesmen whom Gajducek had described and who practiced a ritual in which they ate the brain matter of deceased loved ones at some point prior to the onset of their symptoms. Once the prion protein was imbibed, it combined with the normal PrP C protein to form radiation and heat resistant rods that he called (PrP Sc for Scrapie-affected protein, which it was said, polymerized the endogenous PrPC protein in an unusual conformation). Carlton Gajducek, a member of The National Academy won a Nobel Prize in 1976.

The Nobel committee had recognized his discovery of an unorthodox form of "proteinaceous" replication or polymerization rather, as it was later justified as being because no nucleic acids could be found associated with its seeming replicative proliferation in the brains of its affected victims. These so-called "prion diseases thus were used to suggest that mad cow disease of cattle, scrapie in sheep, kuru in Papua New Guinea aboriginals, Creutzfeld-Jacob disease in Englishmen, and chimpanzees which Gadjucek had injected a 10% solution or slurry of ill-defined brain extracts into their brains all shared a common basis for the violent trembling and shaking Parkinsonian-like affliction that were now subsumed under the disease rubric of spongiform encephalopathies.

The musings of D. Carlton Gajducek and Pruisner, with their Nobel awards, begged the answers to several as yet unanswered questions at that time, as their "insights" as to proteinaceous replicating entities devoid of a nucleic acid cores, still does today, 44 years later, as to how an infectious agent can be transmissible or communicable? The prion era, also begged the question as to how a piece of DNA or RNA wrapped in the case of a "slow virus" as they were called, which was wrapped in a protein, could "wait" for 30-40 years, hiding in the tissues of an infected organism in the cases of other virus entities, and then suddenly explode into a full-blown disease with polymerizing brain tangles (how could a biochemical entity "wait" 40 years to interact with the cellular fluids and tissues of a host? Also, according to the musings of Gajducek and Pruisner, the PrP Sc agent was completely resistant to heat, gamma radiation, or any man-made approaches to sterilize against its activity of initiating polymerization of host endogenous normal PrP C protein, or possibly never be vanquished to the point even using autoclaved equipment and go on to infect any biomedical researchers who happened across a Creutzfeld-Jacob-contaminated blood sample or tissue.

Some years later, a farmer named Mark Purdy wrote an article that solved the riddle of why cattle in Britain were being afflicted by the horrible "new" fatal and neurodegenerative "shaking to their deaths" was due to herbicide poisoning of cattle and other livestock troughs from a new fertilizer that contained a solvent, and proposed that the human "kuru" syndrome seen among the Papua New Guinea tribesmen and the rare Creutzfeld-Jacob syndrome among Europeans were due to a genetically-inherited defect in the endogenous PrPC gene.

The human similar neurodegenerative disease such as kuru and Creutzsfeld-Jacob syndrome, were shown later to have been likely inherited in highly inbred and isolated populations, yet it was argued by the spongiform encephalopathy apologists like Gadjudcek and Pruisner, and most of the virological community, that these proteinaceous prion Sc rods were capable of both infectious and genetic transmission, which defied all rules of infectious diseases.

And also, at that time, the "HIV/AIDS" hysteria began as the invented solution to the determined efforts to justify the fruitless search for a cancer-causing virus by Robert Gallo, and by others in their attempts to constrain the sexual revolutions taking place during those decades. As with the general population, the prion and "HIV" myths were received by the biomedical research community as truths. The specter of prion diseases and "HIV" as slow viruses and virus-like agents generated not only fear of hamburgers, as entire beef herds were slaughtered to combat prions, but the same reasoning ignited terror that if tainted blood were contacted, that "HIV" does not discriminate, resulting in nothing less than a form of terrorism perpetrated not only on average citizens, but also in the steel and glass laboratories housed in the Churches of Modern Biomedical research. The extent to which this distorted logic terrorized many basic and applied biological researchers into quitting their pursuit of a medical research career cannot be underestimated. Both the prescription and illicit drug industries, along with the stigma of possibly acquiring "HIV," literally wiped out a generation of men due to AZT and other toxins, as well as the nitrosamines some of them consumed to "enhance" their "fast-track" lifestyles. It is well known even among pharmaceutical advocates that the high dose and non-cycled usage of AZT caused cancers in less than 3 years, and that the protease inhibitors caused buffalo humps, organ failure, and the sunken wasted faces of the victims of these rank poisons.

THE HUMAN CONSEQUENCES OF FALSE-POSITIVE DIAGNOSES

Direct confirmatory ultrastructural testing following PCR or WESTERN-blot analysis of blood from the same patient's blood draw may help eliminate the problem of false positive pathogen testing in a number of contexts and eliminate medical conundrums wherein indirect protein or nucleic acid testing detects proteins that mimic non-disease-associated proteins or nucleic acids in persons in ill-health, but not infected. Furthermore, an awareness of these issues, it is hoped, will usher in a new conceptual framework regarding all microbial pathogens, but more importantly, help change our entrenched and often erroneous conceptions about causality in human health or disease.

One success I enjoyed which did involve the courts was when I was asked to be the chief scientific advisor to Audrey Serrano- the very-first AIDS patient who had her positive HIV diagnosis and lab test overturned in court by a jury of her peers. She was awarded $2.5 million dollars for the incorrect diagnosis and having to take AIDS drugs for 9 years of her life. She suffers permanent internal health damage from the side effects of the toxic AIDS drugs she took for those 9 years.

Mrs. Audrey Serrano is a 42-year-old woman who had one "HIV" Enzyme-Linked Immunosorbent Assay (EIA) test "lost or misplaced" by her physicians in 1994. Following this "lost or misplaced test," she discovered that her wrong date of birth and social security number was on a subsequent "HIV" EIA report form, and she was never given a confirmatory Western Blot (WB) after the first allegedly positive EIA. She has subsequently tested negative on all EIA's, and repeated Polymerase Chain Reaction (PCR) tests of various types have yielded undetectable levels of "HIV" RNA for the past 9 years. Her T-cell count has hovered around 600-800 for 9 years (which is at the low normal range).

However, from the time that the allegedly positive "HIV" EIA was performed in 1994, and although she was healthy by all criteria,

Mrs. Serrano was immediately prescribed AZT and then HAART (Highly Active Anti-Retroviral Therapy) as though she were "HIV-positive" without informed consent regarding the toxicity profiles of these medications, and even though her T-cell counts were in the low normal range. Upon being placed on HAART after the first allegedly positive "HIV" EIA, she also was simultaneously prescribed bactrim continuously for 9 years, and antidepressants for the first several years after her allegedly positive "HIV" test, despite the fact that similar antidepressant medications had previously generated suicidal thoughts and actions on at least 3 occasions during her interment by DCFS in her youth.

During her "treatment" with the "LIFE-SAVING HAART cocktail" and the antidepressants, she suffered constant diarrhea, muscle wasting, profound fatigue, non-specific skin lesions of various types, bouts of oral thrush (oral candidiasis) herpes outbreaks, severe nose-bleeds, constant gynecological bleeding and pain due to ovarian cysts, fibrocystic breast lesions, hyperplastic pituitary lesions, and severe heart and respiratory difficulties. She has no uterus, as it was removed due to one of her doctor's urging because of her persistent gynecological bleeding and abdominal pain while on HAART and the other medicines.

Since 2003, and after she obtained 6 negative "HIV" EIA's from Bioran Laboratories and from Fallon Clinic, she has refused the "HIV" medications, bactrim, and antidepressant medications. Yet despite her discontinuing all the medications, she has been subsequently diagnosed with irritable bowel syndrome, colitis, and she wakes up most every morning with new bruises on her body. She cannot maintain her weight and is thus still experiencing wasting syndrome.

Because she is unemployed, she cannot currently afford the types of supplements that might help her gain weight or treat her bruising syndrome. The pituitary lesions, ovarian cysts, and fibrocystic breast disease that she developed while on the medications are apparently "in remission." She still experiences severe nosebleeds and angina for which she takes nitroglycerin as needed. In addition, she developed severe asthma and bronchitis while on HAART, for which she takes albuterol and inhalant bronchial medications of various types as needed. Her primary care doctors at U. Mass and elsewhere claimed that Mrs. Serrano knew all along that she was "HIV" negative.

Mrs. Serrano has a High School Diploma, a degree in electronics, a diploma as a paralegal, several certificates in dealing with children with special needs, and has acquired certificates in Special Education, and is currently active in the foundation she has created from ground up, "Families Against Abuse." She maintains a loving household with her mother for her adopted and now teenage daughter Jessica, as she now continues to battle to regain her health. Finally, during Mrs. Serrano's "treatment," her daughter (her adopted niece) was taken from her for 2 years out of fear that Mrs. Serrano would irresponsibly transmit "HIV" to her (despite her negative EIA's and undetectable "viral load" test results throughout).

During this time, Audrey's niece (Jessica) was physically assaulted in the custody of DCFS (Department of Child and Family Services), given 2 documented STD's, and was forced to take Thorazine, Ritalin, Benzedrine, Klonopin, and other medications to control her behavior. Jessica now experiences severe emotional issues.

Despite the fact that all the "HIV" test kits specifically state that, "This test is not intended for use as a diagnostic test to diagnose HIV in any person" (because no HIV test kit has been validated against a pure "HIV" isolate, or even impure isolate without designating it by the electron microscope facility directors as cellular garbage, and thus according to the FDA and rules of classical virus isolation and antibody generation, such non-validated tests cannot and have not be used in any context to proclaim someone as "HIV" positive, and an "HIV-expert's" judgment about the victim's self-reported behavior is still relied upon to obtain an "HIV" or AIDS diagnosis).

All of the following events, and many other more tragic ones not mentioned below have happened to Mrs. Serrano (and her adopted daughter) in the absence of any positive "HIV" test result since the initial 1994 EIA (Enzyme-Linked-Immunosorbent Assay) which was "lost or misplaced."

But to this day, and according to the "AIDS surveillance definitions," Audrey now exhibits a host of AIDS-defining illnesses, without ever having tested positive for "HIV," and without ever presenting an electron micrograph of her "virus."

Audrey's lack of malignant cancer progression also defies theories regarding the initiation, promotion, and development of cancer because of the cancer promoting drug, AZT they made her consume by court order for 9 years. Although these kinds of consequences have not yet visited our COVID-19 Pandemic's victims, there are discussions regarding 14-day quarantines in place in multiple nations (New Zealand, Canada, and the US), and discussions about establishing "internment camps" have recently begun to surface at the highest level of government, and of course, in the media.

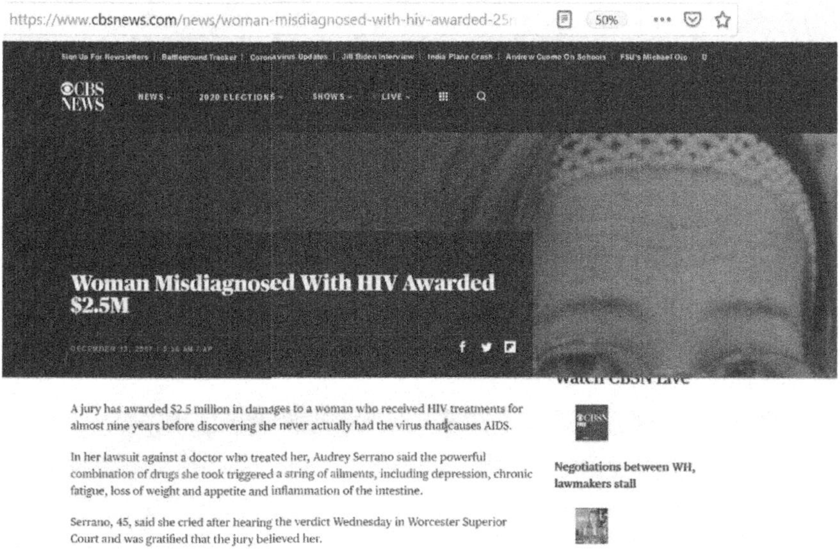

https://www.cbsnews.com/news/woman-misdiagnosed-with-hiv-awarded-25

Sign Up For Newsletters | Battleground Tracker | Coronavirus Updates | Jill Biden Interview | India Plane Crash | Andrew Cuomo On Schools | FSU's Michael Ojo

CBS NEWS — NEWS · 2020 ELECTIONS · SHOWS · LIVE

Woman Misdiagnosed With HIV Awarded $2.5M

A jury has awarded $2.5 million in damages to a woman who received HIV treatments for almost nine years before discovering she never actually had the virus that causes AIDS.

In her lawsuit against a doctor who treated her, Audrey Serrano said the powerful combination of drugs she took triggered a string of ailments, including depression, chronic fatigue, loss of weight and appetite and inflammation of the intestine.

Serrano, 45, said she cried after hearing the verdict Wednesday in Worcester Superior Court and was gratified that the jury believed her.

Negotiations between WH, lawmakers stall

FOX NEWS

Coronavirus U.S. World Opinion Politics More Watch TV

Hot Topics

ANTHONY FAUCI · **Published** 12 hours ago · **Last Update** 9 hours ago

Fauci on US after coronavirus: No shaking hands 'ever again'

By **Dom Calicchio | Fox News**

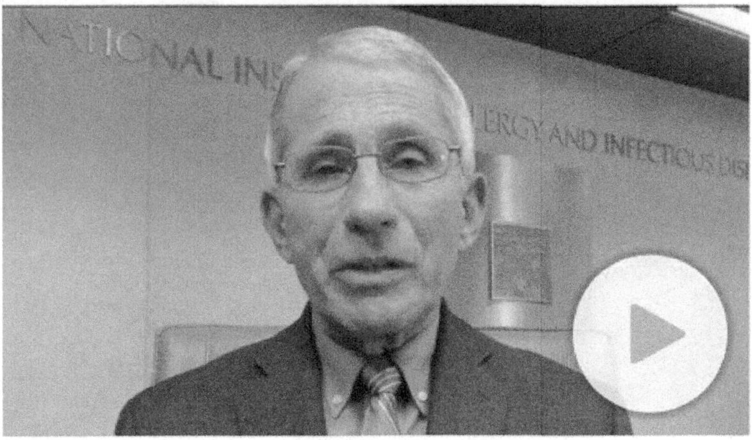

LAB TESTING FOR COVID-19 AND THE PROBLEM OF FALSE POSITIVES AND THE LESSONS LEARNED FROM HIV TESTING MISTAKES WHILE THE WORLD HEALTH ORGANIZATION DELETES NATURALLY ACQUIRED IMMUNITY FROM THEIR WEBSITE AND RECOGNIZES ONLY VACCINATION AS A MEANS OF ACQUIRING TRUE IMMUNITY

On December 23, 2020, Jeffrey A. Tucker, who is Editorial Director for the American Institute for Economic Research published a provocative article entitled **WORLD HEALTH ORGANIZATION DELETES NATURALLY ACQUIRED IMMUNITY FROM THEIR WEBSITE** (The coordinates for Mr. Tucker can be found here https://www.aier.org/jeffrey-tucker-aier-editorial-director/). He paints a frightening picture of how science has been decapitated as if it were a man on a horse without a head:

"As many ecological models are based upon economic ideas, herd immunity is a fascinating observation that you can trace to biological reality or statistical probability theory, whichever you prefer. (It is certainly not a "strategy" so ignore any media source that describes it that way). Herd immunity speaks directly, and with explanatory power, to the empirical observation that respiratory viruses are either widespread and mostly mild (common cold) or very severe and short-lived (Ebola).Why is this?"

"The reason is that when a virus kills its host – that is, when a virus overtaxes the body's ability to integrate it, its host dies and so the virus does not spread to others. The more this occurs, the less it spreads."

"If the virus does not kill its host, it can hop to others through all the usual means. When you get a virus and fight it off, your immune system encodes that information in a way that builds immunity to it. When it happens to enough people (and each case is different so we cannot put a clear number on it, especially given so many cross immunities), the virus loses its pandemic quality and becomes endemic, which is to say predictable and manageable."

"Each new generation incorporates that information through more exposure. This is what one would call Virology/Immunology 101. It is what you read in every textbook. It's been taught in 9th grade cell biology for probably 80 years."

"The WHO's pre-October 12, 2020 definition correctly states the textbook definition of herd immunity in half of the definition, whereas, in the other half of the definition, they evoke vaccination as a condition of generating herd immunity for which there is no evidence that this is the case as will become clear:

Pre-October 12, 2020

"Herd immunity is the indirect protection from an infectious disease that happens when a population is immune **either** through vaccination or immunity developed through previous infection. This means that even people who have not been infected, or in whom an infection has not triggered an immune response, they are protected because people around them who are immune can act as **buffers between them and an infected person."**

Post October 12, 2020

'Herd immunity' also known as 'population immunity,' is a concept **used for vaccination**, in which a population can be protected from certain virus **if a <u>threshold of vaccination is reached</u>.** Herd immunity is achieved by protecting people from a virus, **NOT BY EXPOSING THEM TO IT.** Vaccines train our immune systems to develop antibodies, just as **might happen** when we are exposed to a disease, but-crucially-vaccines work without making us sick..."

THE THRESHOLD FOR ESTABLISHING HERD IMMUNITY FOR SARS-COVID-19 IS NOT YET CLEAR

Although the WHO's pre-October 12 definition includes vaccines as the source and cause of herd immunity, naturally acquired immunity has been deleted in the post of October, 12, 2020 as shown by the two definitions that Tucker presented. Nature's naturally acquired herd immunity loses all importance after October 12, 2020, and in fact is not even mentioned. Herd immunity becomes solely linked to vaccination (which as the WHO asserts "don't of course make us sick like the naturally acquired pathogen would" (unless you belong to the 90-99% majority of the resistant population who would never acquire it in the first place which is not mentioned)!

How could living systems have survived without vaccinations for almost a billion years without being vaccinated, including the 99.999999% of our Hominid past before either the advent of inoculations or vaccines were foisted at us? For a year we have been indoctrinated with the litany that "the FINAL SOLUTION," indeed, the ONLY solution and hope for the COVID-19 pandemic is the Moderna, Pfizer-BioNTech, Bayer, and a blizzard of other vaccines. Seemingly, as it is the case with all diseases, the answer always is vaccination, period.

Some of the same experts of past National and International health "crises" of the bird flu, H1N1, and AIDS era have been beating the drums the loudest, that the final solution to SARS-COVID-19 will be the vaccines currently being cooked against this SARS-CoV-2 coronavirus, and that these vaccines have already been deployed by the tens of millions. Officials believe SARS-CoV-2 is the primary "cause" of the atypical pneumonia because its detection has been linked to an explosion of a cytokine storm host response in < about 0.04-0.1% of "test positives" with morbid symptoms. Yet the SARS-CoV-2 molecular fingerprint is only associated with mild illness in most "positives" or is expressed in a majority of completely asymptomatic "carriers." Among the 0.04-1% who experience the full-blown atypical pneumonia or hypoxemia as it is called, it is believed that the SARS-CoV-2 virus leads to a rapidly progressive and sometimes fatal atypical pneumonia in two to five days, which is "the crisis window" of most concern. However, other coronavirus-like particles have been observed in the gastrointestinal tract, vascular tissues, in the liver, spleen, and in other tissues, suggesting there is much to learn about the dynamics, molecular identity, and various manifestations and tissue tropisms of SARS-CoV-2 and coronaviruses in general. Also, much has been written regarding the phenomenon of "enhancement" due to flu vaccines generally, and certain SARS vaccines specifically, suggesting that caution is warranted in order to avoid killing vaccine recipients with "enhanced" lung infiltrates due to various vaccine's effects that are primarily attributed to eosinophil infiltrates.

These issues have emerged primarily because of modern molecular testing, which is increasingly used and trusted to inform and then to guide critical therapeutic decisions. A more informed awareness needs to be in place that does not exist yet in current standards of care regarding testing. What do positive and negative tests really mean, and how should they be interpreted to better assure the safety and effectiveness of therapeutic interventions in those rare victims of COVID who are symptomatic and have a 12-hour window to somehow acquire enough oxygen to support life (PaO2/FiO2-dissolved oxygen in the blood/amount of available oxygen)?

Although during health crises such as COVID-19 there sometimes is an acute urgency to abandon standards of care and medical intervention successfully used in the past in the hopes that some panacea will emerge to somehow cheat death itself. Direct pathogen testing using EM (electron microscopy to detect actual viremia at high resolution) can be definitive in weeding out the false positive lab test results generated from indirect testing, and with some volunteers willing to pin down the transmissibility issues as Rosenau tried to do, the crisis and profound morbid cases may be better helped therapeutically.

To understand what is wrong with most current, inaccurate,

COVID-19 testing, one must understand that the pathogen isolation protocols themselves are confounded by cellular debris, including breakdown products from sick or dying cells that shed both decaying genomic fragments and proteins, which complex with these nucleic acid fragments to resemble viruses, or they can appear different immunologically to the victim's own immune system, and exacerbate cytokine storms, and massive inflammation, which is what really kills the victims according to the SARS-CoV-2 "experts." Historically since the polio era, whenever baffling conditions or complex health issues arise, objects that are below light's visible wave-lengths are usually blamed. This has been problematic since the time of Koch and Hill, even before the technology of electron microscopy (**EM**) was invented in the late 1930's, and this holds true still today. When it is tacitly assumed that some kind of unfounded faith in biological causality exists in sequence identity comparisons, and the unbridled and undeserved faith in molecular testing warrants anything resembling certainty of function, there clearly has not been sufficient skepticism to be of much use to guide diagnostic interpretations, not to mention therapeutic decision making based on those interpretations.

It is difficult to contemplate how molecular diagnostic detection of entities like "HERVs" ("Human Endogenous Retroviral Sequences," "retroelements," "retroids," "phages") which are normal resident RNA sequences in our genomes can determine the fate of people's lives, or how these molecular sequences are used to incarcerate folks if they were aware they were "positive" for a sexually-transmitted pathogen without telling a partner and proven in court as was the case with "HIV," but this is the current state of affairs. These molecular sequence phenomena could simply represent decay products that mimic nucleic acid sequences of various pathogens. Thus, the need for a direct pathogen detection method is needed.

Are serology-obtained biochemical indicators of nucleic acids or proteins in any way identical to direct measure of actual visible viable pathogens? Let us begin to answer this question and begin this analysis with what a few of the SARS CoV-2 expert testers are reporting.

In one of the more thoughtful analyses of SARS-CoV-2 diagnostic testing, Stites, E.C., Wilen, CB., (The Interpretation of SARS-CoV-2 Diagnostic Tests, Med 2020.08.001) make important observations regarding several aspects of test interpretation that "*are incompletely understood by medical communities and the general population, creating a significant challenge in minimizing the damage caused by disease spread through informed decision making and proper testing utilization.*" Some of these caveats include whether asymptomatic individuals should be tested, what it means to test positive (or negative), and how to interpret tests for "**immunity passports**." Yikes, Orwell is at the door!

They conclude by saying that "***Unexpectedly, the answers seem to run contrary to many of the popular narratives about testing as a tool for managing COVID-19.***"

First it is important to appreciate that there are two classes of tests to detect SARS CoV-2 and viruses in general: a nucleic acid test, which typically is obtained using PCR which detects fragments of stretches of RNA or DNA by first supposedly isolating them and amplifying them using the Polymerase Chain Reaction or PCR, and there are several types of PCR tests. There are also protein tests which will be discussed later. The major point to understand about the ***nucleic acid tests*** is that they are thought to detect *current or very recent infections,* although these tests are worthless during the first days of infection.

Nucleic acid amplification tests (NAAT) that measure viral RNA but do not utilize conventional PCR are also in use to detect the presence of CoV-2 RNA.

Viral antigen tests rely on immunoassays to measure specific viral ***proteins*** and are less sensitive than NAATs but may be faster to perform (NAATs can detect as few as 10 viral RNA fragments in a sample, but it is difficult to see the advantage in having such sensitivity).

However, Stites and Wilen caution that "*testing does not equate to a finer understanding of how testing is used and utilized because physicians struggle with the ability to properly interpret test results.*" A principal reason for this "hedging" is because Stites and Wilen appreciate that tests are not perfect because there are always false positives and false negatives, and as a consequence, test results cannot state definitively whether a disease (or virus) is or is not present. What this means is that tests need to be evaluated ***"probabilistically on the basis of test performance, test characteristics, patient data, and importantly, disease prevalence."***

Based on such measurements (the prevalence of disease in a community for example), the "*positive predictive value*" of a test can be ***"estimated."*** The positive predictive value is a probability that the person who tested positive actually has the disease. Similarly, "*negative predictive values*" can be calculated based on similar information to qualify the chance that someone who tested negative truly does not have the disease.

Stites and Wilen go on to point out that two key metrics that characterize the test are needed to interpret the results of imperfects tests: the diagnostic sensitivity and diagnostic specificity (or commonly just "sensitivity" and "specificity"), and currently, there is limited information on these values for widely used SARS-CoV-2 tests.

The probability of having a disease is a **"fairly subjective estimate" that a health care provider would make on the basis of medical history, presentation, and factors such as known prevalence of the disease in the community**. And the value is never exact.

To make matters worse, there is an extremely important issue to emphasize that has plagued many other so-called viral diseases that rely on indirect tests and molecular assumptions: the fact that there has been rapid development of new tests, and many of these tests have made their way into the clinical arena without the standard preclinical validation processes required by FDA. In other words, in the race to patent test kits, similar to what we are facing with the EUA (Emergency Use Authorization) of CoV-2 vaccines currently (fast-tracking without adequate testing), many small biotech companies see SARS CoV-2 as a golden opportunity to exploit the urgency of the situation, and not subject their tests to appropriate validation standards!

On February 2, 2020, the CDC was the only place in the country that could perform SARS-CoV-2 tests. But on February 12, the CDC announced that the test was providing inconclusive results. By then, The United States had reported 11 cases. In March, the CDC designed its own test, and the Food and Drug Administration picked a conservative testing strategy, allowing laboratories to use only the CDC tests distributed under the Emergency Use Authorization (EUA) authority (Sin Hang Lee. *Testing for SARS-CoV-2 in cellular components by routine nested RT-PCR followed by DNA sequencing*. International Journal of Geriatrics and Rehabilitation, 2 (1): 69-96, July 17, 2020).

One problem with all of this misdirected testing is the fact that instead of relying on direct isolation of virus using centrifuged blood or tissue samples followed by ultra-fine filtration followed by electron microscopic identification of viremia and then followed by re-infection and re-isolation to fulfill Koch's postulates that will show many virus particles/ electron microscope field of view, the testing so far has almost exclusively relied on indirect reverse transcription quantitative polymerase chain reaction (RT-qPCR) sequences published on the Internet. Another assay of these lung aspirates measures fluorescent signal accumulation as a surrogate for direct viral identification and is also known to generate false-negative and false positive results. Although the fluorescent signal accumulation surrogate is typically done with RtPCR product rather than actual virus and using these methods (not direct viral identification), an Australian group reported that the commercial PCR kit they used (RT-qPCR) found its positive predictive value to be only 55.56%, which if you think about it is like flipping a coin. Although this group went on to suggest that any positive results derived from one test should be confirmed using another nucleic acid test, what is the point if no test can be trusted? The gold standard has to be true isolation followed by electron microscopic verification that the chemical measurements are being derived from actual viral particles. Protein testing can be of two types.

The first type detects the protein coat of viruses, which isn't widely used, or used much at all, but the second type is used to determine if you have had a past infection, because it measures the carrier's (the host's) antibodies that are made against the antigen and in response to the [virus], and which requires typically anywhere from several weeks of exposure to the antigen to nearly a month in order to require the body's immune system time to make and begin to amplify the antibody to levels that it can be detected using protein blot tests, or ELISA (Enzyme Linked Immunosorbent Assays). These are the antibody tests.

However, with SARS-CoV-2. we run into some of the same issues as with nucleic acid testing with "HIV" because, for instance, the likely low prevalence of COVID-19 in the general population presents a challenge to protein tests also, and tests without extremely high accuracy could lead to large numbers of incorrect results, resulting in dangerous consequences FOR POPULATIONS. This has particularly disastrous consequences because of the insanity of the RT-PCR cycle debate, which is predicated on the fact that the amplification steps that RT-PCR uses are completely meaningless after about 25 amplifications or "cycles," yet many who have been tested have been diagnosed [and convicted] of harboring SARS-CoV-2 based on more than 35-40 cycles of amplification, again generating many false positives.

The challenge is that when testing for a disease with low prevalence in the tested populations, even a test with relatively high specificity will generate large numbers of false positives. In the case of SARS CoV-2 serology testing, this could mean that many people being told they have protective antibodies do not in fact have them and they are still susceptible to infection.

In the case of SARS-CoV-2, the question of specificity also is a challenging one given that there are several other common and harmless coronavirus-like particles to which many people probably already have antibodies. These existing antibodies can cross react with the antigens used in the SARS-CoV-2 test, leading to false positive results. Even our pet dogs and cats carry coronaviruses, so quit petting your dog and certainly do not teach your dog how to shake hands!

In fact, as it was during the "HIV" hysteria of testing of the 1980's and 1990's in a low prevalence population (which was the case with "HIV" because for one thing it did not exist in the first place), every "positive" result was a false positive. Adam Bonislawski gives a number of cogent examples of what this means, in a piece he wrote on April 16, 2020 for SARS-CoV-2. He interviewed a number of high-ranking officials in public health positions regarding testing, and it is worth reviewing what the gist of some of these Infectious Disease "Specialists" have concluded regarding COVID-19 mass testing. Kaitlyn Sadtier who is the Chief of the section for immunoengineering at the National Institutes of Biomedical Imaging and Bioengineering and a leader of a study launched by the NIH claimed that "*when you are looking at a large sample size with a lower prevalence, those false positives start to become much more of an issue,*" and Robert Garry, professor of microbiology at Tulane University School of Medicine likewise noted the issue about "*potential false positives in the low prevalence populations there will be more false positives than true positives.*"

As of July, 2020, more than **70** serology tests were available in the US under this EUA process for SARS-C0V-2, **and none of these tests are validated for SARS-COVID-19** (although there is at least one report which appeared in Nature in 2002 which did validate a test for 4 macaques using electron microscopic visualization of several viral-like SARS-CoV-2 particles in the monkey's necropsied lungs (Fouchier R et al., *Koch's postulates fulfilled for SARS virus,* Nature Vol 423 15 May 2003), although the authors point out that their study did not rule out other aetiologic agents such as Human metapneumovirus (HMPV) or Chlamydia pneumoniae may have exacerbated the disease in some SARS patients. The real issue is whether any test is of any value with victims with less severe symptoms or who are asymptomatic because The WHO says you do not need to get tested if you are asymptomatic (Katherine J. Wu, *New York Times,* 8/27/2020).

Going back to the Wuhan experience, as they were among the earliest hit and have the most experience, Zhaung GH, Shen MW, Zeng LX, MI BB, Chen FY Liu WJ, Pei LL, Qi X, and Li C. (Potential false-positive rate among the "asymptomatic infected individuals' in close contacts of COVID-9 patients) reported in an ahead of print article (Mar 5; 41 (4): 485-488,2020) that:

"When the infection rate of the close contacts and the sensitivity and specificity of reported results were taken as the point estimates, the positive predictive value of the active screening was only **19.67%,** in contrast the false-positive rate of positive results was **80.33%,** and nearly half or even more of the 'asymptomatic infected individuals' reported in the active nucleic acid test screening might be false positives."

LAB TESTING EPIDEMICS, PREVALENCE, AND FALSE-POSITIVES AND NEGATIVES HAVE PRECEDENTS IN "HIV" TESTING AND THE HUMAN CONSEQUENCES OF FALSE-POSITIVE DIAGNOSES

Direct confirmatory ultrastructural testing following PCR or WESTERN-blot analysis of blood from the same patient's blood draw may help eliminate the problem of false positive pathogen testing in a number of contexts and eliminate medical conundrums wherein indirect protein or nucleic acid testing detects proteins that mimic non-disease-associated proteins or nucleic acids in persons in ill-health, but not infected. Furthermore, an awareness of these issues, it is hoped, will usher in a new conceptual framework regarding all microbial pathogens, but more importantly, help change our entrenched and often erroneous conceptions about causality in human health or disease.

Most modern biochemists and molecular reductionists believe the current SARS-COVID-19 molecular RT-PCR tests directly detect and amplify fragments of the SARS-CoV-2 virus, although this assumption has not been validated with true viral isolation of coronaviruses since 2003, when a published and equivocal experiment was published which performed the necessary technical steps of centrifugal isolation, electron microscope identification, an re-infection of a healthy host.

Viral isolation, purification, electron microscope validation, and re-infection were demonstrated during the 2002-3 SARS CoV-2 crisis by Faucier et al., (Koch's postulates fulfilled for SARS VIRUS. Nature vol 423, 13 May 2003), but a positive signal with PCR depends on the number of cycles used to amplify the suspected sequence sample thought to be derived from a virus (or from anything else), and the morbidity they described in the two macaques that they infected and which showed symptoms of a rash and an influenza-like illness were accompanied by the claim that metapneumoviruses or Chlamydia pneumonia couldn't be ruled out, and also, adequate controls weren't run in their experiments.

For example, it is known that the current PCR tests will yield 100% positive results for any sample when it is amplified between 40-60 cycles, and PCR amplification will yield variable results at or slightly above 30 PCR amplification cycles and will rarely yield a positive result below 15-20 PCR amplification cycles, suggesting that the methodology is equivocal unless there is a gold standard against which it can always with certainty be measured and validated. Kary Mullis authored numerous writings and statements on HIV tests that used his PCR invention however are typically ignored, belittled, and derided by self-proclaimed "HIV experts" and by the promoters of AIDS, and the issues around accuracy of HIV PCR lab tests could be written today about COVID-19 lab tests and for these exact same reasons.

Additionally, false positives not only emerge by the number of PCR amplification cycles used, but by cross reactions with disease states, or with other physiological states such as pregnancy or warts, and from reactions against both benign and potentially pathogenic entities or states that also yield positive signals for a variety of different reasons.

Some of these syndromes that yield false positive test results were compiled during the "HIV" era by Christine Johnson and published in Continuum as shown below.

WHOSE ANTIBODIES ARE THEY ANYWAY? FACTORS KNOWN TO CAUSE FALSE POSITIVE HIV ANTIBODY TEST RESULTS (as the reference list is extensive, it has been made into APPENDIX I).

By Christine Johnson

Continuum Sept./Oct. 1996

The AIDS establishment has managed to convince many people that the HIV antibody tests (ELISA, IFA, and Western blot) are "99.5% accurate". In this article Christine Johnson from HEAL Los Angeles, lists conditions documented in the scientific literature known to cause positives on these tests, and gives her references.

It is expected that this list will generate much discussion and dissension. For the time being, a few clarifications should be made at the outset.

Just because something is on the list does not mean that it will definitely, or even probably, cause a false-positive. It depends on what antibodies the individual carries; as well as the characteristics of each particular test kit.

For instance, some, but not all, people who have had blood transfusions, prior pregnancies or an organ transplant will make HLA antibodies. And some, but not all, test kits (both ELISA and Western blot) will be contaminated with HLA antigens to which these antibodies can react. Only if these two conditions coincide might you get a false-positive due to HLA cross-reactivity.

Some things are more likely than others to cause false-positives. And some things that we are not aware of yet, but which may be documented in the future, may cause false-positives. Some of the factors on the list have been documented only for ELISA, some for both ELISA and Western blot (WB).

Some people may be eager to argue that if a factor is only known to cause false-positives on ELISA, this problem will not be carried over to the WB, so everything should be OK. But remember, a WB is positive by virtue of accumulating enough individual positive bands to add up to the total required by whatever criteria you use to interpret it (39) So the more exposures a person has had to foreign antigens, proteins and infectious agents, the more various antibodies he or she will have in their system, and the more likely it is that there will be several cross-reacting antibodies, enough to make the WB positive.

It is to be noted that all AIDS risk groups (and Africans as well), but not the general US or Western European population, have this problem in common: they have been exposed to a plethora of foreign antigens and proteins. This is why people in the AIDS "risk groups" tend to have positive WBs (i.e., to be considered "HIV-infected") and people in the general population do not. However, even people in the low-risk populations may have false-positive Western blots for poorly understood reasons.(47)

Since false-positives to every single HIV protein have been documented (36), how do you know the positive WB bands represent the various proteins to HIV, or just a collection of false-positive bands reacting to several different non-HIV antibodies?

Factors Known to Cause False-Positive HIV Antibody Test Results

- *Anti-carbohydrate antibodies (52, 19, 13)*
- *Naturally-occurring antibodies (5, 19)*
- *Passive immunization: receipt of gamma globulin or immune globulin (as prophylaxis against infection which contains antibodies)(18, 26, 60, 4, 22, 42, 43, 13)*
- *Leprosy (2, 25)*
- *Tuberculosis (25)*
- *Mycobacterium avium (25)*
- *Systemic lupus erythematosus (15, 23)*
- *Renal (kidney) failure (48, 23, 13)*
- *Hemodialysis/renal failure (56, 16, 41, 10, 49)*
- *Alpha interferon therapy in hemodialysis patients (54)*
- *Flu (36)*
- *Flu vaccination (30, 11, 3, 20, 13, 43)*
- *Herpes simplex I (27)*
- *Herpes simplex II (11)*
- *Upper respiratory tract infection (cold or flu)(11)*
- *Recent viral infection or exposure to viral vaccines (11)*
- *Pregnancy in multiparous women (58, 53, 13, 43, 36)*
- *Malaria (6, 12)*
- *High levels of circulating immune complexes (6, 33)*
- *Hypergammaglobulinemia (high levels of antibodies) (40, 33)*
- *False positives on other tests, including RPR (rapid plasma reagent) test for syphilis (17, 48, 33, 10, 49)*
- *Rheumatoid arthritis (36)*
- *Hepatitis B vaccination (28, 21, 40, 43)*
- *Tetanus vaccination (40)*
- *Organ transplantation (1, 36)*
- *Renal transplantation (35, 9, 48, 13, 56)*
- *Anti-lymphocyte antibodies (56, 31)*
- *Anti-collagen antibodies (found in gay men, hemophiliacs, Africans of both sexes and people with leprosy)(31)*

- *Serum-positive for rheumatoid factor, antinuclear antibody (both found in rheumatoid arthritis and other autoantibodies)(14, 62, 53)*
- *Autoimmune diseases (44, 29, 10, 40, 49, 43): Systemic lupus erythematosus, scleroderma, connective tissue disease, dermatomyositis*
- *Acute viral infections, DNA viral infections (59, 48, 43, 53, 40, 13)*
- *Malignant neoplasms (cancers)(40)*
- *Alcoholic hepatitis/alcoholic liver disease (32, 48, 40,10,13, 49, 43, 53)*
- *Primary sclerosing cholangitis (48, 53)*
- *Hepatitis (54)*
- *"Sticky" blood (in Africans) (38, 34, 40)*
- *Antibodies with a high affinity for polystyrene (used in the test kits) (62, 40, 3)*
- *Blood transfusions, multiple blood transfusions (63, 36,13, 49, 43, 41)*
- *Multiple myeloma (10, 43, 53)*
- *HLA antibodies (to Class I and II leukocyte antigens)(7, 46, 63, 48, 10, 13, 49, 43, 53)*
- *Anti-smooth muscle antibody (48)*
- *Anti-parietal cell antibody (48)*
- *Anti-hepatitis An IgM (antibody)(48)*
- *Anti-Hbc IgM (48)*
- *Administration of human immunoglobulin preparations pooled before 1985 (10)*
- *Hemophilia (10, 49)*
- *Hematologic malignant disorders/lymphoma (43, 53, 9, 48, 13)*
- *Primary biliary cirrhosis (43, 53, 13, 48)*
- *Stevens-Johnson syndrome9, (48, 13)*
- *Q-fever with associated hepatitis (61)*
- *Heat-treated specimens (51, 57, 24, 49, 48)*
- *Lipemic serum (blood with high levels of fat or lipids)(49)*
- *Hemolyzed serum (blood where hemoglobin is separated from the red cells)(49)*
- *Hyperbilirubinemia (10, 13)*

- *Globulins produced during polyclonal gammopathies (which are seen in AIDS risk groups)(10, 13, 48)*
- *Healthy individuals as a result of poorly-understood cross-reactions (10)*
- *Normal human ribonucleoproteins (48,13)*
- *Other retroviruses (8, 55, 14, 48, 13)*
- *Anti-mitochondrial antibodies (48, 13)*
- *Anti-nuclear antibodies (48, 13, 53)*
- *Anti-microsomal antibodies (34)*
- *T-cell leukocyte antigen antibodies (48, 13)*
- *Proteins on the filter paper (13)*
- *Epstein-Barr virus (37)*
- *Visceral leishmaniasis (45)*
- *Receptive anal sex (39, 64)*

The references for these listed false-positive reasons for testing "HIV" positive that have nothing to do with AIDS are listed in **APPENDIX 1.**

IF PCR TEST KIT INVENTOR & NOBEL PRIZE WINNER KARY MULLIS WERE ALIVE TODAY

If PCR test kit inventor Kary Mullis were alive today, he would be sounding the alarms about widespread testing for SARS CoV-2 using the PCR testing technology he invented. Dr. Mullis would certainly reject the paradigm of mass testing of asymptomatic people for SARS CoV-2 using PCR as a way to determine both the infectious status of individuals, or whether or not there is a growing pandemic in populations.

What Dr. Mullis would tell Dr. Fauci is that this public health push to test everyone for SARS CoV-2 will create a majority of false-positive diagnoses, and that the entire premise was scientifically flawed.

Unless electron microscopy of crown shaped viral particles is carried out to verify and confirm a SARS CoV-2 diagnosis, none of these other lab tests can be relied on to be remotely definitive or accurate, whether it is PCR or antibody tests, without electron microscopic verification.

As I said earlier: **Direct confirmatory ultrastructural testing following PCR or WESTERN-blot analysis of blood from the same patient's blood draw may help eliminate the problem of false positive pathogen testing in a number of contexts and eliminate medical conundrums wherein indirect protein or nucleic acid testing detects proteins that mimic non-disease-associated proteins or nucleic acids in persons in ill-health, but not infected. Furthermore, an awareness of these issues, it is hoped, will usher in a new conceptual framework regarding all microbial pathogens, but more importantly, help change our entrenched and often erroneous conceptions about causality in human health or disease.**

This article that I published in 2004 with a group in Perth, Australia explains why (Eleni Papadopulos-Eleopulos, Valendar Turner, John Papadimitriou, Barry Page, David Causer, Helman Alfonso, Sam Mhlongo, Todd Miller, Andrew Maniotis, Christian Fiala. "A critique of the Montagnier evidence for the HIV/AIDS hypothesis." Med Hypotheses. 63(4): 597-601, 2004).Not only are the non-validated, unproven lab tests responsible for fueling the AIDS era and COVID-19 hysteria, but the imagined origins of both viruses and their molecular signatures are in effect delusional hallucinations of partial chemical testing without structural or functional verification. In the context of each one of these syndromes, these "viruses" that are supposedly "jumping" around from monkeys to Africans in the case of AIDS, and with SARS CoV-2, from bats to humans, or with MERS (Middle Eastern Respiratory Syndrome) from camels to humans, nobody to date has observed any leaping viruses. Beliefs regarding leaping viruses are simply tacit unsubstantiated assumptions that are assumed upon DNA and RNA sequence homologies-not because anyone has seen "leaping viruses." From a biological point of view regarding what we know about the function of genomes to maintain invariance over periods of time even in some cases exceeding Earth's geological epoch's, with all these viruses leaping around, how can viruses maintain their phenotypic identity as a taxonomically distinct group based on its primary sequence, and if they cause disease and are mutating every time you look at them, then how can they retain their pathogenicity? Mutation is supposedly a random process leading to random, mostly lethal consequences in all living systems, and probably also with protein-nucleic aggregates which are not living, such as viruses. On September 8, 2011, the British Daily Mail reported that a big group of Chimpanzees who were kept in cages and injected with human HIV repeatedly over decades and tested for AIDS will finally be set free into a sanctuary for traumatized animals in Austria. Not one of the Chimpanzees injected with HIV developed AIDS, even though Chimpanzees have 99% the same genome as humans. Part of the purpose of the experiments was to examine whether an HIV vaccine was viable. It was shown in these experiments over several decades that an HIV vaccine was not viable. If a similar experiment were done with chimpanzees experimentally infected with Covid-19, my speculation is that we would see the same outcomes as the HIV experiments on these Chimpanzees: no illness resulting.

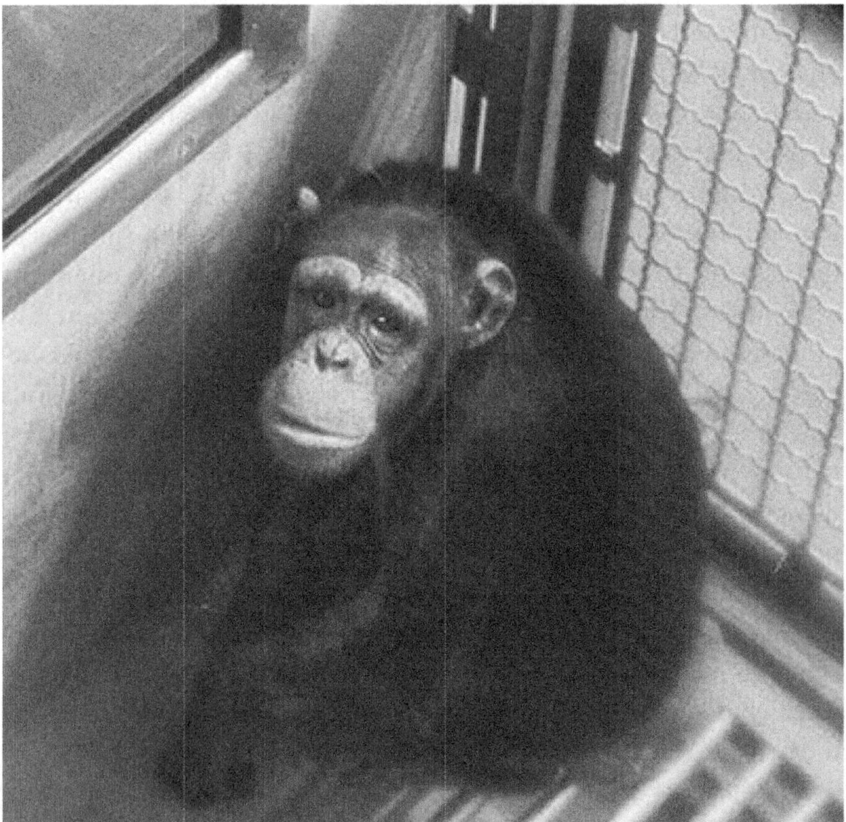

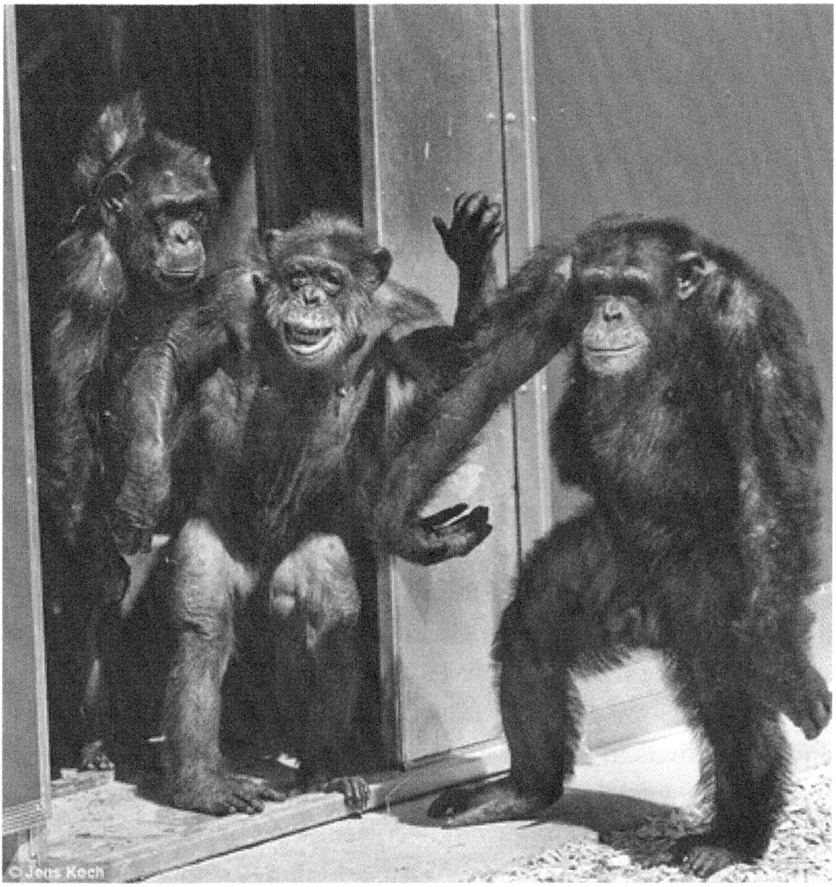

Behind bars: The upper photo, one of the chimps "Locked Down" in the cages that were home to them for many years. This chimp looks sad because of the lock-down. In the bottom photo, these chimps taste freedom for the first time after 30 years in lock-down captivity. The chimps on the right actually look happy and ready to party!

According to the Daily Mail article: "Some chimpanzees were infected with the HIV virus. Of course, they tested HIV positive. But none of them, not here in Austria or anywhere else in the world, developed full-blown AIDS. Therefore, the program was useless. It achieved absolutely nothing… Now, Susi, David, Clyde, Lingoa,

Moritz and all the others will be free to enjoy the remainder of their lives together, thanks to the unstinting efforts of a 59-year-old conservationist named Michael Aufhauser..."

Mr Aufhauser, the founder of an animal charity that operates in four European countries oversaw the construction of the chimp sanctuary outside Vienna, which is built on the site of a defunct safari park. The aim of the firm that bought them was to find a vaccine to combat AIDS. Because chimps share 99 percent of the gene code of man, they seemed natural subjects for study more than 30 years ago.

https://www.dailymail.co.uk/news/article-2034439/Lab-chimps-freed-caged-fior-30-years-injected-HIV.html

The American and European citizens are all being treated today during COVID-19 like these locked-down imprisoned chimpanzees waiting to be experimented on with dangerous drugs and insufficiently tested vaccines by Anthony Fauci and Bill Gates. Our homes have become cages during lock-downs and we are the experimental animals being abused by the WHO, NIH, and CDC.

All of the available data indicate that not only false-positive tests, and the caveats involved with the interpretation of tests are more than simply a conundrum-conceptual and practical problems have emerged because of modern molecular testing because testing is increasingly used and trusted to inform and then to guide critical therapeutic decisions. A more informed awareness needs to be in place that does not exist yet in current standards of care regarding testing. What do positive and negative tests really mean, and how should they be interpreted to better assure the safety and effectiveness of therapeutic interventions in those rare cases of SARS-CoV-2 atypical pneumonia COVID victims who are symptomatic and have a 12-hour window to somehow acquire enough oxygen to support life (PaO2/FiO2-dissolved oxygen in the blood/amount of available oxygen).

Although during health crises such as SARS-COVID-19 there sometimes is an acute urgency to abandon the careful validation of testing needed, and to rush decisions regarding the risks involved in attempting to implement new standards of care and medical intervention in the hopes that some panacea will emerge to somehow cheat death itself, these motives are unwarranted. Direct pathogen testing using EM (electron microscopy) to validate the biochemical indirect tests actually will save vast amounts of time, money, and lives, if it can detect actual viremia at high resolution. Why is PCR needed anyway if viremia (thousands to millions of viral particles) is present in a SARS-CoV-2 victim. EM validation of "the perp" can be unequivocal and definitive in weeding out the false positive lab test results generated from **indirect** testing and identify the legitimate cases from those that may want to stay in bed for a few days, and from those that are asymptomatic (healthy carriers).

To understand what is wrong with most current, inaccurate, COVID-19 testing, one must understand that the pathogen isolation protocols themselves are confronted with a broad range of cellular debris, including breakdown products from sick or dying cells that shed both decaying genomic fragments and proteins, which complex with these nucleic acid fragments to resemble viruses, or they can appear different immunologically to the victim's own immune system, and exacerbate cytokine storms, and massive inflammation, which is what really kills the victims.

Historically since the polio era, whenever baffling conditions or complex health issues arise, objects that are below light's visible wave-lengths are usually blamed. This has been problematic since the time of Koch and Hill, even before this technology (electron microscopy-EM) was invented in the late 1930's, and this holds true still today.

THE REAL FLY IN THE OINTMENT OF SARS-COV-2 TESTING IS CHRISTIAN DROSTEN

The real "fly in the ointment" of SARS-CoV-2 testing is Christian Drosten as described by Wikipedia on 1/4/2021 thus (and all the primary references can be found in the Wikipedia reference list simply by stating Drosten's name on Wiki-there are too many to list here):

"Drosten is one of the co-discoverers of SARS-associated coronaviruses (SARS CoV). Together with Stephan G nther, a few days after identification and before the CDC, he succeeded in developing a diagnostic test for the newly identified virus in 2003. Drosten immediately made his findings of SARS available to the scientific community on the internet, even before his article appear in The New England Journal of Medicine in May 2003. Among others, this was honored by the journal Nature." (Drosten, Christian; *Günther, Stephan*; Preiser, et al, Massachusetts Medical Society. 348(20): 1967–1976. 2003). From 2012, the research group led by Drosten also researched the Middle East Respiratory Syndrome-coronavirus (MERS-Coronavirus)."

"For the coronavirus SARS-Co-V-2 RT-PCR, which first appeared in December 2019, the research group led by Drosten developed a test that was made available worldwide in mid-January 2020. The group also published the sequenced genome from samples obtained in Germany. In the course of the COVID-19 pandemic, Drosten advised politicians and authorities and was invited as an expert in the media, among others in the podcast Das Coronavirus-Update mit Christian Drosten), initially published daily during the week since February 26, 2020…In 2004, Drosten received the GlaxoSmithKline funding award for clinical infectiology, the Abbott Diagnostics Award for Hygiene and Microbiology, and the post-doctoral award for virology from the Robert Koch Foundation. In 2005, he was awarded the Federal Cross of Merit, 2020, for his civil service in time of COVID-19."

Although Drosten and Corman attracted the WHO's and world's attention and admiration, and Corporate Giants like

GlaxoSmithKline and many others even before the work could be reviewed, in the well-chosen words of Journalist Celia Farber who was one of the instigators that broke the AZT story during the AIDS era:

Farber claims that "War has broken out in the scientific literature that strikes at the existential core of Covid-19 and its proposed causative virus. At the heart of the controversy lies the fact that the creators of the most commonly used test, the RT-PCR, published instructions for how to test for SARS-CoV-2 without having virus material available," available," [in their own words], "relying instead on the Chinese scientists' genetic sequence published on the internet."

The paper "*Detection of 2019 novel coronavirus (2019-nCoV) by real-time PCR*, was published 24 hours after it was submitted to Eurosurveillance, clearly evading peer review. Its lead authors were Christian Drosten and Victor Corman, which is how it took on the title "Corman-Drosten paper." It provided the "recipe," or workflow for the Covid-19 diagnostic test, quickly applied all over the world, after it was accepted as the standard of testing by the WHO. They submitted the paper on Jan. 21, it was published in *Eurosurveillance* on Jan. 23, and was immediately accepted as the standard of testing internationally, by the WHO, which began sending test kits to affected regions."

CORMAN-DROSTEN REVIEW REPORT

CURATED BY AN INTERNATIONAL CONSORTIUM OF SCIENTISTS IN LIFE SCIENCES (ICSLS)

"In the harrowing months that followed, amid lockdowns, economic collapse, school closures and widespread panic, few were aware of the immense false positive results, due to a nonexistent gold standard which would be the virus itself. It all came to a head on Nov. 30, when the Corman-Drosten foundation paper was challenged by 22 international scientists who wrote a letter demanding the paper's retraction, along with an extensive critique citing 10 errors in the paper it deemed "fatal."

Titled "External peer review of the RT-PCR test to detect SARS-Cov-2 Reveals 10 Major Flaws at The Molecular and Methodological

Level: Consequences For False-Positive Results," the paper's lead author is Dr. Pieter Borger which tragically offered a testing method that would yield between 80 and 97 percent false positives.

Other issues with the Corman-Drosten's RT-PCR test include the fact that a positive result cannot explain why "asymptomatics" do not get sick, and why in Northern Italy, one of the first epicenters of the SARS-COVID epidemic that began in December, 2019 was associated with two mandated vaccines mandated three months earlier in Italy than the start of SARS-COVID-19, and immediately before the January 2020 SARS-COVID-19 pandemic, by local Italian health departments and Italian Ministry of Health. The first vaccine mandated in northern Italy was an H1N1 vaccine administered to 141,000 persons in September, 2019, and of those, 129,000 were Italians who were over 65 years of age, and of those 129,000, 70% had grave heart problems. This vaccine crusade was followed 2 months later in December, 2019 by an "experimental HEP C vaccine" given to 21,331 persons preceding the explosion of COVID-19 in the Bergano, Italy epicenter a month later (this information was provided by Alexis Gugnolo, an investigative reporter from Rome Info News, and written on March 27, 2020. Alexis Gugnolo does a good job at writing about the US Department of Defense study on influenza vaccines and their ability to facilitate increased risk of coronavirus infections. Here is an excerpt from Gugnolo's article (found here: https://www.fromrome.info/2020/03/27/was-the-winter-flu-vaccine-pre-designed-to-promote-a-coronavirus-epidemic/

about a US Dept. of Defense study proving flu vaccines increase risk of future coronavirus infections by 36% over the unvaccinated:

Dangers of the Winter Flue vaccine

In a study written by Greg Wolf, of the US Armed Forces Surveillance, Airforce Branch, and published in the Journal, Vaccine, on January 10, 2020, and entitled, Influenza Vaccination and respiratory virus interference among Department of Defense personnel during the 2017-2018 influenza season, it was found that U.S. Military personnel who were given the winter flu had a 36% increased chance of contracting a coronavirus infection.

In his conclusion, Greg Wolf wrote:

Receipt of influenza vaccination was not associated with virus interference among our population. Examining virus interference by specific respiratory viruses showed mixed results. Vaccine derived virus interference was significantly associated with coronavirus and human metapneumovirus; however, significant protection with vaccination was associated not only with most influenza viruses, but also parainfluenza, RSV, and non-influenza virus coinfections.

The study included a table which broke down the effects observed:

Table 5
Respiratory viruses and odds ratios by vaccination status.

Virus	Vaccinated (%)	Not Vaccinated (%)	OR (95% CI)	P-Value
Influenza	2058 (31.3)	1289 (44.4)	0.57 (0.53, 0.63)	<0.01
Influenza A	1256 (19.2)	741 (25.3)	0.70 (0.63, 0.78)	<0.01
Influenza A H1N1	205 (3.4)	221 (7.6)	0.42 (0.35, 0.51)	<0.01
Influenza A H3N2	1023 (15.6)	512 (17.5)	0.88 (0.78, 0.98)	0.02
Influenza B	662 (10.1)	474 (16.2)	0.58 (0.51, 0.66)	<0.01
Influenza B Victoria	7 (0.1)	8 (0.3)	0.39 (0.14, 1.08)	0.07
Influenza B Yamagata	85 (1.3)	77 (2.6)	0.49 (0.36, 0.67)	<0.01
Influenza Coinfection	9 (0.1)	9 (0.3)	0.45 (0.18, 1.13)	0.09
Non-Influenza Virus	2096 (31.3)	838 (28.3)	1.15 (1.05, 1.27)	<0.01
Adenovirus	144 (2.2)	78 (2.7)	0.83 (0.63, 1.09)	0.17
Coronavirus	507 (7.8)	178 (5.8)	1.36 (1.14, 1.63)	<0.01
Human Bocavirus	69 (1.1)	34 (1.2)	0.91 (0.60, 1.37)	0.66
Human Metapneumovirus	335 (5.1)	101 (3.5)	1.51 (1.20, 1.90)	<0.01
No Pathogen Detected	2441 (37.3)	799 (27.3)	1.59 (1.44, 1.75)	<0.01
Parainfluenza	139 (2.1)	92 (3.1)	0.67 (0.51, 0.87)	<0.01
RSV	369 (5.6)	203 (6.9)	0.81 (0.68, 0.96)	0.02
Rhinovirus/Enterovirus	875 (13.4)	406 (13.7)	0.96 (0.86, 1.11)	0.71
Non-Influenza Virus Coinfection	226 (3.4)	138 (4.7)	0.72 (0.58, 0.89)	<0.01

Which shows in the third column, the standard deviation increase for viral infection by that species of virus after being vaccinated with the winter flu. Corona is listed as 1.36, that is, an increase of 36%.

The original US Department Of Defense flu vaccine coronavirus study by Greg Wolf referenced can be found here: https://www.sciencedirect.com/science/article/pii/S0264410X19313647?via%3Dihub

Review report Corman-Drosten et al. Eurosurveillance 2020 November 27, 2020

This extensive review report was officially submitted to Eurosurveillance editorial board on 27th November 2020 via their submission-portal, enclosed to this review report is a retraction request letter, signed by all the main & co-authors. First and last listed names are the first and second main authors.

EXTERNAL PEER REVIEW OF THE RT-PCR TEST ADVANCED BY DROSDEN REVEALS 10 MAJOR SCIENTIFIC FLAWS AT THE MOLECULAR AND METHODOLOGICAL LEVEL: CONSEQUENCES FOR FALSE POSTIVE RESULTS: REVIEW REPORT CORMAN-DROSTEN ET AL, EUROSURVEILLANCE, 2020

Pieter Borger, Bobby Rajesh Malhotra, Michael Yeadon, Clare Craig, Kevin McKernan, Klaus Steger, Paul McSheehy, Lidiya Angelova, Fabio Franchi, Thomas Binder, Henrik Ullrich, Makoto Ohashi, Stefano Scoglio, Marjolein Doesburg-van Kleffens, Dorothea Gilbert, Rainer Klement, Ruth Schruefer, Berber W. Pieksma, Jan Bonte, Bruno H. Dalle Carbonare, Kevin P. Corbett, Ulrike Kämmerer

ABSTRACT

In the publication entitled "Detection of 2019 novel coronavirus (2019-nCoV) by real-time RT-PCR" (Eurosurveillance 25(8) 2020) the authors present a diagnostic workflow and RT-qPCR protocol for detection and diagnostics of 2019-nCoV (now known as SARS-CoV-2), which they claim to be validated, as well as being a robust diagnostic methodology for use in public-health laboratory settings. In light of all the consequences resulting from this very publication for societies worldwide, a group of independent researchers performed a point-by-point review of the aforesaid publication in which 1) all components of the presented test design were cross checked, 2) the RT-qPCR protocol-recommendations were assessed w.r.t. good laboratory practice, and 3) parameters examined against relevant scientific literature covering the field.

The published RT-qPCR protocol for detection and diagnostics of 2019-nCoV and the manuscript suffer from numerous technical and scientific errors, including insufficient primer design, a problematic and insufficient RT-qPCR protocol, and the absence of an accurate test validation. Neither the presented test nor the manuscript itself fulfils the requirements for an acceptable scientific publication. Further, serious conflicts of interest of the authors are not mentioned. Finally, the noticeably short timescale between submission and acceptance of the publication (24 hours) signifies that a systematic peer review process was either not performed here, or of problematic poor quality. We provide compelling evidence of several scientific inadequacies, errors, and flaws.

Considering the scientific and methodological blemishes presented here, we are confident that the editorial board of Eurosurveillance has no other choice but to retract the publication.

Another issue to consider is why similar explosions of SARS-COVID-19 do not seem to be occurring with any morbidity or mortality among children and infants, and also only among those with other pre-existing conditions? At least one team of virologists made a legitimate case for the existence of SARS-CoV-2 in 2003 in macaques during the 2002-3 "epidemic."

Much of this madness is reminiscent of the beginnings of "HIV" testing and reportage. Even from the beginning of "HIV" PCR or antibody testing, it had been known that none of the tests detect "HIV" virus particles directly, and that a positive antibody test may occur for more than 100 well-documented reasons that have nothing to do with "HIV" or "AIDS. The situation is different with SARS-CoV-2 because these virus-like particles exist. But some reminder about historical information is important to review.

THE PROBLEMS AND CONSEQUENCES THAT ARE EMERGING WITH FALSE POSITIVE AND FALSE NEGATIVE COVID-19 TESTING HAVE PRECEDENTS IN "HIV" TESTING

It does not even ring any alarms among most people, such as parents, despite package inserts accompanying the products themselves, or which the doctor's never disclose to their "patients," even when the vaccines or drugs include the putrid and often proprietary molecules in vaccines designed to prime the non-immunologically immature immune system. But the gateway problem always will be the testing and our faith and understanding of the testing for disease.

This psychosis dates back to the AIDS era, Fauci, and Robert C. Gallo's "viral-topian" delusions, as it is clear by a few reminiscences of the past. Even from the beginning of "HIV" testing, it has been known that none of the tests detect "HIV" virus particles directly, and that a positive antibody test may occur for more than 100 well-documented reasons that have nothing to do with "HIV" or "AIDS. The first ELISA tests showed for instance, that out of 1.2 million applicants for military service (the Burke study), there were **10,000 out of 12,000** false positives. But this is not the case with SARS CoV-2 because in this case we actually have a real virus that can be visualized, isolated, and which has fulfilled Koch's postulates in 2 macaques, unlike the experience with "HIV" which never has been correctly isolated or visualized.

The "viral load tests" are based on the polymerase chain reaction (PCR) amplification of supposedly specific "HIV" gene sequences, but PCR tests are known to sometimes generate false-positive signals between 40-100% of the time, which is absurd if you consider what this really implies. In a viremic victim, it is a valid question to ask why PCR is even needed if the tissues are teaming with viral particles. Someone with a high "viral load" should have their blood teaming with viral particles, and not need any PCR amplification at all to detect this exponentially high quantity of viral gene sequences or virions. Perhaps this is one reason why the inventor of the PCR technique, the Nobelist, Kary Mullis who invented PCR, once said there is no evidence that "HIV" is the cause of AIDS years ago. A patient with high "HIV" viral load should be able to walk into a physician's office, have their blood drawn, the doctor should be able to send that blood to a lab, and it should be loaded with hundreds of thousands or millions of "HIV" virus particles. But this has not been the case with "HIV." This is the reason why PCR amplification of "assumed" "HIV" viral gene sequences is measured biochemically rather than directly. Chemical amplification of "HIV" gene sequences has to be employed using PCR precisely because there are no detectable viral particles in the blood or tissues, nor have there ever been, in someone who is said to harbor the molecular signature(s) of "HIV" genomic sequences or "HIV's-specific, unique proteins. In an "HIV" serosurvey of out of 20.2 million "HIV" tests done in Russia, only 112 were confirmed and about 20,000 were false positives (Voevodin A. Lancet. 339:1548, 1992). 112 "confirmed" "HIV" molecular signatures out of 20 million negative ones does not constitute the kind of numbers that signal a major AIDS pandemic in Russia. The numbers could represent statistical artifact, or, in the several who seroconverted and showed a positive test result may represent the presence of some kind of auto-immune condition, like psoriasis, arthritis, or warts, or physiological stress, or a genetic polymorphism (human genetic variability).

In 2004, the American Red Cross reported that even after repeated "HIV" testing using different test kit types, that "low-risk" populations, such as blood donors (or military recruits or nuns) will typically yield 12 (PCR) positive or 2 (ELISA) positive results out of 37,000,000 million units of blood, which means that 10 out of 12 were false positives. In a follow-up analysis of this Red Cross study, it was then claimed that 6 of the 12 PCR-positive subjects tests seroconverted within several months, thereby obtaining a "HIV" molecular signature in 8/12 cases, out of 37 million negatives. Again, these numbers could represent statistical artifact, or the several who seroconverted may represent the detection of some kind of auto-immune condition in those who test positive, like psoriasis, arthritis, warts, or physiological stress, or a genetic polymorphism, or a flu recent vaccine which frequently triggers these tests, or pregnancy.

Abbott Laboratory's ELISA test kit package insert says:

"*ELISA testing alone cannot be used to diagnose AIDS.*" (Abbott 1997).

Epitope's (the maker for one of the Western Blot kits) package insert says:

"*Do not use this kit as the sole basis for HIV infection.*" (Epitope 1997).

Roche's "Amplicor test kit's insert states:

"*The amplicor HIV-1 monitor test is not intended to be used as a screening test for HIV, nor as a diagnostic test to confirm the presence of HIV infection.*" (Roche 1996).

Then what in God's name are these tests used for? Perhaps as lie detectors?

Presumably, as grave as an "HIV" or "AIDS" diagnosis is, one might expect there should be awareness generated about the lack of a gold standard (virus isolation) disclosed to the public. Or one might minimally expect, **IF** the test kits predict progression to an "AIDS-defining illness," at least one test kit type or brand available of the 33 or more on the market, that by itself, can serve as a gold standard to identify individuals who carry specific antibodies against the "HIV" virus, or components of the "HIV" virus itself.

All of these same issues need to be addressed with SARS CoV-2 in lung lavages from patients experiencing atypical pneumonias.

Considered alone, it is difficult to contemplate how molecular diagnostics of entities like "HERVs" ("Human Endogenous Retroviral Sequences," "retroelements," "retroids," "phages") determine people's lives, or can be used to justify the incarceration of folks if they were aware, they were "positive" for a sexually-transmitted pathogen without telling a partner, as has been the case with "HIV." The composition and structure of viruses, because they are essentially inert pieces of a nucleic acid wrapped in a proteinaceous and glycoprotein coat, are essentially either a virally—encoded protein expressed by the viral genome, or alternative, they may theoretically also be expressions of normal resident cellularly-encoded RNA or DNA sequences in our genomes that become wrapped in either viral genome-encoded or cell-encoded proteins that are manufactured in the cytoplasm (when of viral origin) or accumulated if of cellular origin during viral budding and other interactions the viral particle has in the cell before or during the intracellular transport and budding process. These molecular sequence phenomena could simply at a cellular level represent decay products that mimic nucleic acid sequences of various pathogens.

Also, any modern analysis of the human genome database will reveal more than 120, 000 full-length retroids containing reverse transcriptase transcripts...See: Marie Dewannieux, Francis Harper Aurelien Richaud, Claire Letzelter, David Ribet, Gerard Pierron, Thierry Heidmann. Identification of infectious progenitor for the multiple-copy HERV-K human endotheous retroelements. Genome Res. Oct 31, 2006;

Also see Marcella A. 316 McClure, Hugh S. Richardson, Rochelle A. Clinton, Crystal M. Hepp, Brad A. Crowther, Eric F. Donaldson. Automated characterization of potentially active retroid agents in the human genome. Genomics 512-523, 2005; David J Griffiths. Endogenous retroviruses in the human genome sequence. Genome Biology 2001,2:reviews1017.1- 1017.5).

http://genomebiology.com/2001/2/6/reviews/1017.

Although "HIV=AIDS" proponents are always saying the "HIV virus's" reverse transcriptase sequence is mutating when patients die on "lifesaving" anti-retroviral drugs that supposedly target this enzyme, genomic analyses show that reverse transcriptase is among the most stable transcripts that make up these retroids, and it is the sequence stability rather than the instability or mutability of the reverse transcriptase sequence itself that make these 120,000 retroid sequences possible to classify. What is also remarkable about the data regarding retroids and HERV's is that reverse transcriptase was once thought by all working in AIDS research to be specific to retroviruses, and this is the enzyme they first measured, and indeed some labs continue to measure, as evidence of "HIV infection." As CoV-2 is also a retrovirus, the same issues apply regarding reverse transcription.

We are all made up partly of "retroviral" components, they are part of us, and these components require reverse transcriptase for normal replication. What they call "HIV" and what they have successfully branded as the most dangerous and infectious virus known to man, is (and can be evoked), and what has been mistaken for these "viruses" are artifacts of the technologies for detecting them, without any of the sober analysis of what those tests are actually detecting or what "HIV's" molecular signature means for a human being. The probable "cause of "HIV" could be these retroids and/or endogenous HERV sequences, that can be evoked, under stress conditions, or which may become expressed in healthy persons as part of a relatively rare genetic polymorphism. Without proper viral isolation and verification with electron microscopy, there is no way of knowing.

Because RNA viruses (retroviruses) are RNA viruses, it should be clearly shown that because of the inherent instability of RNA compared to DNA, it has been proposed that the RNA viruses are not causal of diseases but are byproducts of sick or dying cells. Coronaviruses have fulfilled enough isolation criteria to be considered as distinct virus-like entities, and they even have satisfied several experimental tests that tie their presence to SARS employing Koch's postulates, which was first published in 2003 (Faucier et al. Koch's postulates fulfilled. (Nature Vol 423, p. 240, May, 2003).

But it should be cautioned that all 60-140 nanometer virus-like particles that can be observed with electron microscopes are not viruses despite the fact they are spheres that contain a dark core such as "HIV", or even if they appear as spheres of 60-140 nanometer diameters and sport what appear to be crowns or coronas of spikes of proteins? This is one reason why in tissue sections or serum samples of victims it is so important to document viremia in a victim and show hundreds or thousands of vial-like particles in an electron microscopes field of view at about 7000 diameters magnification (low power) to prove viremia in the blood or in a lymph node or elsewhere. This simple test was never carried out during the entire AIDS era with "HIV" and thus Koch's postulates haven't been fulfilled for "HIV" to this day. In fact, it was claimed by more than one unaccountable "HIV" research group that "HIV" could only be detected in 1 out of 10,000 T-cells, or that despite it being present in samples of sera, it "hides" in lymph nodes so biologists cannot see it in blood. There never was viremia with "HIV," and it would be unfortunate to model the SARS-CoV-2 science that has yet to be carried out, on this tragic science of AID$ and "HIV" research.

Robert Gallo, Anthony Fauci's side-kick who was credited with being the co-discoverer of "HIV" with Luc Montagnier, and although Gallo did not receive any of the Nobel Prize prizes that Montagnier received, used to call me in my office in the afternoons to threaten me over the phone if I did not shut up. He believed that...black slaves caused cancer because art work evidence proved to a scientifically epidemiologically established and on this basis justified a racist construct, that these slaves that were depicted in works of art caught and contagiously transmitted a cancer virus called "HTLV-I" and then HTLV-II in the 16th Century from monkeys during the slave trade, which caused 0.6 % of approximately 330,000 serologically tested Japanese near Nagasaki to develop a leukemia 40 years or so after the atomic bombs were dropped on them. This hypothesis was advanced for the origins of "HIV's" suspected "cancer virus" relative or precursor(s), "HTLV-I and II" by Robert Gallo in 1979-81, to explain why a few (out of hundreds of thousands of) "HTLV-1" seropositive individuals acquired cancer in Southern Japan near Nagasaki. This is also why, a year later, when the announcement was made to the American public by Dr. Gallo and Margaret Heckler in 1984, the phrase, "the probable cause of AIDS has been found...to be "HTLV-III," a known "**cancer virus**" was used. As mentioned, "HTLV-III," was later renamed "HIV" by oncogene Nobelist Varmus's committee (please see National Institute of Health: Gallo R.C., Sliski A., Wong-Staal F. Origin of T-cell leukemia-lymphoma virus. Lancet (ii): 962-963, 1983).

"HIV" is said to have about 9150 base pairs, but this template has not been purified without contaminating cellular nucleic acids. "HIV's" molecular signature could represent a HERV (**H**uman **E**ndogenous **R**etrovirus) nucleic acid sequence, or what is called a 'retroid' of one kind or another. A retroid is a special kind of mobile gene associated with diseases such as multiple sclerosis, and with normal biological functions involving the placenta as well. Unless the rtPCR tests being used for SARS CoV-2 are derived from pure viral isolates, instead of a complex lung aspirate, there is also a particularly good chance that what are being detected are similar RNA sequences or "retroids."

That these endogenous human genetic elements exist and are important has been shown again and again to be likely from studies on HERV's such as "the Phoenix viruses," that can be produced by infecting cells with certain sequences of DNA, which then is replicated and packaged by the cells into ***virus-like*** particles. Any modern analysis of the human genome database will reveal more than 120,000 full-length retroids containing reverse transcriptase transcripts.

Although "HIV=AIDS" proponents are always saying the "HIV virus's" reverse transcriptase sequence is mutating when patients die on "lifesaving" "anti-retroviral" drugs that supposedly target this enzyme, genomic analyses show that reverse transcriptase is among the most stable transcripts that make up these retroids, and it is their sequence stability rather than their instability or mutability of the reverse transcriptase sequence itself, that make these 120,000 retroid sequences possible to classify in a genomic analysis. What is also remarkable about new data regarding retroids and HERV's is that reverse transcriptase was once thought by all working in AIDS research to be specific to retroviruses, and this is the enzyme they first measured, and indeed some labs continue to measure, as evidence of "HIV infection." We are all made up partly of "retroviral" components, they are part of us. What they call "HIV" and what they have successfully branded as the most dangerous and infectious virus known to man, is and can be evoked under both stress and physiological conditions-(pregnancy and the trophoblast). In many, whose lives have been terminally stigmatized, and their lives ruined, and what we have told to accept as a lethal "virus," are the flawed technologies and reasoning used to detect it, and without any of the sober analysis of what those tests are actually detecting or what "HIV's" molecular signature means for a healthy or sick human being. Without true viral isolation and viremia, retroid or HERV molecular fragments cannot be assumed to be of viral origin, nor can the proteins they may make as detected on ELISAs or WESTERN BLOTS. The probable "cause of "***HIV***" could be these retroids and/ or endogenous HERV sequences, that can be evoked, under stress conditions, or which may become ex-pressed in healthy persons as part of a statistically small and rare genetic polymorphism.

A more likely explanation of the origin of "HIV's" molecular signature comes instead not from academically institutionalized racist notions, but from recent studies in genomic research that suggests that the so-called template for the protein molecular signatures of "HIV" may derive from endogenous DNA sequences (coming from cellular origin instead of viral origin). It is known that these cellular proteins are expressed under certain conditions by normal uninfected yeast, insects, dogs, rhesus monkeys, chimps, and humans.

"HIV's" molecular signature could represent a HERV (Human Endogenous Retrovirus) nucleic acid sequence, or what is called a 'retroid' of one kind or another. A retroid is a special kind of mobile gene associated with diseases such as multiple sclerosis, and with normal biological functions involving the placenta [3]. That these endogenous human genetic elements exist and are important has been shown again and again to be likely from studies on HERV's such as "the Phoenix viruses," that can be produced by infecting cells with certain sequences of DNA, which then is replicated and packaged by the cells into virus-like particles.

Also, any modern analysis of the human genome database will reveal more than 120,000 full-length retroids containing reverse transcriptase transcripts [1]. Although "HIV=AIDS" proponents are always saying the "HIV virus's" reverse transcriptase sequence is mutating when patients die on "lifesaving" anti-retroviral drugs that supposedly target this enzyme, genomic analyses show that reverse transcriptase is among the most stable transcripts that make up these retroids, and it is the sequence stability rather than the instability or mutability of the reverse transcriptase sequence itself that make these 128,000 retroid sequences possible to classify.

There may indeed be a relationship between "HIV's" molecular signature and immune disorder in some individuals, but the hundreds of billion-dollar question science has not been permitted to ask about these individuals is: which comes first? Which is cause and which is effect, and what is the meaning of the molecular signature of "HIV" in a healthy person who tests "HIV-positive?"

Other so-called "HIV-specific" sequences, such as those that give rise to the so-called GAG, PR, RT, ENV molecules are also found in the normal human genome database. In gene bank searches, one can find 16 samples of Spumavirus transcripts, 6 examples of snake-head virus, 16 samples of FIV (feline immune deficiency virus), 60 examples of detecting one or more HBV (hepatitis B virus) genes, and at least 11 cases of "HIV" sequences that are said to be scattered throughout the normal human genome, according to the analyses of McClure and other modern human Genome Database analyses [1].

The confusing thing may be that some of these endogenous cellular DNA or RNA sequences are only expressed rarely, or in response to physiological stresses: they are not infectious, and they may represent as much a 17% of the normal human genome according to some scientists.

"HIV's" molecular signature may have nothing to do with a specific virus: the molecular signature thought to be a virus may in fact be generated also in response to previously latent real viruses that at some point of physiological stress provokes a new and complex immune response, which is read as "HIV's" molecular signature. The immune system of a person so infected by multiple or numerous latent real viral infections could be perpetually generating new immunogens, which is read by AIDS scientists as an ever changing and mutating "HIV." In theory, such an immune chain reaction caused by multiple real viral, or bacterial or fungal infections would be progressively more debilitating for the stability and effectiveness of immune function, and a vaccine against any specific virus or other pathogen would be ineffective against the development of AIDS. If this hypothesis is correct, then an experimental animal model of AIDS should be induced in laboratory animals by infecting them at a low multiplicity with an exceptionally large number of diverse viruses, as was suggested one by Nobelist, and PCR-inventor, Kary Mullis, in a Genetics paper he wrote in 1995.

Most importantly, the nature and plasticity of potentially stereotypic signals of especially the immune cells or cancer cell's genomes under various stressful and even normal states are not yet known. Despite "AIDS establishment" claims that the whole human genome has been sequenced and is known, and that "HIV's" molecular signature is not found in the normal human genome, or in stadiums full of "HIV-negative" people, the nature of some immune cells is their unique ability to re-arrange their genomes to produce antibodies to new agents. Therefore, all possible or even stereotypic re-arrangements of the genomes of immune cells is not yet sequenced, because the antigens (foreign molecules from outside the organism) that would evoke new antibodies have not yet plagued Mankind yet, or such novel sequences may only be assembled or evoked in immune cells when certain stresses are placed on the individual. The human genome project did not sequence all human genomes, or even genomes from different "representative individuals." We have no idea what these so-called genes do, or how they function.

Thus, the need for a direct pathogen detection method becomes urgent. Are serology-obtained biochemical indicators of nucleic acids or proteins in any way identical to a direct measure of actual visible viable pathogens? Let us begin to answer this question and begin this analysis with what a few of the SARS CoV-2 expert testers are reporting.

In one of the more thoughtful analyses of SARS-CoV-2 diagnostic testing, Stites, E.C., Wilen, CB., (The Interpretation of SARS-CoV-2 Diagnostic Tests, Med 2020.08.001) make important observations regarding several aspects of test interpretation that "are incompletely understood by medical communities and the general population, creating a significant challenge in minimizing the damage caused by disease spread through informed decision making and proper testing utilization." Some of these caveats include whether asymptomatic individuals should be tested, what it means to test positive (or negative), and how to interpret tests for "immunity passports."

They conclude by saying that… "***unexpectedly, the answers seem to run contrary to many of the popular narratives about testing as a tool for managing COVID-19.***"

First it is important to appreciate that there are two classes of tests to detect SARS CoV-2 and viruses in general: a nucleic acid test, which typically is obtained using PCR which detects fragments of stretches of RNA or DNA by first supposedly isolating them and amplifying them using the Polymerase Chain Reaction or PCR, and there are several types of PCR tests. There are also protein tests which will be discussed later. The major point to understand about the ***nucleic acid tests*** is that they are thought to detect *current or very recent infections,* although they are worthless during the first days of infection.

Nucleic acid amplification tests (NAAT) that measure viral RNA but do not utilize conventional PCR are also in use to detect the presence of CoV-2 RNA.

Viral antigen tests rely on immunoassays to measure specific viral ***proteins*** and are less sensitive than NAATs but may be faster to perform (NAATs can detect as few as 10 viral RNA fragments in a sample, but it is difficult to see the advantage in having such sensitivity).

However, Stites and Wilen caution that "testing does not equate to a finer understanding of how testing is used and utilized because physicians struggle with the ability to properly interpret test results." A principal reason for this "hedging" is because Stites and Wilen appreciate that tests are not perfect because there are always false positives and false negatives, and as a consequence, test results cannot state definitively whether a disease (or virus) is or is not present. What this means is that tests need to be evaluated "probabilistically on the basis of test performance, test characteristics, patient data, and importantly, disease prevalence."

Based on such measurements (the prevalence of disease in a community for example), the "positive predictive value of a test can be ***"estimated."*** The positive predictive value is a probability that the person who tested positive actually has the disease. Similarly, "negative predictive values" can be calculated based on similar information to qualify the chance that someone who tested negative truly does not have the disease.

Stites and Wilen go on to point out that two key metrics that characterize the test are needed to interpret the results of imperfects tests: the diagnostic sensitivity and diagnostic specificity (or commonly just "sensitivity" and "specificity"), and currently, there is limited information on these values for widely used SARS-CoV-2 tests. It gets worse. Probability of having a disease is a "**fairly subjective estimate that a health care provider would make on the basis of medical history, presentation, and factors such as known prevalence of the disease in the community**." And the value is never exact.

Finally, in this context, there is an extremely important issue, in addition, to emphasize that has plagued many other so-called viral diseases that rely on indirect tests. And this issue is the fact that there has been rapid development of new tests and many have made their way into the clinical arena without the standard pre-clinical validation processes required by FDA. In other words, in the race to patent test kits, similar to what we are facing with the EUA (Emergency Use Authorization) of CoV-2 vaccines currently (fast-tracking without adequate testing), many small biotech companies see SARS CoV-2 as a golden opportunity to exploit the urgency of the situation, and not subject their tests to appropriate validation standards!

On February 2, 2020, the CDC was the only place in the country that could perform SARS-CoV-2 tests. But on February 12, the CDC announced that the test was providing inconclusive results. By then, The United States had reported 11 cases.

In March, the CDC designed its own test, and the Food and Drug Administration picked a conservative testing strategy, allowing laboratories to use only the CDC tests distributed under the Emergency Use Authorization (EUA) authority (Sin Hang Lee. Testing for SARS-CoV-2 in cellular components by routine nested RT-PCR followed by DNA sequencing. International Journal of Geriatrics and Rehabilitation, 2 (1): 69-96, July 17, 2020).

One problem with all of this misdirected work is the fact that instead of relying on direct isolation of virus using centrifuged blood samples following by electron microscopic identification of viremia (many virus particles/ electron microscope field of view), the testing so far has almost exclusively relied on indirect reverse transcription quantitative polymerase chain reaction (RT-qPCR) on cell-free fluid samples of respiratory tract specimens. Also, another assay of these lung aspirates measures fluorescent signal accumulation as a surrogate marker for direct viral identification and which also is known to generate false-negative and false positive results. The fluorescent signal marker is typically done with PCR product rather than actual virus, and one Australian group, using this methodology (not direct EM viral identification), reported that the commercial PCR kit they used (RT-qPCR) found a positive predictive value to be only 55.56%, which if you think about it, is like flipping a coin. Although this group went on to suggest that any positive results derived from one test should be confirmed using another nucleic acid test, what is the point if no test can be trusted or has been validated against the gold standard of viral isolation, purification, and electron microscopic verification?

So far, we have primarily discussed nucleic acid testing. Protein testing can be of two types. The first type detects the protein coat of viruses, which isn't widely used, or used much at all, but the second type of protein test is used to determine if you have had a past infection, because this test measures the victims antibodies made against the antigen (virus), and which requires typically anywhere from several weeks to nearly a month in order for the body's immune system time to make enough antibody t0 detect with protein blot tests, or ELISA tests (Enzyme Linked Immunosorbent Assays). These are antibody tests which checks if the host has had a response to a pathogen.

However, with protein testing of either type (proteins from the virus or proteins made by the host in response to the virus), we run into some of the same issues that confound nucleic acid testing. For instance, the likely low prevalence of COVID-19 in the general population presents a challenge to the interpretation of protein tests also, and tests with lower specificity or sensitivity, the prevalence of the pathogen in the population, the health of the test subject, etc. all still confound a certain diagnosis, and could lead to dangerous consequences.

The challenge is that when testing for a disease with low prevalence in the tested population, even a test with relatively high specificity will generate large numbers of false positives. In the case of SARS- CoV-2 serology antibody testing, this could mean that many people who are being told they have protective antibodies do not in fact have them and they are still susceptible to an infection.

In the case of SARS-CoV-2, the question of specificity is a challenging one given that there are several other common coronaviruses to which many people probably already have antibodies, and these harmless viral-like coronaviruses can cross react with the SARS-CoV-2 strain, or its surrogate markers. These existing antibodies can cross react with the antigens used in the SARS-CoV- test, leading to false positive results.

In fact, as it was during the "HIV" hysteria of positive "HIV" test results during the 1980's and 90's which always remained high in high prevalence populations (which always was and has been the case with "HIV" because for one thing, the virus never existed in the first place and what was being measured for the most part were the effects of IV drug abuse, nitrosamine usage, and as Christine Johnson's list of false positives indicates, a plethora of non-virus-caused syndromes such as pregnancy or warts). With "HIV" testing, every "positive" result was and is a false positive because what is being biochemically measured is "junk" or cellular debris (see the Gonda Letter to Robert C. Gallo in which he said "[to Robert Gallo):

> **"If this assumption is based on the cultures being antigen positive, I would like to point out that the "particles" in micro- graph 0905 are the debris of a degenerated cell. No other extracellular "virus-like particles" were observed free between cells anywhere in the pellet. The small extracellular vesicles in 0904 are at least 50% smaller than HTLV mature particles seen in type I, II, or III" ("HIV, or the cellular garbage Gonda was referring to from Gallo's cultures was called HTLV-III before it was renamed by the Varmus committee "HIV"-see page 154, 1984 in Part II). Again, these vesicles can be found in any cell pellet. I do not believe any of the particles photographed are HTLV I, II, or III."**

Also it is important to remember what Luc Montagnier said, who received the Nobel Prize for discovering "HIV", and Gallo had been chasing "HIV" as a cancer virus "variant" for more than a decade before Montagnier's 1983 report about LAV (another previous name for "HIV," and who sadly received no credit as a co-discoverer of cellular garbage, and thus Montagnier and Bar Sinoussi received the credit., and for which received no credit by the Nobel committee.in 2008.

Adam Bonislawski gives a number of cogent examples about the pitfalls of testing for SARS-CoV-2 in a piece he wrote on April 16, 2020. He interviewed a number of high-ranking officials in public health positions regarding testing, and it is worth briefly reviewing what the gist of some of these Infectious Disease Specialists have concluded regarding COVID-19 mass testing.

Kaitlyn Sadtier who is the Chief of the section for immuno-engineering at the National Institutes of Biomedical Imaging and Bioengineering, and a leader of a study launched by the NIH claimed that "when you are looking at a large sample size with a lower prevalence, those false positives start to become much more of an issue." Robert Garry, a professor of microbiology at Tulane University School of Medicine likewise noted the issue of potential false positives in the low prevalence populations is a major problem because there will be more false positives than true positives."

To make testing matters worse, as of July, 2020, there were more than 70 serology tests available in the US that were sanctioned using the EUA process (rather than through obtaining FDA approval), and none of these tests have been or are validated with electron micrographic evidence of isolation, purification, and SARS-CoV-2 viremia in a victim's tissue(s). The real issue is, was, and always will be- whether any test is of any value with victims with less severe symptoms or who are asymptomatic.

Going back to the Wuhan experience, as they were among the earliest hit and have the most experience, Zhaung GH, Shen MW, Zeng LX, MI BB, Chen FY Liu WJ, Pei LL, Qi X, and Li C. (Potential false-positive rate among the "asymptomatic infected individuals' in close contacts of COVID-19 patients) reported in an ahead of print article (Mar 5; 41 (4): 485-488, **2020**; doi 10.3760/cma.j.cn 112338-200221-00144)... that.

> *"When the infection rate of the close contacts and the sensitivity and specificity of reported results were taken as the point estimates, the positive predictive value of the active screening was only 19.67%, in contrast the false-positive rate of positive results was 80.33%, and nearly half or even more of the 'asymptomatic infected individuals' reported in the active nucleic acid test screening might be false positives." In a "Morning Briefing Newsletter," which is available online, for the past several months, the CDC has been saying that people without symptoms do not need testing."*

Yet most of the so-called positive test results, as shown by a focus here of a specific example or two of what are taught as distinct diseases, appear to be mostly the result of medicine's and pharma's continued propaganda campaign to convince people that they are inherently ill, as the following references demonstrate in the context of one of these "political" diagnoses (**13-100**).

To understand what is wrong with most current, inaccurate, SARS CoV-2 testing:

Most pathogen isolation protocols themselves are confronted with a broad range of cellular debris, including breakdown products from sick or dying cells that shed both decaying genomic fragments and proteins, which complex with these nucleic acid fragments to resemble viruses, mycoplasma, or appear different immunologically to the victim's own immune system. This is especially the case with cryptic forms of bacteria, and especially "viruses" (or autoimmune artifacts) such as "Hepatitis C." Historically since the polio era, whenever baffling conditions or complex health issues arise, objects that are below light's visible wave-lengths are usually blamed, since the time of Koch and Hill, before this technology (electron microscopy-EM) was invented (in the late 1930's), and this holds true still today.

When these uncertainties are added to other contexts such as transfusion medicine, tissue transplantation, and most egregiously when it is tacitly assumed that some kind of unfounded faith in biological causality has been deserved by those who do not know or accept the profound limitations of sequence identity comparisons and the unbridled and undeserved faith in molecular testing, there clearly hasn't been sufficient time or sober skepticism to incorporate all of the new work on the Human genome.

For example, considered alone, it is difficult to contemplate when molecular diagnostics of entities like "HERVs" determine people's lives or even are used to incarcerate if they were aware they were positive for a sexually-transmitted pathogen without telling a partner and proven in court ("Human Endogenous Retroviral Sequences," retroelements, "retroids," phages), when these phenomena could simply at a cellular level represent decay products that mimic nucleic acid sequences of various pathogens, then the need for a direct pathogen detection method becomes urgent. Therefore, we began with a specific case and we asked the question whether or not serology-obtained biochemical indicators of nucleic acids or proteins were in any way identical to a direct measure of actual visible viable pathogens?

With such philosophical biases in mind, it should be amply stressed that the problems with the current medical paradigms are not only financial in nature. Nor are the problems inherent in medicine associated with profit motives the most egregious and dangerous current threats. During periods of critical or chronic illness, everyone at some point can find fault with procedural blunders that invariably occur to carry out standards of care, or issues raised about how and when a therapeutic intervention is or is not provided. What is not clearly obvious is that there are larger and far graver issues to be illuminated.

However, as it is with any darkness before a storm, our best improvements might soon begin to be set into motion, because we are becoming more aware of what these shortcomings involve, and we can and will eventually implement needed changes, simply because of increasing needs. These needs can be outlined as generalizations by simply examining in detail several specific examples. Therefore, how molecular testing can lead to stigmatization of victims should be emphasized.

This conundrum can be avoided by direct confirmatory ultrastructural testing following PCR or WESTERN-blot analysis of blood from the same patient's blood draw, because this classic virological isolation process may help eliminate the problem of false-positive pathogen testing in a number of contexts, and eliminate medical conundrums wherein indirect protein or nucleic acid testing detects nucleic acids or proteins that mimic non-disease-associated proteins or nucleic acids in persons not infected. Furthermore, an awareness

of these issues, it is hoped, will usher in a new conceptual framework regarding any pathogen, but more importantly, our conceptions about causality in human health or disease.

A few notable observations should have emerged this month and in the months before that should be presented regarding testing for COVID-19 or coronaviruses more generally, asymptomatic "carriers," and also, what "experts" have published regarding potentially disastrous therapeutic interventions. Below the entire abstracts have been presented. From a group in China who published on COVID-19 patients and then withdrew the article sometime between now and then, we read: Zhuang GJ, Shen MW, Zeng LX, Mi BB, Chen FY., Liu WJ, Pei LL, Qi X, Li C. 2020 Mar 5;41(4):485-488. **Potential false-positive rate among the asymptomatic infected individuals' in close contacts of COVID-19 patients**.

Results: When the infection rate of the close contacts and the sensitivity and specificity of reported results were taken as the point estimates, the positive predictive value of the active screening was only 19.67%, in contrast, **the false-positive rate of positive results was 80.33%.** The multivariate-probabilistic sensitivity analysis results supported the base-case findings, **with a 75% probability for the false-positive rate of positive results over 47%.**

Conclusions: In the close contacts of COVID-19 patients, nearly half or even more of the 'asymptomatic infected individuals' reported in the active nucleic acid test screening might be false positives.

The Editor office's response for Ahead of Print article was withdrawn because:

"The article [paraphrased because of bad English] "**Potential false-positive rate among the 'asymptomatic infected individuals in close contacts of COVID-19 patients** were under strong discussion after pre-published questions from the readers focused on the [fact that the] article's results and conclusions were dependent on theoretical deduction, but that the field epidemiology data were valid. Reviewers suggested that further research was needed to prove the current theory. Based on these criticisms, it was decided by the editorial board to remove the article from 'prepublished' lists."

Although this article is available still on The National Library of Medicine's free website library, the initial acceptance and publication of the data by Zhuang et al. is at a minimum, suspicious because it is not clear if it was withdrawn purely on in lack of merit as the editors claim, or whether the retraction was due to some kind of political correctness and the official party line with respect to COVID-19 currently unfolding, insecurity about sources such as fish markets versus homologies to bat nucleic acid sequences suggesting a different "official story," or if it really is detectable in the first place.

In support of the idea that the nucleic acid tests do not work in the case of the current COVID-19 epidemic, whereas the original isolation and characterization of SARS CoV-2 by 1.Tyrrell DA, Bynoe ML in 1966 was definitive, and fulfilled Koch's postulates in their paper; "**Cultivation of viruses from a high proportion of patients with colds.** Lancet 1:76–77, 1966. Many other groups too numerous to list here also have recently published that frequent false negatives and false positives are being found with nucleic acid testing (which supposedly tests for CoV-2 SARS viral sequences although this is doubtful because of the manner by which recent sputum samples have been characterized without the use of electron microscopy to confirm isolation, and despite evidence of CT-confirmed pulmonary improvements regardless of the detection of nucleic acid positivity persisting, and other inconsistencies as well.

One group suggested that they found evidence that some 33,000 of the confirmed cases as of April 7 2020 are not showing consistent testing results for CO-2 SARS "RNA," and this group did not even withdraw their manuscript: (https://www.ncbi.nlm.nih.gov/pubmed/32270882):

Wang X**1**., Tan L **2**., Wang X1, L1 W,**1** Wang X1, Tan L**2**, Wang X1[3], Liu W,**1**. Lu Y**3**, Cheng L**4**, Sun Z**5**. Int J Infect Dis. 2020 Apr 18. pii: S1201-9712(20)30235-6. doi: 10.1016/j.ijid.2020.04.023. [Epub ahead of print] **Comparison of nasopharyngeal and oropharyngeal**

swabs for SARS-CoV-2 detection in 353 patients received tests with both specimens simultaneously.

1. Department of Laboratory Medicine, Tongji Hospital, Tongji Medical College, Huazhong University of Science and Technology, Wuhan, China.
2. Department of Infection Control, Tongji Hospital, Tongji Medical College, Huazhong University of Science and Technology, Wuhan, China.
3. Department of Laboratory Medicine, Tongji Hospital, Tongji Medical College, Huazhong University of Science and Technology, Wuhan, China. Electronic address: junyanlu_2000@163.com.
4. Department of Laboratory Medicine, Tongji Hospital, Tongji Medical College, Huazhong University of Science and Technology, Wuhan, China. Electronic address: chengliming2015@163.com.
5. Department of Laboratory Medicine, Tongji Hospital, Tongji Medical College, Huazhong University of Science and Technology, Wuhan, China. Electronic address: zysun@tjh.tjmu.edu.cn.

BACKGROUND: *Since the outbreak of coronavirus disease (COVID-19) in Wuhan in December 2019, by March 10, 2020, a total of 80,932 confirmed cases have been reported in China. Two consecutively negative RT-PCR test results in respiratory tract specimens are required for the evaluation of discharge from hospital, and oropharyngeal swabs were the most common sample.* ***However, false negative results occurred in the late stage of hospitalization, and avoiding false negative result is critical essential."***

METHODS: *We reviewed the medical record of 353 patients who received tests with both specimens simultaneously and compared the performance between nasopharyngeal and oropharyngeal swabs.*

RESULTS: *Of the 353 patients (outpatients, 192; inpatients, 161)* *studied, the median age was 54 years, and 177 (50.1%) were women. Higher positive rate (positive tests/total tests) was observed in nasopharyngeal swabs than oropharyngeal swabs, especially in inpatients. Nasopharyngeal swabs from inpatients showed higher positive rate than outpatients. Nasopharyngeal swabs from male showed higher positive rate than female, especially in outpatients. Detection with both specimens slightly increased the positive rate than nasopharyngeal swab only. Moreover, the consistency between from nasopharyngeal and oropharyngeal swabs were poor (Kappa=0.308).*

CONCLUSION: *In conclusion, our study suggests that nasopharyngeal swabs may be more suitable than oropharyngeal swab at this stage of COVID-19 outbreak.*

And, in the Journal of Medical Virology we read:

False-negative of RT-PCR and prolonged nucleic acid conversion in COVID-19: Rather than recurrence. Xiao AT[1], Tong YX[1,] Zhang S2. J Med Virol. 2020 Apr 9. doi: 10.1002/jmv.25855.

Abstract

> *"A novel coronavirus (COVID-19) pandemic cause by Severe Acute Respiratory Syndrome Coronavirus-2 (SARS-CoV-2) threatens the world. We read with interest the recent report by Li et al. that included 610 patients with Coronavirus Disease 2019 (COVID-19). They reported a high false-negative rate of real-time reverse transcription polymerase chain reaction (RT-PCR) results for SARS-CoV-2 detection. In addition, recent report regarding SARS-CoV-2 "turn positive" in recovered cases with COVID-19 were published. Here, we studied the characteristics of nucleic acid conversion for SARS-CoV-2 from 70 COVID-19 patients.* ***We found that 15 (21.4%) patients experienced a "turn positive" of nucleic acid detection by RT-PCR test for SARS-CoV-2 after two consecutive negative results,*** *which may be related to the false negative of RT-PCR test and prolonged nucleic acid conversion."*

A SOLUTION TO THE TESTING MADNESS

Direct confirmatory **ultrastructural testing** following PCR or WESTERN-blot analysis of blood from the same patient's blood draw may help eliminate the problem of false positive pathogen testing in a number of contexts and eliminate medical conundrums wherein indirect protein or nucleic acid testing detects proteins that mimic non-disease-associated proteins or nucleic acids in persons in ill-health, but not infected. Furthermore, an awareness of these issues, it is hoped, will usher in a new conceptual framework regarding all microbial pathogens, but more importantly, help change our entrenched and often erroneous conceptions about causality in human health or disease.

The most heinous consequence of this unforgivable and unspeakable testing delusion are mandated vaccines. Fierce objections have been forcefully and articulately advanced toward policy changes regarding over-vaccination and re-vaccination schedules and antibiotic over-prescription during infancy, childhood, adolescence, middle age, and old age. An entire spectrum of what amounts to even costlier and problematic and highly adverse event-inducing life-long maladies and endemic illnesses are increasing exponentially, and when drugs are given to treat the side effects of previous drugs, these arguments have been ignored and censored and veer off toward insanity.

Too much profit is made by the medical system treating their own mistakes and treating endemic iatrogenic diseases caused by the medical system itself. Consider the invitations, advertising, and even legally enforced mandates to herd our children and seniors into the slaughter-house of ever more drugs and vaccines that continues to this day. Almost each month there are new so-called "preventive" vaccines and drugs that are being aggressively advertised and marketed for new ailments you have never heard of or have never known that you or your children are suffering from, without your awareness. When obedience is not willingly provided to the agenda of Big Pharma, even by the asking of a simple question about seeing the safety data for such "staples" as the hepatitis B vaccine, some parents have been threatened with incarceration by governmental agencies at the insistence of certain factions of the medical establishment. Children in fact have been illegally prevented from attending school, and in other situations, parents have been incarcerated until they "listen" to doctor's orders and force their children to follow "standards of care" rather than try alternative therapeutics they want to explore that involve no toxicity and can do no harm. Yet we are forced to accept that these medicines do no harm and are beneficial. We are counseled that we should blindly accept them without a discussion, or without harboring any concerns for the long-term effects they may have and which they could potentially unleash on entire populations because of an "impassioned crusade" to vaccinate and medicate the entire human race to establish "herd immunity" and to accomplish disease "eradications" through vaccines ONLY, and to the exclusion of naturally acquired populational immunity otherwise known as natural herd immunity.

But are these projections really true, or are they simply cruel violations of human potential and the common good? Vaccine makers in some cases have admitted or include on the package inserts page-long lists of adverse reactions associated with many vaccines prescribed to children, teens, adults, and seniors. A common but not exhaustive list of these maladies include arthritis, asthma, seizures, ADD, shingles, AIDS and other ill-definable autoimmune syndromes, diabetes, meningitis, pneumococcal illnesses, hypertension, and a plethora of "pulmonary hypertensive disorders," and cancers. Yet healthy children, adolescents, and young adults in fact appear in many statistical surveys to becoming "sicker" without any concerns raised about the long-term effects on health of preventative interventions such as the so-called "hepatitis B" and "HPV" vaccines that supposedly protect against cancers that will occur 50 years later, with these vaccine's > 10% severe and often life-long adverse event profiles.

Regarding **"How Inaccurate Viral Lab Tests Can Create and**

Inflate the Illusion of a Pandemic by Creating Millions of False-Positive Virus Tests," there are several important issues to emphasize.

First: It should be clear that testing constitutes a kind of gate to hell in the first place, because if you are asymptomatic and test positive, you could easily be rewarded as being a false positive and come to enjoy the worry, fear, stigma, possible government penalization (internment camps) and other unspeakable medical terrorism, even when CDC has warned against testing for asymptomatics! In fact, after appreciating the caveats involved in testing that have been reviewed above, one may ask oneself if it is even worth it ever to be tested...how do you know what the prevalence is in the location you are in if the population you are in depends on these tests (or the government depends on these tests) to determine prevalence in the first place, even after the CDC itself has said for months that asymptomatics need not even bother with getting tested? It is a tautology of illogic.

Second: With all of the caveats of sensitivity and specificity and with the current blizzard of small biotech companies (and large) raining down tests that are not validated against the gold standard of true virus isolation, how can one ever be sure the test kit type one is given even works?

Third: Regarding high and low "prevalence," it should be clear that the numbers of "cases" we have been told are completely fictitious, and that of those truly sick individuals that are/are not filling up hospital wards (depending on what media news reports you believe), COVID-19 has remained from the beginning an atypical pneumonia syndrome (with gastrointestinal and cardiovascular comorbidities of pathological expression that shows objectively detectable symptoms in approximately less than 0.1% of those groups carefully followed, suggesting that there is nothing but low prevalence for COVID-19 diseases.

I have not tripped over any bodies on the sidewalks since February 2019, have you? If you go with the higher numbers we are sometimes told are accruing by the media, suggesting 5%-10%-15%

of the population of the world are cases, then there is a logical contradiction (or lie) in the works. People have been subsumed under the COVID-19 "case" classifications for a variety of reasons to inflate numbers since the beginning of this "Global Pandemic."

The spinners of the lie cannot have it both ways. Either the numbers of morbidly ill people are as high as they say, in which case where are the bodies to avoid stumbling over on the sidewalks and where are the funeral pyres burning, or are atypical pneumonia SARS-CoV-2 victims almost negligible (as is probably the case), again because the "prevalence" determines in part if a test is positive in the first place and no validated tests have yet been in widespread usage, according to the CDC, because clearly, a tautology emerges with testing using non-validated tests to determine prevalence in a population in order to diagnose a victim to the SARS-CoV-2, COVID-19 disease designation.

Fourth: If you are asymptomatic, testing will not save you…it will damn you, as it did during the "HIV-AIDS" era, for which we have those same persons to thank: Fauci, Birx, Redfield, Gallo, etc. If you should happen to test positive, you could be "convicted" of having SARS-CoV-2 viruses (or conservatively, some cross-reactive endogenous and harmless coronavirus that cross reacts with the probe being used) and then be quarantined by THE STATE, or worse, be placed in an "internment camp" as some recent reports have suggested are "just around the corner." You could be kept against your will in that internment camp until you submit to a PCR nucleic test and test negative, and/or register a negative PCR signal for CoV-2 after 40 PCR amplification cycles, and as determined by an EUA non-FDA approved test in the growing arsenal of non-validated dozens of non-gold standard validated tests that are now flooding the market. You probably will not be tested using an antibody test to demonstrate proof of past infection, but if you are, and do test positive, the prevalence issue still is in place, and a positive protein antibody test is evaluated using the same constraint that PCR testing is constrained by the prevalence of positive tests in a population as shown by a test that is interpreted based on prevalence-a tautology.

Fifth: The "positive predictive value of a test can only be *"estimated."* The positive predictive value is a probability that the person who tested positive actually has the disease. Similarly, "negative predictive values" can be calculated based on similar information to qualify the chance that someone who tested negative truly does not have the disease.

INACCURATE VIRAL LAB TESTS CREATE AND INFLATE THE ILLUSION OF A PANDEMIC BY CREATING MILLIONS OF FALSE-POSITIVES

Today in medical schools and elsewhere, the Great 1918-19 Influenza "pandemic" always is attributed to a viral cause, despite the fact that in 1918 viruses weren't yet discovered as there were no electron microscopes yet invented (until the mid to late 1930's and which weren't really deployed for biological investigation until 1939). Although even back in Rosenau's day, a variety of ingenious filter types were used to strain out bacteria (and mycoplasmas?) to assess transmissibility and determine modes of transmission. If and until the indirect approach of "reverse genetics" can substitute for the actual synthesis of infectious viral particles and then Rosenau- like functional criteria are met, we will be in the dark as to the cause of influenza.

Taubenberger, Hultin, and Morens are aware of the potential influence of environmental factors as they mention this in their work. But Rosenau's functional characterization that even though direct exposures of infected sera and lung aspirates of dying or dead patients to healthy volunteers, even in the form of IV injections, shaking hands, talking 2 inches from a face, coughing of an infected person to a healthy one didn't induce any illness in 1918, the review paper of Jeffery Taubenberger, Johan V Hultin, and David M. Morens is worth an open minded read (Discovery and characterization of the 1918 pandemic influenza virus in historical context. Antivir Ther. 2007; 12 (4 Pt B): 581-591, 2007).

The discordance caused by the non-harmony created between modern reverse genetics, molecular biology, and Rosenau's functional characterization regarding the transmission of The Great "H1N1" "Spanish flu" are alive and well in SARS-CoV-19 today. Until our technology fits common sense, we will be left out in "the deep cold, "perhaps not as cold as the foreboding permafrost from which the Hultin expedition sought and obtained the RNA to "reconstruct" the Great Influenza "virus," but the cold that descends around sciences based on assumptions, nevertheless. Perhaps it was best expressed by Rosenau when he stated, "*I think we must be very careful not to draw any positive conclusions from negative results of this kind.*"

It is interesting to note, or at least be aware, that at the time the Rosenau influenza experiments were being designed and carried out and ever since, the cancer virus conundrum also was being born in the hands of Payton Rous, as shown in his 1966 Nobel Prize acceptance speech when he said: "no human cancer has ever been linked to a viral cause." This will become extremely important during the era of AIDS in the 1980's, and still today in 2021.

The consequences of these hypotheses that begin with the "tarot cards" of molecular testing need to be reevaluated in light of the fact that that an entire planet has been sequestered without the electron microscopic visualization of SARS CoV-2 viral-like particles in a single asymptomatic "healthy carrier" of the RT-PCR-positive accused, and because a 350 year-old technology known as hyperbaric oxygen therapy (HBOT) has been reported to have reversed or saved 100% of morbidly ill SARS-COVID-19 victims. After the first year of social distancing and mask wearing, or in some countries no mask wearing or lockdowns, it now appears that more than 90+ % of SARS-CoV-2 symptomatic individuals recovered or will recover with a minimum of intervention, and for those who go on to develop lung consolidation, atelectasia, or induration, or kidney damage, the only rational method of therapy is hyperbaric oxygen combined with specific nutrients. Another consequence of these developments and ideas is that our perception of SARS-COVID-19 and influenza in general must change. Influenzas must be viewed not so much as a medical crisis, but more as a philosophical, psychological, and political crisis. Specifically, in the realm of philosophy and human psychology, SARS-COVID-19 is and has been a crisis of epistemology, which is a branch of philosophy that asks, "how do we know what we think we know?"

In the realm of international politics, and the politics of science and medicine, SARS-COVID-19 is a crisis of how the people have been manipulated to regard other people and society using forecasts of the future which is not a science. This is because all of vaccinology and much of virology are at their basis are predicated on the assumption that when nothing happens, nothing happens. To explain this claim, a hypothetical example might suffice. Let us assume that: "The reason the Greeks and the Americans didn't get sick in 2011 with an epidemic of cholera is because all of them were vaccinated with the cholera vaccine in 2010."

This hypothetical statement reveals this null assumption in vaccinology, that when nothing happens, nothing happens. The reasons that are believed to support such a hypothetical proclamation by vaccinologists and other people who try to advance preventative medicine is that, as a hypothetical example, let us assume that the Greeks or Americans did not get sick in 2011 because they all were vaccinated with a cholera vaccine in 2019, or had somehow achieved "herd" immunity previously to the introduction of the 2011 cholera "epidemic." This kind of reasoning does not consider the simple fact that there may have been no conditions for cholera to flourish, or no introduction of cholera into their water supplies, or no co-morbidity such as an epidemic of influenza descending on the Americans and the Greeks in 2011. In other words, vaccinologists, and infectious disease investigators, as well as many microbial pathologists, tacitly assume that the absence of evidence (when nothing happens), does not mean the absence of evidence (then nothing happens), but instead, means their intervention "worked."

A science must be based upon things or events that do happen. In this context we are told to believe that if we are not accepting of a vaccination, or if society is not vaccinated, we are doomed.

THE HEALTHY SICK PEOPLE

During the insanity of SARS-COVID-19 reign of terror, certain destructive ideals and behaviors of ancient human history have been codified as would an illusion about witches and sorcerers magical powers being real, and because of the way the SARS-COVID-19 pandemic has become manifested, it truly has been a delusion, ushered along by the promise of vaccines which are pharmaceuticals, which as pointed out earlier, in Greek, (pharmakaia) means sorcery or witchcraft.

Virological and vaccinology wellsprings of delusion are predicated on a fear of the invisible…a fear of contagion, and the attribution of malevolent forces to wraiths and things that are not there, or that do not exist in the material world. This conclusion was reached because of forty years spent working daily in level 3 and level 4 biocontainment labs and laminar flow hoods. These types of sterile lab conditions tend to foster an awareness of what hygienic and aseptic (sterile) procedures and techniques really require and underscore the futility and insanity of mask-wearing as if it were Halloween, or social distancing, as a means to controlling microbial pathogens, instead of relying on an 800-million-year legacy of acquired immunity naturally and our immunological diversity.

When entire nations or a planet of organisms is exposed to a foreign protein via inoculation or vaccination, the intervention qualifies as a selective force on our future evolutionary path, and natural selection does not anticipate future events.

Furthermore, an awareness of aseptic practices juxtaposed against the current dictums and warnings of Pharma and the Public Health Service regarding mask wearing and social distancing harken back to holy waters besprinkled during baptisms, and the crucifixes dangling about the necks of black-robed priests of the past, which have now been forged into stethoscopes, should the heart suddenly stop pumping the four humors Aristotle had wrongly surmised comprised the center of human consciousness, and the way consciousness was distributed in the body. Aristotle surmised that the heart was the location of human consciousness because he saw a chicken running around after its head was cut off.

Shortly thereafter, a 1,500 year-long ban on human dissection was launched by the Christian Church because the location of human consciousness was believed to be in the heart because Aristotle saw and wrote about a chicken running around a barnyard after its head was cut off, and concluded that consciousness was not in the head but in the heart, and despite the fact that previously, Hippocrates correctly had surmised that human consciousness was situated somewhere in the head (instead of the heart) because he had doctored soldiers injured on one side of the head during battle, and he noted that their motor movements or sensation on the opposite side of their bodies were diminished or completely compromised. Hippocrates also discovered that ketogenic dietary regimens were an effective therapeutic management for epilepsy, and ketogenic diets are still used today for hospitalized epileptics when all the anti-seizure drugs fail (Jim Robins. A symphony in the brain. Grove Press, New York, 2000).

Following the Christian era, the black robes of the clergy were bleached white, and the potions of toads feet and tinctures of dragon tails become lifetime prescriptions of cardiac medications, and methamphetamines given to children who were too active. The white robes conveyed to the pious and the masses alike the impression of sterility, and purity.

In this unspeakable alliance of the past practices of witchcraft and sorcery, only the scenery, costumes, and communion rituals were changed, yet the potions, drugs, and especially the vaccines concocted by biotechnology, biomedical researchers, also without scientific evidence, replaced the witches brews of previous superstitious eras. Reason prevailed in some quarters, which became evident after each and every vaccine in history including the fabled polio vaccines were immediately halted because they caused paralysis. Similarly, some of the SARS-COVID vaccines have been withheld or withdrawn because they induce death and clotting, as with the Astra Zeneca and Moderna vaccines pulled from distribution in Nordic countries recently. Contemporary pharmaceutical witches, and pharmaceutical sorcerers that practice the modern "practice of medicine" often have no better scientific evidence and track records and no better outcomes to the sorcerers and witches of the middle ages that used medieval potions not based on scientific evidence. In inoculations and vaccines, they are blended from vile harmful extracts of puss and other putrid, rotting dead materials extracted from the diseased, and from fetal embryonic tissues, cadavers, and even the germs of human excrement as with the first polio vaccines. Now they are derived from RNA. It may be the case that modern pharmaceutical potions are in fact more deadly, and dangerous than the potions used by witches in the middle ages! Regardless, modern medicine is all too often indistinguishable from magic and witchcraft, lacking any scientific evidence, and more akin to a religion than a science

For example, these kinds of reports are a dime-a-dozen in the vaccinologist's universe:

Pfizer drops India vaccine application after regulator seeks local trial https://www.reuters.com/article/health-coronavirus-india-pfizer/pfizer-drops-india-vaccine-application-after-regulator-seeks-local-trial-idUSKBN2A50GE, February 5, 2021

THE ACCURACY PROBLEMS WITH COVID-19 & ALL OTHER VIRAL TESTING: MULTIFACTORIAL SINGULARITIES AND 20,000 BIRDS

Due to the multifactorial singularity type of logic that advanced the much-cherished cancer biology and virology of the 1970's & 1980's, and indeed today, we can now say that to advance the idea that the so-called cancer-associated virus can cause cervical cancer or liver cancer or leukemia in humans at a rate of 0.06% out of 600,000 "carriers" in 25-40 years, is like saying:

"I have 20,000 birds. 10,000 of these birds molt once a year. The other 10,000 molt 3 times a year. Now, none of the 10,000 birds that molt once a year died by flying into utility poles. However, 6 of the 10,000 birds that molt 3 times a year died by flying into utility poles. Therefore, among these birds, molting 3 times a year CAUSED them to hit utility poles and die."

Molting 3 times annually —> hitting utility poles —> death.

This is a purely hypothetical and statistical argument, but it demonstrates how worthless such arguments are that claim that events such as cancers or deaths via influenzas occur at vanishing low rates justify a failed vaccine-fought war on influenza viruses, or other viruses such as the alleged cancer viruses, hepatitis B viruses, HPV viruses, the fabled "Hep C" viruses and others. These putative viral diseases such as the hepatitis C virus have been used to justify the roll-out of vaccines in Italy and elsewhere that precisely preceded a huge explosion of influenza there last December, 2019, which was preceded 2 months earlier on more than 400,000 Northern Italians centered around Bergano Italy and have justified the trillions of dollars spent on vaccine development.

How does this delusion about the 20,000 birds and utility poles work? Let us suppose that an ill-defined molecular marker occurs at a frequency of 0.06% of those hundreds of thousands who carry the identical molecular marker called a cancer virus without acquiring cancers or influenzas? With this type of multifactorial singularity-style of logic, rare events can be named and justified. It is an inevitable consequence of statistics that happen at low frequency that are thought to cause something to happen.

Multifactorial singularities like these arise and become institutionalized as causal forces or processes despite the contradiction of simple logic: if a virus X causes cancer in 1 in a million who also have that virus or its markers, then 999,999 times out of a million it does not cause cancer. Therefore, virus X causes cancer! In simple language, a multifactorial singularity is "a cause" confounded by many factors that influence statistics. Although they frequently employ math and numerical data, multifactorial singularities have no predictive power for determining if any individual will become ill or develop a syndrome.

When multifactorial singularities like "HPV and cancer, or "HBV and cancer" or "HIV/AIDS" or "HIV" and cancers arise (such as Kaposi's sarcoma), and when their pathogenesis is unknown (exactly how they cause illness), all that becomes relevant is the imagined cause, and everyone is unequivocally assured that it is deterministic or causal that "HIV" causes AIDS, except of course, in the minds of the hypotheses' initial framers, like Luc Montagnier, or Rous who received Nobel Prizes based on this reasoning.

For instance, Luc Montagnier said in a recent documentary following his Nobel acceptance that: "*you can catch it* ("HIV") *many times and if your immune system is strong you can get rid of it no problem!*" (This specific interview with the Nobelist, Luc Montagnier, discoverer of "HIV" can be watched online at http://www.youtube.com/watch?v=WQoNW7lOnT4l) ...

Luc Montagnier:

> ***"...I believe HIV, we can be exposed to HIV many times without being chronically infected. Our immune system will get rid of the virus in a few weeks, if you have a good immune system; and this is also the problem with African people; their nutrition is not very equilibrated, they are in oxidative stress, even if they are not infected with HIV, so their immune system does not work well***

> ***already, so it is prone, you know, to allow HIV to get in and persist. So, there are many ways, not the vaccine, many ways to decrease the transmission, just by simple measures of nutrition, giving anti-oxidants, proper anti-oxidants-hygiene measures, fighting the other infections."***

Interviewer:

> *"If you have a good immune system, then your body can naturally get rid of HIV?"*

Luc Montagnier:

> ***"Yes."***

And yet these kinds of statements are only a glimpse of similar thoughts and statements of those to whom we bestow our trust and science's highest Nobel awards. Yet we are repeatedly deluged with misinformation by the media, medical "authorities", and government about how we need to persistently live in fear with statements like: "*Everyone is at risk;" you can catch* "it" *through just one contact; "you don't need co-factors;" "Africa's population is being decimated by an "HIV" virus* (although it's population has doubled or increased by more people that live in the U.S. during the so-called 30+ year AIDS pandemic); "that an antibody positive test is something to fear;" "that sexually-transmitted viruses jumped from non-human primates to black persons because phylogenetic sequence homologies in favor of racist thinking backed by phony science is believed and promoted without discussion;" "that viruses leap from camels to humans," or from bats to pangolins to civets to humans;" "that PCR detects viral load;" and as of this year, by the science fraud and scaremongering of Dr. Prof. Christian Drosten and his rapidly globalized PRC test of the 2019- nCOV sequence, which was renamed SARS-CoV-2 on February 7, 2020- that the Chinese had actually discovered **a new** virus (From: "The Science Fraud by Prof. Christian Drosten Corona_Facts July 10, 2020-Original German article https://telegra.ph/Der-Wissenschaftsbetrug-durch-Prof-ChristianDrosten-07-10).

The reasons for this fraud are because on 1.24.2020 and on 3.2.2020:

"...The authoritative virologists of the Chinese disease authority (CCDC) published their results on 24.01.2020 and 03.02.2020. They report on the isolation of "many" short gene sequences, which, when strung together, could represent a genetic strand of a new type of virus. The authors explicitly pointed out (as well as all other virologists involved to date "as of 10.07.2020") that the absolutely necessary experiments have not yet been carried out which would make it possible to claim that this is indeed a genetic strand of a pathogenic virus. On the contrary: Chinese virologists even explicitly point out that the constructed genetic strand bears up to 90% similarity to genetic strands of harmless and for decades known, claimed corona viruses in bats. This is what is stated in the study of 24.01.2020 under discussion, "our study does not fulfill Koch's postulates."(From: "The Science Fraud by Prof. Christian Drosten Corona_Facts July 10, 2020-Original German article https://telegra.ph/Der-Wissenschaftsbetrug-durch-Prof-ChristianDrosten-07-10)

As longtime investigative journalist John Rappoport writes: (Vicious criminal Neil Ferguson playing key role in new lockdowns https://blog.nomorefakenews.com/2020/12/24/neil-ferguson-playing-key-role-in-new-lockdowns/)):

Neil Ferguson: the ghost in the machine

Why do governments salute when he predicts a pandemic and tells them to lockdown their countries?

Does anyone care about his past?

Why does he still have a prestigious job?

Who is he connected to?

Neil Ferguson, through his institute at London's Imperial College, can call the shots on a major percentage of the global population.

He's Mr. Genius, when it comes to projecting computer models of epidemics. Fellow experts puff up his reputation. According to the Business Insider (4/25), "Ferguson's team warned Boris Johnson that the quest for 'herd immunity' [letting people live their lives out in the open in the UK] could cost 510,000 lives, prompting an abrupt U-turn [massive national lockdown in the UK]...

His simulations have been influential in other countries as well, cited by authorities in the US, Germany, and France." Not only cited, not only influential, but swallowed whole.

Business insider continues:

"On March 23, the UK scrapped 'herd immunity' in favor of a suppression strategy, and the country prepared for weeks of lockdown. Ferguson's study was responsible."

"Dr Deborah Birx, coronavirus response coordinator to the Trump administration, told journalists at a March 16 press briefing that the Imperial paper [Ferguson's computer projection] prompted the CDC's new advice to work from home and avoid gatherings of 10 or more.

Ferguson, instigator of **LOCKDOWN.**

"Stripping away of basic liberties. Economic devastation. So, let us look at Ferguson's track record, spelled out in the BI piece: "Ferguson co-founded the MRC Centre for Global Infectious Disease Analysis, based at Imperial, in 2008. It is the leading body advising national governments on pathogen outbreaks."

"It gets tens of millions of dollars in annual funding from the Bill & Melinda Gates Foundation, and works with the UK National Health Service, the US Centers for Disease Prevention and Control (CDC), and is tasked with supplying the World Health Organization with 'rapid analysis of urgent infectious disease problems'."

"Gates money goes to Ferguson. Ferguson predicts dire threat from COVID, necessitating lockdowns–thus preparing people to accept a vaccine. The vaccine Gates wants. Ferguson supplies a frightening computer projection of COVID deaths–to the CDC and WHO."

F*erguson thus communicates a rationale for the Gates vaccine plan. National governments surrender to WHO and CDC.*

LOCKDOWNS

> *Business Insider: "Michael Thrusfield, a professor of veterinary epidemiology at Edinburgh University, told the paper he had "déjà vu' after reading the [Ferguson] Imperial paper [on COVID], saying Ferguson was responsible for excessive animal culling during the 2001 Foot and Mouth [mad cow] outbreak." "Ferguson warned the government that 150,000 people could die. Six million animals were slaughtered as a precaution, costing the country billions in farming revenue. In the end, 200 people died."*
>
> *"Similarly, he [Ferguson] was accused of creating panic by overestimating the potential death toll during the 2005 Bird Flu outbreak. Ferguson estimated 200 million could die. The real number was in the low hundreds."*
>
> *"In 2009, one of Ferguson's models predicted 65,000 people could die from the Swine Flu outbreak in the UK — the final figure was below 500." "So, you have to ask yourself, why would anyone believe what Ferguson has been predicting in this COVID hustle? Are his fellow experts that stupid? Are presidents and prime ministers that stupid? And the answer is: This is a monumental covert op; some people are that stupid; some are caught up in the op and are afraid to say the emperor has no clothes; some are aware of what is going on, and they want to destroy national economies and lead us into, yes, a new world order."*
>
> *"Gates knows he has his man: Ferguson. As the recipient of tens of millions of dollars, a year from the Gates Foundation, Ferguson is not about to issue a model that states: COVID is nothing to worry about, let people live their lives and we will be all right. The chance of that happening is on a par with researchers admitting they never properly identified a new virus as the cause of illness in 2019, in Wuhan."*

When you check the primary sources of various health organizations and Nobel Prize-awarded discoverers as they recount their glory, their hard-won hypotheses, and listen to them candidly discuss their caveats, it becomes clear that forces other than science and reason are at work in most if not all of our Public Health Directives, in higher educational systems, medical schools, and indeed, in even in elementary school science and health classes. In these contexts, apparently the views of Payton Rous, Luc Montagnier, and many others are worth careful consideration and intense questioning, and for many of the reasons they themselves provide. With these Nobel prize-worthy suggestions, Dr. Montagnier, so-called co-discoverer of the "HIV"-AIDS ruse, as quoted above, also has in effect dusted off the Century-old argument of his own country's biomedical forerunners, Louis Pasteur, and Antoine Bechamp, regarding the supremacy of soil or terrain versus the seed, microbe, or toxin in the development of clinically visible disease. But the fear of "seeds" guides most of the decision making that happens still at the highest levels of The Public Health Agencies. For example, without any evidence of improved efficacy or indeed any evidence at all except for the gathering reports of vaccine adverse events and an increasing VAERS payout program for vaccine damaged kids, the June 2006 recommendation from the Advisory Committee on Immunization Practices was to provide a second dose of varicella vaccine to children aged 4 to 6 years.

(March 2007) **MMR, Chicken Pox Vaccines Work for Preemies.** Main Category: Pediatrics News Article Date: 08 Mar 2007 – 11:00 PDT.

> *"Exogenous re-exposure to varicella virus has probably helped in maintaining immunity to this pathogen. Given the ongoing decline in varicella incidence, and thus in opportunities for community exposure to the virus, a second dose of vaccine may also be needed in the future for high-risk populations such as healthcare workers." If it is not enough to introduce vile poisons into our infants and children: doctors also want to inject premature infants who possess no immune system. Vaccines for measles-mumps-rubella and varicella, or chicken pox, are effective in extremely preterm infants, even though preemies'*

immune systems are not as developed as full-term babies. This confirms a long-held assumption by pediatricians and neonatologists across the country."

"The assumption has always been that it would be OK, that very early babies would have enough immunity, but no one had formally researched the subject," said Carl D'Angio, M.D., associate professor of Pediatrics at the University of Rochester Medical Center, and author of a paper on the subject in Pediatrics this month. "I'm happy be able to reassure my colleagues and parents that it is OK."

"The study, which included 16 term and 16 extremely preterm (born before about 6 1/2 months of pregnancy) infants born between May 2002 and May 2005, is the first of its kind to examine the antibody levels of measles, mumps, rubella and varicella in this population before and after vaccination. It was published in this month's Pediatrics. The same number of preterm infants and full-term infants in the study reached a level of immunity considered protective against the diseases."

"This positive outcome, however, was not guaranteed because preemies' immune systems do not always react the same way as full-term infants [**No kidding**]!

"For instance, a change in the types of vaccine used in the UK apparently resulted in an increase in Haemophilus influenzae type b infections, like bloodstream infection or meningitis, in children. Children born prematurely appeared to be particularly at risk for this, alluding to potential problems this population may have with responding to vaccines. That is not the case for the MMR and chicken pox vaccines. Now we can all breathe a sigh of relief.

"We were right," D'Angio said. Although not generally life-threatening, measles, mumps, rubella, and chicken pox can all have serious complications. While many adults contracted chicken pox as a childhood rite of passage, the varicella "virus" killed 100 and hospitalized 11,000 people every year before the vaccine became available."

"The mumps virus causes fever, headache and swollen glands,

> *but it may also cause deafness, meningitis, painful swelling of the testicles or ovaries, and death! The rubella virus causes a rash, mild fever, and arthritis, but in pregnant women, it can lead to a miscarriage or birth defects, according to the CDC. D'Angio's study was funded by the National Institute of Allergy and Infectious Diseases and the National Center for Research Resources, both part of the National Institutes of Health. D'Angio is finishing a similar study on the pneumococcal conjugate vaccine, which helps prevent meningitis and blood and ear infections, and is in the process of studying the influenza vaccine."*

Generally, "the virus" causes a rash, itching, fever, and fatigue, but it can also cause severe skin infections, scars, pneumonia and brain damage. And a person who has had chicken pox can get a painful rash called shingles years later (only apparently if they obtained a chickenpox vaccine as children), according to the Centers for Disease Control and Prevention. The measles virus causes a rash, cough, runny nose, eye irritation and fever, but it can [could] also lead to ear infections, pneumonia, seizures, brain damage, and rarely, death" (if it existed, which it doesn't according to a fresh German High Court Ruling in favor of Dr. Stephan Lanka, a virologist who recently won a law suit challenging the existence of any measles virus-(see German Supreme Court Upholds Biologist's Claim that Measles Virus Does Not Exist (vaccineimpact.com).

See Gary Goldman's detailed discussion about the chickenpox vaccine, and shingles, a topic that he is spent the better part of his career analyzing:

Gary S. Goldman, Ph.D., began to report an unexpectedly high shingles incidence rate among children while serving as Research Analyst for the Varicella Active Surveillance Project (VASP), one of three sites selected by the CDC to study the effect of the varicella vaccine on the population.

"When Goldman sought to independently publish several manuscripts

following his resignation, Dr. Laurene Mascola, Acute Communicable Disease Control Unit, Los Angeles Department of Health Services, had the Los Angeles legal department issue Goldman a notice to "Cease and Desist Publication" in a medical journal.

> ***RE: Varicella Active Surveillance Project***
>
> *Dear Mr. Goldman,*
> *"This letter is notice to you to cease and desist in your efforts to publish or disseminate any information gathered as part of your participation on the VASP. 316 404 0 100 200 300 400 500 2006 2007 4 12."*
>
> *Goldman's attorney responded to this notice, firmly stating Goldman's intention to proceed with publication in the best interest of public health and safety. The Los Angeles legal department did not respond further to Goldman's attorney. Additionally, there seemed to be conflicts of interest: the CDC vaccine preventable disease group that promoted vaccination was the same group that oversaw vaccine monitoring of safety."*

"Goldman independently published three manuscripts after overcoming the notice to "Cease and Desist" initiated by Dr. Laurene Mascola, Acute Communicable Disease Control Unit, Los Angeles Department of Health Services. Since VASP with funding from CDC was a public-funded study, data was not confidential and was available to any citizen through the Freedom of Information Act (FOIA), and which inspired the following paper: Goldman G. **Incidence of herpes-zoster among children and adolescents in a community with moderate varicella vaccination coverage** Using capture-recapture methods to assess varicella incidence in a community under active surveillance. Vaccine, Oct. 1; 21(27- 30):4243–9. (3) 2003, and also, Vaccine, 2003 Oct 1; 21(27-30):42, 50–55. 14."

"Some of the same authors that attempted to have Goldman "Cease and Desist" publication and who wrote a "Scientific

Commentary" explaining (incorrectly) why Goldman's analysis of incidence rates (published in 2005) were in error, wrote a paper in 2009 using methods similar to what Goldman outlined and derived nearly the same shingles incidence rates that Goldman derived in 2002."

How many are currently hospitalized or killed/year in American hospitals alone from iatrogenic (medically-caused) interventions? Almost 2,000,000 are the current estimates? Montagnier at least, among other Nobelists are increasingly becoming ever more vocal and widely acknowledged that the soil or terrain of the organism, and not the "seeds" or germs, ultimately determines if and how much illness will result from any seed, imagined or real. The evidence shows that Montagnier is right about this "soil" or so-called victim's resistance being the primary concern that needs to be better understood, not the "seed" or the multifactorial singularity, which is forced into a 1-fits-all-causal delusion that has destroyed millions of lives through history.

And because Montagnier is now claiming that "we can be exposed to HIV many times without being chronically infected...because *"our immune system will get rid of the virus in a few weeks, if you have a good immune system,"* then clearly, Montagnier has sided with Antoine Beauchamp's argument, and not Pasteur's in the context of "HIV" and AIDS.

The gene revolution has essentially come and gone-leaving us with extraordinarily little to show for such awesome support, continuing investment, and initial promise. Its failure has been the result of tacit assumptions about Nature that proved to have been incomplete. A new revolution in the biological sciences is currently taking shape along with the discovery of epigenetic, and now extracellular matrix influences forces that control the genes (Tone Sandal, Klara Valyi-Nagy, Robert Folberg, Mina Bissell, Virginia Spensor, Andrew Maniotis. Epigenetic reversion of breast carcinoma phenotype and DNA sequestration. American Journal of Pathology, Vol 170 (5): 1739-49. May 2007). These matrices constitute key epigenetic and extracellular factors that control the genes and their expression. If these ideas and discussion are at this point insufficient to at least stimulate a long-needed reappraisal wherein we "didn't talk then but need to know now," then a few examples of more familiar vaccines designed to thwart these common childhood illnesses are all easily obtained from Medline, as are these vaccines' rates of protective immunity (if any). Medline. The SARS-CoV-2 virus has been shown to be a real viral-like particle in many contexts: however, its pathogenicity is not yet established. Its role in the immune response of eosinophil enhancement, ground-glass pathology, ciliary destruction, or other possible physiological sequalae to infection are still under intense investigation.

CHAPTER II

THE GREAT TIMELINE OF VACCINE EXPERIMENTATION ON HUMAN BEINGS: SPECIFIC DATA FROM MANY SOURCES

LEGENDS DESCRIBE HOW CHINESE PARENTS would blow year-old dried, ground up, and powdered disease effusions into the noses of children to protect them from these diseases.

Similar legends from the Middle East describe how The Persians would "purchase the pox" and then take these disease effusions home, and then would cut the arm of the inoculation recipient and smear the purchased material on the cut.

Various poorly documented plagues and poorly recorded "pestilences" occurred during the early Christian era, and most of these pestilences were linked to periods of warfare, and mass migrations, and conquest.

Again, the great student of both modern and past vaccinology, Eleanor McBean, has surmised a different account of the origins of inoculations and vaccinations than is presented in most textbooks or historical accounts:

WHO STARTED VACCINATION AND WHY, by Eleanor McBean, from "**The Poisoned Needle:**"

It has been claimed, by an unenlightened few, that vaccination is based on scientific principles and is of comparatively recent origin. But these claims have been proved false, first, because inoculation was practiced and abandoned as useless by primitive tribes many centuries ago, and second because Jenner and the modern experimenters in vaccination were not scientists and did not test and prove their theories by any scientific criteria before launching the hazardous practice on the public.

For many years Edward Jenner was acclaimed a hero for what was thought to be his discovery of cow-pox vaccination. But this dubious honor was later admitted belonging to Benjamin Jesty, whom all the chroniclers name as the one responsible for the original discovery of cow-pox inoculation. Jesty, a farmer, Plett, a teacher and Jensen, a farmer, were named as 'successful experimenters" in the field of cow-pox vaccination several years before Jenner's first inoculation These and all subsequent vaccination experiments were then, and still are, haphazard and unscientific attempts at solving the problem of disease prevention.

Before we trace the ancient history of vaccination let us review some of the outstanding authorities who recognized that:

VACCINATION IS NOT SCIENTIFIC

Many of the world's greatest thinkers, scientists, statesmen and even doctors have condemned vaccination as being a crime against humanity, a fraud promoted for private gain, an insult to the race and a blot upon the name of civilization Yet, this treacherous practice of blood pollution, which was cradled in the lap of. ignorant savage tribes have been adopted by, supposedly, enlightened government of the present day and forced on the protesting population—for profit.

M.M. Gernerd in his book "The Vaccination Imposture" says:

"Vaccination is not in any sense scientific; doctors never know what the result will be in any case; they don't absolutely know that it ever prevented smallpox; they never know when they have pure vaccine; the practice is born of pure superstition; and it has been a breeder of many kindred fallacies."

Florence Nightingale, the world's most famous nurse and an authority on smallpox by right of extensive experience, said:

"Everyone who knows anything about public health questions will agree

to the practical unity of epidemics, and the determining causes, and that exemption from... disease must be sought not by any one thing, such as vaccination, but by inquiring into and removing the causes of epidemic susceptibility generally."

Alfred Russell Wallace, in his famous book, "The Wonderful Century (p. 314) says:

"The successive Vaccination Acts were passed by means of allegations which were wholly untrue and promises which have all been unfulfilled. They stand alone in modern legislation as a gross interference with personal liberty and the sanctity of the home; while as an attempt to cheat outraged nature, and to avoid a zymotic disease without getting rid of the foul conditions that produce or propagate it, the practice of vaccination is utterly opposed to the whole teaching of sanitary science, and is one of those terrible blunders which, in their far-reaching evil consequences, are worse than the greatest of crimes."

Among our best authoritative sources of information are the actual government records showing the INCREASED DEATH-RATE AFTER VACCINATION WAS ESTABLISHED!

The following entries are what most believe were the origins of modern inoculations and vaccinations:

1717 The Jesuits who had been sent to India were sent for in order to introduce inoculation from India to England with the help of Lady Montague who was a respected and influential member of England's upper class.

1767 Dr. J.Z Holwell sends back a report back from India describing the inoculation techniques of the Brahmans entitled: "*An Account of the Manner of Inoculating for the Smallpox in the East Indies, London, 1767.*"

1796 It has been widely documented and in the public record that James Phipps, the 8-year-old vaccinated by William Jenner, was revaccinated 20 times. He died at age 20. There also are rumors that Jenner's own son, who was also vaccinated more than once, died at 21.

1797 Edward Jenner sent a paper to the Royal Society about variolae vaccinae or smallpox of the cow and its potential similarities to human smallpox and tried to popularize the folklore that: exposure to inflamed cow utters with corresponding inflammation or eruptions on milk-maids hands is the cow form of human smallpox. The paper is rejected and returned with a warning *"He had better not promulgate such a wild idea if he valued his reputation."*

1798 Edward Jenner publishes his Inquiry variolae vaccinae, or smallpox of the cow.

1799 THE JENNARIAN DOCTRINE AND THE PRACTICE OF VACCINATION SPREADS ALL OVER ENGLAND

1800 The Jennerian vaccination doctrine spreads all over Europe, while Benjamin Waterhouse of Harvard University who has faked his medical credentials is credited (cursed) as the man who brought vaccinations to the U. S.

1803 Baron, in his "Life of Jenner" recounted how a Mr. Allen who was Secretary to Lord Holland, wrote to Jenner from Madrid in 1803 pointing out that: *"There is no country likely to receive more benefits from your labours than Spain; for, on the one hand, the mortality among children from small-pox has always been very great; and, on the other hand, the inoculation for the cow-pox has been received with the same enthusiasm here as in the rest of Europe."* ....*"The result, however, was the reverse of satisfactory; the inoculation of the spurious sort has proved fatal to many children at Seville, who have fallen victims to the small-pox after they had been pronounced secure from that disease."* ("Life of Jenner" Vol i., p. 604, 1893).

1809 Massachusetts passed the first mandatory vaccination law in the U.S.

1824 English scientist John Cooke observed: *'The fumes from these metals, or the receptance of them in solution into the stomach, often causes paralysis. Metal workers had suffered for centuries from a paralysis similar to polio caused by the lead and arsenic in the metals they were working with."*

1839 Smallpox epidemic sweeps England and kills 22,081 people.

1840 Mandatory vaccination is outlawed by the British Parliament.

SMALLPOX TRAVELS TO THE AMERICAS

1850 In 1850, in the U.S. frigate Independence, with a ship's company of 560 people aboard, there were 116 cases of smallpox, seven fatal. Fleet-surgeon Whelen wrote: *"The crew of this ship almost universally presented what are regarded as genuine vaccine marks. The protection, however, proved to be quite imperfect."*

1850 The New Orleans Medical and Surgical Journal 1880, published a communication from Dr. T. H. Bemiss, Lahaina, Hawaii, on the introduction and spread of leprosy in these islands. "Alarmed," says the writer, "by an invasion of small-pox in 1853, a general vaccination of the whole population was ordered, and physicians being at that time very few on the islands, non-professionals aided in the work. It is charged by some that, as a natural result of the labours of the heterogeneous force so appointed, not only syphilis but also leprosy was greatly increased. In my last circuit trip in my district, I found very few adults who had never been vaccinated. This involves the question of inoculability (of leprosy), in my opinion the main, if not the only means of propagation, other than inheritance."

1850 Massachusetts is the first state to require vaccination for school attendance.

1853 In England, Parliament passes The Compulsory Vaccination Act stating that every parent is required to have their baby vaccinated within 3 months of birth or face a fine of 20 shillings.

1855 Massachusetts is the first state to form a Medical Inquisition in the U. S. and adopt mandatory vaccination laws.

1860 The following is part of a letter which appeared in the Lancet on July 7th, 1860, signed a "Military Surgeon:" "VACCINATION AT SHORNCLIFFE.— SIR,— Having seen in the Lancet of last week an article commenting on a return moved for by Mr. DUNCOMBE, respecting those who have died from Vaccination, the number of amputations required to save life at the camp at Shorncliffe, I can only say that it would be advisable to extend this return, and ask for the number of those who have died or had their arms amputated since the promulgation of an order from the late Director-General

ALEXANDER, limiting the performance of the operation to a particular part of the arm, viz., two inches above the elbow-joint in front, immediately over the insertion of the deltoid muscle. The results from this unfortunate erroneous rule, have, I fear, produced an amount of injury that will never be known, as it will be exceedingly difficult, even in the present day, to procure an accurate return, as military medical men are too fully alive to the injury likely to occur to their future prospects of promotion in the service, were they found ready and willing to expose such mistakes. The irritation, inflammation, and consequent loss of limb, and in some cases of life, from adopting this rule, I myself am practically acquainted with, as I was on board, not exceptionally long since, in a case where a fine healthy young soldier had his arm amputated at the shoulder-joint to save his life, in consequence of mortification supervening upon erysipelatous inflammation of the forearm after Vaccination."

1864 A US Department of Navy record was found stating: "Upon the U.S. steamship Jamestown, serving in Japanese waters, there occurred, in 1864, among a ship's company of 212 persons, 31 cases of small-pox, with four deaths. The entire crew had been vaccinated after leaving the United States."

1867 Nonpayment of fines for skipping smallpox vaccination result in harsher penalties. Thousands defied the **Medical Inquisition** and left Britain rather than submit their children to the practice.

THE CONDITIONS UNDER WHICH THE ANTI-COMPULSORY VACCINATION LEAGUE WAS FORMED IN BRITAIN, AND WHEN "THE SMALL-POX" WAS INTRODUCED FROM SAN FRANCISCO

1868 "Small-pox was introduced from San Francisco in the year 1868. In that year, a general vaccination took place, spring lancets being used, which the President of the Board of Health (Mr. David Dayton) informed me were difficult, if not impossible, to disinfect—the operation causing irreparable mischief. The synchronicity of the spread of leprosy with general vaccination is a matter beyond discussion, and this terrible disease soon afterwards obtained such a foothold amongst the Hawaiians that the Government made a first attempt to control it by means of segregation. Another outbreak of smallpox occurred in 1873, and yet another in 1881, both followed by general arm-to-arm vaccination and a rapid and alarming development of leprosy, as may be seen in successive reports of the Board of Health. While the preponderance of medical and scientific opinion is against the theory that leprosy is, in the ordinary sense of the word, a contagious disease, the evidence in favour of its being communicable by inoculation is overwhelming."

1868 The excessive mortality among the prisoners at Andersonville, in the American Civil War, has been mainly attributed to the general re-vaccination, practiced upon them under conditions of severe morbidity. JOSEPH JONES, M.D., Professor of Physiology and Pathology, University, Nashville, U.S.,1868, wrote: "The Federal prisoners confined in Camp Sumpter, Andersonville, Georgia, were vaccinated, and, in a number of cases, large gangrenous ulcers appeared at the points where the vaccine lymph had been inserted, causing extensive destruction of tissues, exposing arteries, nerves and bones, and necessitating amputation in more than one instance. From the establishment of the prison, on February 24th, 1864, to October 1st, over 10,000 Federal prisoners died, i.e., near one-third of the entire number perished in less than seven months. These accidents led to the belief among some of the prisoners that the surgeons had intentionally introduced poisonous matter into their arms during vaccination. No wonder they had such a persuasion, seeing that about 100 of them lost the use of their arms, and about 200 were so injured that they soon afterwards died. Though some medical officers were tried before a special military commission, convened in accordance with orders from the War Office at Washington, on the charge of having willfully poisoned the Federal prisoners with vaccine lymph, it was shown that the unhappy consequences of vaccination at Andersonville were paralleled in the Northern prisons. 'After careful inquiries,' says Dr. JONES, 'among returned Confederate prisoners,

I am convinced that the accidents attending Vaccination were quite as numerous and severe in Northern prisons as in Southern."

1870 In 1870 sixty-one cases [of smallpox] occurred on the United States steam ship Franklin. "The disease first appeared on a sailor with 'an excellent vaccine scar.' The officers and crew were immediately vaccinated with fresh vaccine matter obtained at Lisbon, this vaccination being the third one during the cruise. Nineteen days later, the second case occurred. The disease has been epidemic in many places in Europe during the past season, but I hoped our vaccinations would prevent trouble with-it on-board ship. In a cruise of the North Carolina up the Mediterranean, she shipped at Norfolk a crew of 900 men, most of whom had been vaccinated, or had the small-pox, but were nevertheless twice vaccinated prior to the ship sailing, a third time at Gibraltar, and a fourth time at Port Mahon." Dr. Hendersen, who reported these facts, noted that despite vaccinations and revaccinations, "157 men of the crew had varioloid.

1870 Outbreak of smallpox all over Europe.

1871 Smallpox continues to rage all over Europe.

1871 "Europeans resolutely object to be vaccinated with lymph from native sources; and, notwithstanding the law, when imported lymph cannot be obtained, they and their children remain unvaccinated. As a consequence, the population of Europeans attacked with leprosy is comparatively small and, indeed, of rare occurrence, except in the case of soldiers who are subject to the military regulation of revaccination. This repugnance to native lymph on the part of Europeans in the West Indies was pointed out by Dr. R. Hall Bakewell, Vaccinator – General, Trinidad, in his remarkable evidence before the Select Parliamentary Committee of 1871, and has been referred to by Dr. Castor, of British Guiana, and other authorities."

1876 The famous London physician, medical journal editor, author, and harsh critic of vaccines, Dr. Charles Creighton worked in London as a hospital registrar until his appointment in 1876 as demonstrator of anatomy at the University of Cambridge. Over the next five years he wrote his first book, Bovine Tuberculosis in Man (1881), and published several articles on anatomy in the Journal of Anatomy and Physiology. He became co-editor of the journal in 1879. He devoted most of his later career to exposing vaccines as dangerous and useless as an active member of the London Society of the Abolition of Compulsory Vaccination.

1879 Mr. P. A. TAYLOR reveals his intention to introduce a Bill during the next Session for the Repeal of the Compulsory Clauses of the Vaccination Acts, and told the House of Commons, in April, 1879, that he had "seen dozens and scores of persons who had stated to him that they honestly believed that their children had died from vaccination. They took perfectly healthy children to be vaccinated, an incision was made in the arm, in a few days a sore appeared on the arm, from thence it spread all over the body, and finally the children died in agony" (Lancet, August 21st, 1881).

1880 Mr. J. T. HIBBERT, M.P., then Parliamentary Secretary to the Local Government Department, written in June, 1880: "The Return (433) shews an increase of deaths from syphilis of infants under one year from 255, in 1847,—to 1,554, in 1875,—which, in my opinion, is one of the most unsatisfactory features in connection with vaccination, and one which leads me to support the proposed modification of the Vaccination Law now before the House of Commons."—Lancet, July 17th, 1880.

THE MEAN ANNUAL RATE OF MORTALITY IN ENGLAND FROM SMALL-POX IN 1880 (P. lxxix., Table 34, of the 43rd Annual Report of the Registrar-General, 1882) N.B.—Vaccination made compulsory, 1853; more stringently so, 1867. "Small-pox vaccination was made compulsory by an Act of Parliament in the year 1853; again in 1867; and still more stringent in 1871. Since 1853, we have had three epidemics of small-pox, each being more severe than the one preceding."

1st 1857	14,244 deaths
2nd 1863—64—65	20,059 deaths
3rd 1870—71—72	44,840 deaths

1883 1883 PASTEUR MAY (or may not) HAVE CURED ONE BOY OF HYDROPHOBIA PASTEUR'S ANTHRAX VACCINE DESTROYED HERDS OF CATTLE, ALMOST GOT PASTEUR THROWN OUT OF FRANCE, AND HOW PASTEUR DEFINED THE PROBLEM OF VACCINE ATTENUATION, BUT NOT THE VIRULENCE PROBLEM

1885 (July 6) It was widely acknowledged that Pasteur's vaccination of the nine-year old boy, Joseph Meister, whom Pasteur injected with the "weakened microbes" of hydrophobia (rabies) 2 days after the boy had been bitten 14 times by a rabid dog, " saved the boy, and heralded a true revolution in Europe against the rabies virus (hydrophobia was what rabies was called at the time because dogs infected with it acted as if 'afraid of water').

1885 "The earliest record of an epidemic caused by Hepatitis B was made by Lurman in 1885. An outbreak of smallpox occurred in Bremen in 1883 and 1,289 shipyard employees were vaccinated with lymph from other people. After several weeks, and up to eight months later, 191 of the vaccinated workers became ill with jaundice and were diagnosed as suffering from serum hepatitis. Other employees who had been inoculated with different batches of lymph remained healthy. Lurman's paper, now regarded as a classical example of an epidemiological study, proved that contaminated lymph was the source of the outbreak" (Lurman A. (1885) Eine icterus epidemic. (In German). Berl Klin Woschenschr 22:20–3).

1886 Dr. Charles Creighton's The History of Epidemics sponsored by the Royal Commission on vaccination was published in the Encyclopedia Britannica regarding Jenner's contribution: "that he had no doubt about the value of vaccination, that it never occurred to him to question the thing at all, and that he took it as one of the things he had been taught as a student." He left the Commission in no doubt as to the result of his studies in preparation for writing the piece: "In my opinion," Dr. Charles Creighton said, "based on an extended study of the original data, I conclude that] Jenner's work was incorrect, and that cowpox was not, as Jenner stated, 'Variola

Vaccinse,' and cowpox has nothing to do with variola and was not a protective against variola, and vaccination affords no protection against smallpox."

1886-1892 In Australia when a few children died as a result of smallpox vaccinations, the government abolished compulsory vaccination in that country and smallpox suddenly declined to the vanishing point. Australia had only three cases of smallpox in 15 years as compared with Japan's record of 165,774 cases and 28,979 deaths from this cause in only 7 years under compulsory vaccination and re-vaccination.

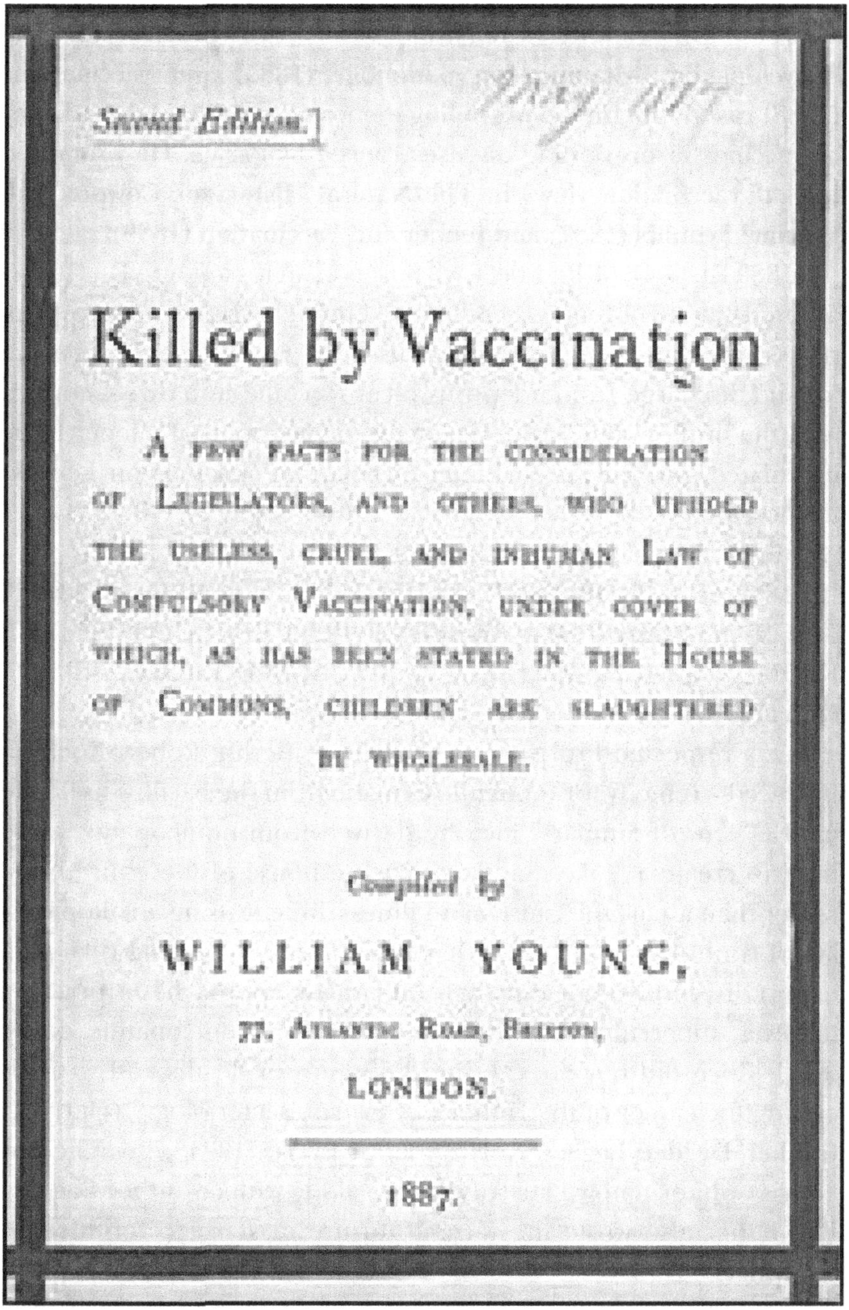

[*Second Edition.*]

Killed by Vaccination

A FEW FACTS FOR THE CONSIDERATION OF LEGISLATORS, AND OTHERS, WHO UPHOLD THE USELESS, CRUEL, AND INHUMAN LAW OF COMPULSORY VACCINATION, UNDER COVER OF WHICH, AS HAS BEEN STATED IN THE HOUSE OF COMMONS, CHILDREN ARE SLAUGHTERED BY WHOLESALE.

Compiled by

WILLIAM YOUNG,

77, ATLANTIC ROAD, BRIXTON,

LONDON.

1887.

1888 Dr. Charles Creighton wrote two articles for the Encyclopædia Britannica on pathology (1885) and vaccinations (1888) cast doubt on the prevailing theory of germs and the efficacy of vaccines in preventing diseases caused by germs. He promoted his anti-vaccination views in The Natural History of Cowpox and Vaccinal Syphilis (1887) and Jenner and Vaccination (1889).

1889 Dr. G. D. M'Reddie, Civil Surgeon, in his letter to Dr. Ghose, on the 18th of February, 1888, states: "From observations I know leprosy is hereditary. It is also contagious in the sense that it is necessary for the discharge from a leprous ulcer to come into direct contact with the broken skin of the recipient, or the blood of a leper to be inoculated into the system, as in vaccination." (Report on Leprosy to the Hon. H. Beverley, MA., by Madhub Chunder Ghose, Leper Asylum, Calcutta, August 27th, 1889).

1890 AS A PROFESSOR OF HYGIENE IN BERLIN, ROBERT KOCH INTRODUCED A REMEDY FOR TUBERCULOSIS MADE FROM THE BACILLIS ITSELF...AND CAUSED THOUSANDS OF DEATHS

As a respected Professor of Hygiene in Berlin, Robert Koch introduced a remedy for tuberculosis made from the bacillus itself. He used a "Law of Similars" idea he derived from homeopathy, as he tried to create a "Like-stimulates-like" response of the entire body, rather than attack the cause of an illness directly using an allopathic law of contraries approach with a toxic substance or drug (like penicillin). To implement the "Law of similars approach" in practice, however, tuberculin had to be employed in homeopathic doses, which Koch did not do, causing thousands of deaths and virtually ending the career of the Father of German Bacteriology" (Harris L. Coulter, Divided Legacy, North Atlantic Books, 1994; researched by Harris Coulter, a now Late friend, who along with co-author Barbara Loe Fisher also wrote the vaccine torture masterpiece entitled,**"A Shot In The Dark"**).

1892 In an article on Keanu's inoculation, the Occidental Medical Times, April, 1892, Dr Sidney Bourne Swift intimates that:

"It must not be forgotten that the leprosy was first discernible at the points of inoculation. Nor can it be considered remarkable, knowing how the disease had been propagated by the vaccination lancet. In one instance reported to Queen Liliuokokalani, an entire school in Hawaii was swept away, with the exception of a single survivor, by this means."

1892 Hawaiian Legislature, June 25, 1892. DAVID DAYTON, Esq., President, Board of Health, wrote: "SIR,—An effort is being made in the Legislature to repeal or amend the law relating to vaccination; the object being to leave vaccination optional with parents and individuals. The chief objection raised against the present compulsory system appears to be the belief of some that leprosy, and other diseases, have been propagated by means of vaccination."

1892 The Honolulu Board of Health documents that: "Resistance to vaccination is spreading in many districts in these islands, and at the same time there is observed a sensible diminution in the number of lepers. In New Zealand, prosecutions for non-vaccination have for some time been abandoned. In the South African Colonies of Natal and Cape Colony the vaccination laws are enforced only during outbreaks of small-pox, and vaccination is everywhere regarded with mistrust. In the Transvaal and Orange Free State vaccination is entirely optional. In England there are about one hundred towns and poor law unions where the vaccination laws are a dead letter. In several of the Swiss cantons compulsory vaccination has been tried and abolished, and in no canton is there any penalty for non-vaccination. An attempt was made to pass a federal vaccination law in 1881 and was defeated in a Referendum by 253,968 votes against 67,820. In the Australasian Colony of Tasmania, the compulsory law has been suspended by reason of its deleterious effects on the health of the people. In the Colonies of New South Wales. and Queensland, Australia, the people have successfully resisted every attempt to impose the hotly-disputed Jennerian dogma upon them."

PARALYSIS OUTBREAKS BEGAN TO OCCUR IN VERMONT, AND IT WAS NON-CONTAGIOUS IN FAMILIES, AND IT WAS ASSOCIATED WITH COTTON FARMING, APPLE FARMING, AND ARSENATE RESIDUES

1892 Paralysis outbreaks began to occur in Vermont, in an apple growing region. In his report the Government Inspector Dr. Charles Caverly noted that parents reported that some children fell ill after eating fruit. He stated that: '"infantile paralysis usually occurred in families with more than one child and in which paralysis wasn't contagious, and so no efforts were made at isolation of the victims as it was very certain it was non-contagious'" (with only one child out of many in the family afflicted according to Caverly). This epidemic and others that occurred that were less well documented were most likely due to arsenate banned by the British some years later, as it was a pesticide poison used for the orchards in Vermont's cotton and apple-producing farms. Records in Vermont also chronicled that dogs and fowl in the area were also stricken, and that humans with the lowest fevers died more often.

An excellent account of the polio era leading up to the Great 1916 "polio epidemic" can be found in "Infantile Paralysis in Vermont," published in 1924 by The Burlington Vermont State Department of Public Health. This "record" is a collection of yearly maps of Vermont, compiled by Dr. Charles Solomon Caverly. The book begins with a description of a paralytic outbreak that took place in the summer of 1894, and a series of maps of Vermont then is provided where each recorded case was marked on the map with a red dot to note the location of the victim. Not only did each year's map record every reported case of paralysis that occurred, and where in the state each case occurred (by county), detailed information about each case was also provided by Dr. Caverly-the ethnic background of the family, the employment status and line of work of the head of the household, the time of year it was reported, the temperature and weather at the time of diagnosis, the amount of rainfall measured, how the paralysis became manifested (and in which limb(s), how many days the incubation period likely lasted before paralysis was first observed (typically no longer than several days), and dozens of other interesting facts that Caverly recorded about each case.

At the end of each chapter in The Record, Caverly speculated about each year's case clusters, as to how paralysis and reported cases could possibly "travel" infectiously from county to county from the previous year, in an attempt to discover how "paralysis" cases spread (along train routes, roadway routes, water routes, etc.). But there appeared to be no railroad lines, or roads, rivers, natural barriers such as mountains, or any other reason to account for how one year, 1910 for instance, higher clusters of paralysis occurred on one side of a mountain valley while the next year, the other side of the mountain and across the state was where the new cases occurred, while no new cases occurred again in the first place, and even though the mountains would have restricted spread, by limiting travel of "infected healthy carriers" or paralyzed individuals alike.

1894 Those who opposed vaccination were blasted in the New York Times as engaging "in a futile attempt to head off human progress and to reopen a question about which pretty much all of the world has made up its mind." (REF: Cited in Brooklyn Medical Journal. 8(1894):576 and reference in Colgrove, p.14).

1894 In an inaugural Address to Medical Society of King's College, October 26th, Dr. Edward Crookshank claimed that: "That vaccination is capable of extirpating the disease or of controlling epidemic waves is absolutely negated by the epidemic in 1825, and the epidemics which followed in quick succession in 1838, in 1840, 1841, 1844-5, 1848, 1851-2. Vaccination was made compulsory in 1853, but epidemics followed in 1854, 1855, and 1856, culminating in the terrible epidemic in 1871-72 with more than 42,000 deaths. Epidemics followed in 1877 and 1881." en.wikipedia.org//index.php?title=Edgar_Crookshank&action=edit§ion=2>

1896 A Final report of the Royal Commission on vaccination is submitted. The commission could not ignore the evidence against vaccination, so they recommended that mandatory vaccination should be stopped.

1896 Walter Robert Hadwen, MD, a vocal, late nineteenth century anti-vaccination reformer wrote:

"The very moment you take a medical prescription, and you incorporate it into an act of Parliament, it passes beyond the confines of a purely medical question and becomes essentially a social and political one." REF: Hadwen, W.R. "The Case Against Vaccination." Gloucester: Gloucester Anti-vaccination League, 1896. p 5.

1898 In England, a Royal Commission is appointed to inquire into certain aspects of the vaccination question. The committee would be in session for 7 years and would issue 6 reports, with the final report in 1896. The result of the final report was the Vaccination Act of 1898. Vaccination Act removes penalties from vaccination law.

1898 Dr. William Tebb, MD, MA, DPH, publishes: "**A Century of Vaccination and What It Teaches,**" "The most distinguished names in the profession have testified to vaccination being the certain vehicle for the dissemination of leprosy. These names include Sir Erasmus Wilson (sometimes called the father of dermatologists); Dr. John D. Hillis; Dr. Liveing; Sir Ranald Martin; Professor W. T. Gairdner; Dr. Tilbury Fox; Dr. Gavin Milroy; Dr. R. Hall Bakewell, formerly Physician to the Leper Asylum, Trinidad; Dr. A.S. Black, of Trinidad; Dr. Edward Arning; Dr. Walter M. Gibson, late President of the Honolulu Board of Health; Professor H. G. Piffard, New York; Dr. A. M. Brown, London; Dr. Frances Hoggan; Dr. Blanc, Professor of Dermatology, University of New Orleans; Dr. Bechtinger, of Rio; Professor Montgomery, of California; Dr. Sidney Bourne Swift, late Medical Director, Leper Settlement, Molokai, Hawaii; Dr. P. Hellat, St. Petersburg; Professor Henri Leloir, Lille; Dr. Mouritz; Surgeon Brunt; Dr. John Freeland, Government Medical Officer, Antigua; Dr. S. P. Impey, Superintendent Leper Asylum, Robben Island, Cape Colony; and many others. On the subject of leprosy there are no higher authorities."

1900 A claim is published that the Rockefeller-backed University of Chicago buys the Encyclopedia Britannica and all derogatory references to vaccination are removed.

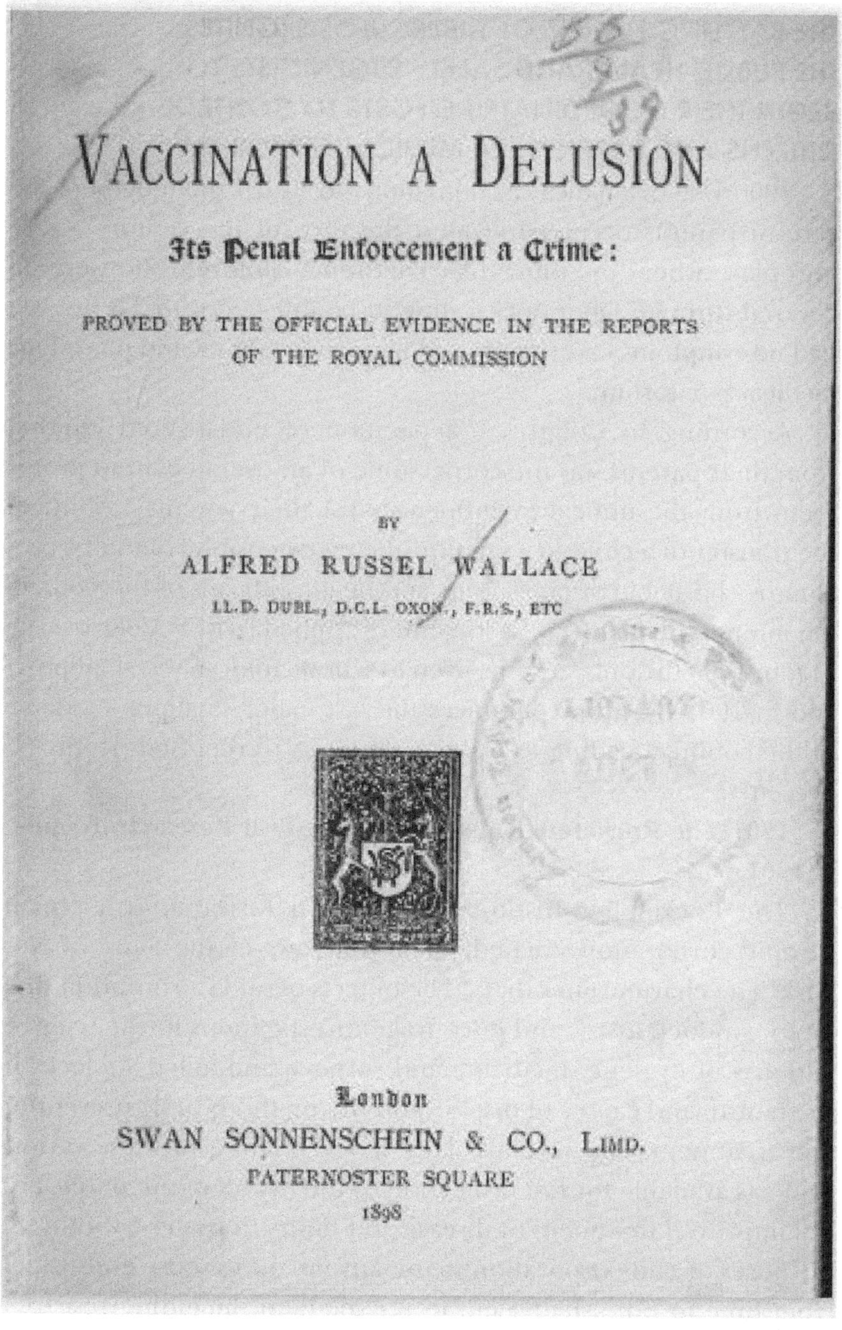

VACCINATION A DELUSION

Its Penal Enforcement a Crime:

PROVED BY THE OFFICIAL EVIDENCE IN THE REPORTS
OF THE ROYAL COMMISSION

BY

ALFRED RUSSEL WALLACE

LL.D. DUBL., D.C.L. OXON., F.R.S., ETC

London
SWAN SONNENSCHEIN & CO., LIMD.
PATERNOSTER SQUARE
1898

THE BAFFLING NATURE OF TUBERCULOSIS IGNITES THE PUBLIC HEALTH AND SAFETY EUGENICISTS TO BEGIN THEIR COORDINATED EFFORTS TO CONTROL CITIZENS AND PARENTS VIA MEDICAL TERRORISM

1900 Use of medical examinations to usurp the judgment and care of parents occurred around the turn of the century are set into place when 'pre-tubercular children'—children who were discovered through laboratory testing to be infected with TB but who had no symptoms—were removed from their homes and placed in a medical sanatorium.

According to Colgrove: "Separation of endangered children from their parents was the cornerstone of an overall plan to protect them from the unhealthy influences [of their parents]. Although the transfer of a child to a sanatorium was ostensibly voluntary, coercion by charitable organizations and health officials of the poor, often immigrant, families was sometimes applied." (REF: Colgrove, pg. 51). In 1900 the only vaccine given to schoolchildren was smallpox.," and in 1901 Boston experiences the last major smallpox epidemic in the country, leading to 1,596 cases and 270 reported deaths (17 percent).

1901 The Rockefeller Institute for Medical Research, founded in 1901.

The Rockefeller Institute for Medical Research is a philanthropic corporation created under the laws of the State of New York. The charter states that; "The objects of said Corporation shall be to conduct, assist, and encourage investigations in the sciences and arts of hygiene, medicine and surgery, and allied subjects, in the nature and causes of disease and the methods of its prevention and treatment, and to make knowledge relating to these various subjects available for the protection of the health of the public and the improved treatment of disease and injury. It shall be within the purposes of said corporation to use any means to those ends which from time to time shall seem to it expedient, including research, publication, education, the establishment and maintenance of charitable or benevolent activities, agencies or institutions appropriate thereto, and the aid of any other such activities, agencies, or institutions already established or which may hereafter be established." **ENDOWMENT**- The Institute has been generously endowed by Mr. John D. Rockefeller by a series of gifts which have from time to time capitalized its growing needs. A special fund supports a system of pensions for members of the Scientific Staff. The Institute's endowment also includes a legacy from the late Henry Rutherford for the promotion of cancer research. **https://digitalcommons.rockefeller.edu/cgi/viewcontent.cgi?article=1005&context=rockefeller-institute-descriptive-pamphlet**

1901-2 "A Massachusetts state statute granted city boards of health the authority to require vaccination when necessary for public health or safety. For example, the Cambridge Board of Health adopted an ordinance requiring all residents to be vaccinated or to pay a fine of five dollars, the equivalent of $118 today. During the 1901-02 outbreaks, Boston public health officials dispatched teams of physicians and police officers to administer vaccinations, by force. Even though outbreaks occurred across all ethnic and economic classes, efforts were concentrated on neighborhoods populated by immigrants and ethnic minorities." REF: Lawrence H. Officer and Samuel H. Williamson, "Purchasing Power of Money in the United States from 1774 to 2006," Measuring Worth.Com, 2007.

"One of four Massachusetts residents who resisted the ordinance was Rev. Henning Jacobson, who asserted that he and his son had developed serious reactions to previous vaccinations and refused to be revaccinated during the epidemic. State law permitted a medical exemption for children at risk from vaccination but held no exclusions for adults. Jacobson argued that the compulsory vaccination law was "…unreasonable, arbitrary and oppressive, and therefore, hostile to the inherent right of every freeman to care for his own body and health in such a way as to him seems best; and that the execution of such a law against one who objects to vaccination, for whatever reason, is nothing short of an assault upon his person."

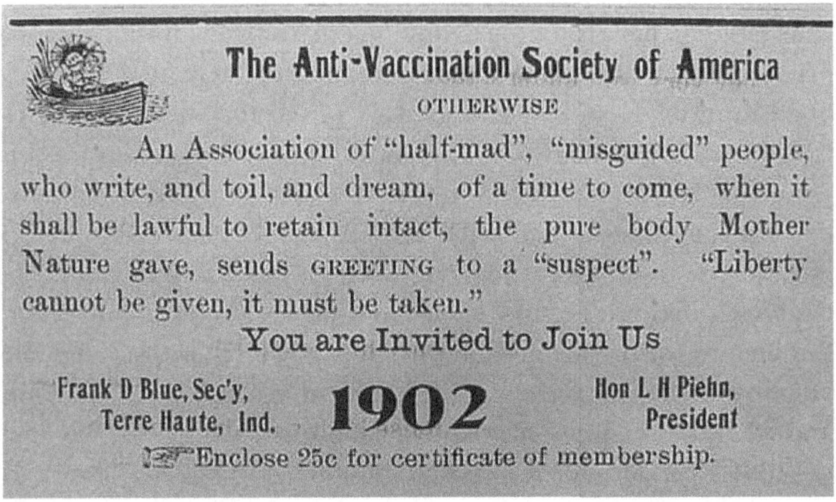
The Anti-Vaccination Society of America

OTHERWISE

An Association of "half-mad", "misguided" people, who write, and toil, and dream, of a time to come, when it shall be lawful to retain intact, the pure body Mother Nature gave, sends GREETING to a "suspect". "Liberty cannot be given, it must be taken."

You are Invited to Join Us

Frank D Blue, Sec'y, Terre Haute, Ind.

1902

Hon L H Piehn, President

☞Enclose 25c for certificate of membership.

THE SUPREME COURT HANDS DOWN ITS RULING IN THE JACOBSON CASE: JACOBSON VS COMMENWEALTH OF MASSACHUSETTS DOCKET 197 US 11 IN 1905

"Failing three times in the lower courts, Jacobson took his case to the U.S. Supreme Court in 1905. The question before the Court was whether the state had overstepped its authority and whether the sphere of personal liberty was protected by the due process clause of the 14th Amendment. In making their ruling, the justices no doubt considered the difficulty Boston had experienced containing the smallpox outbreak in 1901-02.

Perhaps the justices had family members who had been vaccinated or had experienced smallpox. Perhaps they considered the lack of standardized public health programs. Whatever criteria were used, the Supreme Court handed down its landmark ruling in 1905: States were given the right to coerce vaccinations on their citizens if they deemed vaccination to be the best way to protect the community from disease."

"As a result, the Jacobson decision has defined the central

relationship between the rights of the individual vs. the role of the government to protect its citizens against infectious diseases and epidemics to the present day. Jacobson is the first case in U.S. history to deal with the right of self-determination regarding one's own body. The Court affirmed that it was the prerogative of each state legislature to determine how to control an epidemic, including the use of police powers if deemed necessary. Because the federal judiciary could not usurp the role and powers of the states, each state was given the right to decide its own vaccination laws and mandates.

The only stipulation given by the Court was that states were to ensure that enforcement must not be "unreasonable, arbitrary or oppressive."

The Court clearly stated that protection of the public would supersede individual interests for the "**greater good**." REF: Mariner, Wendy K. JD, LLM, MPH, et al. 'Jacobson v Massachusetts It's Not Your Great-Great-Grandfather's Public Health Law.' American Journal of Public Health. April 2005, Vol 95, No. 4: it stated that:

"The issues in Jacobson are enduring because they arose from the fabric of American democracy and our Constitution.

(Jacobson was one of the few Supreme Court cases before 1960 in which a citizen challenged the state's authority to impose mandatory restrictions on personal liberty for public health purposes. Jacobson laid the foundation for U.S. public health officials to mandate vaccination by law. REF: Jacobson v. Massachusetts and Public Health Law: Perspectives in 2005. http://www2.cdc.gov/phlp/jacobson/pdfs/public_health_guide.pdf).

1906 to 1928 Vaccines against pertussis and diphtheria developed.

1906 – Rockefeller Institute for Medical Research, New York.

J Exp Med 1906 Dec 21;8(6):707-12. doi: 10.1084/jem.8.6.707. J W Jobling

THE OCCURRENCE OF SPECIFIC IMMUNITY PRINCIPLES IN THE BLOOD OF VACCINATED CALVES

Enforcing the Vaccination Laws.

Photo of an abortive Sale at East Croydon, May 3rd, 1907.

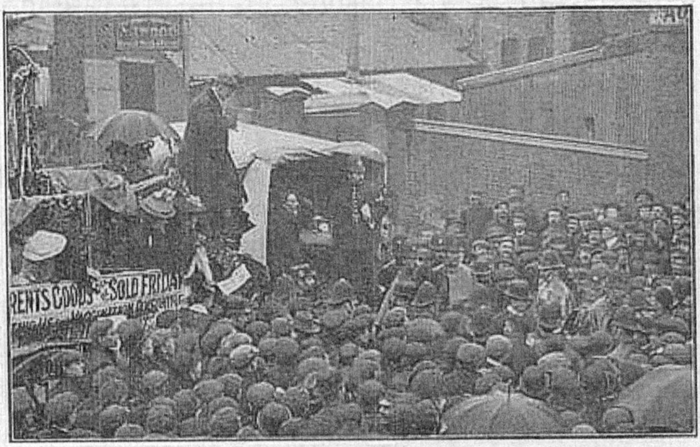

The Clerk to the Croydon Magistrates stated that over two thousand Vaccination Summonses had been applied for in Croydon. During recent years, six distress sales and attempted sales have been held, involving hundreds of cases of Fines and Costs. About fifty Croydon fathers have gone to prison rather than have their children vaccinated, or pay monetary penalties imposed.

1907 CALCIUM ARSENATE COMES INTO USE PRIMARILY ON COTTON CROPS AND ORCHARDS

1908 A Massachusetts town with three cotton mills and apple orchards recorded that 69 children suddenly fell ill with infantile paralysis, and in 1909 The UK bans apple imports from the States because of heavy lead arsenate residues.

1909 Numerous outbreaks of "serum hepatitis" and jaundice now attributed to hepatitis B virus were reported following the introduction, in 1909, of hypodermic needles that were used, and more importantly reused, for administering salvarsan for the treatment of syphilis.

1910 Flexer and Lewis ground up human spinal cord of a paralysis victim, and as Pasteur had done in the context of rabies, injected the suspension directly into a monkey's brain. That (one) monkey became paralyzed, then they extracted some fluid from its brain, and injected it into another monkey's brain, and so on through a series of monkeys paralyzing all of them in the process [with the foreign proteins of other monkeys directly injected into the brains and nervous systems of the recipients]. But making the monkeys drink the liquid or injecting into their arms, the suspension did not paralyze them.

BOTH SIDES

OF THE

VACCINATION QUESTION

THE FALLACY OF VACCINATION

By JOHN PITCAIRN

PRESIDENT OF THE ANTI-VACCINATION LEAGUE OF AMERICA

WHAT VACCINATION HAS REALLY DONE

By JAY FRANK SCHAMBERG, M.D.

PROFESSOR OF DERMATOLOGY AND OF INFECTIOUS ERUPTIVE DISEASES, PHILADELPHIA POLYCLINIC AND COLLEGE FOR GRADUATES IN MEDICINE; DIAGNOSTICIAN TO THE BUREAU OF HEALTH AND CONSULTING PHYSICIAN TO THE MUNICIPAL HOSPITAL, PHILADELPHIA

With References and Bibliographies

THE ANTI-VACCINATION LEAGUE OF AMERICA

517–518 CROZER BUILDING 1420 CHESTNUT STREET

PHILADELPHIA, PA.

1911

1912 – Laboratories of The Rockefeller Institute for Medical Research, New York. J Exp Med Sep 1;.16(3):315-24, 1912. doi: 10.1084/jem.16.3.315.

THE DURATION OF IMMUNE BODIES IN THE BLOOD AFTER ANTI-TYPHOID

1912 Most states in the U.S. had passed laws permitting or requiring medical examinations before school matriculation. (REF: Colgrove, p 49).

"Throughout the twentieth century, public education became widespread, and cities quickly realized that the schoolhouse served as a locus of prevention. James Colgrove, author of State of Immunity: The Politics of Vaccination in Twentieth-Century America defined the evolution this way: 'Although controversy over public health regulations was not uncommon during this period, vaccination provoked an especially vociferous response. Other regulations that limited individual liberty in order to protect the common good generally required that people refrain from an action or behavior. Vaccination, in contrast, required people to submit to a procedure, one that involved discomfort and whose safety and efficacy remained uncertain in the minds of many.' (REF: Colgrove. p. 10). The balance between the right of the individual and the good of the whole has long been a difficult dance. Since the beginning of mandatory vaccination programs, health officials have pressed individuals to participate through the use of several scripted arguments. These have included: Promoting the concept of herd immunity (an entire community will be protected if everyone is vaccinated); citing large epidemiological studies to minimize the number of injured in proportion to the numbers who have been vaccinated; and framing vaccination as a necessary act of a good citizen. Sometimes the arguments have been presented civilly, encouraging compliance through cooperation. But far too often, the approach has been forced. At the turn of the twentieth century, medical education began to shift toward an emphasis on sickness. The belief was fostered that only experts could legitimately make health decisions and physicians were positioned as better qualified than parents to judge the well-being of children. One of the best opportunities for the state to intervene and assess children was prior to attending school, and by 1912 most states had passed laws permitting or requiring medical examinations before school matriculation." REF: Colgrove, p 49.

1912 Parliamentary records of 1912 show that in New Zealand, the following vaccines and serums were used (Peter and Hilary Butler: "Just a little prick," ISBN 0473 10844 5):

Acne Vaccine (Mixed);Acne Bacillus vaccine;
Coley's Fluid;
Colt Bacillus Vaccine;
Combined Vaccines for colds;
Catarrhalis Micrococcus Vaccine;
Diptheria Anti Sera;
Friedlander Bacillus Vaccine;
Gonococcus Vaccine;
Influenza Bacillus Vaccine;
Meningococcus Anti Serum.;
Plague (Haffkine's Prophylactic) Pituitary Extract (Valporole);
Pneumococcus Vaccine;
Staphylococcus vaccine (mixed);
Staphylococcus Vaccine (Aureus);
Staphylococcus Anti Serum, (Polyvalent);
Staphylococcus Anti Sera;
Puerperal Fever Staphylococcus Anti Sera;
Pyogenes Staphylococcus Anti Sera;
Rheumatic Fever;
Staphylococcus Anti Sera;
Erysipelas; New Tuberculin T.R. (Koch);
New Tuberculin T.R. (Azoules);
New Tuberculin T.R. (Koch); (Lucius and Bruning) Tuberculin for Von Piquet's reaction; Tuberculin (Old) Human (Koch);

Tuberculin (Old) Bovine (Koch);
Tubercle Emulsion (Lucius and Bruning);
Tubercle Vaccine 0.0005 mgm;
Tubercle Vaccine 0.0001 mgm;
Normal Horse Serum;
Moist Tubercle, for "opsonic estimation" (the linking of antigen and antibody entities with an intermediary molecule that has a free end for each;
Staphylococcus Albus Vaccine;
Tubercle for conjunctival test;
Typhoid Bacillus Vaccine

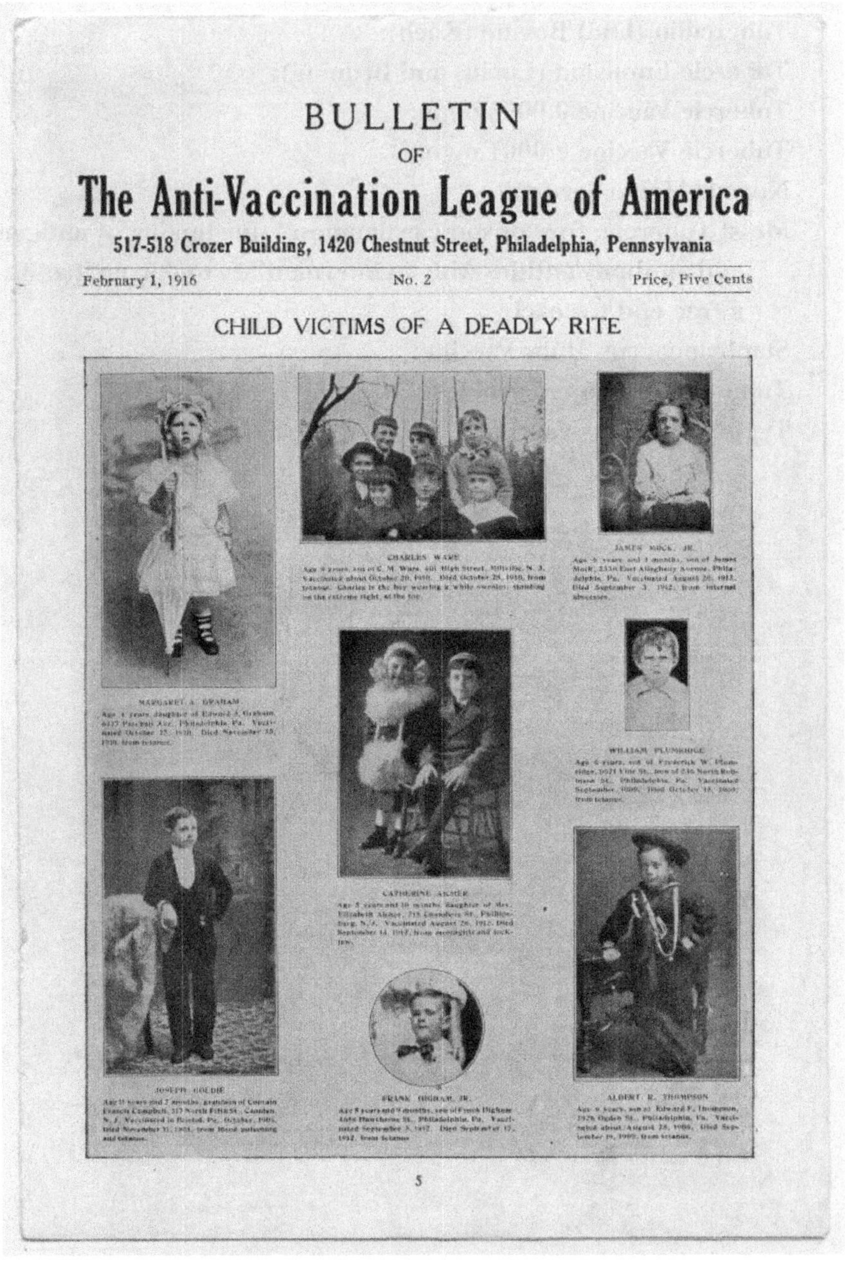

BULLETIN
OF
The Anti-Vaccination League of America
517-518 Crozer Building, 1420 Chestnut Street, Philadelphia, Pennsylvania

February 1, 1916 | No. 2 | Price, Five Cents

CHILD VICTIMS OF A DEADLY RITE

CHARLES WARE

JAMES MOCK, JR.

MARGARET A. GRAHAM

5

1915-1918 Massachusetts legislators, brag about having the most forceful mandatory vaccine laws in the country, and they rejected annual appeals from 1915 to 1918 to repeal mandatory requirements. REF: "State of Immunity," by James Colgrove. University of California Press, 2006. p. 64.

1916 – THE FIRST AMERICAN PUBLIC HEALTH CONTROL PROGRAMS BEGIN IN FORCES DURING AND FOLLOWING A GREAT 1916 PARALYSIS EPIDEMIC, AND THE CONCEPT OF "THE HEALTHY CARRIER STATE" WAS A RESULT OF THE NON-CONTAGIOUS NATURE OF PARALYSIS

During this great and feared 1916 "polio epidemic" that began only five years after mandatory vaccinations were implemented for the military in the United States in 1911, in retrospect we see the fears of contagion and catechisms regarding failure to vaccinate arrogantly being asserted as fact for the first time in its recognizable modern form. For example, both before and during the 1916 epidemic, and still today, nobody could figure out why both rich and poor individuals contracted paralysis. Nobody could explain why both the well-fed and the hungry became paralyzed, or why acute flaccid paralysis prevalence was higher among gentiles than the "unwashed immigrants," or why both those who swam in public pools, and those who did not, contracted paralysis.

Fear turned into public health campaigns to enforce quarantines and fines for those who kept their windows open or who failed to maintain their living quarter environs as clean as possible to ward off an imagined fly vector.

Public health officials, and medical "scientists" (like Flexner who believed polio to be spread through the air) could not explain why rich Philadelphia playboys and orphans of the state would both contract paralysis, and how only one individual out of a family of many children acquired paralysis. It was written by some historians that more spinal taps were performed during that era than could be counted, and "exsanguinations" of cerebral spinal fluid, or mercury injected into the spinal fluid were thought to reduce the symptoms of paralysis.

For lack of a consistent causal association for transmission of paralysis, and the fact that many more folks also appeared to "have it" or "carry it" that never so much as developed the sniffles-the only thing that was left for public health authorities, and the academic scientists and physicians to hypothesize, after all of these hypotheses (and others) failed to quell the occurrence of paralysis during the summertime, was the idea of a "healthy carrier state."

THE CAUSE OF THE GREATEST DISEASE IN HUMAN HISTORY: 20,000,000 LIVES ARE ESTIMATED TO HAVE DIED, BUT THE "SPANISH FLU" WASN'T FROM SPAIN AND IS NOW BELIEVED TO HAVE BEEN PARTLY CAUSED BY AN INTERNATIONAL VACCINATION CAMPAIGN, WAR, AND NOT PFEIFFER'S BACTERIAL BACCILIS

Pfeiffer isolated an organism in 1892 variously referred to as Pfeiffer bacillus or influenza bacillus which was accepted by many as the causative agent of influenza. However, in 1918, various observers failed to find this organism in many cases of influenza, antemortem or postmortem. A report on sputum cultures taken from 47 individuals in Baltimore during the epidemic showed that streptococci were present in 24 sputums, staphylococcus in 1, pneumococcus in 15, and the influenza bacillus in 8.

In cultures taken in various Army camps prior to and during the epidemic of influenza in the fall of 1918, varying proportions of persons were found to carry streptococci, pneumococci, and the Pfeiffer's bacillus. Such variations were also found in cultures from the bronchi or lungs at autopsy, and differences were found from camp to camp. The proportion of persons carrying streptococci, or some other secondary invader did not remain constant, being replaced from time to time by another bacterium.

It was the impression of many in 1918 that an unrecognized and unknown type of agent of some kind was the primary cause of influenza and that the streptococci, pneumococci, and influenza bacilli were secondary invaders which might be termed "bacterial hitch-hikers." Attempts by two groups of investigators to transmit the infection by nasal instillation of filtered and unfiltered secretions from influenza cases in human volunteers were not successful. Nor could they produce influenza in the volunteers by nasal swabs with Pfeiffer's bacillus.

1917 U.S. soldiers are vaccinated prior to going overseas to fight in WW I. They soon begin to "drop dead by the thousands" from a strange syndrome that preferentially attacked young adults.

1918 ROCKEFELLER INSTITUTE REPORT ON ANTI-MENINGITIS VACCINATION AND OBSERVATIONS ON AGGLUTININS IN THE BLOOD OF CHRONIC MENINGOCOCCUS CARRIERS

A meningococcus vaccine suspended in salt solution has been given subcutaneously as a prophylactic to about 3,700 volunteers in three injections of 2,000 million, 4,000 million, and 4,000 or 8,000 million cocci at weekly intervals. These doses rarely caused more than the mildest local and general reactions. Exceptionally a more severe reaction emphasized the presence of an unusual individual susceptibility to the vaccine. In such instances the symptoms were in part those of meningeal irritation and **sometimes simulated the onset of meningitis.**

Frederick L Gates J Exp Med 918 Oct 1;28(4):449-74. doi: 10.1084/jem.28.4.449. Base Hospital, Fort Riley, Kansas, and The Rockefeller Institute for Medical Research, New York.

1918 DEPARTMENT OF THE NAVY — NAVAL HISTORICAL CENTER 805 Kidder Breese — Washington NAVY Yard, Washington, DC in a report entitled, "THE PANDEMIC OF 1918-1919" prepared by the US Department of Health, Education and Welfare Public Health Service National Office of Vital Statistics stated that the extraordinary feature of "the Great Spanish flu" was that it attacked young people in the prime of life after they had been recently vaccinated.

The pandemic of influenza in 1918-19 which swept over nearly every continent and island of the whole globe has been described as one of the great human catastrophes. There are excellent descriptions of epidemics and pandemics as far back as the year 1500, and various records of epidemics since the 1918-19 **potential vaccine-induced iatrogenocide.**

Many of the other historic epidemics and pandemics were relatively mild infections, while others were more severe, but none of the other epidemics showed the extraordinarily high mortality rate in young adults that characterized the 1918-19 pandemic and its aftermath in 1920. This is also one of the first epidemics, besides several earlier smallpox outbreaks, that clearly followed a mass-vaccination campaign. The greatest amount of mortality in epidemics prior to and subsequent to 1918-19 was found in children under 1 year of age and in persons 65 years and over.

Frost, in one of his reports, pointed out that influenza and pneumonia mortality rose sharply in some cities in the United States in December 1915 and January 1916, which may or may not have been related to the 1918 epidemic. In January 1916, influenza was reported to be epidemic in 22 States, but it was described as a mild type of illness.

As early as December 1917, influenza was prevalent in Camp Kearny, California, and in other Army camps in January 1918, but the disease was said to be mild. In the spring, localized outbreaks occurred in the civilian population of the United States, and mortality from pneumonia rose sharply in certain cities. In March and April, Camp Funston, Kansas, experienced three waves of influenza. The first two affected all types of personnel, and the third, which occurred late in April, was predominantly in recruits who arrived shortly after the second wave. Mild epidemics of influenza were reported in various localities in Western Europe in April and May of 1918, and in June and July more extensive outbreaks occurred in Great Britain and in Europe, China, India, the Philippine Islands, and Brazil. In these countries, mortality rose moderately. The 1918-19 epidemic was often referred to in the United States as "Spanish influenza," but there is no reason to believe that it originated in Spain. Indeed, the occurrence of influenza in the United States in the spring of 1918 may have preceded that which occurred in Spain.

During August 1918, epidemics of influenza were reported in Greece, Sweden, Switzerland, Spain, the West Indies, and late in the month it appeared almost simultaneously in Camp Shelby, Mississippi, and Boston, Massachusetts. In September, it appeared in rapid succession in other Army camps and in the civilian population along the Atlantic seaboard and the Gulf of Mexico and spread rapidly westward over the country. By October, the epidemic had involved the entire United States, except isolated places and some mountain areas. The interval between the peaks of the epidemic in Boston and San Francisco was about 4 weeks, and the peaks in the number of deaths usually were reached in about 1 month following the beginning of the epidemic in a community or area. As a rule, epidemics affected rural areas later than cities in the same sections. In some areas there was a recrudescence of the epidemic in January and February 1919, which was most marked in cities where the autumn epidemic was less severe. Thus, the influenza epidemic of 1918-19 in the United States was characterized by a relatively mild phase in the spring of 1918, an explosive outbreak with high mortality in the fall, and a third phase or recrudescence early in 1919.

The incidence and mortality of influenza in military personnel in 1918-19 has been described in great detail in Epidemiology and Public Health by Vaughan, and in Volume 9 of the history of the Medical Department of the United States Army in the World War. [See also the Surgeon General's account in Annual Report of the Secretary of the Navy, 1919 — Miscellaneous Reports]. About 90 percent of the men in military service in World War I were young adults between 20 and 35 years of age. Consequently, the Armed Forces were seriously affected, as were the same age groups in the civilian population. In the Army over a million men were hospitalized for influenza and pneumonia, and of these there were more than

44,000 deaths. There were approximately 5,000 deaths among Navy personnel. Hospital admission rates and death rates for American troops stationed in Europe were lower than for troops in the United States. The large number of recruits concentrated in close quarters probably accounted for higher rates in the latter. In the camps having the larger numbers of recently vaccinated trainees incidence and mortality was highest, and in all camps the rates were higher in recruits than in seasoned troops. The crowding in camps probably favored the spread of secondary invading organisms as well as the etiologic agent of influenza. The peak of the epidemic was reached in September in Navy personnel and about the middle of October in the Army. A secondary rise in incidence of these respiratory diseases occurred in the Army in January and February 1919, but it was limited to troops stationed in Europe.

When appropriate adjustments are made for differences in the age and sex distribution of military and civilian populations, it appears that the death rate was about one-fourth higher in the Army than in the civilian population of the United States.

It is reasonable to assume that this difference was largely due to greater crowding in the recruit population of the Army, but as mentioned, over-vaccination and re-vaccination of armed forces also could have accounted for the observed increase.

Collins showed mortality rates from influenza and pneumonia by age in 1918 as compared with certain other years. The relatively high mortality in young adults in 1918 and the 2 years immediately following seems to have been characteristic of that period and was not found in epidemics prior to or subsequent to this 3-year period.

1918 – Did An International Vaccine Campaign Gone Bad Start and Spread the So-Called & Misnamed "Great Spanish Influenza"?

In the account of survivor of the "Great Spanish Flu," Eleanor McBean, the following is claimed: E. McBean (Vaccination the Silent Killer p28) (Source: Dr. Rebecca Carley):

Eleanor McBean writes: "Very few people realize that the worst

epidemic ever to hit America, the Spanish Influenza of 1918 was the after effect of the massive nation-wide vaccine campaign. The doctors told the people that the disease was caused by germs. Viruses were not known at that time or they would have been blamed. Germs, bacteria, and viruses, along with bacilli and a few other invisible organisms are the scapegoats, which the doctors like to blame for the things they do not understand. If the doctor makes a wrong diagnosis and treatment, and kills the patient, he can always blame it on the germs, and say the patient did not get an early diagnosis and come to him in time.

If we check back in history to that 1918 flu period, we will see that it suddenly struck just after the end of World War I when our soldiers were returning home from overseas. That was the first war in which all the known vaccines were forced on all the servicemen. This mish-mash of poison drugs and putrid protein of which the vaccines were composed, caused such widespread disease and death among the soldiers that it was the common talk of the day, that more of our men were being killed by medical shots than by enemy shots from guns. Thousands were invalided home or to military hospitals, as hopeless wrecks, before they ever saw a day of battle. The death and disease rate among the vaccinated soldiers was four times higher than among the unvaccinated civilians. But this did not stop the vaccine promoters. Vaccine has always been big business, and so it was continued doggedly.

It was a shorter war than the vaccine-makers had planned on, only about a year for us, so the vaccine promoters had a lot of unused, spoiling vaccines left over which they wanted to sell at a good profit. So, they did what they usually do, they called a meeting behind closed doors, and plotted the whole sordid program, a nationwide (worldwide) vaccination drive using all their vaccines and telling the people that the soldiers were coming home with many dread diseases contracted in foreign countries and that it was the patriotic duty of every man, woman and child to get "protected" by rushing down to the vaccination centers and having all the shots.

Most people believe their doctors and government officials and do what they say. The result was that almost the entire population submitted to the shots without question, and it was only a matter of hours until people began dropping dead in agony, while many others collapsed with a disease of such virulence that no one had ever seen anything like it before. They had all the characteristics of the diseases they had been vaccinated against, the high fever, chills, pain, cramps, diarrhea, etc. of typhoid, and the pneumonia like lung and throat congestion of diphtheria and the vomiting, headache, weakness, and misery of hepatitis from the jungle fever shots, and the outbreak of sores on the skin from the smallpox shots, along with paralysis from all the shots, etc. The doctors were baffled and claimed they did not know what caused the strange and deadly disease, and they certainly had no cure. They should have known the underlying cause was the vaccinations because the same thing happened to the soldiers after they had their shots at camp.

The typhoid fever shots caused a worse form of the disease, which they called para-typhoid. Then they tried to suppress the symptoms of that one with a stronger vaccine, which caused a still more serious disease, which killed and disabled a great many men. The combination of all the poison vaccines fermenting together in the body, caused such violent reactions that they could not cope with the situation. Disaster ran rampant in the camps. Some of the military hospitals were filled with nothing but paralyzed soldiers, and they were called war casualties, even before they left American soil. I talked to some of the survivors of that vaccine onslaught when they returned home after the war, and they told of the horrors, not of the war itself, and battles, but of the sickness at camp.

The doctors did not want this massive vaccine disease to reflect on them, so they agreed among themselves to call it Spanish Influenza. Spain was a faraway place and some of the soldiers had been there, so the idea of calling it Spanish Influenza seemed to be a good way to lay the blame on someone else. The Spanish resented having us name the world scourge on them. They knew the flu didn't originate in their country." "20,000,000 died of that flu epidemic,

worldwide, and it seemed to be almost universal or as far away as the vaccinations reached. Greece and a few other countries, which did not accept the vaccines, were the only ones that were not hit by the flu. Doesn't that prove something?

"At home (in the U.S.) the situation was the same; the only ones who escaped the influenza were those who had refused the vaccinations. My family and 1 were among the few who persisted in refusing the high-pressure sales propaganda, and none of us had the flu not even a sniffle, in spite of the fact that it was all around us, and in the bitter cold of winter."

Everyone seemed to have it. The whole town was down sick and dying. The hospitals were closed because the doctors and nurses were down with the flu. Everything was closed, schools, businesses, post office everything. No one was on the streets. It was like a ghost town. There were no doctors to care for the sick, so my parents went from house to house doing what they could to help the stricken in any way they could. They spent all day and part of the night for weeks, in the sick rooms, and came home only to eat and sleep. If germs or viruses, bacteria, or any other little organisms were the cause of that disease, they had plenty of opportunity to latch onto my parents and 'lay them low' with the disease that had prostrated the world. But germs were not the cause of that or any other disease, so they did not 'catch' it. I have talked to a few other people since that time, who said they escaped the 1918 flu, so I asked if they had the shots, and in every case, they said they had never believed in shots and had never had any of them. Common sense tells us that all those toxic vaccines all mixed up together in people, could not help but cause extreme body-poisoning and poisoning of some kind or another is usually the cause of disease."

Whenever a person coughs or sneezes, most people cringe, thinking that the germs are being spread around in the air and will attack people. There is no need to fear those germs anymore because that is not the way colds are developed. Germs cannot live apart from the cells (host) and cannot do harm anyway, even if they wanted to. They have no teeth to bite anyone, no poison pouches like snakes, mosquitoes, or bees, and do not multiply, except in decomposed substances, so they are helpless to harm. As stated before, their purpose is useful, not destructive.

The 1918 flu was the most devastating disease we ever had, and it brought forth all the medical bag of tricks to quell it, but those added drugs, all of which are poisons, only intensified the over-poisoned condition of the people, so the treatments actually killed more than the flu did.

These excerpts were taken from Vaccination the Silent Killer: Honor of Ida and McBean, E.: Vaccination the silent killer (U.S.A.) Honor Publications, P.O. Box 346, Cutten, CA 95534, U.S.A.

Other accounts and records recorded the following information regarding the so-called Great "Spanish Flu" (a flu that was neither Spanish nor originating from Spain):

It has been estimated that there were about 20,000,000 cases of influenza and pneumonia in the United States in 1918-19, with approximately 850,000 deaths. In 1918 alone, 464,959 deaths from influenza and pneumonia were registered in the registration States and the District of Columbia as compared with 115,526 in 1917. This includes deaths in the Army, Navy, and Marine Corps which occurred in registration States. Eighty percent of the deaths in 1918 occurred in the last 4 months of the year.

The numbers of deaths from influenza and pneumonia by age in registration States in 1917, 1918, and 1919 are shown in the table below. A number of States in which Army camps were located are not included in this table, so a considerable number of deaths of civilians and of military personnel for 1918-19 are missing which accounts for the difference in an estimated total of 850,000 for the United States and the figure of 650,399 for the registration States. In 1918 the death rate for males was 669.0 per 100,000 population; for females, 507.5. At ages 25 to 34, the rate was 1,216.6 for males and 781.4 for females. These excessively high mortality rates profoundly influenced the estimated average length of life calculated for the year 1918. It was reduced 24 percent from 1917 to 1918 for males and 22 percent for females. However, these estimated average lengths of life in years returned to their previous trends in 1920.

Because the so-called epidemic did not behave according to rational "medical or biological rules" or hypotheses, an imagined filter-passing entity, called viruses, were proposed, but really never became established accept until decades later. They were perhaps best described as "rumor viruses" then, as they still are today.

Unlike any influenza or disease in history, the so-called "Great Spanish Flu," whatever caused these numbers to occur, killed young male adults preferentially in their prime (as designated by question marks) similar to the so-called AIDS epidemic of the 1980's, sparing infants and the aged, the typical targets of seasonal influenza-like syndromes. Could the compulsory vaccine campaigns upon entering the military account for these numbers?

PREVENTION, SOCIAL DISTANCING, AND LOCKDOWN CONTROL OF THE GREAT FLU DIDN'T WORK

"It often happens that when a severe outbreak of a disease occurs many measures are applied, some of which appear to be extreme and dictated by panic. In 1918, which was no exception, isolation of cases and quarantine of contacts were applied vigorously in some areas, but there is little evidence to indicate that these measures were successful in preventing introduction or spread of the disease. Closure of schools and prohibition of public gatherings likewise were of doubtful value. The use of face masks to protect the wearer against infection had its advocates. The use of germicidal gases to destroy the organism was suggested. The use of a vaccine containing the influenza bacillus was advocated, but as one would expect, no value could be demonstrated. If a vaccine containing the viruses now known to cause the disease had been made available early in the epidemic, it is doubtful whether it would have been effective, since the epidemic in the fall of 1918 spread with great rapidity."

Victor Gaughan stated in 1922 about the so-called Spanish Flu in retrospect that the most reasonable administrative action that could have been taken was to direct efforts toward relief measures, namely, medical and nursing care and hospitalization.

Much of the descriptive material and charts on the 1918-19 epidemic used in this comprehensive Department of Navy report were obtained from published reports or books by W.H. Frost, Edgar Sydenstricker, Victor Vaughan, and Eugene Opie. The publications of Selwyn Collins were a valuable source of information on characteristics of epidemics of influenza in the United States prior to and subsequent to 1918.

1918 ROCKEFELLER INSTITUTE RESULTS OF PROPHYLACTIC INOCULATION AGAINST PNEUMOCOCCUS IN 12,519 MEN PMID: 19868242 PMCID: PMC2126122 DOI: 10.1084/jem.28.1.19

The local and general toxic reaction varies greatly in different individuals. The smaller the individual doses, the fewer are the severe reactions. This makes it desirable to divide the total dosage into as many inoculations as circumstances make practicable. **At Camp Upton 12,519 men** have been vaccinated against Pneumococcus Types I, II, and III. Three or four doses were given at intervals of 5 to 7 days.

1918 Pathologists became intimately familiar with the condition of lungs of victims of bacterial pneumonia at autopsy. But the viral pneumonias caused by the influenza pandemic were so violent that many investigators said 'the "only lungs they had seen that resembled them were from victims of poison gas! '

1919 Despite the Supreme Court's emphasis on protecting the "greater good," North Dakota enacted laws expressly forbidding the passage of any mandatory vaccination requirements.

1919 Washington and in 1920 Wisconsin repeal mandatory requirements and replace them with personal belief exemptions.

1919 A series of studies was undertaken on the occurrence and characters of hemolytic and other streptococci which had been found to be of serious importance in certain pneumonias, complicating measles, and influenza, especially in military establishments. Research on pneumococci and meningococci vaccine and on meningitis carriers were carried on in the Institute in New York or in field studies in various military camps and cantonments.

SERUM PRODUCTION: In order to help meet the suddenly increased demand for the curative serums worked out at the Institute, a special stable for horses was quickly erected and a special and suitable laboratory staff assembled at the Department of Animal Pathology. In undertaking serum manufacture on a large scale, the officers of the Institute had another object in view; namely, the standardization of the product.

THE ROCKEFELLER INSTITUTE FOR MEDICAL RESEARCH latter consideration became of high importance in establishing standards for the commercial producers. Three kinds of curative serums were manufactured in quantity; namely, antimeningococci, antipneumococcic Type I, and antidysenteric (polyvalent). Other serums intended for diagnostic purposes, such as Types I, II, III, and IV antimeningococcic, and Types II and III antipneumococcic serums were produced in smaller amounts. The quantities of the several kinds of serums distributed are as follows: 939.40 liters, or 46,970 bottles (20 cc.) of antimeningococcic serum; 344.79 liters, or 3,447 bottles (100 cc.) of antipneumococcic serum; 78 .36 liters, or 3,918 bottles (20 cc.) of antidysenteric serum. The amounts partially include the various diagnostic serums issued. Reference should be made to the fact that before the United States entered the war, the Institute had resumed the preparation of antimeningococcic serum, in order to meet the requests from England, France, Belgium, Italy, and other countries.

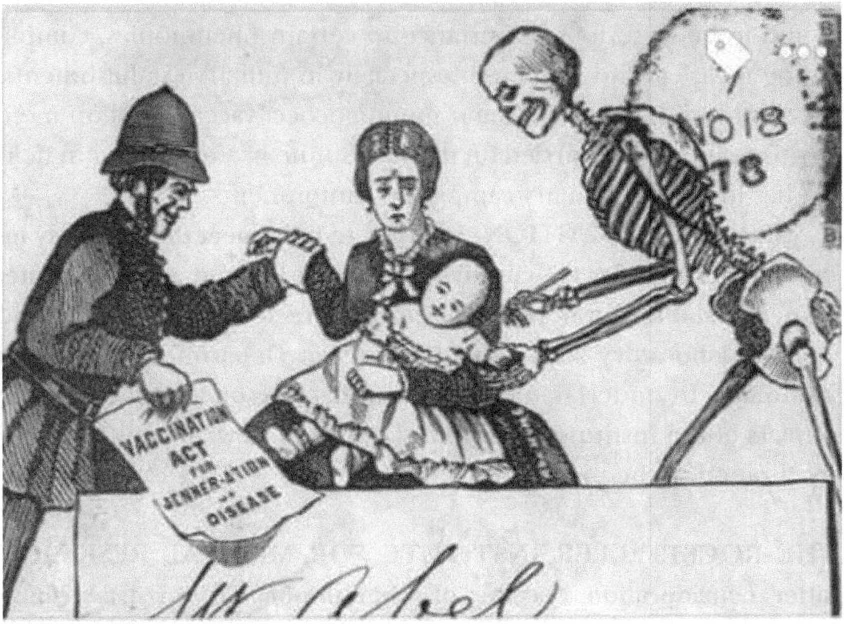
VACCINATION
ACT
FOR
JENNER-ATION
DISEASE

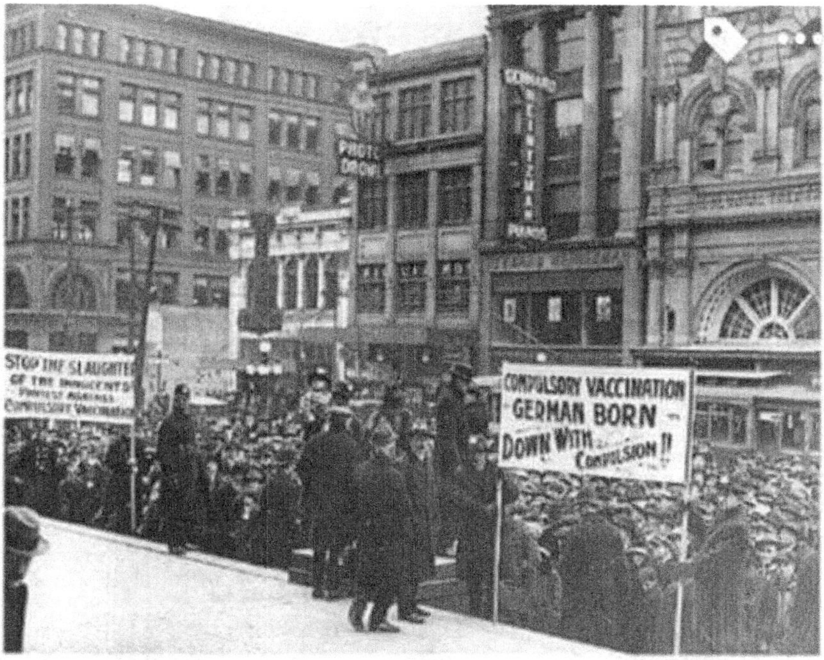

Rally of the Anti-Vaccination League of Canada, Old City Hall
November 13, 1919
Photographer: William James
Thanks to the City of Toronto Archives

1920 Charles M Higgins from The Horrors of Vaccination Exposed and Illustrated: Petition to the President to Abolish Compulsory Vaccination in Army and Navy:

STOP COMPULSORY VACCINATION

All Together Now---Quick!

Public Demonstration

A public demonstration against compulsory vaccination will be held on the

CITY HALL STEPS

12 NOON

Thursday, November 13

COME IN YOUR THOUSANDS—MAKE YOUR VOICE HEARD—80% of Toronto people know vaccination to be ineffective as a preventive of smallpox and that it is a positive menace to health—especially to the health of children. The death rate from vaccination is actually greater than the death rate from smallpox. Our motto is "No Compulsory Vaccination." Let us have the British—not the German—way in matters of public health.

COME, VETERANS!

You have had recent experience—you have seen comrades well enough to pass the doctor sicken and some die after vaccination. This is your fight for Medical Freedom.

SEND A CONTRIBUTION TO PAY FOR PUBLICITY.

The Anti-Vaccination League

ARTHUR BLACK FARMER,

378 Markham Street, Secretary-Treasurer.

"GOD SAVE THE KING."

GREAT EPIDEMICS OF DEADLY DISEASE, IN ANIMALS AND MANKIND, CAUSED BY VACCINATION: LETTERS

Now, not only is vaccination extremely dangerous to health and life in many individual cases and frequently causes more deaths every year than smallpox, particularly in little children, as already clearly proved, but another shocking fact is that vaccination has been proved to be the cause of several great epidemics of deadly disease among mankind and domestic animals and has probably also been the cause of many other serious epidemics whose origin has not yet been proved.

This shocking fact of vaccine epidemics in recent times is readily proved by current medical works, by Government Reports, and by notorious public facts occurring within the last few years, as I will now show.

I may first refer on this point to one of the strongest pro-vaccination works now published, viz., "Acute Contagious Diseases," by Drs. Welch and Schamberg, Lea Brothers & Co., Philadelphia, 1905. On page 65, in this work, the following serious admission is made:

"Several appalling epidemics of septicemia after vaccination are on record; one occurred in the United States, one in Germany, and one in France."

These epidemics are shown to have caused many deaths in children and adults, the fatal effect being very rapid, the deaths occurring in one or a few days after vaccination.

On page 74, in the same work, this clear admission of an epidemic of that most awful and fatal disease, lockjaw, caused by vaccination, is made as follows:

"In October, November, and December, 1901, there was a small epidemic of tetanus after vaccination in Camden, Philadelphia, and to a certain extent in near-by towns. "Camden had eleven cases, and Philadelphia even more than this number."

It is to be here noted, however, that, bad as this last admission is, the pro-vaccinators did not give the public the whole truth in this last statement, but which I will now add here, viz., that in these epidemics the deaths from the lockjaw infection in the vaccination wounds exceeded by manifold the deaths from smallpox at the same time and locality! Here is another great proof of the medical and statistical truth to which I have repeatedly called attention, viz., that vaccination is frequently a much more dangerous and fatal disease than natural smallpox, and, therefore, obviously, for this reason alone, should not be forced on any person against free will and consent.

VACCINATION BOTH A THEORETICAL AND A PROVED CAUSE OF EPIDEMICS AND NOW PANDEMICS

In a previous letter to the Secretary of War, dated October 14, 1918, and published in the Washington Herald of November 20, 1918, I have pointed out the dangerous nature of vaccination, particularly during epidemics, and the hygienic importance of suspending all vaccination during our recent epidemic of influenza and pneumonia, and the further desirability of making all vaccination strictly free and voluntary. I also then called attention to the probability that the repeated and multiple vaccinations of millions of men, in this country and Europe, with various septicemic infections for the last two years, may have had some relation to this epidemic, which seems to have been more severe among the vaccinated men in the military camps and hospitals than among the rest of the population. And I would now like to repeat here some of the important facts which I have stated in said letter as to both the probable and the proved relation of vaccination to many deadly epidemics.

GRAVE NATURE OF RECENT EPIDEMIC OF INFLUENZA AND PNEUMONIA

From the rapidity, severity, and mortality of this disease, it would seem not to be a true influenza, as heretofore known, and as its worst cases are characterized by a rapid and fatal ending, with a few days' sickness, in malignant or septic pneumonia, with abscesses in the lungs, it seems more related to the very fatal "Pneumonic Plague' which raged in Manchuria after the Japanese war. This suspicion is strengthened by the fact that the chief germ found in the fatal cases is the "streptococcus," which is found in the worst forms of "blood poisoning" or "septicemia," and also in vaccination. Now, the act of ordinary vaccination, as already proved, is, in itself, an act of blood poisoning, pure and simple, and it is so classed in medical and statistical works as a form of "septicemia," and one disease germ commonly found, with many others, in vaccine virus is the streptococcus, which is the chief germ found in all bad pus infections and abscess formations. Therefore, as the act of vaccination is simply the impregnation of the body and blood with a pus infection identical with "septicemia" or "pyemia," and as this infecting process has been repeated at wholesale in the bodies of thousands and tens of thousands of men closely massed in camps, should it be any wonder if an epidemic of some sort of "septicemia" should crop out at some time under such conditions?

In leading medical and statistical works, both influenza and pneumonia and typhoid fever and vaccination are all classed as different forms of "septicemia," and while I do not, of course, know, and do not say, that the recent epidemic of influenza and pneumonia was actually caused by vaccination, yet I repeat that when the body and blood of millions of men all over this country and Europe are deliberately impregnated with various septic diseases, or septicemic infections, can any reasonable person, whether doctor or layman, be surprised if such world-wide, and million times repeated, acts of septicemic infection should be ultimately proved to have some causative or conditional relation to the recent world-wide epidemic of septicemic disease? Is it physically or medically possible to go on sowing and spreading some known and unknown septic diseases at wholesale, within human bodies, without reaping some big harvest of deadly septic diseases as a necessary consequence? In the words of Scripture, can we keep on "sowing" the "winds" of infection without ultimately "reaping" the "whirlwind" of epidemics?

It has been suggested that this epidemic originated in the multi-vaccinated and diseased or impoverished German army and has traveled one-quarter round the earth from that focus of infection.

It has also been suggested that this epidemic originated from a regiment of coolies or native Hindoo troops brought from India to France who were infected with a severe disease like Pneumonic Plague, and from them this disease spread to the other soldiers in camp and field and thence over the world.

It has been further suggested that this disease should not be called a true influenza or pneumonia at all but is essentially a most virulent form of general septicemia, and that it originated from the frightfully infected soil of the battle-fields, which, in addition to the ordinary deadly soil infections, contains virulent septicemic and cadaveric infections from the great mass of buried and unburied bodies. And as the soldiers in camp and field were already impregnated with several septicemic infections in the multiple vaccinations of five or six kinds to which they have been almost universally subjected, their systems thus became "sensitized" or highly susceptible to further infection, particularly to what was evidently a new and very severe type of soil and cadaveric infection. This, theory seems to fit the present known facts and would explain the probable origin of this very severe type of virulent septicemic plague, which shows itself in this mysterious and deadly epidemic with its mortality of thirty to sixty per cent, which we have been improperly regarding as ordinary influenza and pneumonia.

In my letter to the Secretary of War I proved that there was a distinct medical and logical relation between influenza and vaccination, and that many serious diseases, including smallpox and cowpox, commence like influenza and may be mistaken for it, but I do not need to go into proof of that point here, but can now say that this point further strengthens the suspicions stated that the recent epidemic of influenza and septicemia or septic pneumonia may have had some causative relation to the extensive wholesale and repeated vaccinations in the military camps throughout the world, and would indicate, according to another theory, that this vaccine infection had escaped from and overflowed its usual bounds and was running wild as a world-wide epidemic infection; and hence the positive and compelling reasons for checking this overflowing infection by suspending all vaccination while this epidemic and infecting condition exists, and making all vaccination voluntary instead of compulsory as heretofore. (See U. S. Naval Medical Bulletin, Oct., 1914, page 591, Smallpox on Battleship Ohio confounded with Influenza).

EPIDEMICS ARE ACTUALLY CAUSED BY VACCINATION

That the hypothetical condition suggested in the preceding paragraph, that the wholesale and world-wide vaccine infection going on for the past few years had possibly escaped from its usual bounds and has been overflowing and running wild and thus causing epidemics in mankind, or animals that this, I say, may be no mere hypothesis or theory, but rather a hard fact, is proved by the frightful epidemics of "foot and mouth disease" in the United States in 1902, 1908, and 1914, some of which originated from two of the largest vaccine factories in this country, one in Philadelphia and the other in Detroit, and were widely distributed to cattle and mankind in several of our States. See reports of U. S. Bureau of Animal Industry, 1902 and 1908. Also, Yearbook of U.S.A. Department of Agriculture, 1914, page 20. See also page 96 in Supplement.

It is clearly shown in these reports that vaccine infection was the direct cause of these epidemics in 1902 and 1908; but the cause of the epidemic of 1914 and 1915 is not so clearly proven, although there is a strong suspicion that it was caused by vaccine infection, like the two others, and, as a matter of fact, it originated in the same State Michigan here the epidemic of 1908 originated and where one of the largest vaccine factories in the country is located.

These vaccine epidemics caused the destruction of hundreds of thousands of cattle and other domestic animals in over a score of States, at a loss of many millions of dollars to the Government and people of this country. See page 102. Surely, Mr. President, any medical operation so inherently dangerous and capable of inflicting such injury on animals or man should not be forced on any person against conscientious objection or without free will and consent and should not be required by our enlightened democratic Government in our Army or Navy in any form except purely voluntary, like all other medical remedies and operations.

There is an attempt made in some of the official reports to deny that these epidemics of "foot and mouth disease" were caused by vaccination or could be transmitted or were transmitted to mankind via a virus and were limited to domestic animals, but this may be a grave mistake. The most convincing evidence that this disease was transmitted to many human victims, both child and adult, with most awful effects in 1902 and 1908, and is frequently transmitted to mankind in vaccine virus.

VACCINE FACTORIES A POSSIBLE AND PROVED SOURCE OF EPIDEMICS AND SHOULD BE INVESTIGATED BY CONGRESS AND THE GOVERNMENT (in a democracy, the people-us-are the government)

This foot and mouth disease is a horrible eruptive fever, a kind of "cowpox," or something like a mongrel smallpox and diphtheria combined, or also like an awfully bad chickenpox, with successive crops of vesicles, blisters or blotches, something like cold sores, large and small, breaking out all over the body, but chiefly on the hoofs, or hands and feet, lips, and nostrils, also inside the mouth and throat as is common in smallpox. Sometimes these blotches become confluent and pustular and continue for months, but, usually, the eruption ends in a few weeks in recovery or death. In the worst cases, with internal eruptions and pus infection, affecting vital nerve centers, the end comes in a few days by the victim choking to death from paralysis of the heart and breathing organs like what happens in infant paralysis, rabies, and lockjaw. For effects on cattle and mankind, see Figs. 7, 8, 9, 11, 12 and 13 in Supplement.

Now here we see that at least two and probably three great epidemics of fatal disease have originated from vaccine factories and this raises the serious question as to how far other epidemics, or even the recent epidemic of influenza and pneumonia, may have originated from some vaccine factory or from some of their products extensively or carelessly used. Surely the places where dangerous infectious diseases are constantly propagated on a gigantic scale and disseminated therefrom into the bodies of millions of animals and mankind, should be the very possible or probable source of epidemic disease. Obviously, therefore, this entire subject of the present extensive manufacture and distribution of diseases or disease cultures or products and its relation to epidemics and public health should be thoroughly investigated by Congress and the Government at an early date. To show you what a gigantic and dangerous medical interest this vaccine manufacture has become, it may be sufficient to state that there are now about 100 concerns licensed by the U. S. Government to manufacture vaccines and serums for animal and human uses. This is one of the great medical interests supporting compulsory vaccination, which is a grave medical malpractice, and should be abolished wherever it exists and replaced by wholly voluntary vaccination as already shown.

1918 – EPIDEMICS AND HIGH DEATH RATES IN THE ARMY PROBABLY CAUSED BY WHOLESALE AND REPEATED VACCINATIONS. DEATH RATE OF ARMY FROM DISEASE MUCH GREATER THAN THAT OF CIVIL POPULATION

After careful study of this subject for years I passionately believe that, with the excellent sanitary and hygienic conditions now used in our Army, the dangerous system of disease inoculations, whereby the blood of every man is impregnated with multiple and repeated vaccinations of several diseases, such as smallpox, typhoid, para-typhoid, etc., is a system, to say the least, that is neither necessary nor ultimately useful for army health. And it is probable that this system produces far more disease than it prevents. For example: For one death which naturally occurs in the whole population from smallpox or typhoid fever, ten to one hundred deaths occur from the far more frequent and fatal diseases of tuberculosis, measles, pneumonia, and meningitis. And let us here ask, what is the use of having soldiers forced to submit to a whole series of disease infections, if these infections, at best, given immunity only for a little while from such diseases as smallpox and typhoid and make the system more susceptible to the far worse diseases of measles, pneumonia, and meningitis, which actually seems to be the possible effects of vaccination from the recurring epidemics of these dangerous diseases in our heavily vaccinated camps?

As a matter of fact, my studies of deaths from vaccination for many years past show that meningitis and pneumonia are some of the most frequent complications; and these two diseases seem to have a certain relation to vaccination and seem to be very fatal where vaccination precedes them, and thus acts in what is called a "double" or "mixed infection," which is known to be extremely dangerous to health and life.

Another most significant fact in this connection is the high death rate from disease in the Army, as compared with the civil population, which I will now consider.

On page 18 in the Report of the Secretary of War for 1918 the death rate of the Army in the United States from disease for the year ending August 30, 1918, is given as 6.4; that is, about 6 1/2 deaths for every thousand men in the Army. The age-groups composing the Army are, of course, on the general average, between twenty and forty, inclusive. In the same Report it is admitted that the male civilian death rate for the same ages as in the Army (twenty to forty) was about 4.7, which is a difference of 1.7 or nearly 2 per 1000 in favor of the civil population or civilian males! This civil death rate is thus, actually, and relatively, much lower than the army death rate, and this fact is incredibly significant as positively indicating some serious cause at work to lower greatly the vitality and resistance and increase the death rate in the army! Now what is that cause?

The figures 6.4 per thousand for the Army and 4.7 per thousand for the civil population of the same ages is a great actual difference, but, of course, means, relatively, a much greater total difference against the Army because the army population is made up of "hand-picked" men selected for their nearly perfect health and physique and the absence of all serious constitutional diseases such as tuberculosis and others, which are all excluded from the army group. On the other hand, the civil population of the same age-group of twenty to forty includes the healthy and diseased, and particularly those afflicted with tuberculosis, which constitute a big fraction, and which disease is most prevalent and fatal in this very age-group of twenty to forty! Yet this civil population, containing all the diseased at the most fatal adult ages, has a much lower death rate than the "hand-picked" physically perfect army group! Now what is the cause of this much higher death rate in men of the most physically perfect class, and who are now treated with the best sanitary and hygienic living conditions, and where the death rate should be the lowest? What is the cause of this difference if it is not that extraordinary medical practice, or malpractice, which deliberately impregnates the bodies of these exceptionally healthy and "hand-picked" men with a whole series of the worst type of disease infections known that is, septicemic infections, like the typhoids and the variolas, etc.? And should anyone wonder, therefore, if the death lists of the army should show plainly in the blood poisoning diseases of pneumonia, meningitis, etc., which are known to follow frequently after vaccination? See pages 139 to 142 for a convincing proof of this point. Surely no person of ordinary sense or even an extreme vaccinator can presume to seriously tell us that impregnating the human body and blood with several disease cultures and infections is a purely healthy practice per se. And surely no person of ordinary sense can come to any other conclusion except this: that such operations must be dangerous and unhealthy per se.

In all this contention, Mr. President, there is, surely, something which is especially important, which should be most carefully considered and fully investigated by the Commander-in-Chief, by Congress and the Departments, at an early day.

1920's by the 1920s, health officials began to use newly developed marketing techniques to promote the importance of vaccination and encourage cooperation. Vaccination programs appealed to the emotions of parents to motivate them to comply. Fear and guilt were used to characterize parents who did not vaccinate as nonconformists and neglectful. Charged language emphasized, and often magnified, the risk of the illness to convince of the benefit of vaccines. These techniques were successful: During this period, roughly 80 percent of all students received all doses of recommended vaccines prior to school entry—an all-time high. (REF: CDC. Estimated Vaccination Coverage with Individual Vaccines and Selected Vaccination Series. US, National Immunization Survey, 2006).

1921 Franklin D. Roosevelt develops paralysis after swimming in Bay of Fundy, New Brunswick.

1928 The question of encephalitis following vaccination was investigated by the health organization of the League of Nations in 1928, and on August 27 that year, at Geneva, the League published a report on the situation. Says the report: "The post-vaccinal encephalitis with which we are dealing has become a problem of itself mainly in consequence of the events of the last few years in the Netherlands, England and Wales. In each of these countries, the cases which have occurred have been sufficiently numerous and similar to require them to be considered collectively. Their occurrence has led to the realization that a new, or at least previously unsuspected or unrecognized risk attaches to vaccination… the risk has, in the Netherlands, been considered of sufficient gravity to cause the temporary suspension of the administrative measures by which the vaccination of children has been secured, while in England the subject has already received the attention of two expert committees, appointed by the Ministry of Health."

1928 British Medical Journal, Page 74 Dr. RP Garrow: FATALITY RATE OF SMALL-POX IN THE VACCINATED AND

UNVACCINATED. "SIR,-It is an almost universal medical belief (and I share this belief) that the fatality rate among persons attacked by small-pox is much greater, age for age, among the unvaccinated than among the vaccinated. An interesting contradiction is furnished in the smallpox statistics of England and Wales for the four years 1923-26. The following table furnishes the numbers of cases of " small-pox " in vaccinated and unvaccinated persons over 15 years of age, together with the numbers of deaths and the fatality rate per cent for each of these years and for the whole period. ... It will be observed that in each year the fatality rate was greater among the vaccinated than among the unvaccinated. In a total for these years of 11,019 cases, 4,010 occurred among the vaccinated, -with 13 deaths-a fatality rate of 0.3 per cent,-and 6,915 -occurred among the unvaccinated with 4 deaths -a fatality rate of 0.06 per cent. That is to say, the fatality rate among vaccinated cases was just five times as great as among unvaccinated cases."

1928 Dr L. A. PARRY writes in the British Medical Journal 1/21/1928: "SIR,-The letter of Dr. Garrow raises a remarkably interesting question, one of many which have been vexing the minds of those who have watched events in connection with smallpox and vaccination in recent years. I, in common with all others of our profession, was educated medically in the orthodox fashion: small-pox was a disease which was contracted by unvaccinated persons and was with them a terrible amid fatal malady; in the rare event of a vaccinated person being attacked, the disease was a trifle and of no importance. Here are a few of the questions in connection with vaccination which are worrying me. Will any of our members who have studied the subject give me answers? (1) That raised by Dr. Garrow: How is it that small-pox is five times as likely to be fatal in the vaccinated as in the unvaccinated? (2) How is it that as the percentage of people vaccinated has steadily fallen (from about 85 in 1870 to about 40 in 1925) the number of people attacked with variola has declined pari passu and the case mortality percentage has progressively lessened? The years of least vaccination have been the years of least small-pox and of least mortality. (3) How is it that in some of our best vaccinated towns-for example, Bombay and Calcutta-small-pox is rife, whilst in some of our worst vaccinated towns, such as Leicester, it is almost unknown? (4) How is it that something like 80 per cent. of the cases admitted into the Metropolitan Asylums Board small-pox hospitals have been vaccinated, whilst only 20 per cent. have not been vaccinated? (5) How is it that in Germany, the best vaccinated country in the world, there are more deaths in proportion to the population than in England-for example, in 1919, 28 deaths in England, 707 in Germany; in 1920, 30 deaths in England, 354 in Germany. In Germany in 1919 there were 5,012 cases of small-pox with 707 deaths; in England in 1925 there were 5,363 cases of small-pox with 6 deaths. What is the explanation? (6) Is it possible to explain the lessened incidence and fatality of small-pox on the same grounds as the lessened incidence and fatality of other infectious fevers-namely, as due to improved hygiene and administrative control? These are just a few points in connection with the subject which are puzzling me, and to which I want answers. I am in doubt, and I want to know the truth.' Will some of the experts help me?"

1929 THE EFFECT OF EXTRACTS OF CERTAIN ORGANS FROM NORMAL AND IMMUNIZED ANIMALS ON THE INFECTING POWER OF VACCINE VIRUS. Laboratories of The Rockefeller Institute for Medical Research. J Exp Med 1931 Feb 28;53(3):387-98. doi: 10.1084/jem.53.3.387.

Experiments on the Nature of the Enhancement.—The enhancement is not species specific, as the tests show that rabbits injected with neurovirus plus rat or guinea pig testicle extract, prepared and used as the rabbit extract, exhibit typical enhanced lesions. All animals injected became sick and some died on about the 8th day, with the usual general signs especially in lung and kidney. The age of the animal from which the organs for the extracts are taken, as well as the age of the injected animal, has no influence on the phenomenon of enhancement. That, at least, the action of the extracts is directed toward the cell is shown by the occasional observation that some rabbits having pronounced lesions from pure neurovirus showed a typical vaccinal eruption in spots injected only with testicle extract.

Extracts of normal testicles from susceptible animals enhance to an extraordinary degree the infectivity of both the neuro and dermal strains of vaccine virus. The Noguchi virus is not affected by testicle extracts when injected into the skin, but kidney extract has a definite enhancing power on the strain when injected into either skin or testicle. The effect of tissue extracts seems to be on the cells of the host rather than on the virus. This is indicated by the fact that virus injected intravenously localizes most readily in an area of skin previously injected with testicle extract. Furthermore, an enhanced lesion results if the virus is injected into an area as long as 3 days after the area has been injected with testicle extract. The augmenting substance of the tissue extracts is little affected by high dilutions, passes through a Berkefeld V candle and is carried down with the proteins precipitated by weak acids. Rabbits with enhanced lesions show general symptoms and about 25 per cent die with generalized vaccinia. Kidney, and probably skin, brain and liver extracts possess enhancing properties, but to a much less degree than the testicle. On the other hand, spleen, blood and probably lymph nodes and bone marrow not only fail to produce enhancement, but actually restrain or even suppress entirely the vaccinal skin infection.

1929 Dr. Morris Kharasch, a chemist and University of Chicago researcher develops and files patent for the controversial mercury preservative used in vaccines known today as thimerosal. Then it was called Merthiolate.

1929 Eli Lilly & Company commercializes thimerosal as Merthiolate.

1931 Lubeck, Germany, 75 children died in from pediatrician's experiment with tuberculosis vaccine.

1931 The first North American electron microscope was constructed in 1938, at the University of Toronto, by Eli Franklin Burton and students Cecil Hall, James Hillier, and Albert Prebus. Siemens produced a transmission electron microscope (TEM) in 1939. Although current transmission electron microscopes are capable of two million-power magnification, as scientific instruments, they remain based upon Ruska's prototype.

1937 The official Journal of the American Medical Association on April 2, 1937: "A multiplicity of untoward sequelae have been observed in patients treated with immune serum. The common symptomatology includes fever, urticaria, erythema, oedema, lymphadenoma, arthralgia, smothering sensations, headache, nausea, and vomiting. Occasionally there are more serious and lasting manifestations such as peripheral neuritis, epididymitis and orchitis."

1937 The Philippines had the worst smallpox epidemic ever in the early 1900s after a vaccination rate of 95 percent. Physician William Howard Hay's address of June 25, 1937; The Congressional Record, June 25,1937.

WEST NILE VIRUS IS SAID TO ORIGINATE FROM A HEALTY BLACK WOMAN IN 1937 BEFORE ELECTRON MICROSCOPES COULD CONFIRM IT WAS A VIRUS

1937 West Nile virus is said to originate from a black woman from the south Nile river delta in 1937 (Smithburn KC, Hughes TP, Burke AW, Paul JH. A neurotropic virus isolated from the blood of a native of Uganda. Am J Trop Med Hyg; 20:471-92, 1940), before the days of sucrose density gradient centrifugation combined with EM in order to demonstrate viral particles. This would be the first of many viruses said to emerge from black persons...without any evidence...others would later include hepatitis B, "HIV," and even "HPV."

1938 the prestigious British medical journal Lancet publishes a piece arguing: "That diphtheria can be prevented by immunization no more implies a command to immunize people than the fact that nitric acid and glycerin make an explosive mixture implies a command to blow up our neighbors. Yet the immunization of the masses is undertaken with almost religious fervor. The enthusiast rarely stopped to wonder where it would all finish or whether the fulsome promises made to the public in the form of 'propaganda' would ever be honored. Those who have had to take detailed notice of immunization accidents of the past few years know that to get the truth of what really went wrong generally calls for the resources of something like a secret service. Immunization surely should remain a matter of private, not of public venture—a question for the individual to decide on personal grounds and in term of his own risks, fears and prejudices."

1939 THE TOBACCO MOZAIC VIRUS IS PHOTOGRAPHED WITH AN ELECTRON MICROSCOPE & PROOF OF THE EXISTENCE OF VIRUSES ARE MADE POSSIBLE FOR THE FIRST TIME. BY THE ULTRA-SHORT WAVELENGHS OF LIGHT THE ELECTRON BEAM GUN PRODUCES BELOW THE WAVELENGTHS OF VISIBLE LIGHT SEEN THROUGH THE BEST OPTICAL MICROSCOPES

1940's During the 1940's, advertisements appeared in American magazines showing cartoons of huge house-flies attacking babies as they slept in their cribs, as it was still thought in the 1940's that flies were still perhaps the most likely source of paralysis. DDT was then developed to spray everything, including the household kitchen and the food supply, when it was not yet appreciated that DDT and other pesticides such as arsenic used at the turn of the century in the orchards scattered throughout New England induced the same pathological damage to the same areas of nerve tissue that was and is characteristic of that now assumed to be infection-acquired paralysis from a virus.

1941 In the April, 1941, issue of the Naval Medical Bulletin, reporting on the results of tests on 20,000 recruits at the Naval Training Station at San Diego, California, between July, 1939, and January, 1941, Captain G. E. Thomas of the Medical Corps of the Navy tells the story. He describes an experiment on these men. "All had been checked by all known means and found free of syphilis and were then confined. These men were vaccinated against smallpox. Those who did not show 'successful' vaccination were re-vaccinated. The experiment showed that more of this developed syphilis from the smallpox vaccination than the percentage who developed syphilis from all causes in the civilian population in the United States."

1941 "On the eve of US entry into World War II, concern about a repeat of the 1918 influenza pandemic and its effect on armed forces led the US military to establish the Commission on Influenza (later combined with other commissions to become the present Armed Forces Epidemiological Board) and place high priority on developing a vaccine" (Woodward TE, editor. The histories of the commissions. Washington: Office of The Surgeon General; 1992). "Pandemic influenza did not materialize, but the vaccine did. The first successful large-scale influenza vaccine field trials were completed in 1943" (Francis T. Vaccination against influenza. In: World Health Organization. Influenza, a review of current research. Geneva: The Organization; 1954. p. 689–740). "In 1947, failure of the vaccine to provide protection against the epidemic influenza type A antigenic variant confirmed concerns of vaccine obsolescence and led to the term 'antigenic shift' " (von Magnus P. The influenza virus: its morphology, immunology, and kinetics of multiplication. Bull World Health Organ. 1953;8:647–60)"and designation of the 1947 FM1 strain by the Commission on Influenza as subgroup A on the basis of the hemagglutination inhibition (HI) test."

1942 A report of the US Secretary of War, Henry L. Simpson regarding the deaths from yellow fever shots stated that: "Recent Army experience with yellow fever vaccine resulted in 28,505 cases of hepatitis with 62 deaths."

1944 Pertussis vaccine recommended for universal use in infants.

1944 M. Meadow Bayly, M.R.C.S., British authority on immunology, and author of the book, The Schick Inoculation Against Diphtheria, writes in 1944:

"Perhaps the greatest evil of immunization lies in its diversion of public attention from true methods of disease prevention. It encourages public authorities to permit all kinds of sanitary defects and social problems to remain undressed, particularly in schools. It ignores the part played by food and sunlight and many other factors in the maintenance of health. It exaggerates the risk of diphtheria and works upon the fear of parents. The more it is supported by public authorities, the more will its dangers and disadvantages be concealed or denied. The pitfalls connected with a comparison of inoculated with uninoculated groups are well known to statisticians and have been emphasized in the medical press; the importance of seeing that the two groups are comparable in all other respects has been entirely ignored in the official statements issued. Our belief that we can attain prevention from diseases originating in filth by injecting toxic substances into the body, has made public authorities in many American cities callous to the demands for ordinances and regulations providing pure milk, ice cream, meat, and other foods."

1944 Albert Sabin reports that a major cause of sickness and death of American troops based in the Philippines was poliomyelitis. US military camps there were sprayed daily with DDT to kill mosquitoes. Neighboring Philippine settlements were not affected.

1944 NIH reports that DDT damages the same anterior horn cells that are damaged in infantile paralysis.

1946 Gebhaedt shows polio seasonality correlates with fruit harvest.

1947 MacCallum publishes research suggesting a virus is the causative agent for serum hepatitis (MacCallum, F.O., Homologous serum hepatitis. Lancet 2, 691, (1947).

1947 DPT (tri-valent diphtheria/pertussis/tetanus) recommended by the AAP (American Association of Pediatrics) for routine use.

1948 The Vaccination Inquirer reports that the English and Scottish Health Ministers acknowledged more than 25,000 cases of diphtheria in immunized children from 1941 to 1945, with nearly 200 deaths in immunized children. The clinical picture of diphtheria immunization is brought up-to-date by the Journal of the American Medical Association for June 5, 1948, in an article entitled, "Danger of Vaccination and Inoculation:"

If intradermal tests are used, one should be sure that the tests are preceded by a negative reaction to a scratch test in order to avoid generalized reactions, which may be serious and which may even, on rare occasions, result in the death of an overly sensitive child. Allergic children should be given prophylactic treatment for diphtheria, pertussis, and tetanus...Hypo-immunization against pertussis (whooping cough) is important because respiratory allergies are likely to develop in an allergic child. If whooping cough does develop, it should be combated with human immune globulin or hyper-immune human serum.

1948 Dalldorf and Sickles took excrement from a paralysis victim and prepared a 20% suspension with ether and centrifugation, then they injected it directly into the living brains of suckling mice that were 3-7 days old. They caused the mice to become paralyzed.

ONE PARTICLE FROM A TURD LAUNCHES THE POLIO ERA

1949 Enders of Harvard claims he can make this 'virus' from human embryonic cells, making it far easier to make a vaccine. Their conclusion was that this was the successful isolation of a virus that must be causing polio paralysis in humans. But all they proved was that a feces-derived suspension of human cellular material caused illness in lab animals when injected into their brains. They called this suspension 'poliovirus' and it was to become a 'vaccine seed' for modern polio vaccines. Enders received the 1954 Nobel Prize.

1949 Endocrinologist Dr Morton Biskind, a practitioner and medical researcher, found that DDT causes 'lesions in the spinal cord similar to human polio.'

1950 Dr. Joseph Stokes of the University of Pennsylvania infects 200 women prisoners with viral hepatitis.

1950 A small nanometer-sized ball-like particle, 24-30 nm in size, was isolated from human excrement, and made visible for the first time with an electron microscope. It was named the 'poliovirus.'

There was and still is no evidence that the ball-like particle causes paralysis.

1950 US Public Health Industrial Hygiene Medical Director, J.G. Townsend, notes the similarity between parathion poisoning and polio and believes that some polio might be caused by eating fruits or vegetables with parathion residues.

BETWEEN THE 1950's AND 1980'S, 12 MILLION VACCINES CAUSE YAWS, "HIV," SHISTOSOMIASIS, AND HEPATITIS C

Starting in the 1950s Africans experienced a massive increase in medical injections associated with mass injection campaigns targeted at yaws, with introduction and spread of parenteral therapies to treat other diseases, and with plummeting prices for antibiotics and injection equipment. For example, UNICEF administered 12 million injections for yaws in Central Africa alone during 1952-57. From the 1950s into the 1980s, unsafe injections may have contributed to the silent spread of HIV in Africa in much the same way that unsafe injections for schistosomiasis and other treatments in Egypt established hepatitis C as a major blood-borne pathogen, infecting about 15% to 20% of the general population at the end of the 1990s" (Editorial with Gisselquist, statistics quoted from: International Journal of STD & AIDS Royal Society of Medicine, October 2002 Africa HIV/AIDS through unsafe medical care. Also available: Africa Policy E-Journal. http://www.africaaction.org/docs02/hiv0210t.htm).

1950s –1972 Mentally disabled children at Willowbrook School (NY) were deliberately infected with hepatitis in an attempt to find a vaccine. Participation in the study was a condition for admission to the institution, typical of widespread experimentation on vulnerable populations by the vaccinologists.

1950 (September) Ralph R. Scobey, M.D., president of the Poliomyelitis Research Institute. Inc. Syracuse, New York (Archives of Pediatrics, Sept. 1950) lists 170 of polio-like symptoms and effects but with different names such as: epidemic cholera, cholera morbus, spinal meningitis, spinal apoplexy, inhibitory palsy, intermittent fever, famine fever, worm fever, bilious remittent fever, ergotism, and others.

There are also such common nutritional deficiency diseases as beriberi, scurvy, Asiatic plague, pellagra, prison edema, acidosis, and others. "No drugs, medicines or medical treatments have ever been able to cure any of these diseases and no germs have been isolated as the cause. But they all respond to fasting, cleansing, proper diet and improved circulation. The similarity of these diseases to polio is too obvious to go unnoticed. They are, in reality, all one disease with varying stages of intensity and different names.

It is ridiculous to assume that polio is caused by a virus and the rest of them are caused by nutritional deficiency. Inasmuch as nerve cells react in much the same way to various poisons, further research will probably show that in these cases polio micro-organisms are not always present, but intoxication (poisoning) may be produced through faulty metabolism or by the absorption of poisons from without" (Ralph Scobey, 1950).

THE DAYS OF INNOCENCE ARE OVER: HOW CERVICAL CANCER CELLS CHANGED THE WORLD AND HELPED WIN THE BIOLOGICAL ARMS RACE

1950's and early 60's During the 1950's, the third major push for a polio vaccine that might prevent rare childhood paralysis became coupled to the unsubstantiated belief that a virus also must be a cause of human cancers with renewed vigor after the Second World War. Oddly, some of the cells first used to try to grow the intestine-derived polio "agent" were cancerous cervical tissue cells, cells that became to be known as HeLa cells.

The idea also was advanced at about this time that suspected human cancer viruses also could be immunized against to rid cancer from the face of the world via vaccinations made against them.

This belief in the existence of human cancer viruses during

the 1950's polio era helped shape a campaign to launch a "War on Cancer" during the 1960's and 1970's. This initiative was begun by Mary Lasker, Mathilde Krim, and others. They had close personal connections to the most powerful political circles inside of Washington, and also to Hollywood and to the Hollywood stars. Mary Lasker was the wife of a prominent New York businessman who had died of cancer, Albert D. Lasker, while Mathilde Krim had married the director of Orion Pictures who also had developed countless connections in both Hollywood and in Washington D.C.

In 1956, the Albert and Mary Lasker Foundation, Inc., along with George Gund, the George Gund Foundation, and David M. Levy, funded the James Stevens Simmons Memorial Fund at the Harvard School of Public Health. (Gifts to Harvard, January 1 to March 31, 1956. Nathan March Pusey. ctr/50001545-1580.) Simmons was the Dean of the Harvard School of Public Health from 1946 to his death in 1954. From 1940 to 1946, he was a founder of "The Armed Forces Epidemiological Board," with then-Colonel Stanhope Bayne-Jones as his executive assistant. (The Genesis of the Board for the Investigation and Control of Influenza and Other Epidemic Diseases in the Military. US Army-History of the National Cancer Institute's Viruses and Cancer Programs / National Institutes of Health (pdf, 379pp).

Members of the NACC in 1958 were Lane Adams of the American Cancer Society; Dr. Murray M. Copeland; Dr. Charles A. Evans; Dr. Henry S. Kaplan; Mrs. Mary W. (Albert D.) Lasker; Dr. Robert A. Moore; Dr. Isidor S. Ravdin; Dr. Leo G. Rigler; Dr. Joseph F. Ross; Dr. Harold P. Rusch; Dr. Richard S. Schreiber; Dr. Howard E. Skipper; Dr. Warren Weaver; Mr. James E. Webb; and Dr. Sidney Weinhouse. Bayne-Jones was a member of the National Advisory Cancer Council from 1959 to 1961 and had maintained ties with his Yale "skull and cross-bones" connections thereafter for many years, such as some of the members of the President's Cancer Panel, 1976, and National Advisory Cancer Council, 1957-71 (J Natl Cancer Inst 1977 Aug;59 (2suppl):763), and The President's Cancer Panel (J. Natl. Cancer

Inst 1977 / tobacco document). Colonel Bayne-Jones was appointed to the Surgeon General's Advisory

Committee on Smoking and Health (US Department of Health, Education, and Welfare, Press Release, Nov. 11, 1962). Colonel Bayne-Jones acted as their quasi-chairman and was senior most member, and he'd been administrator as Yale medical school dean: he was 'the father figure' for the group" (Richard Kluger's notes for "Ashes to Ashes," interview of SGAC member Leonard M. Schuman, public health epidemiologist from University of Minnesota; July 15, 1988). Mary W. Lasker's friend Florence Mahoney had close ties to President Kennedy.

These people, and their connections and beliefs served to codify much of what has become the modern "science" and views of cancer viruses that still are prevalent today. Study of their initiatives and world views reveals that their sociological, militaristic, philanthropic, and cultural views were of influence equal to, and arguably far exceeding, any scientific hypotheses or theories about cancer biology, as will become clear by consideration of the following information.

"Scientifically," there was a strong influence from Dr. Mathilde Krim, who was not only instrumental in establishing a "war on cancer" but also among the first and most vocal to found AmFAR during the AIDS era (the American Foundation for AIDS research that was ideologically conceived of and begun under similar pretenses and fanfare as the launching of the War on Cancer, including the recruitment of Hollywood stars and producers). Along with Mary Lasker, Krim first convinced Lyndon Johnson of the importance of defeating the virus she believed might cause human cancers based on no evidence that one existed in the first place, as Rous recounted in his 1966 Nobel lecture. Early in Nixon's regime, Lasker and Krim finally triumphed and convinced the president, and other heads of State, to direct hundreds of millions of dollars of taxpayer money to rid the world of cancer. (It is interesting to note that AmFAR is similarly now directed by the shoe-salesman and fashion magnate, Richard Cole).

With her "Human Cancer Virus Program" now funded and erected to identify and contain the first imagined "human cancer virus" believed to transform normal cells into cancerous ones, and then to develop a vaccine against it, Krim and her cancer virus theorizing promised to make the world cancer free. Nixon's administration then erected the intensely funded Special Cancer Virus Program, along with its special buildings created to contain that cancer virus when, and if, it ever was found. It was a venture Christened by Nixon as an initiative similar to splitting the atom or putting men on the moon. These political maneuvers also helped launch a new biological arms race during The Cold War between the Soviet Union and the U.S. About the same time, the Soviets were given a small collection of what the Americans believed were animal tumor viruses during a visit by a Soviet-American scientific delegation, and thus the Soviets were thus made aware that the race was on to find "the first Human tumor virus" with all it could mean in terms of a biological arms race, or Sputnik-like competition.

1950 Dr. Morton Biskind presents evidence to the US Congress that pesticides were the major cause of polio epidemics. He is joined by Dr. Ralph Scobey who reported he found clear evidence of poisoning when analyzing chemical traces in the blood of polio victims.

1951 Scientists report they cannot find the designated polio virus in many polios (paralysis) victims.

1951 Dr. Morton Biskind treats his polio patients as poisoning victims, removing toxins from food and environment, especially DDT contaminated milk and butter. Dr. Biskind writes: "Although young animals are more susceptible to the effects of DDT than adults, so far as the available literature is concerned, it does not appear that the effects of such concentrations on infants and children have even been considered."

1951 Doctors report they are having success treating polio (paralysis) with anti-toxins used to treat poisoning, dimercaprol and ascorbic acid.

Dr. F. R. Klenner reported: "In the poliomyelitis epidemic in

North Carolina in 1948 60 cases of this disease came under our care… The treatment was massive doses of vitamin C every two to four hours. Children up to four years received vitamin C injection intramuscularly… All patients were clinically well after 72 hours."

1951 The man who became most responsible for the view that poliomyelitis was contagious was Dr. Simon Flexner, author of the famous (or infamous) Flexner Report, which led the way to the closing of the naturopathic and homeopathic colleges in the United States. Said Flexner: "It was not easy to establish in an individual case precisely how the disease was acquired; it was difficult to bring evidence that was not at all convincing that this disease was contagious." In discussing Flexner's report, L. Emmett Holt stated: "Even five years ago, if anyone had suggested that the disease under discussion was an infectious or contagious one, it would have been looked upon as a joke" (Scobey, Archives of Pediatrics, May 1951).

1952 Prof Konstantine Vinodouroff of the Institute of Neurology, Russian Academy of Medical Science, tells the Americans that Russia has never had an outbreak of polio. The Americans are amazed.

1952 George Bernard Shaw said, "During the last considerable epidemic at the turn of the century [1900], I was a member of the Health Committee of London Borough Council, and I learned how the credit of vaccination is kept statistically by diagnosing all the revaccinated cases [of smallpox] as pustular eczema, varioloid or what not—except smallpox." Further Extracts from His Writings, The Vaccination Inquirer, Sept. 1952.

1953 Dr. Kumm was appointed Director of Research of the National Foundation for Infantile Paralysis (NFIP). The NFIP was funded by its "March of Dimes" program, and it sponsored the hasty development of the Salk vaccine in the early 1950s, at the height of the DDT/polio controversy. Dr. Kumm also "served as a civilian consultant to the Surgeon General … directing field studies of the use of DDT…" (American Journal of Digestive Diseases, 20:330, 1953).

1953 Clothes are moth-proofed by washing them in EQ-53, a formula containing DDT.

1953 In a letter a Dr. Biskind wrote: It was known by 1945 that DDT was stored in the body fat of mammals and appears in their milk... yet far from admitting a causal relationship between DDT and polio that is so obvious, which in any other field of biology would be instantly accepted, virtually the entire apparatus of communication, lay and scientific alike, has been devoted to denying, concealing, suppressing, distorting and attempts to convert into its opposite this overwhelming evidence. Libel, slander, and economic boycott have not been overlooked in this campaign.

1954 Legislation recognizing the dangers of persistent pesticides is enacted, and a phase out of DDT in the US accelerates along with a shift of sales of DDT to third world countries. DDT is phased out at the same time as widespread polio vaccinations are about to begin.

1954 Dr. Jonas Salk developed the first commercial polio vaccine with a virus found **"in the pooled feces of three healthy children in Cleveland"** (not paralysis victims). The 'polio vaccine' was shortly thereafter administered to 400,000 US children. The official safety report stated that it protected '30-90 percent' of recipients. This was a vague statistic. However, manufacturers could make a 300% markup on the vaccine.

1955 The inactivated polio vaccine (IPV) is licensed but would be modified in 1987.

1955 On April 24, 1955, an infant with paralysis was admitted to Michael Reese Hospital in Chicago, Illinois. The patient had been inoculated in the buttock with Cutter 'polio' vaccine on April 16 and developed flaccid paralysis of both legs on April 24.

1955 (May) "With the announcement that Cutter was withdrawing its vaccine, there ensued a nationwide panic. The AMA put out the warning to all its members to stop using Cutter's 'polio' vaccine, although regrettably some doctors never received word. Many states and cities announced immediate cessation of mass immunizations, even though their vaccine had come from manufacturers other than Cutter. Local health departments began to track down every single dose of Cutter vaccine, which, it was soon discovered, had traversed the entire country.

Throughout May and June, cases of polio caused by Cutter's vaccine spread beyond the Far West and began to appear in every region of the country. The epicenter of the devastation was in California and the rural state of Idaho. Ninety-nine cases of polio would eventually be attributed to Cutter vaccine in California, with the incidence of polio among Cutter vaccinees exceeding the textbook definition of a wild polio epidemic by nearly threefold. In Idaho, with eighty-eight polio cases attributed to Cutter vaccine, the rate was fifteen times greater. Before it was over, the 'Cutter incident,' as it was euphemistically called in scientific circles, resulted in 260 people contracting polio and almost 200 cases of paralysis. Eleven people died. A devastating epidemic had been caused by two particularly bad batches of vaccine" (Many of the extracts have come from an excellent book: The Virus and The Vaccine-The True Story of a Cancer -Causing Monkey Virus-Contaminated Polio Vaccine, And the Millions of Americans Exposed, by Debbie Bookchin and Jim Schumacher, St. Martin's Press, 2004).

1955 President Dwight Eisenhower awarded Salk the Congressional Medal declaring the polio vaccine a great victory for American science.

1956 Dr. Albert Sabin tests experimental polio vaccine on 133 prisoners in Ohio.

1956 Health Authorities change the rules for defining polio. Doctors are instructed to diagnose polio only if the patient has paralytic symptoms for 60 days or more. Milder cases of polio are no longer reported.

1957 "Canada suspended its distribution of Salk's vaccine. By November, all European countries had suspended distribution plans, apart from Denmark. By January 1957, 17 US states had stopped distributing the vaccine. The same year The New York Times reported that nearly 50 per cent of cases of infantile paralysis in children between the ages of five and 14 had occurred after vaccination" (Bookchin and Schumacker, 2004: This book is among the most outstanding of its kind, and most of the preceding chapter 4 was derived directly from their work).

1957 Asian flu pandemic is claimed to kill 100,000 people, due **to the "H2N2 influenza virus."**

CDC CHANGES THE RULES FOR DEFINING POLIO AGAIN

1958 Cases of inflammation of the membrane that protects the brain and spinal neuron cells, causing muscular weakness and pain, but not paralysis, are no longer to be classified as polio. These cases must now be called "viral or aseptic meningitis." Non-paralytic cases were now to be re-named meningitis even if the poliovirus is present. The reported figures for polio were officially to exclude 'cases of aseptic meningitis due to poliovirus or other enteroviruses. "Reported cases of aseptic meningitis went from near zero to thousands, and polio cases dropped the same amount (following the introductions and widespread use of polio vaccines."

1958 Toward the end of the 1950s, after many discussions behind closed doors, vaccine officials alter the definition of polio again. After this period, all cases with classic polio paralytic symptoms are to be diagnosed initially as Acute Flaccid Paralysis (AFP). To determine if a person were infected, two stools are taken from the patient and sent to the CDC to see if they could find polio in the sample(s). If not, they were declared as not polio, even if the children have all the classic symptoms, which after many victims had been processed according to this protocol, the number of cases of polio rapid "declined," by changing the disease's definition. This "slight of the disease definition was a fraudulent way to make it appear as if polio vaccinations were working.

1958 Officials triumphantly declared large parts of the world polio free, even while the newly defined **Acute Flaccid Paralysis (AFP)** suddenly became common. Credit for this great victory over disease was given to Salk, Sabin and the vaccine manufactures.

1959-1968 Quadrigen that is in routine use is pulled off the market in 1968 for safety and efficacy reasons (DPT-IPV combo).

1961 The oral (live)virus Salk polio vaccine (OPV) is licensed.

1961 On February 25, The Journal of the American Medical

Association published that: "It is now generally recognized that much of the Salk vaccine used in the U.S. has been worthless." Live strains produced by Sabin and put in sugar cubes were adopted instead."

1961 "MERCK STOPPED SHIPPING PURIVAX (ITS 'PURIFIED' VERSION OF THE SALK VACCINE) AS SOON AS ITS OWN TESTS IN MAY 1961 CONFIRMED THAT THE VACCINE WAS CONTAMINATED WITH SV40... Its unilateral withdrawal of vaccine from the market had not been well received by the DBS (Division of Biological Standards). If Merck recalled vaccine, then everyone else would have to. That would have resulted in public panic and would have run counter to the Technical Committee's May 18 directive that polio vaccination 'continue to be pursued with vigor with the materials presently available."

"In June, after the Girardi cancer results had come in, Hilleman (Merck's science director) had tried one more time to get all vaccine production halted. That suggestion was rebuffed. Merck had already suspended production and was trying to figure out how to screen SV40 out of the vaccine when DBS tests on vaccine samples indicated that Parke-Davis supplies were also badly contaminated. Parke-Davis now also stopped vaccine manufacture. The truth was that by the time the Associated Press reported the 'news' in late July, both companies had not produced vaccine for several weeks. Parke Davis eventually resumed production, but Merck would soon decide that producing a polio vaccine that at times might be contaminated was not worth the risk." (Bookchin and Schumacker, 2004).

1961 In 1961, the Food and Drug Administration ordered all vaccine manufacturers to screen out the SV40. One study suggests that Lederle did not do so. Kops, S.P., "Oral polio vaccine and human cancer: a reassessment of SV40 as a contaminant based upon legal documents, Anticancer Res 2000 Nov-Dec; 20(6C): 4745-9.

1962 The Wistar human tissue study appeared in midsummer 1962, shortly before the human tissue study that Enders had completed at Hilleman's urging. Enders and his collaborator, another Harvard researcher, Harvey Shein, reached essentially the same conclusions as the Wistar group, with a different kind of tissue, human kidney cells. Koprowski had rushed the Wistar study into press hoping to scoop Enders and gain some publicity for Wistar. But in the end, despite being second, the Enders study attracted a good deal more attention because it was published in the prestigious Proceedings of the National Academy of Sciences. A lengthy New York Times story on August 10, 1962, reported the Enders study: 'A cancer-causing virus has for the first-time produced cancer like changes in human cells… Changes that the virus produced in cultures of human kidney cells included greatly accelerated growth patterns and chromosomal aberrations…'

By the fall of 1962, as news of the most recent SV40 research spread, the anxiety that had been growing in scientific circles about the simian virus reached its zenith. 'It was the worst thing in the world,' Hayflick recalls of the news. 'Please tell me: What else could we find worse in monkey kidney cells?' In Britain, Wellcome Laboratories decided to stop inactivated vaccine production and switch entirely to live polio vaccine production.

As in the United States, however, both the British and Canadian governments decided not to recall old stocks of Salk vaccine. Britain had a surplus of 6 million injections in 1961. In Sweden, the concern was about Sabin-type vaccine. There were plans to give monkey gamma globulin to four thousand children who had received oral vaccine in the belief that it would contain antibodies against any simian viruses, including SV40, which might have contaminated the oral doses. In the Soviet Union, site of the most extensive use of Sabin's vaccine, tests were conducted to determine the spread of SV40. Many of the technicians and scientists involved in Chumakov's massive vaccination trial proved to have been infected by the virus, and the Soviets were now fearful of SV40's possible long-term effects. Among American research and health officials, a joke with gallows-type humor began to make the rounds: The Soviets would lose the 1964 Olympics because their athletes would all have tumors thanks to SV40"(Bookchin and Schumacker, 2004).

1963 The measles vaccine was licensed.

1963 The use of coercion begins in force to compel parents to vaccinate their children became particularly prevalent. A 1963 publication by the federal Communicable Disease Center, the original name for the CDC, contended that "the use of the word epidemic itself in public statements is the most effective single means of simulating the public to action." That same year, the measles vaccine was approved for use in children. Shortly thereafter, a nationwide campaign to eradicate a national measles "epidemic" was spearheaded by the president of the Joseph P. Kennedy Foundation, Massachusetts Senator Ted Kennedy. To implement the vaccination strategy, a mixture of cooperative appeals and coercive school mandates were set in motion. REF: Achieving Public Response to Immunization Programs. (Referenced by Colgrove, pg 12).

1965 Baruch Blumberg working at the National Institutes of Health (NIH), discovered the Australia antigen (later known to be Hepatitis B surface antigen, or HBsAg) in the blood of healthy black Australian aboriginal people. (Alter HJ, Blumberg BS (1966). "Further studies on a "new" human isoprecipitin system (Australia antigen)". Blood 27 (3): 297–309).

1968 QUADRIGEN VACCINE (DPT-IPV COMBO) USED ROUTINELY PULLED OFF THE MARKET IN 1968 FOR SAFETY AND EFFICACY REASONS.

BIRDS START SWAPPING GENES WITH HUMANS AFTER ABOUT 100 MILLION YEARS

1968 Hong Kong flu pandemic is claimed to kill 700, 000 people, due to the "H3N2 virus". Both "H2N2" (1957 pandemic) and H3N2 are said to have likely arisen by exchange of genes between avian and human flu viruses, possibly following dual infection in humans.

1968 About half of the states had laws requiring vaccination for school attendance, but they were inconsistently enforced.

1969 Rubella vaccine is licensed.

1970 The HEW reported in 1970 that as much as 26 percent of children receiving rubella vaccination, in national testing programs, developed arthralgia or arthritis. Many had to seek medical attention, and some were hospitalized to test for rheumatic fever and rheumatoid arthritis. (Science, US, March 26, 1977.)

1970 Dane and others describe "virus-like particles" in serum of patients with Australia-Antigen-associated hepatitis. (Dane DS, Cameron CH, Briggs M (1970). "Virus-like particles in serum of patients with Australia-antigen-associated hepatitis". Lancet 1 (7649): 695–8. doi:10.1016/S0140-6736(70)90926-8 discovered the virus particle in 1970 by electron microscopy.

1972 U.S. ended routine use of smallpox vaccine.

1972 Jonas Salk, inventor of the IPV (inactivated polio vaccine), testified before a Senate subcommittee that nearly all polio outbreaks since 1961 were caused by the oral polio vaccine.

1974 NSSM [National Security Study Memorandum] 200 drafted by Henry Kissinger, was based on a classified memo sent by Kissinger to select cabinet officials of the Nixon Administration in 1974, titled: Implications of Worldwide Population Growth for US Security and Overseas Interests (THE KISSINGER REPORT)

Sterilization of men and women has received wide-spread acceptance in several areas when a simple, quick, and safe procedure is readily available. Female sterilization has been improved by technical advances with laparoscopes, culdoscopes, and greatly simplifies abdominal surgical techniques. Further improvements by the use of tubal clips, trans-cervical approaches, and simpler techniques can be developed. For men, several current techniques hold promise but require more refinement and evaluation. Approx. Increased Cost $6 million annually.

Injectable contraceptives for women which are effective for three months or more and are administered by pare-professionals undoubtedly will be a significant improvement. Currently available methods of this type are limited by their side effects and potential hazards. There are reasons to believe that these problems can be overcome with additional research. Approx. Increased Cost: $5 million annually

https://pdf.usaid.gov/pdf_docs/PCAAB500.pdf

THE ERA OF "HEPATITIS B, "AIDS," "SLOW" VIROLOGISTS, AND BELIEFS REGARDING BLACKS AS THE ORIGINS OF ALL PANDEMICS BEGINS WHILE DR. ROBERT GALLO THINKS VIRUSES CAUSE CANCERS AND NOT ATOMIC BOMBS

1975 Robert Gallo published a paper saying he had isolated a new human virus – human leukemia virus 23. "Gallo was jubilant, it was the justification for years of dedication. 'We got permanently growing cell lines eventually, and it was a great eureka. We succeeded ten times in ten different cell lines, and we thought we had made the discovery, the genuine article, that retroviruses exist in humans. A year or more of analysis went by. We thought it was a triumph." This period of research turned from being Gallo's greatest triumph to date into his greatest disaster. When other scientists looked at this virus, they discovered it was a mixture of three animal viruses: from a gibbon, a baboon and a woolly monkey." Virus Hunters by Jad Adams, 'AIDS; The HIV myth' Macmillan London UK, St. Martin's Press New York USA 1989, ISBN -333-48930-6

1976 Baruch Blumberg is credited with the discovery of the Au (Australia) antigen, HbsAg in the blood of a black Australian aboriginal, and was awarded the Nobel Prize that he shared with NIH's former Neurobiology Program director, D. Carlton Gajdusek—the discoverer of the so-called "slow virus" prion diseases, such as "kuru." According to most historical accounts, pediatrician and virologist Carlton Gajdusek became head of the laboratories for virological and neurological research at the NIH in 1958 and was inducted to the National Academy of Sciences in 1974 in the discipline of microbial biology. In the course of his research trips in the South Pacific, Gajdusek had brought 56 mostly male children back to live with him in the United States. As a strong proponent publicly of incest, Gajdusek was later accused by one of these boys he brought back, now an adult man, of molesting him as a child. Four of seven other boys now turned men recounted their relationships with Gadjusek on a 2009 BBC documentary as "the sex was untroubling" while for three of them they testified that "the sex was a shaming, abusive and a violation." Gajdusek was charged with child molestation in April 1996, based on incriminating entries in his personal diary and statements from a victim. He pleaded guilty in 1997 and, under a plea bargain, was sentenced to 12 months in jail. After his release in 1998, he was permitted to serve his five-year unsupervised probation in Europe, and never returned to the U.S.

Despite the subtle character defects of Blumberg, with his obsession with transfusions and the blood of black persons, or Gajdusek and his love for young boys and public advocacy of incest, the doctors were jointly given The Nobel Prize in Physiology or Medicine in 1976 "for their discoveries concerning new mechanisms for the origin and dissemination of infectious diseases," because the infectious agents and mechanisms of disease causation were believed not to conform to the standards of accepted pathogen isolation or of distinctive genetic (nucleic acid) identity in the case of both hepatitis B viral isolations or prions, or in the context of the timing of infection to demonstrable cell pathology or morbidity in the case of both prions and neurological syndromes, and hepatitis B in the context of liver cancer.

The classic proofs of pathogenicity worked out by Koch were thrown out the window. For instance, Blumberg in a Proceedings of the National Academy of Sciences (PNAS) paper he wrote admitted not ever being able to isolate viral particles at the ultrastructural level or even transmit the disease in an animal model, while D. Carlton Gajducek championed the idea that "infectious proteins" devoid of nucleic acids were at the basis of his slow, debilitating neurodegenerative disorders (e.g., kuru, CJD, Mad Cow, scrapie in sheep).

Importantly, both hepatocellular carcinoma and kuru-like

syndromes were first characterized by an imagined but scientifically unproven extremely long latency periods after initial "infection." In this regard, both liver cancers in the case of hepatitis B, or destruction of the brain tissue years or decades after "infection" with prion agents could "incubate" for as much as 30-40 years, before symptoms developed.

Although both the concepts of slow viruses, and pathogens devoid of nucleic acids were vigorously challenged and rejected by many in the scientific establishment during the 1980's because these fantasies challenged the established biochemical chain of events worked out for all other known and well characterized infectious agents, and because these syndromes were touted by different studies to be both infectious and (genetically) run in families, Stanley Pruisner (in the context of prions) believed Gajducek's hypotheses to be plausible anyway, and found that the hypothesized and molecularly unusual and difficult to detect disease-causing PRP protein was present in both diseased and healthy hamsters (for which another Nobel Prize was awarded to Pruisner).

1976 –STERILIZATION VACCINES TESTED ON HUMAN SUBJECTS CONTAINING HCG, THE HUMAN PREGNANCY HORMONE INCLUDED INSIDE OF A TETANUS TOXOID VACCINE USED TO INDUCE ANTI-HCG ANTIBODIES TO THWART PREGNANCY

Antibody response to Pr-beta-HCG-TT vaccine in human subjects Contraception 1976 Feb;13(2):237-43. doi: 10.1016/0010-7824(76)90037-8. G P Talwar, S K Dubey, M Salahuddin, C Das https://pubmed.ncbi.nlm.nih.gov/1245129/

Abstract

PIP: Antibody response to processed beta human chorionic gonadotropin tetanus toxoid vaccine (Pr-beta-HCG-TT) was investigated in 4 human subjects who were in reproductive age and of proven fertility and had undergone tubal ligations. The subjects responded by producing detectable anti-HCG antibodies after a lag period of 6-8 weeks and plateau levels at about 5 months after primary immunization with the vaccine. Anti-HCG antibody titers were still high in 3 subjects after nearly 11 months of immunization. The titers declined to near 0 after 16 months in 1 subject indicating the reversibility of antibody response with this vaccine. The antibodies reacted immunologically with the HCG molecule and were competent to neutralize the biological activity of HCG in the radioligand receptor assay.

1976 In a published report of the April 7, 1976, WHO meeting of international experts, the final paragraph urged extreme caution in developing live vaccines from a New Jersey strain, (H1N1) because of the possible danger of spread to susceptible human or animal hosts (World Health Organization. Influenza. Wkly Epidemiol Rec. 1976;51:123). That paragraph was written specifically to respond to reports that several investigators outside Western Europe had plans to develop and test such vaccines. One year later, an H1N1 virus, said to be identical to the laboratory strain from 1950–1951, swept the world.

1976 During the great swine flu hoax, President Ford is vaccinated before a TV audience of millions. More than 500 people receiving flu vaccinations become paralyzed with Guillain-Barre Syndrome who had been given a so-called swine flu vaccine that never was tested even in animals.

1979 A 16-minute segment of 60 minutes with Mike Wallace about the adverse effects and propaganda of the 1976 swine flu campaign is aired in which the then CDC Head, Dr. David Sencer, is interviewed (Dr. Sencer is now retired from working for a private industry job he obtained after being fired from the CDC: he can be heard defending his actions here

(http://www.cnn.com/2009/HEALTH/04/30/swine.flu.1976/index.html),

and he maintains as of April 2009 that he believed he "was doing the right thing" when he urged widespread vaccinations with an untested vaccine after an unconfirmed flu-like illness broke out among 5 soldiers at Fort Dix, New Jersey, after one of the 14 eventually diagnosed with the illness at the military base, a Private Lewis, died several days after he collapsed during a marching exercise. Sencer's program was suspended after at least 25-32 people died from vaccine reactions, while about 500 others later suffered from Guillain-Barre syndrome. In this 60 Minutes Mike Wallace interview, it is clearly presented that although the initial "swine flu" vaccine was tested, the X53-a vaccine given to more than 40 million Americans never was tested. In the 16 minute documentary, a GBS patient also is interviewed whose life was ruined by the shot, footage is presented regarding the 1 soldier, Private Lewis, who collapsed while marching and who was revived by his commanding officer without that officer contracting any flu, and the statement is made that no confirmed cases of a flu variant was reported anywhere in the world before the CDC and the Federal Government decided to launch its vaccine campaign on some 40 million American lab rat recipients using an untested vaccine.

1976 Bassili WR, Stewart GT. Published, "Epidemiological evaluation of immunization and other factors in the control of whooping-cough." Lancet 1976 Feb 28;1(7957):471-4: "The general incidence of whooping-cough is lower in fully immunized children, but present immunization schedules do not adequately protect the infant below 1 year of age either from contracting infection or from its complications. In a recent outbreak in Glasgow, nearly one-third of notified cases were fully immunized. In Glasgow and probably in the U.K. as a whole, the persistence of whooping-cough in some areas is more strongly correlated with adverse socio-economic conditions than with lack of immunization. The decline in recent years could be attributable to improvement in these conditions at least as much as to immunization. There is no epidemiological justification for continuing mass immunization, but there is a strong case for an intensified eradication policy which might include selective immunization in high-risk groups and areas.

1977 Vaccination against whooping-cough. Efficacy versus risks (The Lancet, vol. 1, January 29, pp. 234-7, 1977): "Calculations based on the mortality of whooping-cough before 1957 predict accurately the subsequent decline and the present low mortality... Incidence [is] unaffected either by small-scale vaccination beginning about 1948 or by nationwide vaccination beginning in 1957... **No protection is demonstrable in infants.**"

1978 Several scientific reports published in medical journals were linking the smallpox vaccine to a broad spectrum of increasingly common diseases and disorders. Autism, diabetes, neuromyelitis, other neurological diseases, tuberculosis, chromosome damage and sudden infant death were being associated with the smallpox vaccine. References to those reports, as published in leading primarily.

foreign medical journals between 1960 and 1978, are available at http://www.vaclib.org/basic/smallpoxindex.htm*.

1978 Experimental "hepatitis B" vaccine trials were conducted by the CDC, in New York, Los Angeles and San Francisco, and the ads for research subjects specifically asked for promiscuous homosexual men, while there is also evidence that the first "hepatitis B" vaccines were also tested on Blacks in Central Africa, and mentally retarded children. (Leonard G. Horowitz, "Hepatitis B Vaccine and the Origin of HIV/AIDS: Perspectives on a Possible Vaccine Induced Pandemic" Les Premieres Recontres Medicales, May 29, 2001).

Baruch Blumberg touts the Hepatitis B vaccine as the first anti-liver cancer vaccine.

1979 Bulletin No. 6, March 30, Wyeth DPT Vaccine Recall. "Between August 1978 and March 1979, 77 infants in Tennessee died suddenly from unexpected causes – compared with 74 during the same period in 1977-78. These deaths were diagnosed as sudden infant death syndrome, or crib death. Of these 77 infants, eight died within a week of being vaccinated against diphtheria, tetanus and pertussis (whooping cough) using the same lot of DTP vaccine."

1979 Dr. Robert S. Mendelsohn, who was the National Medical Director of the US federal government "Head Start Program" and a syndicated columnist who wrote "The People's Doctor," and the chairman of the Medical Licensure Committee for the State of

Illinois. He also held a position as an Associate Professor at The University of Illinois, Chicago, and Medical Director of Chicago's Michael Reese Hospital. Dr. Mendelsohn was once quoted as saying:

"My suspicion, which is shared by others in my profession, is that the nearly 10,000 SIDS deaths that occur in the United States each year are related to one or more of the vaccines that are routinely given children. The pertussis vaccine is the most likely villain, but it could also be one or more of the others" (See Mendelsohn's book: "Confessions of a medical heretic," Contemporary Books, 1997).

1979 A 16-minute segment of 60 minutes with Mike Wallace and Robert K. Ditchburn reviewed a paper from the British Medical Journal 1, 1601-1603, June 16, 1979 entitled: "Whooping Cough after stopping pertussis immunization;": "Summary and Conclusions. This study investigated "An epidemic of whooping cough [that] occurred in a rural practice in Shetland, containing 144 children under 16."

"The finding of that study was that "before July 1974, all children were immunized against pertussis, but after that date immunization was stopped. Of the 134 children studied, 93 had been immunized and sixty-five of the children developed whooping cough. The incidence of infections was similar in those who had and had not been immunized. The incidence was also similar in those born before and after July 1974. There was no evidence to support the routine use of pertussis immunization in rural Shetland."

1978-9 Robert C. Gallo claimed that he discovered the first tumor retrovirus because he discovered statistics which had claimed that 0.06 per cent (339 cases) of T-cell leukemia among 600,000 Japanese subjects who are antibody-positive for "HTLV-I" had been reported. It escaped his attention, however, that many of those 600, 000 individuals tested were living within 175 miles from Nagasiki.

"Gallo is credited with isolating and describing the first human retrovirus. Japanese and American researchers confirmed by analyzing the RNA of both isolates that the Japanese and American viruses were related strains of the same virus. They could never be exactly the same because of the mutations which occur as the virus replicates, but the RNA sequence was close enough in the two isolates." "Once the virus (REVERSE TRANSCRIPTASE AND ANTIBODY POSITIVE SERUM SAMPLES-no virus was identified) had been described, other laboratories looked for it (biochemically not with an electron microscope). "It" was found in black patients born in the US, Caribbean countries, or South America; Caribbean-born black people in England, Africans and Japanese. What could tie these disparate regions together mused Gallo." "The answer he came up with was the slave trade. Miyoshi in Japan found Japanese macaques had antibodies to HTLV-I and he suggested the monkeys had the disease first and infected people. Researchers at Gottingen, Germany, and in Gallo's lab found that many species of African monkeys had antibodies which reacted with HTLV-I. African green monkey and chimpanzee viruses were most closely related to the virus Gallo had found in leukemic cells." "Gallo suggested: 'HTLV-I originated in Africa where it infected many species of Old-World primates including human beings. It reached the Americas along with the slave trade.' Curiously, it may well have arrived in Japan the same way. In the sixteenth century Portuguese traders traveled to Japan and stayed specifically in the islands where HTLV-I is now endemic. Along with them they brought both African slaves and monkeys, as contemporary Japanese works of art show, and either one or the other may have carried the virus.'

"The discovery of HTLV-I infection on Hokkaido, one of the northern islands of Japan, immediately challenged this view of events but Gallo and his colleagues have remained attached to the monkey-virus (BLACK-SLAVE PERSON TRANSMITTED) theory."

"So, why is it thought that this virus causes the leukemia? 'First because of the coincidence between virus and leukemia – find one and you will find the other,' Gallo says." "The incidence of adult T-cell leukemia in Japan (175 miles from Nagasiki) is estimated to be only 0.06 per cent based on 339 cases of T-cell leukemia among 600,000 subjects who are antibody-positive for HTLV-I. Why is this?"

"Because of the latency period, responds Gallo. It will cause leukemia, **but it may take as long as forty years.**"

INTERPRETATION: Thus Gallo's believed, and the scientific world and U.S. Government accepted that Japanese art work evidence proved that black slaves caught a cancer virus ("HTLV-1") from monkeys on those lonely long ocean voyages during the slave trade, which caused Japanese living near Nagasaki to catch cancer centuries later after atomic bombs were dropped on their civilian populations to "save lives," and that it may take as long as 40 years for the so-called "retrovirus" to emerge from cells to causes cancer.

Other "top AIDS scientists," "experts," and medical journals even have advanced the idea that Africans must have smeared monkey blood on their loins to enhance their sexual experience, or engage in "dry sex," further promoting the racist theory of the origin of "HIV," having been transferred to blacks from non-human primates SOMEHOW, and that these Africans continue to even acquire new AIDS viruses from non-human "contacts" to this day:

"Sir: The isolation from monkeys of retroviruses closely related to HIV strongly suggests a simian origin for this virus... Several unlikely hypotheses have been put forward... In his book on the sexual life of people of the Great Lakes area of Africa Kashamura wrote: "pour stimulerintense, on leur inocule dans les cuisses, la region du pubis et le dos dusang preleve sur un singe, pour un homme, sur une guenon, pour ne femme" (to stimulate a man or a woman and induce them to intense sexual activity, monkey blood [for a man] or she-monkey blood [for a woman] was directly inoculated in the pubic area and also the thighs and back). These magic practices would therefore constitute an efficient experimental transmission model and could be responsible for the emergence of AIDS in man" (Noireau F. The Lancet, "HIV transmission from monkey to man").

1980 (December 20) O. Tonz and S. Bajc, "Convulsions or status epilepticus in 11 infP ants after pertussis vaccination" (Schweiz. Med. Wochenschr., vol. 110, no. 51, pp. 1965-71): In three of 11 cases, grand mal epilepsy persisted, and two children developed infantile epileptic encephalopathy (Lennox Syndrome). "The following conclusions are drawn from these observations: 1) In view of the usually benign course of whooping cough today, current vaccination is hardly satisfactory. Improvement of the available vaccines is an urgent necessity… 2) Parents should be better informed about the risks involved in pertussis vaccination. 3) Booster inoculations should be abandoned. 4) Health authorities should decide whether the current pertussis vaccination program should be abandoned. 5) Complications following vaccination should be registered…."

1980 Anti-Pregnancy Vaccine – Observations on the antigenicity and clinical effects of a candidate antipregnancy vaccine: beta-subunit of human chorionic gonadotropin linked to tetanus toxoid https://pubmed.ncbi.nlm.nih.gov/7418885/

Abstract

Observations on the antibody response and clinical effects of injection of purified beta-subunit of human chorionic gonadotropin covalently linked to tetanus toxoid were made in 15 healthy young women who had previously undergone tubal ligation. Antibodies detectable by radioimmunoassay were found in 14 of the women. Clinical surveillance and immunologic, hematologic, and biochemical tests indicated excellent local and systemic tolerance to the antigen. No significant adverse effects on menstrual function, endocrine status, or health were found.

PIP: A vaccine for pregnancy prevention made of purified beta-subunit of human chorionic gonadotropin (hCG) covalently linked to tetanus toxoid was tested in 15 healthy women who had previously undergone tubal ligation. The objectives of the trial described were to 1) evaluate the magnitude, constancy, and duration of the antibody response; 2) to determine whether immunization gave any evidence of toxicity or unwanted side reactions; 3) to determine whether the antibodies neutralized the biologic activity of hCG in vitro and in vivo test systems; and 4) to examine the cross-reactions between the antibodies and other glycoprotein hormones. This was a multicentered clinical trial with 1 clinic each in Sweden, Finland, Chile, and Brazil participating. 14 of 15 women had antibodies detectable by radioimmunoassay, the longest response lasting 400 days after injection. Duration of response to hCG antibody varied among participants. Clinical and immunological, hematological, and biochemical surveillance of the study participants lasted over 2 years, and during that time no significant signs of local or systemic intolerance to the vaccine were noted. Menstrual and endocrine changes were evaluated, and, aside from 1 case of 120-day amenorrhea post injection, menstrual and endocrine changes were judged insignificant or unrelated to the vaccine. Body weight increase was the single greatest complaint among the women involved, followed by breast and adnexal tenderness, and in a few cases colostrum development. In vitro, antisera were capable of neutralizing the activity of hCG in stimulating testosterone production in Leydig cell cultures.

1981 All 50 states had enacted legislation demanding measles vaccination as a prerequisite for enrolling in school. During that 13-year period, legislators characterized their sweeping changes regarding vaccination requirements as giving parents "helpful prompts to action." The belief by public health officials that parents needed a push toward social responsibility provided the justification for increasingly coercive measures to force vaccination. Since the 1980s, regulations for daycare and health care institutions and recommendations for colleges regarding "vaccine-preventable diseases" have been added. In fact, more than 200 vaccination laws, appropriations bills, and policies are considered during each state legislative session across the nation. Funding for vaccination programs is a substantial part of every state's annual budget. As the number of mandates increased, every state retained clauses within their statutes to exempt children from vaccination for medical reasons. Every state, except West Virginia and Mississippi, currently allows parents to refuse vaccinations if they have significant religious objections to the procedure.

THE PRE-AIDS RUMOR VIRUS ERA FORMALLY BEGINS

1981 June 5th. "Pneumocystis Pneumonia–Los Angeles," by Dr. Michael Gottlieb and colleagues of University of California at Los Angeles, appeared in Morbidity and Mortality Weekly Report (vol. 30, pp. 250-52), a Centers for Disease Control and Prevention (CDC) publication. This was the first article about AIDS in the medical literature. By the end of the year, Gottlieb and colleagues had published two reports (the first MMWR and the second in the NEJM) that detailed nine case studies, noting the commonalities among the cases, such as sexual preference and quick development of a rare form of pneumonia. All (100%) of the patients were claimed to be previously healthy individuals who had laboratory-confirmed cytomegalovirus (CMV) infection within five months of PCP diagnosis and candida mucosal infection, according to the report.

http://www.infectiousdiseasenews.com/200606/discovery.asp.

Because CMV is found in every "AIDS" patient, Gottlieb suggests it is the cause of the syndromes, despite the fact that his patients never came into contact with each other. Gottlieb is never given tenure at UCLA despite years of lecturing and work on discovering the "Gay Plague, and opportunistic infections that come to characterize the beginning of the AIDS era.

1981 Japan licenses "safer" DPT vaccine, the acellular DTaP. 1982 In 1982, Maryland health officials blamed a pertussis epidemic on parents' fears of the dangers of DPT vaccine; but when former top virologist for the U.S. Division of Biological Standards, Dr. J. Anthony Morris, analyzed the 41 cases, he confirmed only 5, and all had been vaccinated.

1983 to 1985 First Hib (Hemophilus influenza B) vaccine (taken off the market in 1985 for safety and efficacy reasons).

1983 "LAV" (Lymphadenopathy-Associated Virus" (A REVERSE TRANSCRIPTASE-POSITIVE SERUM SAMPLE USING GALLO'S APPROACH AND CHARACTERIZATION OF THE CANCER VIRUSES, "HTLV-I AND II") is "isolated" from a young male homosexual, with a previous history of two treatments for gonorrhea, one treatment the year before for syphilis, and antibodies against Herpes I and II, Epstein-Barr virus, and cytomegalovirus are reported to be present in this young man by Luc Montagnier's Pasteur group. The paper is rejected but shepherded through to publication the next year by Robert Gallo, to be awarded eventually with the Nobel Prize in 2008 for the first isolation of "The AIDS virus."

1984 (February) Severity of whooping cough in England before and after the decline in pertussis… (Archives of Disease in Childhood, vol. 59, no. 2, pp. 162-5): "Since the decline of pertussis immunization, hospital admission and death rates from whooping cough have fallen unexpectedly… The severity of attacks and the complication rates in children [who were] admitted to hospital were virtually unchanged.

1984 March 29 A letter by Gallo is written, dated one day before he submitted his papers to Science, in which Gallo states:

"It's extremely rare to find fresh cells [from AIDS patients] expressing the virus… cell culture seems to be necessary to induce virus," a statement which raises the possibility he was working with a laboratory artifact.

http://sciencefictions.net/pdfdoc/

1984 (March) Mathew Gonda, who heads the EM facility at the National Cancer Institute claims there is no "HTLV-I, HTLV-II, or HTLV-III in the Gallo lab's HTLV-IIIB isolate electron microscopy samples, and that only cellular garbage can be seen in the Papovic/Gallo samples. Because Gonda is the Head of the Electron Microscopy Lab at the NCI, the document is significant, because it was apparently sent to Gallo days before the Heckler-Gallo Press release several weeks before the Papovic/Gallo et al., publications would appear in Science, claiming that "HTLV-IIIB" was the cause of AIDS (later renamed "HIV" by a secret committee organized by former Nobelist and NIH head, Harold Varmus). Here it is shown in full, as provided by the investigative medical journalist, Janine Roberts: March 26, 1984 (Received March 27:

Letter_from_R_Gallo_to_J_Minowada_03.29.84.pdfPersonalCorrespondence. Mar 29, 1984

Dr. Mica Papovic Laboratory of Tumor Biology NIH Building 37,

Dear Mica
I am sending you 4 extra copies of results requested by Betsy Read. She said Dr. Gallo wanted these micrographs for publication because they contained HTLV particles. If this assumption is based on the cultures being antigen positive, I would like to point out that the "particles" in micro- graph 0905 are in debris of a degenerated cell. No other extracellular "virus-like particles" were observed free between cells anywhere in the pellet. The small extracellular vesicles in 0904 are at least 50% smaller than HTLV mature particles seen in type I, II, or III. Again, these vesicles can be found in any cell pellet. I do not believe any of the particles photographed are HTLV I, II, or III.
cc Robert Gallo
Betsy Reed
Best regards,
Mathew Gonda, PhD. **Head, Electron Microscopy Lab**

1984 (April) Announced in a media press release by Dr. Robert Gallo and Health and Human Services Secretary Margaret Heckler, "HIV" is named as "the probable cause of AIDS" and is thought to be "a variant of a known human cancer virus." Dr. Gallo rushes that same day to patent the first "HIV" test kit, and was subsequently brought up on charges of scientific misconduct by the Dingell Commission and the Office of Scientific Integrity of the NIH (John Crewdson: Gallo Case, Truth Termed A Casualty Report: Science Subverted in AIDS Dispute; Chicago Tribune (CT) – SUNDAY, January 1, 1992), for accusations that Gallo attempted to steal from Dr. Luc

Montagnier's group at the Pasteur their so-called "LAV-BRU-virus," which the Pasteur group had "isolated" the year before from a young male homosexual, with a previous history of treatment for gonorrhea, syphilis, Herpes I and II, and EBV. At the Gallo/Heckler "HIV causes AIDS" press release, an "HIV" vaccine is promised in 2 years by Secretary Heckler. Like "The Great Spanish Flu of 1918 (following the vaccination of the military), the so-called "HIV" virus is said to attack mostly people in the prime of their young lives.

1984 (April) Evidence is presented in 4 Science articles by Gallo's group that "HIV" causes AIDS. As reviewed by Michael Gieger, Executive Director of HEAL San Diego: "Robert Gallo's claim that HIV is the cause of AIDS was first put forward on the basis of four papers he published in Science, May 4 1984 issue. (Popovic M, Sarngadharan MG, Read E, et al. Detection, Isolation,and Continuous Production of Cytopathic Retroviruses (HTLV-III) from Patients with AIDS and Pre-AIDS. Science 1984;224:497-500.; Gallo RC, Salahuddin SZ, Popovic M, et al. Frequent Detection and Isolation of Cytopathic Retroviruses (HTLV-III) from Patients with AIDS and at Risk for AIDS. Science 1984;224:500-502; Schupbach J, Popovic M, Gilden RV, et al. Serological analysis of a Subgroup of Human T-Lymphotrophic Retroviruses (HTLV-III) Associated with AIDS. Science 1984;224:503-505; Sarngadharan MG, Popovic M,Bruch L, et al. Antibodies Reactive to Human T-Lymphotrophic Retroviruses (HTLV-III) in the Serum of Patients with AIDS. Science 1984:224:506-508)."

"The New York Times (Lawrence K. Altman) reported the news of the claim, but his article contained six or seven caveats to the effect that the claim might not bear out. Gallo's team were unable to demonstrate the presence of the virus in two thirds – 64 per cent – of the AIDS patients sampled. As noted in the article: As summarized in Table 1, we found HTLV-III in 18 of 21 samples from patients with pre-AIDS, from three of four clinically normal mothers of juvenile AIDS patients, 13 of 43 adult AIDS patients with Kaposi's sarcoma, and 10 of 21 adult AIDS patients with opportunistic infections." As analyzed by Michael Geiger, Board of Directors, Health Education Men's Liason, San Diego (HEAL): This result partly veiled the stark failure of the sampling to identify persuasively HIV as a cause of AIDS. For the sum total of AIDS patients with symptoms of AIDS – the groups in bold in the table above – was that in ONLY 26 (3 +13 +10) out of 72 (8 + 43 + 21) cases was the Gallo lab able to show HTLV-III virus detected and isolated. 26 of 72, or 36%, was insufficient to demonstrate that HIV was the plausible cause of the AIDS symptoms or their underlying immune deficiency. If anything, the testing demonstrated that HTL-III was certainly not a plausible cause of AIDS."

The heavily edited Gallo group papers claimed, however: These studies of HTLV-III isolates from patients with AIDS and pre-AIDS and from healthy individuals at risk for AIDS provide strong evidence of a causative involvement of the virus in AIDS. Thus, contrary to subsequent headlines the paper did not state firmly that HTLV-III (later renamed Human Immunodeficiency Virus) was the cause or even a "probable" cause of AIDS, only that there was evidence of a "causative involvement of the virus in AIDS.

In another paper of the four (Sarngadharan MG, Popovic M,Bruch L, et al. Antibodies Reactive to Human T-Lymphotrophic Retroviruses (HTLV-III) in the Serum of Patients with AIDS. Science 1984:224:506-508), however, the claim was bolder: The data presented here and in the accompanying reports suggest that HTLV-III is the primary cause of AIDS.

The low figure of only 36% of AIDS patients with symptoms that had HTLV-III virus present was excused in an accompanying news report in a Science Research News column by Jean Marx as possibly due to deterioration of the samples.

When the investigators calculated the percentage, they used the total of all the AIDS samples sent to them, even though some had deteriorated to the point where they were of questionable value for analysis.

The paper itself had noted: The incidence of virus isolated

reported here probably underestimates its true incidence since many tissue specimens were not received or handled under what we now recognize as ideal conditions. This is particularly so for the samples received from late-stage AIDS patients. That is to say, 26 of the 72 with AIDS tested positive for the virus, 22 of the 47 who did not have AIDS (asymptomatic or pre-AIDS (i.e., mild, and non-AIDS specific symptoms), suggesting that HTLV-III positivity was a poor guide as to who would develop AIDS symptoms. Later, this problem was solved by counting as AIDS only those who were HTLV-III positive.

The initial description and press release by Margaret Heckler of "HIV" as a known variant of a cancer virus in retrospect was perhaps unfortunate, because as stated by Gallo and Montagnier in a 2003 New England Journal of Medicine article (Gallo RC., Montagnier LM. The discovery of HIV as the cause of AIDS. NEJM Vol. 349:2283-2285, December 2003), the molecular (biochemical) profile that was associated with "HIV," was derived from the same techniques used to characterize the molecular signatures of Gallo's previous putative and doubtful "cancer viruses," "HTLV-I" and "HTLV-II" he envisioned jumping from monkeys to black slaves during the slave trade as was revealed to him in art works, and by using his strange, indirect, non-specific reverse transcriptase, or antibody detection methods, and of course, the detection of reverse transcriptase, later became known to be ubiquitous in nature and not specific to any viruses.

But at the press conference, the team formed by Gallo and the U.S. Government then claimed that "HTLV-III ("HIV") was distinctly different from Gallo's own leukemia-associated retroviral signatures of "HTLV-I" and "HTLV-II" in that it attacked and killed lymphocytes, rather than induced them to proliferate as would leukemic cells (if "HTLV-I or HTLV-II" actually caused leukemia, for which today as of 2012, there still is no evidence to support this claim).

The patent and intellectual property issues of the U.S. and French governments surrounding the creation of an "AIDS" blood test to protect the blood supply also proved to be an unfortunate series of confusing and hateful events that made possible accusations against the American-French collaboration that virtually insured suspicion of the "HIV=AIDS" hypothesis, and served, it could be argued, to derail progress toward defining AIDS and immune suppression. But because Robert Gallo became a shepherd and scientific peer review was avoided with respect to the 1983 Barre-Sinoussi/Montagnier et al. paper, and although it was claimed that there was an initial molecular concordance between the Montagnier's "LAV-BRU" isolate, and Gallo's "HTLV-IIIB isolate (later called "HIV"), nobody could "amplify Montagnier's "LAV-BRU isolate" (later called "HIV) or "grow" it on either sides of the Atlantic, and the Gallo group pooled their "isolate" from the sera of twenty persons said to have AIDS (naming it the "HTLV-IIIB isolate"), and they amplified the molecular signature thought to be associated with AIDS in cancer cells instead of normal lymphocytes, to avoid Montagnier's problem of not being able to "grow" (detect) the LAV-BRU" isolate in the cord sera of normal lymphocytes treated with "AIDS-patient" sera.

The "HTLV-IIIB" molecules discovered in this Gallo group "isolate" from what were then defined as 20 different ARC or AIDS patients, and despite "a laboratory accident" whereby it was claimed that a different contaminated isolate was sent from The Pasteur Institute to Bethesda which "infected" the cultures of the Gallo group, Robin Weiss's group in England, and at least several other laboratories, research in these labs was thus confounded for at least the next year (Robert Gallo, personal communication). And despite the fact that Gallo shepherded through the 1983 Barre-Sinnousi et al. paper the year before through to publication because it did not pass initial review, the patent on the blood test was filed by Dr. Gallo the day of the press release. This patent filing was from henceforward destined to be plagued by numerous accusations of stealing, deception, misconduct, and fraud. However, shepherding of papers occurs frequently among cooperating scientific groups, and as such, such papers are not rigorously "peer-reviewed."

The interests of the U.S. and French governments, and especially the Pasteur Institute regarding the patenting of an AIDS blood test, fear of contagion, religious views regarding morality, sex, and drugs, and politics began an era that perhaps should be characterized as the most politicized disease in history. And even though it was finally concluded that there was no misconduct or steeling of the "HTLV-IIIB" or LAV-BRU reverse-transcriptase positive "viral isolates" found in the Gallo/Papovic case, the numerous accusations, and the lengthy and costly investigations of misconduct and blame only served to polarize those involved and those critical of them, and the charges of wrongdoing only fueled bitter rivalry and criticism that has lasted for more than two decades.

Yet the ill-defined, and according to Gonda, non-existent viral particles, and the molecular markers in these samples that became known as "HIV" in isolates that Montagnier's and Gallo's group claimed to have tied to a clinical syndrome in "pre-AIDS" and AIDS patients and in one putative ARC patient as the Pasteur had intensively studied (Patient One), constituted a strong motive for many to pursue in depth, the nature and meaning of that molecular signatures of "HIV" in persons said to have immune suppression. Then, in November, of 1984, the Pasteur Institute investigators published "the genetic sequence" of "LAV," and because no two "HIV" samples have ever been the same, many scientists and doctors were critical of the strength of Montagnier's and Gallo's correlation between "HIV's" molecular markers and the disease syndromes to which these signatures were associated because of documents that became available during the numerous investigations. And when the papers were published for all to see, it turned out to be insufficient to demonstrate the claim. Gallo had found the virus in too few of the AIDS patients with actual AIDS symptoms.

1984 THE CENTERS FOR DISEASE CONTROL (CDC) REPORTED A MEASLES OUTBREAK IN A DOCUMENTED 100% VACCINATED POPULATION (MORBIDITY AND MORTALITY WEEKLY REPORT (MMRW) 33 (24), 6/22/84.Morbidity and Mortality Weekly Report (MMRW) 33 (24),6/22/84.

1985 Flossie Wong-Stall and Robert Gallo publish: "The association of Kaposi's sarcoma with AIDS deserves special mention.

This otherwise extremely rare malignancy occurs predominantly in a restricted group, that is, the homosexuals, and can occur in the absence of any T-cell defect in the patients." (Flosie Wong-Staal & Robert C. Gallo. Nature Vol 317, 3 Oct 1985). Kaposi's sarcoma as one of the first two AIDS-indicator diseases becomes no longer is an AIDS-indicator disease.

Note: In other words, Kaposi's sarcoma, as one of the first two types of AIDS-indicator illnesses occurred among homosexuals only, without any detectable defect in T-cell counts or physiology due to "HIV."

1985 Professor G. Stewart claims that: "There is no doubt in my mind that in the U.K. alone some hundreds, if not thousands, of well infants have suffered irreparable brain damage needlessly" (due to being vaccinated). Prof. G. Stewart, Dev. Biol. Stand. Vol. 61: pp 395-405. 1985.

1985 Vaccines required for school included polio, tetanus, and pertussis (DTP), as well as measles-mumps-rubella (MMR).

1985 (Development of Biological Standards, vol. 61, 1985, pp. 395-405):Whooping cough and pertussis vaccine: a comparison of risks and benefits in Britain the period 1968-83: "Since 1975, acceptance of pertussis vaccine has fallen from over 70% to 50% or less in most parts of Britain. This permits evaluation of a continuing natural experiment in which the frequency and severity of whooping cough can be compared [with] those of adverse events following injections of pertussis vaccine... There is a significant correlation between vaccine-acceptance and hospital admission by District of residence... It is concluded that, in children living in non-deprived circumstances in Britain, the risk of pertussis vaccine during the period 1970-83 exceeded those of whooping cough. In some deprived sectors, the risks from whooping cough might have been marginally higher but there was no evidence that this was associated with any increase in deaths or permanent disabilities."

1985 Vaccine Supply and Innovation: From the National Research Council; Institute of Medicine; Division of Health Promotion and Disease Prevention Identifying Individuals at High Risk of Adverse Effects

"The effort to prevent adverse reactions by identifying high-risk individuals before immunization also is complicated by the time element. For example, live viral vaccines are contraindicated in children with certain immunodeficiency syndromes, but these hereditary syndromes are rarely recognized before 2 months of age (unless a sibling has been affected), the time at which routine immunization usually begins.

Summary

Vaccines licensed in the United States provide excellent protection to society against their target diseases and are safe for an overwhelming proportion of recipients. They are not, however, universally effective, or completely safe. The judgment as to what is adequately safe is difficult, and decisions on the urgency with which improvement of vaccines needs to be pursued depends on the undesirability of the risks of vaccination in relation to the risks of disease, and on other health needs.

Adverse events following immunization are reported to the FDA by manufacturers, pharmacists, physicians, and the military, and to the CDC by the parents or guardians of children who receive federally funded vaccines. Although these reporting systems are useful, neither of them provides an adequate basis for estimation of the total number of events that occur, in part because reporting is voluntary. Even if reporting were mandatory, however, the data would not allow determination of the number of events actually caused by, rather than coincidental to, the administration of vaccines because information on similar events in unvaccinated individuals is not collected. Conclusions about cause and effect and rates of adverse reactions to vaccines should be drawn only from carefully designed, well-controlled epidemiological studies.

Responsibilities for identifying vaccine-associated risks, promoting awareness of contraindications to vaccination, and completing all of the steps required for vaccine improvement are now poorly defined and coordinated. Proposals outlined elsewhere in this report should ensure greater cooperation among the multiple public and private components of the vaccine innovation and immunization effort."

1986 US CONGRESS ACKNOWLEDGES VACCINE INJURY AND PASSES AND RONALD REAGAN SIGNS THE NATIONAL CHILDHOOD VACCINE INJURY COMPENSATION ACT- ELIMINATES TRADITIONAL PRODUCT LIABILITY FOR VACCINE INJURIES

which acknowledges vaccine injury as a regular occurrence that deserves federal taxpayer compensation and its own court outside of the normal judicial process. A tax is placed on every vaccine which is paid into a fund to pay out damages for physical injury from vaccination. Billions of dollars in lawsuits over vaccine injury are removed from the US court system into the special federal court where final court financial damages are capped at $250,000 per vaccine injury, including cases of severe brain damage. Over $4 billion dollars has been paid out by the National Vaccine Injury Court with taxpayers, instead of pharmaceutical companies, paying the bill.

1986 VAERS system begins (Vaccine Adverse Events Reporting System), that chronicles, and then provides today compensation for approximately 1 out of 3 cases of vaccine damage of individuals.

1986 Recombinant Hepatitis B vaccine licensed.

1986 – STERILIZATION ANTI-HCG VACCINE TESTED ON MONKEYS WITH SUCCESS. HCG IS THE PREGANCY HORMONE IN HUMANS AND SUCCESS IS ACHIEVED IN DEVELOPING AUTOIMMUNITY ANTIBODIES TO HCG HORMONE IN FEMALE MONKEYS

Enhancement of antigonadotropin response to the beta-subunit of ovine luteinizing hormone by carrier conjugation and combination with the beta-subunit of human chorionic gonadotropin by G P Talwar, O Singh, V Singh, D N Rao, N C Sharma, C Das, L V Rao Fertil Steril 1986 Jul;46(1):120-6. doi: 10.1016/s0015-0282(16)49469-0. https://pubmed.ncbi.nlm.nih.gov/2424791/

Abstract

Previous studies have demonstrated the control of fertility in monkeys on immunization with the beta subunit of ovine luteinizing hormone (beta-oLH) along with Freund's complete adjuvant (CFA). An eventual birth control vaccine would demand immunization without CFA. Beta-oLH linked to tetanus toxoid (TT) adsorbed on alum-induced antibody response in bonnet monkeys with detoxified sodium phthalyl derivative of Salmonella enteritidis lipopolysaccharide added only in the first injection. The antibodies reacted with both LH and human chorionic gonadotropin (hCG). A higher immune response was obtained with the use of a conjugate of beta-oLH and beta-hCG linked to a common carrier (TT) or with a mixture of beta-hCG/TT and beta-oLH/TT. In both cases, the antibodies were of high affinity with Ka ranging from 5 X 10(9) to 6 X 10(10) M-1. The antibodies were devoid of reactivity with human thyroid-stimulating hormone and human follicle-stimulating hormone. Monkeys with titers above 120 ng/ml hCG binding capacity (greater than 60 ng/ml in most cases) were protected from becoming pregnant during repeated mating with males of proven fertility in ovulatory cycles.

PIP: The potential for immunizing against gonadotropins without using Freund's complete adjuvant was explored in bonnet monkeys by using tetanus toxoid (TT) as carrier and Salmonella lipopolysaccharide (LPS) as adjuvant. Pure hCG beta subunit and or sheep LH beta subunit was coupled with TT by employing N-succinimidyl-pyridyl-dithio-propionate reagent. Fertile female bonnet monkeys were injected with 50 mcg gonadotropin equivalent monthly. 1 mg sodium phthalyl derivative of LPS was added to the 1st injection. Animals with low titers were also given a booster on Day 145 with Leiras adjuvant. 3 of 5 monkeys immunized with ovine beta-LH subunit bonded to TT had strong responses, and 2 produced high antibody titers after a booster with Leiras adjuvant. A 2nd group of 3 monkeys treated with both ovine beta LH and beta hCG conjugated to a common carrier, TT, showed high titers, between 750 and 1300 ng/ml, which were sustained for nearly a year.

Scathard analysis indicated that the combined antigens raised antibodies of high affinity, with Ka values ranging from 5 x 109 to 6 x 1010 per M. There were no cross reactions with either human FSH or TSH. 2 of the monkeys immunized against the combined antigens remained infertile for 6 and 3 cycles respectively, or until their antibody titers fell to 35 and 5 Monkeys in the 1st group also were infertile for several cycles before their antibody levels fell below 120 ng/ml against hCG.

1986 In 1986, 90% of 1,300 pertussis cases in Kansas were "adequately vaccinated." In Chicago, 72% of pertussis cases were up-to-date with their vaccinations. Neil Miller, Vaccines: Are They Safe and Effective? p. 33.

1987 Hib vaccine is licensed.

1987 DEVELOPMENT OF IMMUNOLOGICAL METHODS OF FERTILITY REGULATION

https://pubmed.ncbi.nlm.nih.gov/3124969/

Abstract: Birth control vaccines both would increase the choice of methods open to women and men and additionally would offer specific advantages, including the development of vaccines that are unlikely to disrupt the menstrual cycle or cause the side-effects associated with oral contraceptive (OC) use. For a birth control vaccine to be acceptable for use in human beings, it must meet several criteria: the antigen must be unique to the reproductive target; the antigen must have a fertility-related function that can be blocked by antibody or is susceptible to cell-mediated immunity, and alternatively, the function should be located on a cell that can be lysed by complement; an acceptable level of effectiveness should be achieved by no more than 1 or 2 injections for the primary immunization, with booster injections at intervals of no less than 6-12 months; and the vaccine must undergo sufficient testing in animals to ensure its safety for long-term use. For the vaccine to be widely acceptable, its effects need to be reversible. Before a fertility-regulating vaccine can be envisaged for widespread use in men or women, animal models must be found for thorough testing of toxicity, teratogenicity, effectiveness, duration, and reversibility of immunity and specificity for the target. Theoretically, the mammalian reproductive system is susceptible to immunological intervention at several points. Many reproductive hormones, as well as several antigens could be isolated from the ovum, sperm, embryonic tissue, and fetal tissue, could be candidate targets. Human chorionic gonadotropin (hCG) is a major candidate for vaccine development. The World Health Organization's (WHO) Special Program of Research, Development and Research Training in Human Reproduction, through its Task Force on Vaccines for Fertility Regulation, has been supporting research on a synthetic vaccine directed against the last 37 amino acids of the C-terminal end of the beta hCG molecule. A 2nd approach, being followed by the National Institute of Immunology, New Delhi, and the Population Council, New York, involves developing a vaccine against the entire beta chain of the hCG molecule. A prototype vaccine using the beta subunit of ovine luteinizing hormone emulsified with Freund's complete adjuvant has been studied extensively in female primates by the Population Council, but as yet there is no evidence of acute or chronic health hazards in this heterologous immunization model. The development of a vaccine based on sperm antigens will require considerable basic research. Interference with fertility could occur at several points: during sperm production in the testes, during sperm maturation in the epididymis, or during interaction with the egg in the female reproductive tract. Most research on ovum antigens is directed towards the zona pellucida, the acellular, gelatinous layer surrounding the ovum. It is estimated that vaccines that interfere with sperm function and fertility will be available for human testing by the early 1990s **(J. Spieler)**.

1987 Nobelist, Howard Temin who discovered reverse transcriptase (RT), and Nobelist and former NIH head Harold Varmus, claimed that reverse transcriptase "is a normal protein found in the uninfected cells of yeasts, insects and mammals, after the scientific community had accepted that reverse transcriptase was specific for retroviruses" (Varmus H. Reverse transcription Sci. Am. 257:48-54, 1987).

1987 National Academy of Sciences member Peter Duesberg publishes a monumental review article in the journal Cancer Research demonstrating that "HIV" is a harmless passenger virus that cannot possibly cause the symptoms attributed to AIDS (Peter H. Duesberg, "Retroviruses as Carcinogens and Pathogens: Expectations and Reality. Cancer Research 47, 1199-1220, March 1, 1987).

SMALLPOX VACCINE TRIGGERS AIDS?

1987 (May) London Times Edition Smallpox vaccine 'triggered Aids virus.' BY PEARCE WRIGHT, SCIENCE EDITOR

The Aids epidemic may have been triggered by the mass vaccination campaign which eradicated smallpox. The World Health Organization, which masterminded the 13-year campaign, is studying new scientific evidence suggesting that immunization with the smallpox vaccine Vaccinia awakened the unsuspected, dormant human immune-deficiency virus infection (HIV).Some experts fear that in obliterating one disease, another disease was transformed from a minor endemic illness of the Third World into the current pandemic. While doctors now accept that Vaccinia can activate other viruses, they are divided about whether it was the main catalyst to the Aids epidemic. But an adviser to WHO who disclosed the problem, told The Times: 'I thought it was just a coincidence until we studied the latest findings about the reactions which can be caused by Vaccinia. Now I believe the smallpox vaccine theory is the explanation to the explosion of Aids.' 'In obliterating one disease, another was transformed.'

Further evidence comes from the Walter Reed Army Medical Centre in Washington. While smallpox vaccine is no longer kept for public health purposes, new recruits to the American armed services are immunized as a precaution against possible biological warfare. Routine vaccination of a 19-year-old recruit was the trigger for stimulation of dormant HIV virus into Aids. This discovery of how people with subclinical HIV infection are at risk of rapid development of Aids as a vaccine-induced disease was made by a medical team working with Dr Robert Redfield at Walter Reed. The recruit who developed Aids after vaccination had been healthy throughout high school. He was given multiple immunizations, followed by his first smallpox vaccination. Two and a half weeks later he developed fever, headaches, neck stiffness and night sweats. Three weeks later he was admitted to Walter Reed suffering from meningitis and rapidly developed further symptoms of Aids and died after responding for a short time to treatment. There was no evidence that the recruit had been involved in any homosexual activity.

In describing their discovery in a paper published in the New England Journal of Medicine a fortnight ago, the Walter Reed team gave a warning against a plan to use modified versions of the smallpox vaccine to combat other diseases in developing countries. Other doctors who accept the connection between the anti-smallpox campaign and the Aids epidemic now see answers to questions which had baffled them.

How, for instance, the Aids organism (?), previously regarded by scientists as 'weak, slow and vulnerable,' began to behave like a type capable of creating a plague. Many experts are reluctant to support the theory publicly because they believe it would be interpreted unfairly as criticism of WHO. In addition, they are concerned about the impact on other public health campaigns with vaccines, such as against diphtheria and the continued use of Vaccinia in potential Aids research. The coincidence between the anti-smallpox campaign and the rise of Aids was discussed privately last year by experts at WHO.

The possibility was dismissed on grounds of unsatisfactory evidence. Advisors to the organization believed then that too much attention was being focused on Aids by the media. It is now felt that doubts would have risen sooner if public health authorities in Africa had more willingly reported infection statistics to WHO. Instead, some African countries continued to ignore the existence of Aids even after US doctors alerted the world when the infection spread to the United States.

However, as epidemiologists gleaned more information about Aids from reluctant Central African countries, clues began to emerge from the new findings when examined against the wealth of detail known about smallpox as recorded in the Final Report of the Global Commission for the Certification of Smallpox Eradication.

The smallpox vaccine theory would account for the position of each of the seven Central African states which top the league table of most-affected countries; why Brazil became the most afflicted Latin American country; and how Haiti became the route for the spread of Aids to the US. It also provides an explanation of how the infection was spread more evenly between males and females in Africa than in the West and why there is less sign of infection among five to 11-year-olds in Central Africa. Although no detailed figures are available, WHO information indicated that the Aids league table of Central Africa matches the concentration of vaccinations.

The greatest spread of HIV infection coincides with the most intense immunization programmes, with the number of people immunized being as follows: Zaire 36,878,000; Zambia 19,060,000; Tanzania 14,972,000; Uganda 11,616,000; Malawai 8,118,000; Ruanda 3,382,000 and Burundi 3,274,000. Brazil, the only South American country covered in the eradication campaign, has the highest incidence of Aids in that region. About 14,000 Haitians, on United Nations secondment to Central Africa, were covered in the campaign. They began to return home at a time when Haiti had become a popular playground for San Francisco homosexuals.

Dr Robert Gallo, who first identified the Aids virus in the US, told The Times: 'The link between the WHO programme and the epidemic in Africa is an interesting and important hypothesis.' I cannot say that it actually happened, but I have been saying for some years that the use of live vaccines such as that used for smallpox can activate a dormant infection such as HIV. 'No blame can be attached to WHO, but if the hypothesis is correct it is a tragic situation and a warning that we cannot ignore.' Aids was first officially reported from San Francisco in 1981 and it was about two years later before Central African states were implicated. It is now known that these states had become a reservoir of Aids as long ago as the later 1970s. Although detailed figures of Aids cases in Africa are difficult to collect, the more than two million carriers, and 50,000 deaths, estimated by the World Health Organization are concentrated in the Countries where the smallpox immunization programme was most intensive. The 13-year eradication campaign ended in 1980, with the saving of two million lives a year and 15 million infections. The global saving from eradication has been put at dollars 1,000 million a year. Charity and health workers are convinced that millions of new Aids cases are about to hit southern Africa. After a meeting of 50 experts near Geneva this month it was revealed that up to 75 million, one third of the population, could have the disease within the next five years. Some organizations which have extensively studied Africa, such as War on Want, believe that South Africa's black population, so far largely protected from the disease, could be most affected as migrant workers bring it into the country from the worst hit areas further north. The apartheid policy, they predict, will intensify its outbreak by confining the groups into comparatively small, highly populated towns where it will be almost impossible to contain its spread.

1988 In Clinical Investigative Medicine, (Vol. 11, no. 4, August 1988, pp. 304-9), it says that: 17 had been vaccinated for measles. All 17 experienced measles again, showing IgM antibodies indicating acute infection. A history of prior vaccination is not always associated with immunity nor with the presence of specific antibodies.

1988 A serological survey was performed on 573 subjects aged 3-80 years or older to evaluate presence of neutralizing antibodies for types 1,2,3 Sabin vaccines strains as well as a wild strain of poliovirus type 1 isolated in France (Virologie. 1988 Oct-Dec;39(4):241-5) reported that: "The results obtained indicate a satisfactory polio immunity level in all the 4 groups: seropositives, 96.7%-98.9% for type

2, 91.8%-98.2% for type 1 (Sabin vaccine strain), 89.3%-96.6% for type 3 and 84.2%-96.4% for type 1 wild strain. The highest immunity levels were found in group D (children with recorded history of complete polio vaccination) and in group A (unvaccinated people but contemporary with the past polio epidemics). A special comment is made with respect to 14 subjects showing satisfactory antibody titres for all the three types of Sabin-vaccine strains but who have proved to be seronegative (less than 4) for the wild type 1 poliovirus strain.

Translation: The best "neutralizing" antibody levels were found in groups A and D: the completely vaccinated (having had all their shots), and group D, the non-vaccinated who never received vaccine, but who were said to have lived during past polio epidemics-and who are said by doctors to have acquired polio naturally and overcome it naturally. Moral of the story: either get completely vaccinated, or do not bother, and you will end up in either group A or D with the highest neutralizing antibody levels.

1988 Birth Control Vaccines Baillieres Clin Immunol Allergy 1988 Oct;2(3):759-74.

The status and prospectus of developing birth control vaccines, that is vaccines against hormones, sperm or pre-embryonic structures that may confer temporary infertility, are reviewed. An acceptable vaccine must be directed against an antigen that is ephemeral, specific, and preferably protein, and the vaccine itself must be 90% effective, consistent, reversible, free of side effects, and preferably a single injection. Chorionic gonadotropins are the most successful antigens so far. Phase I clinical trials have been conducted in India and Scandinavia, sponsored by the Population Council, of anti-beta-hCG- tetanus toxoid, combined alpha-ovine-LH-beta-hCG bound to tetanus toxoid and cholera toxin chain B, and a combined ovine and human antigen in an alum and LPS adjuvant. Trials of a CTP-beta-hCG-diphtheria toxoid in Australia sponsored by WHO resulted in titers deemed high enough to neutralize functional hCG levels. Research on nonhormonal antigens currently involves several sperm antigens, trophoblast antigens, and most successful to date, zona pellucida antigens. A purified porcine sperm receptor has been used to produce antibodies effective against pregnancy in laboratory animals. Another aspect of research on antifertility vaccines is the search for the best vaccine delivery system, especially on formulations that permit stable vaccines with single injections. Best hopes focus on microsphere systems. Future research may look into possible T-cell-mediated responses.

1988 CRIB DEATH AND INFANTILE CONVULSIONS VIRTUALLY DISAPPEAR WHEN JAPAN MOVED THE VACCINATION AGE TO TWO YEARS OLD IN 1975

Cherry, et al., Pediatrics Supplement, p. 973, 1988.

When Japan moved the vaccination age to 2 years old in 1975, crib death and infantile convulsions virtually disappeared.

1988 Hib added to vaccine immunization schedule. 1988 Cherry, James D., MD, Brunell, Philip A. MD, Golden, Gerald A., MD, and Karzon, David T., MD. Report of the Task Force on Pertussis and Pertussis Immunization – 1988,."(Pediatrics, June 1988, Volume 81, Number 6, Part 2, Supplement, p. 955 "Reported cases and outbreaks in older children and young adults may reflect a less durable vaccine-induced protection than seen in natural disease. The duration of protection has varied in several studies, depending on the epidemiological setting, ie, prevalence of natural disease as well as the vaccine product used.

A study in Michigan showed an efficacy of 80% 3 years after the last dose, 50% between 4 and 7 years, and virtually none after 12 years. Breakthrough disease noted in this study was usually mild." 1988 Vaccine Injury Compensation Program Funded. 1988 JAMA publishes a report claiming that a case-control study has shown that 41 percent of meningitis occurred in children vaccinated against the disease." The vaccine's protective efficacy was minus 58 percent. This means that children are much more likely to get the disease if they are vaccinated. (JAMA, 1988, Osterholm et al., 260: 1423-1428.)

1988 Several other important events occurred in 1988. In January, The CDC updated the International Classification of Diseases codes for HIV infection for use with U.S. morbidity and mortality data, and in June, the brochure "Understanding AIDS," prepared by Surgeon General C. Everett Koop in collaboration with the CDC, was mailed to every household in the United States. In August, NIAID's AIDS Vaccine Evaluation Units initiated their first study of an experimental AIDS vaccine.

In September, NIDR investigators reported that saliva inhibits transmission of HIV, and in October, AIDS protestors, demanding a quicker approval process for drug treatments, shut down the FDA. In October, NIAID established three programs: The Centers for AIDS Research (CFARS) to improve the diagnosis, treatment, and prevention of AIDS; the Pediatric AIDS Clinical Trials Units (Pediatric ACTUs), a network of clinical sites to test experimental drugs on children; and the Programs for Excellence in Basic Research (PEBRA), to develop novel strategies to determine how HIV causes disease [From "In their own words).

1989-1990 Shyh-Ching Lo finds Mycoplasma incognitos in 22/34 AIDS patients and in non-AIDS patients. Mycoplasma are found by EM to be enriched in affected tissues.

The finding is ignored by Anthony Fauci-Czar AND Robert Gallo of the AIDS funding racket debacle.

AUTISM EXPLODES IN THE UNITED STATES

1989- 2003. The incidence of autism (and other related disorders) went from about 1 in 2,500 children to 1 in every 166. Up until about 1989 pre-school children got only 3 vaccines (polio, DPT, MMR). By 1999 the CDC recommended a total of 22 vaccines to be given before children reach the 1st grade, including Hepatitis B, which is given to newborns within the first 24 hours of birth. Many of these vaccines contained mercury. MMR is particularly worrisome, but health officials censor all concerns or criticisms even by well-known doctors and scientists, and congressional hearings. In the 1990s approximately 40 million children were injected with mercury-containing vaccines. The cumulative amount of the potent neurotoxin mercury being given to children in this number of vaccines in many cases would be an amount 187 times the EPA daily exposure limit. It becomes not OK for your fish to have some mercury in them, but OK to put it directly into your infant's bloodstream.

1989 In 1989, the country of Oman experienced a widespread polio outbreak six months after achieving a complete vaccination rate.

1990 Relevance of Immuno-Contraceptive Vaccines for Population Control.

I. Hormonal immunocontraception Arch Immunol Ther Exp (Warsz) 1990;38(1-2):47-60. https://pubmed.ncbi.nlm.nih.gov/2126920/

Abstract

Human chorionic gonadotropin—subunit beta (beta-hCG) has been so far most extensively studied antigen for immuno-contraceptive properties. Studies of vaccination of non-human primates has been so far controversially reported since some antisera obtained from baboons immunized with beta-hCG had shown cross-reactivity to other tissues. Despite these problems and concerns about the complete safety of this first-generation vaccine, a decision has been made to proceed with a limited clinical trial with this vaccine. Results from these trials are encouraging and indicate that contraceptive antibody titers can be achieved with permissible adjuvants. Neutralization of LH and/or FSH by circulating antibodies may impede their action and interfere with the maturation of gametes. Gonadotropin releasing hormone can be also a suitable target for immunological attack.

PIP: The human reproductive process entails numerous possible sites for immunological intervention aimed at controlling fertility. Currently under investigation are a vaccine based on gonadotropin releasing hormone (GnRH) interception, regulation of male fertility by immunointerception of follicle-stimulating hormone (FSH), vaccines based on the neutralization of human chorionic gonadotropin (hCG), and anti-hCG immunization. In Phase I clinical trials, passive transfer of anti-GnRH antibody has produced short-term infertility; long-term infertility has been achieved through active immunization against the decapeptide. In terms of FSH, the research has failed to demonstrate how long-term neutralization brings about male infertility. Before immunization against FSh is considered further as a means of immunocontraception, further studies are needed on the required levels of physiological FSH and testosterone for normal testicular functions to be maintained. 4 other Phase I clinical trials in this area involve vaccines based on the beta subunit of hCG or its fragment. Preliminary results from these trials suggest that contraceptive antibody titers can be obtained with permissible adjuvants, especially tetanus toxoid.

1990 Conjugate Hib vaccine licensed. 1990-1993 The National Vaccine Information Center (NVIC) operated by Dissatisfied Parents Together (DPT) says that a new Institute of Medicine (IOM) reports an association between DPT vaccine and permanent brain damage: "confirms that the vaccine can cause children to suffer acute brain inflammation which sometimes leads to death or permanent neurological damage. The parent consumer activist group also charges that they have obtained evidence through the Freedom of Information Act that the Department of Health and Human Services (DHHS) is failing to properly monitor reports of death and injuries following vaccination and that doctors around the country are failing to report deaths and injuries which occur after vaccination to DHHS." "In a year-long investigation of the Vaccine Adverse Reaction Reporting System (VAERS) operated by the Food and Drug Administration, NVIC/DPT analyzed VAERS computer discs used by the FDA to store data on reports of deaths and injuries following DPT vaccination. A total of 54,072 reports of adverse events following vaccination were listed in a 39-month period from July 1990 to November 1993, with 12,504 reports being associated with DPT vaccine, including 471 deaths." "A wide variation in the numbers of reports associated with different lots of DPT vaccine were discovered, with some lots listing many more deaths and injuries than others. In one DPT vaccine lot, there were 129 adverse events and 9 deaths reported between September 1992 and September 1993. Most adverse events occurred within a few days of vaccination and many reports also contained descriptions of classic pertussis vaccine reaction symptoms. This particular lot met the FDA's criteria for triggering an "investigation" (ie., report of one death or two serious injuries within a seven-day period) 11 times within a 12-month period." "There are some lots of vaccine which are associated with many more deaths and injuries than other lots. These lots are often referred to as 'hot lots.' Even though the FDA's criteria for an investigation was triggered 11 times within a 12-month period on just one of the many lots we looked at, we know for a fact the lot was never recalled. The FDA has not recalled a suspicious lot of DPT vaccine because of high numbers of deaths and injuries associated with it for at least 15 years," said Kathi Williams, NVIC/DPT co-founder and Acting Director. "That is because the position of those who operate VAERS is that the DPT vaccine does not cause death or injury. So, the death and injury reports are ignored. It is a shocking example of how little we know about the true extent of vaccine-associated injuries and deaths.

1990 THE FDA GRANTS DEPARTMENT OF DEFENSE WAIVER OF NUREMBERG CODE FOR USE OF UNAPPROVED DRUGS AND VACCINES IN DESERT SHIELD AND HEPATITIS B VACCINE IS RECOMMENDED FOR ALL NEWBORN INFANTS AND CHILDREN: PREDICTIONS OF VACCINE-INDUCED DISEASES AND SYNDROMES ARE REALIZED

1991 The WHO Task Force on Vaccines for Fertility Regulation. Its formation, objectives, and research activities

Hum Reprod 1991 Jan;6(1):166-72. doi: 10.1093/oxfordjournals.humrep.a137252.

https://pubmed.ncbi.nlm.nih.gov/1874951/

Abstract

Over the past 18 years, the WHO Task Force on Vaccines for Fertility Regulation has been supporting basic and clinical research on the development of birth control vaccines directed against the gametes or the preimplantation embryo. These studies have involved the use of advanced procedures in peptide chemistry, hybridoma technology and molecular genetics as well as the evaluation of a number of novel approaches in general vaccinology. As a result of this international, collaborative effort, a prototype anti-HCG vaccine is now undergoing clinical testing, raising the prospect that a totally new family planning method may be available before the end of the current decade.

PIP: The WHO Task Force on Vaccines for Fertility Regulation is one of several Task Forces, consisting of international, multidisciplinary groups of scientists and clinicians collaborating in research on specific goals, established in 1972. Its accomplishments are reviewed here. The Task Force convened a meeting in 1974 to select criteria for tissues and molecules capable of mounting antifertility responses. These molecules had to be restricted to the target tissue, sequestered in the reproductive tract, present transiently, and chemically characterized. Some of the antigens considered were sperm enzymes and membranes, as well as a data bank of sera naturally immunized against sperm. Other were anti-ovum and placenta molecules such as zona pellucida, the SP-1 placental antigen, and the placental hormones chorionic somatotrophin and human chorionic gonadotropin (hCG). Trophoblast-derived monoclonal antibodies and gene libraries are being screened. Anti-hCG is the vaccine composed of a portion of the beta subunit complexed to a carrier antigen, diphtheria toxoid, in a water- oil emulsion with an adjuvant has been tested in a phase I clinical trial in 1986-1988. A Phase II trial is being planned to see if the immune response in women is large enough to be capable of preventing pregnancy. Further improvements in the vaccine are being envisioned, such as incorporation of the peptide carrier conjugate and immune stimulant into biodegradable microspheres, hopefully to produce a longer-lasting immunity and a more stable vaccine. While the WHO Task Force on Vaccines for Fertility Regulation has been forced to cut back on some avenues of research, its success has stimulated other centers to take up several important projects, e.g., the sperm LDH and zona pellucida vaccines.

1991 Recombinant Hepatitis B recommended for all newborn infants and children. In 1991 there were 210 REPORTED cases of hepatitis B vaccine injury from 1991 – 1998 in Illinois, and 5 deaths. The hepatitis B vaccine is arguably perhaps one of the single largest disasters in the history of vaccination terrorism and insanity. Hepatitis B is typically found in IV drug addicts, and a few other sub-populations. How it became a mandated infant vaccine defies all comprehension and the story of this tragedy deserves some pause and careful recounting.

Other FDA licensed vaccines have been FDA approved and extensively used before they even had been tested in animals, because there never has been, nor is there currently an animal model for such diseases as "hepatitis B" in the first place as reported in characteristically dense scientific language or stated indirectly as in this Science article published in 1999, and in a Gastroenterology, article published in 1990:

"Viral clearance without destruction of infected cells during acute HBV infection." Science Apr 30;284(5415):825-9, 1999):

"Viral clearance during hepatitis B virus (HBV) infection has been thought to reflect the destruction of infected hepatocytes by CD8(+) T lymphocytes. However, in this study, HBV DNA was shown to largely disappear from the liver and the blood of acutely infected chimpanzees long before the peak of T cell infiltration and most of the liver disease.These results demonstrate that noncytopathic antiviral mechanisms (i.e. viral mechanisms that do no harm to cells) contribute to viral clearance during acute viral hepatitis by purging HBV replicative intermediates from the cytoplasm and covalently closed circular viral DNA from the nucleus of infected cells."

In other words, there is no liver destruction observable even after exposure to hepatitis B in chimps.

From (Yamamura et al., HBV production in transgenic mice. From: Gastroenterol. 1990 Sep;25 Suppl 2:49-53):

The founder mouse is now 19 months of age but shows no clinical or pathological change, suggesting that HBV itself is not cytopathic.

But these published facts, even though accepted in the world's and medical profession's most prominent journals, the carnage of the hepatitis B vaccine proceeded with renewed vigor during the 1990's, nor did these and many other disturbing facts stop the FDA from licensing vaccines and imposing universal forced hepatitis B vaccines on infants hardly several hours old, or for day care and school-entering populations, and indeed, in 48 states and numerous foreign countries.

BLUMBERG'S FRANKENSTEIN AND-THE HOMICIDE OF HEPATITIS B VACCINE

The earliest record of an epidemic caused by hepatitis B virus was made by Lurman in 1885. An outbreak of smallpox occurred in Bremen in 1883 and 1,289 shipyard employees were vaccinated with lymph from other people. After several weeks, and up to eight months later, 191 of the vaccinated workers became ill with jaundice and were diagnosed as suffering from serum hepatitis. Other employees who had been inoculated with different batches of lymph remained healthy. Lurman's paper, now regarded as a classical example of an epidemiological study, proved that contaminated lymph was the source of the outbreak (from Wikipedia). (Lurman A. (1885) Eine icterus epidemic. (In German). Berl Klin Woschenschr 22:20–3).

From the 1950s –1972: Mentally disabled children at Willowbrook School (NY) were deliberately infected with hepatitis in an attempt to find a vaccine by one of Baruck Blumberg's collaborators, Klugman. Participation in the study was a condition for admission to the institution.

In 1965, Baruch Blumberg working at the National Institutes of Health (NIH), thought he discovered the "Australia antigen" (later known to be Hepatitis B surface antigen, or HbsAg), and he found it of course (could not you guess) in the blood of healthy black Australian aboriginal man's blood he kept in his refrigerator. (Alter HJ, Blumberg BS (1966). "Further studies on a "new" human isoprecipitin system (Australia antigen)". Blood27 (3): 297–309).

In 1976, Baruch Blumberg was then credited with the discovery of the Au antigen, HbsAg in the blood of a black Australian aboriginal, and was awarded the Nobel Prize that he shared with NIH's former Neurobiology Program director, D. Carlton Gajducek—the discoverer of the so-called "slow virus" prion diseases and convicted child rapist. The doctors were jointly given The Nobel Prize in Physiology or Medicine in 1976 "for their discoveries concerning new mechanisms for the origin and dissemination of infectious diseases," because the infectious agents and mechanisms of disease causation were believed not to conform to the standards of accepted pathogen isolation, the idea of distinctive genetic (nucleic acid) identity in the case of prions, the timing of infection to demonstrable cell pathology or morbidity in the case of prions and hepatitis B in the context of cancer, or to the classic proofs of pathogenicity worked out by Koch. For instance, D. Carlton Gajducek championed the idea that "infectious proteins" devoid of nucleic acids were at the basis of slow, debilitating neurodegenerative disorders (e.g., kuru, CJD, Mad Cow, scrapie in sheep)—syndromes that are characterized by extremely long latency periods after initial "infection," and destruction of the brain tissue years or decades after "infection." In 1905, the U.S. Supreme Court upheld state laws mandating smallpox vaccinations and in 1906 to 1928 the vaccines against pertussis. Records show that in 1907, the neurotoxin calcium arsenate came into use primarily on cotton crops, and in 1908 in a Massachusetts town with three cotton mills and apple orchards, 69 children suddenly fell ill with infantile paralysis. And in 1909, the UK banned apple imports from the States because of the heavy lead arsenate residues.

The effects on cattle and sheep on the "slow viruses" in absurdities such as the Mad Cow Diseases of Gajducek has been now attributed to toxins by British farmers like Mark Purdy.

Although the concept of slow viruses, and pathogens devoid of nucleic acids were vigorously challenged and rejected by many in the scientific establishment during the 1980's because the idea challenged the established biochemical chain of events worked out for all other infectious agents, and because these syndromes appeared to be both infectious and run in families, Stanley Pruisner believed Gajducek's hypotheses to be plausible, and found that the hypothesized disease-causing PRP protein was present in both diseased and healthy hamsters (for which another Nobel Prize was awarded to him). A similar sequence of events unfolded in the quest to isolate the hepatitis B "virus." A few examples may be helpful:

According to some reports, in 1970, Dane and others describe "virus-like particles" in serum of patients with Australia-Antigen-associated hepatitis. (Dane DS, Cameron CH, Briggs M (1970). "Virus-like particles in serum of patients with Australia-antigen-associated hepatitis". Lancet1 (7649): 695–8.doi:10.1016/S0140-6736(70)90926-8discovered the virus particle in 1970 by electron microscopy.

Yet according to the Nobelist, and so-called discoverer of hepatitis B, Baruch Blumberg himself, there was considerable difficulty in linking any nucleic acid-containing viral particle to the syndrome of hepatitis B, which spontaneously resolves without any medication or vaccine in more than 95% of those who acquire the syndrome:

"Hepatitis B virus" is now thought to be transmitted primarily through sex, dirty needles and perinatal transmission, or transfusions, and it is present in the blood of black men who are Australian aborigines, and occasionally, Micronesians, Vietnamese, Taiwanese, and with higher frequency, patients with leukemia or Down syndrome, who either all share these risks or risk behaviors, or as could be argued convincingly, are detected in these groups because it is a rare genetic polymorphism that can be induced in hepatitis patients because of tissue destruction, and perhaps, from many other causes. The HPsAG antigen represents a simple and relatively rare (in the West-not so rare in Asia or Australia or Africa) blood polymorphism because most people (>95%) who harbor the HBsAG molecular signature never become sick, develop hepatitis, or cancer of any kind. Moreover, the hepatitis B era constituted the basis or foundation upon which "molecular recombinant vaccines," as well as many of the mistaken theories of the AIDS era were based upon.

1991 (June) Nature publishes claim that fish farming causes influenza pandemics 351, 527 (13 Jun 1991) doi:10.1038/351527a0.

1992 (February 28) "The epidemiology of pertussis in the Republic of Ireland" (Communicable Disease Report[:] CDR Review, vol. 2, no. 3, pp. R31-3): Following adverse publicity in 1973, uptake of the vaccine fell to 30% in 1976. In recent years, it has leveled out at only 40-45%. Yet when large epidemics of pertussis occurred in 1985 and 1989, mortality from pertussis fell to almost negligible levels.

1992 BIRTH CONTROL VACCINES: THE "PROGRESS" CONTINUES

From Prog Hum Reprod Res https://pubmed.ncbi.nlm.nih.gov/12286012/

Abstract:

During 1986-1988, the WHO Special Programme of Research, Development and Research Training in Human Reproduction used the diphtheria toxoid as a carrier for a fragment of the human chorionic gonadotropin (hCG) molecule (a conjugate immunogen) and an immunostimulant in a phase I clinical trial of this prototype antifertility vaccine in sterilized women.

Between 1990 and 1991, it conducted teratology studies in rats and rabbits to determine whether the vaccine causes fetal abnormalities. The vaccine did not adversely affect either the animals or their fetuses. Clinical trials of the vaccine's effectiveness (phase II trials) are scheduled for 1992. At least 2 injections several weeks apart, are needed to produce an anti-hCG immune response which is only effective for 3-6 months, however. So, the same components of the original vaccine were placed in a polymer to deliver the vaccine slowly over a prolonged and predetermined time frame. WHO hoped that this advanced vaccine would raise effective immunity levels long enough to last for at least 1 year after 1 injection? WHO is conducting dose-response and toxicity studies of this prototype vaccine in rabbits and baboons to identify the optimal dose which would elicit an effective immunity level over a desired period of time and would be safe for testing in humans? WHO hopes to begin a phase I clinical trial with this advanced anti-hCG vaccine in late 1992? WHO anticipates that the preclinical and clinical trials will reveal a need for further modifications and improvements? WHO is supported multicenter research on antitrophoblast vaccines which target membrane cells of the preimplantation embryo since 1985? It uses monoclonal antibodies (MABs) and recombinant DNA technology to identify and isolate surface molecules. So far, this research has tested 15,000 MABs but is centering on 9 MAbs. A study in baboons showed that 1 MAB reduced fertility, even though researchers could only use minute amounts of the protein in the injection.

1992 ANTI-SPERM AND ANTI-OVUM VACCINES: THE SELECTION OF CANDIDATE ANTIGENS AND THE OUTCOME OF PRECLINICAL STUDIES

M A Isahakia 1, C S Bambra Scand J Immunol Suppl 1992;11:118-22. doi: 10.1111/j.1365-3083.1992.tb01633.x.

Abstract

A clear conceptual basis for anti-sperm and other modes of immunological birth control exists in spite of the limited basic research done on surface antigens of sperm or egg. In the normal physiological condition, the immune system does not respond to sperm, egg, or fetus. Compared with anti-egg or anti-fetus immunocontraception, an anti-sperm vaccine has two theoretical advantages. First it would work in both males and females; second, it would not raise problems of autoimmunity in the female if a sperm-specific protein is used. However, for the development of such contraceptive vaccines the following scientific questions need to be resolved: (1) what surface protein to use as an antigen; (2) what adjuvant to use in humans for an anti-fertility vaccine; (3) how to maintain a high titre; (4) how the contraceptive effect will be terminated; and (5) what the potential side-effects are.

PIP: Certain sperm antigens are auto- or isoimmunogenic, and naturally occurring sperm antibodies have been implicated in 10-15% of unexplained human infertility. Thus, efforts to develop an immunocontraceptive for human application have targeted sperm antigens. The World Health Organization Task Force on Contraceptive Vaccines designated the human sperm SP-10 as a primary vaccine candidate. The presence of SP-10 mRNA was demonstrated in baboons and macaques, and it is an ideal primate model for evaluating human efficacy. At a workshop on worldwide research on all monoclonal antibodies against sperm, HS-11 and HS-63 were selected for further evaluation because of their high specificity and significant anti-fertility effects. Isoenzyme LDH-C4 is a primary sperm antigen: it provokes antibodies that are absolutely cell specific and do not cross-react with somatic LDH isozymes. Immunization of both males and females with purified LDH-C4 results in an immune response and antibodies suppress fertility in female mice, rabbits, and baboons. The PH-20 protein from guinea pigs has a required function in sperm-zona binding, and a 100% effective contraception is obtained when either male or female guinea pigs are immunized with purified PH-20. Regarding zona pellucida antigens (ZP), the porcine zona pellucida contains the major glycoprotein families identified as ZP1, ZP2 and ZP3. In a human in vitro fertilization system, only antibodies against ZP3 completely suppressed sperm-egg interaction. Passive administration of anti-zona pellucida antibodies results in long-term reversible contraception. The development of antigens capable of evoking an immune response, thereby preventing fertility without ovarian histopathology, is under way. A zona pellucida contraceptive vaccine containing 8-cell, but not T-cell, zona pellucida epitopes may prevent ovarian pathology.

1992 Alfred Hassig, former 35-year Director of the Swiss Red Cross Transfusion Service, and President of the Board of Trustees of the International Society of Blood Transfusion stated:

"The sentence of death accompanying the medical diagnosis of AIDS should be abolished. In the virological research, so much money is invested, and the research people want to stay in that area because if you deviate to research in other directions probably other people come in and must be funded. Virologists have nothing new to offer. They keep coming up with excuses, they find constant growth and change in the virus structure, it evades, attacks, strange things, but none of them has the courage to explain properly how these things could possibly be so. AZT (anti-viral AIDS medicine) has, in countless cases, brought about the inevitable and slow asphyxiation of the patient's body cells. The doctors wrongly diagnose the fatal consequences of AZT medication as AIDS following a prior HIV infection. Treatment with AZT and allied toxic substances may be equivalent to joining a suicide squad with a time fuse. It is the duty of every doctor to preserve life at any cost — and not death-curse people based on any test, so they are so frightened they kill themselves. I am sad to say that these voodoo methods were practiced despite there never being any proof that the detected antibodies are an indication of mortality in all diagnosed people. I consider it medical malpractice to push patients into dying by prophesying an early death. We are medical scientists, not prophets!" (Meditel 1992;Continuum Jan/Feb 1996).

1992 Institute of Medicine releases report presenting evidence indicating that there is: "a causal relation between DTP vaccine and anaphylaxis and between the pertussis component of DTP vaccine and extended periods of inconsolable crying or screaming.

The committee also reported that the evidence indicates a causal relation between the rubella vaccine and acute arthritis in adult women. The committee found the available evidence weaker but still consistent with a causal relation between DTP vaccine and two conditions–acute encephalopathy and hypotonic, hyporesponsive episodes–and between rubella vaccine and chronic arthritis in adult women. Estimated incidence rates of these adverse events following vaccination are provided, where possible. The committee found that the evidence does not indicate a causal relation between the DTP vaccine and infantile spasms, hypsarrhythmia, Reye's syndrome, and sudden infant death syndrome. The committee found insufficient evidence to indicate either the presence or absence of a causal relation between DTP vaccine and chronic neurologic damage, aseptic meningitis, erythema multiforme or other rash, Guillain-Barre syndrome, hemolytic anemia, juvenile diabetes, learning disabilities and attention-deficit disorder, peripheral mononeuropathy, or thrombocytopenia, and between rubella vaccine and radiculoneuritis and other neuropathies or thrombocytopenic purpura."(C.P. Howson and H.V. Fineberg, Adverse events following pertussis and rubella vaccines. Summary of a report of the Institute of Medicine. JAMA Vol. 267 No. 3, January 15, 1992).

1992 "The hepatitis B vaccine causes positive HIV test results." (Lee, D, Eby W, Molinaro, G. HIV false positivity after Hepatitis B vaccination. Lancet 339: 1060, 1992).

1992-2006 In 1992 The Lancet publishes the first article describing idiopathic CD4+ T-lymphocytopenia (ICL-AIDS), and 199 more articles appear describing this disease with designation and title in the following years. CD4+ T-lymphocytopenia is one of the 40 or more AIDS-indicator diseases in a patient without "HIV" proteins or nucleic acids detectable despite repeated efforts. Essentially, ICL is AIDS without "HIV."

1992 Minnesota researchers report that "HIV-sequences" exist in normal in human, chimpanzee, and rhesus monkey DNAs" (Horwitz MS, Boyce-Jacino MT, Faras AJ. Novel human endogenous sequences related to human immunodeficiency virus type 1. J Virol. Apr; 66 (4):2170-9, 1992).

1992 AMERICA'S CENTERS FOR DISEASE CONTROL (CDC) IN ATLANTA ADMITS THAT THE POLIO LIVE-VIRUS VACCINE HAD BECOME THE MAIN CAUSE OF POLIO IN THE UNITED STATES

1992. Specifically, the CDC asserted that, from 1973 to 1983, 87% of all (non-imported) cases of polio resulted directly from vaccine administration. Even more amazingly, it was asserted that every non-imported case of polio in the United States from 1980 to 1989 was vaccine-induced (Strebel, P. M., et al., Epidemiology of Poliomyelitis in the U.S. One Decade after the Last Reported Case of Indigenous Wild Virus Associated Disease, Clinical Infectious Diseases, CDC, February 1992, pp. 568-579).

1992 JM Fine, LC Chen "Confounding in studies of adverse reactions to vaccines," American Journal of Epidemiology, 136 (1992), pp. 121-35. Studies show that children die at a rate eight times greater than normal within three days of getting a DPT shot.

1993 DPTH (DPT-Hib combo) licensed.

1993 BIRTH CONTROL VACCINE RESEARCH-WORLD HEALTH ORGANIZATION FORUM – 1993;14(1):90-1.

https://pubmed.ncbi.nlm.nih.gov/8439385/

The WHO Special Program of Research, Development, and Research Training in Human Reproduction has developed a prototype antifertility vaccine. The vaccine is directed against human chorionic gonadotrophin (hCG) and consists of a conjugate immunogen, formed from a synthetic fragment of the beta subunit of hCG joined to diphtheria toxoid and mixed with an immunostimulant. After 4 years of extensive preclinical safety and efficacy studies, the Program conducted a Phase I clinical trial between 1986 and 1988, using the vaccine in sterilized women to assess its safety. Teratology studies were carried out in rats and rabbits in case it failed to prevent pregnancy; the results showed that the WHO prototype vaccine had no adverse effects either on the pregnant animals or on the fetuses.

The Program is now planning to conduct Phase II clinical trials to assess the effectiveness of the vaccine. The studies done so far have shown that the prototype anti-hCG vaccine is well tolerated, safe, and immunogenic in humans, but this version requires at least 2 injections, at an interval of several weeks, to elicit an anti-hCG immune response lasting for 3-6 months. Therefore, the Program has been developing an advanced prototype vaccine designed to elicit effective levels of immunity which will last for 12-18 months following a single injection. The advanced prototype anti-hCG vaccine consists of the same immunogen conjugate and immunostimulant used in the prototype version, but they are incorporated into a polymer designed to release the vaccine slowly over an extended and predetermined period of time. Dose-response and toxicity studies are currently under way in rabbits and baboons to determine the optimal dose of the vaccine and to see if this vaccine is safe for testing in humans.

1993 It is reported that half of infants that test "HIV" positive at birth serorevert (reverse) their "HIV-positive status within 18 months (Parekh BS, Shaffer N, Coughlin R, et al. Dynamics of maternal IgG antibody decay and HIV-specific antibody synthesis in infants born to seropositive mothers. The NYC Perinatal HIV Transmission Study Group. AIDS Res Hum Retroviruses 9:907-12, 1993).

1993 MMWR November 05, 1993 / 42(43);840-841,847 Diphtheria Outbreak — Russian Federation, 1990-1993 Despite high levels of vaccination coverage against diphtheria, an ongoing outbreak of diphtheria has affected parts of the Russian Federation since 1990 (1); as of August 31, 1993, 12,865 cases had been reported. This report summarizes epidemiologic information about this outbreak for January 1990- August 1993 and is based on reports from public health officials in the Russian Federation. Within the report is also says: "an estimated 90% of children were fully vaccinated with four or more doses of diphtheria toxoid by the time they entered school."URL: http://www.cdc.gov/epo/mmwr/preview/mmwrhtml/00022128.htm.

1994 The Lancet publishes claims that "The incidence of asthma has been found to be five times more common in vaccinated children." –The Lancet, 1994.

1994 p24, another protein once thought to be unique to "HIV" is known to be expressed in the thymus glands of "HIV-negative children (Dura WT, Wozniewicz BM. Expression of antigens homologous to human retrovirus molecules in normal and severely atrophic thymus. Thymus 22 (4):245-54, 1994). 1994 D. C. Christie, et al., "The

1993 Epidemic of Pertussis in Cincinnati: Resurgence of Disease in a Highly Immunized Population of Children," New England Journal of Medicine (July 7, 1994), pp. 16-20.

1994 Failure to reach the goal of measles elimination. Apparent paradox of measles infections in immunized persons. Mayo Vaccine Research Group, Archives of Int. Medicine 154(16):1815-20, 1994 Aug. 22. "The apparent paradox is that as measles immunization rates rise to high levels in a population, measles becomes a disease of immunized persons."

1995 Varicella licensed.

1995 It was confirmed again that about half of infants that test "HIV" positive at birth serorevert (reverse) their "HIV-positive status by 18 months Chantry CJ, Cooper ER, Pelton SI, Zorilla C, Hillyer GV, Diaz C. Seroreversion in human immunodeficiency virus-exposed but uninfected infants. Pediatr Infect Dis J 14:382-7, 1995).

1995 CONGRESS OF THE UNITED STATES: OFFICE OF TECHNOLOGY AND ASSESSMENT OF THE FAILURE OF THE FIRST 33 "HIV"-VACCINE TRIALS: ADVERSE REACTIONS TO "HIV" VACCINES: MEDICAL, ETHICAL, AND LEGAL ISSUES. (Roger C. Herdman, Director). Below are excerpts from this important milestone document, and some comments regarding the status of "HIV" vaccines since Margaret Heckler in 1984 announced that one would be available in 2 years:

From page 1, 2: "A number of vaccines are being developed that use new strategies and each of these strategies carry special risks:"

Vaccines using live vectors, such as the vaccinia virus shown to be attenuated in laboratory animals, may prove to be inadequately attenuated, producing the disease caused by the unattenuated vector.

2. Naked DNA vaccines have been shown to create potent immune responses, but there are theoretical reasons to be concerned that they might produce tumors or autoimmune diseases or be transmitted from mother to fetus.

Although inactivated whole virus vaccines have generally been successful in protecting from infection with other viral diseases, it would be difficult to assure that all HIV particles in such a vaccine were inactivated.

Live attenuated virus vaccines have also been successful in protecting from other viral diseases, but there is the potential for the viruses to be inadequately attenuated, for an adequately attenuated viral vaccine to cause disease in immunocompromised individuals (Read AIDS patients), and for an adequately attenuated virus to revert to virulence.

There is also concern that a live attenuated vaccine could induce tumors. "A number of social harms-non-medical adverse consequences-may result from vaccination:"

Vaccines may cause a false-positive HIV screening testing test… resulting in discrimination against vaccine recipients in, for example, military service, health insurance, life insurance, employment, and travel.

Participation in an HIV vaccine trial, itself, may result in stigmatization, as others may assume that all vaccine trial participants are members of groups, such as injection drug users and men who have sex with men, who are at increased risk for HIV infection.

Vaccinees, relying on the protection afforded by an experimental vaccine, may engage in behaviors that increase their risk for HIV infection.

In June, 1994, the AIDS Research Advisory Committee (ARAC) of the National Institute of Allergy and Infectious Diseases (NIAID) recommended that Phase III clinical trials with enveloped vaccines should not proceed in the United States. Factors contributing to the decision included scientific, political, and ethical issues, and the significant level of scientific uncertainty about the wisdom of immediate trials. Phase I and II clinical trials of HIV will continue."

From page 2,3. There are 15 ethical issues in HIV vaccine development. The last one states: # 15. "Although vaccine sponsors have no legal obligation to provide compensation to subjects for injuries incurred as a result of their participation, there is an ethical obligation to do so."

From page 3. Liability and Compensation for Adverse Reactions:

Any system that limits compensation to injuries from one specific cause, like an HIV vaccine, raises questions of fairness to people with similar injuries from a different vaccine.

A compensation system limited to persons with adverse reactions to an HIV vaccine invites the question why people living with injuries from other vaccines or from other causes should not be compensated as well.

More companies are engaged in HIV vaccine research than in research for any other type of vaccine. Potential liability may have discouraged some companies, but it has not stopped HIV vaccine development.

From page 4. "Given the need for an HIV vaccine, it appears unlikely that a manufacturer would be held responsible for distributing a vaccine with a risk of development of cancer that could not be verified at the time it was released." "The decision whether or not to invest in the development of a vaccine depends on complex financial considerations of a number of factors, including the scientific obstacles to vaccine development, the potential market for the vaccine, the price at which the vaccine could be sold, and the potential liability for vaccines. The major factor influencing vaccine development is the expected return on investment or profitability, and the major obstacles to developing an HIV vaccine are scientific."

Vaccine manufacturers are not likely to be responsible for harms resulting from the bigotry of others. Physicians who administer HIV vaccines may be the more likely targets for any claim that a vaccine recipient was not adequately warned about possible discrimination.

From page 9: Adverse reactions to HIV vaccines: Ten vaccinees developed a rash to several products, and one also developed joint pain. A few individuals developed a positive test result." IV vaccine could induce tumors.

These paragraphs are from page 48 and constitute double-speak (ie. Lies that are cloaked in fancy science-speak:

Some experts have questioned whether priming with an HIV vaccine can potentiate subsequently acquired natural HIV infection. The historical prototype giving rise to this concern is dengue virus, a tropical viral disease. The presence of serum antibodies induced by a first attack of mild dengue can facilitate the development of severe disease on subsequent infection with a related dengue virus. This "antibody-dependent enhancement" (ADE) of infection can be demonstrated in the laboratory by an increase in growth of virus in cell culture in the presence of antibodies from the serum of exposed individuals. Recipients of envelope vaccines have been shown to develop small amounts of enhancing antibodies. The clinical significance of HIV vaccine-induced ADE is unclear. No direct evidence exists at this time that ADE has any clinical significance. Many scientists consider it to be an unrelated laboratory phenomenon only. Enhancement of disease has not been duplicated with HIV-1 or SIV in primate experiments, although it has been recommended that studies in primate models should continue."

"Other mechanisms of Enhanced Disease: Historically, two other vaccines have been associated with an accompanying subsequent natural infection that is atypically severe: an experimental respiratory syncytial virus (RSV) vaccine and a licensed measles virus vaccine. Both were vaccines composed of whole virus inactivated by formalin (like the Salk vaccine). While the mechanisms of disease enhancement remain unclear, they both appear to occur by mechanisms unrelated to ADE of the dengue fever type. The enhance disease experiences with these vaccines were wholly unexpected and have had a significant effect on further vaccine development. For measles, a live attenuated vaccine has supplanted the inactivated vaccine, and currently there is no licensed RSV vaccine. It has been suggested recently that inactivated RSV vaccine may induce inappropriate cytokines, or cell-to-cell communication substances, that are responsible for enhancement."

Translation: These vaccines cause the diseases for which they are meant to prevent. This is what is called "enhancement.'

From page 50:

"There is a narrow margin between surviving virus and the destruction of viral immunogenicity; this was highlighted early in the use of licensed polio vaccine when a number of vaccinated individuals developed paralytíc poliomyelitis from vaccine lots containing residual live virus. The safety problem was resolved by simple refinements in the inactivation process. By contrast, assuring inactivation of all HIV particles could prove difficult. In particular, concern exists as to whether cell cultures or animal models are sufficiently sensitive to detect the minimal residual live virus capable of infecting humans. There has also been theoretical concern regarding residual reactive viral DNA in the product."

In addition, the safety of the "lymphoblastoid" cell lines used to prepare the virus is unknown. "Adventitious agents," that is, unwanted agents growing silently in the cell cultures used to prepare vaccine stock, have posed safety problems in the past. As an example, SV40, a monkey tumor virus, contaminated early lots of inactivated polio vaccine prepared in monkey cells.

"Live attenuate vaccines using live attenuated virus, exemplified by polio or measles vaccines, are capable of producing immune responses that closely mimic the solid, long-term protective immune response afforded by natural viral infection. In addition to a more vigorous and broader antibody response, attenuated virus vaccines may more effectively induce cytotoxic T-lymphocytes and mucosal immunity compared with vaccines composed of inert antigens, such as envelope protein vaccines."

(**Comment: We see from the past how well this has worked out... e.g. The polio era as described earlier in this book**).

On page 33, however, it is claimed that:

"The number of infectious agents for which we have failed to develop a satisfactory vaccine, even those targeted as high priority (49), is far greater than the number for which we have been successful. Examples of VIRUSES for which we have failed include the viruses Herpes simplex, infectious mononucleosis, cytomegalovirus, respiratory syncytial virus, and rotavirus; vaccines against many sexually-transmitted disease agents, such as syphilis and gonorrhea (which aren't due to viruses); vaccines against parasitic diseases, such as malaria and schistosomiases; and vaccines against numerous bacterial infections, including tuberculosis."

Original antigenic sin (OAS).HIV infection induces an abundance of antibodies, including neutralizing antibodies: however, several groups have shown that the generation of neutralizing antibodies tends to lag behind the generation of viral escape mutants by several months or even years. One explanation for this observation involves the phenomenon of original antigenic sin (OAS)_, the fixing of an immune response in a non-adaptive pattern.

Translation: By evoking the concept of "a non-adaptive pattern" is begging immunology to break the rules of what we understand about the immune response. It is interesting it is couched in the term, ORIGINAL SIN!"

Here is the bottom line as to why <u>they</u> <u>think</u> this happens:

"Vaccine-induced OAS may occur when a vaccinated individual is exposed to a non-cross-reactive strain of HIV that induces the production of antibodies specific for the vaccine strain that are unable to neutralize the newly encountered strain."

Translation: When exposed to HIV, however, vaccinated individuals exhibiting OAS may be no worse off than unvaccinated individuals because unvaccinated individuals also have a lag in generation of antibody to HIV because their immune response has not been "primed" by vaccination. It is not known whether the lab in antibody production in unvaccinated individuals is greater than the lab in the production of antibody directed by contemporaneous HIV strains in vaccinated individuals exhibiting OAS. In other words, neither "HIV-positives, or "HIV" vaccinated individuals show the fallacies of both vaccines and the **scam** of the AIDS era.

1995 In Rev. Soc. Bras. Med. Trop., vol. 28, no. 4, Oct-Dec pp. 339-43, 1995, we read:

"The history of previous vaccination [in very early childhood] did not diminish the number of complications of the cases studied." Then why vaccinate?

1995 DOES MEASLES VACCINE SPREAD THE MEASLES VIRUS?

Detection of Measles Virus RNA in Urine Specimens from Vaccine Recipients

JOURNAL OF CLINICAL MICROBIOLOGY, Sept. 1995, p. 2485–2488 Vol. 33, No. 9 0095-1137/95/$04.0010 Copyright q 1995, American Society for Microbiology PAUL A. ROTA,* ALI S. KHAN, EDISON DURIGON,† THOMAS YURAN, YVONNE S. VILLAMARZO, AND WILLIAM J. BELLINI

"...In our study, individuals received the Moraten strain of measles vaccine as measles-mumps-rubella vaccine. Measles virus RNA was detected by RT-PCR in the urine specimens from several of the vaccinated children as late as 14 days after vaccination. Because our research protocol was limited to only 14 days of specimen collection, we were unable to determine the upper limit for the duration of viral RNA in urine. In the previous study by Llanes-Rodas and Liu (19), measles virus antigen was detected in urine as late as 16 days after vaccination. The finding that several of the urine samples were positive for measles virus RNA as early as 1 day after vaccination was surprising. In the previous study (19), none of the urine specimens were positive by immunofluorescence before day 4. Since a single cycle of viral replication would be expected to take 17 to 24 h, it is unlikely that the RT-PCR detected the progeny of virus replicating in the urinary tract. Rather, this observation suggests that shortly after vaccination the input virus or viral antigen, in the form of nucleocapsids, is deposited directly into the bladder via interstitial fluid. This finding also demonstrates the increased sensitivity of RT-PCR compared with the immunofluorescence techniques that were used in earlier studies(18). Unfortunately, most of the specimens were of such poor quality that cytological studies or resolution of vaccine virus was not attempted. In the previous study (19), attempts to isolate vaccine virus on cell culture were unsuccessful. The changing epidemiology of measles, in the form of mild measles cases in previously vaccinated individuals (1, 11, 20), suggests that more asymptomatic or subclinical cases might be occurring. The frequency of such infections, which would not meet the standard case definition of the Centers for Disease Control and Prevention, is not known. Also, it is not known whether individuals who do not display the full range of clinical signs characteristic of measles infection are capable of transmitting the virus to other susceptible individuals. In one previous study, urine samples from 5 of 12 measles case contacts were positive for measles virus antigen even though only 1 of these 5 contacts developed clinical signs (5). In general, RT-PCR has proven to be a rapid and sensitive method to detect measles virus RNA in a variety of clinical specimens (13, 15, 21, 24, 26, 28). Successful RT-PCR amplification of measles virus RNA from urine samples now allows the detection of measles virus RNA from a specimen that can be obtained from a large number of individuals by noninvasive means. We plan to use this assay to determine further the extent of asymptomatic or mild infection in case contacts during an outbreak, to determine the role that these cases play in the transmission of measles, and to measure the shedding patterns of vaccine recipients. In future surveys, more care will need to be taken to obtain and process the specimen in a manner that minimizes RNA degradation."

1995 – From 1995's United States Congressional Record regarding at that time the failure of the first 30 Human "HIV" vaccine trials, due to what was called, Original Antigenic Sin (OAS).

"HIV infection induces an abundance of antibodies, including neutralizing antibodies (neutralizing antibodies are those antibodies that inactivate "HIV"): however, several groups have shown that the generation of neutralizing antibodies tends to lag behind the generation of viral escape mutants by several months or even years (DAMN SNEEKY MUTANTS AGAIN)! One explanation for this observation involves the phenomenon of original antigenic sin (OAS), the fixing of an immune response in a non-adaptive pattern. When exposed to HIV, however, vaccinated individuals exhibiting OAS may be no worse off than unvaccinated individuals because unvaccinated individuals also have a lag in generation of antibody to HIV because their immune response has not been "primed" by vaccination. It is not known whether the lag in antibody production in un-vaccinated individuals is greater than the lag in the production of antibody directed by contemporaneous HIV strains in vaccinated individuals exhibiting OAS," because again:

"Vaccine-induced OAS may occur when a vaccinated individual is exposed to a non-cross-reactive strain of HIV that induces the production of antibodies specific for the vaccine strain that are unable to neutralize the newly encountered strain."

A more Biblical translation: Original (antigenic) sin sometimes may occur in "HIV" vaccine trials in either experimental or placebo groups because the antigen(s) injected are different than the antigens that supposedly make up "HIV" and because there is a lag time in antibody production. It should be clearly noted in this context, however, that this explanation by the AIDS vaccinologists makes as much sense as the story that "original antigenic sin" is God's punishment for seeking the knowledge of good and evil through vaccine experimentation on human beings.

It should be recalled that after Adam and Eve realized they were naked, God decided to push his children out of the sterility of Eden. Because he loved them, God decided to protect his children from the vile germs of the world he had created on the second day, by vaccinating them. In his divine wisdom, God provided Adam and Eve with "a

choice," which is why God sent his servant, The Snake (the vaccination devil) to tempt Eve to either receive the vaccine poison from the snake's bite, or as with Sabin's sugar cubes, to receive the poison orally after putting it into The Apple. Although the serpent's bite was meant to hurt to remind all of the generations of Adam and Eve of their fundamental sinful, vile, germ-ridden wretched nature, redness and tenderness only occurred at the snake-bite injection site. God's vaccine worked so well that in all the generations of Adam and Eve (who were related genetically), molecular mimicry did not occur, and, thus demyelination syndromes, peripheral neuropathies, Crohn's disease, arthritis, shingles, seizures, insulin-dependent diabetes, autism spectrum disorders, and other adverse reactions did not occur in the many generations that followed. And God saw that it was good. Also, unlike today's vaccines, there were no impurities in God's vaccine such as the following list on WAVE's website presents-"World Association of Vaccine Education: (http://www.novaccine.com/vaccine-ingredients/).

It should be emphasized here that squalene (MF-59) among other adjuvants, toxins, fixatives, antibiotics, neurotoxic metals, and other compounds listed above, has been used in "HIV" vaccines to "boost" the immune system non-specifically [1]. Unfortunately, the same substance is used in arthritis research, and in animal models of other autoimmune diseases to cause those diseases. There also is evidence that adjuvants like squalene (MF-59), when they have been added to certain lots of anthrax (and perhaps "HIV") vaccines given to soldiers on threat of court martial if they do not roll up their shirt on command [2], have induced autoimmune syndromes in almost 100% of every sick Gulf-War I veteran tested, and have evoked antibodies to squalene in their blood [3,4]. This type of promising vaccine experimentation on our young soldiers who are spreading democracy and freedom throughout the world is particularly disturbing in light of the fact that squalene and other adjuvants have been used by scientists for many years to induce rodents to develop arthritis, macrophagic myofasciitis, multiple-sclerosis (demyelinating syndromes), and lupus [5, 6].

Finally, "original antigenic sin, if it is a distinct and important immunological mechanism that accounts for vaccine trial failures, should not be confused with past suggested mechanisms as "antigenic shift" that also have been proposed to account for past vaccine trial failures. For instance, the phrase "antigenic shift" was used to describe the failure of the flu vaccine to protect soldiers entering World War II:

1941 "On the eve of US entry into World War II, concern about a repeat of the 1918 influenza pandemic and its effect on armed forces led the US military to establish the Commission on Influenza (later combined with other commissions to become the present Armed Forces Epidemiological Board) and place high priority on developing a vaccine (Woodward TE, editor. The histories of the commissions. Washington: Office of The Surgeon General; 1992). Pandemic influenza did not materialize, but the vaccine did. The first successful large-scale influenza vaccine field trials were completed in 1943 (Francis T. Vaccination against influenza. In: World Health Organization. Influenza, a review of current research. Geneva: The Organization; 1954. p. 689-740). In 1947, failure of the vaccine to provide protection against the epidemic influenza type A antigenic variant confirmed concerns of vaccine obsolescence and led to the term "antigenic shift" (von Magnus P. The influenza virus: its morphology, immunology, and kinetics of multiplication. Bull World Health Organ. 1953;8:647-60) and designation of the 1947 FM1 strain by the Commission on Influenza as subgroup A´ on the basis of the hemagglutination inhibition (HI) test).

Question: Is this hemagglutination inhibition test or its interpretation infallible and specific only for flu viruses?

As a slight digression, it is an interesting historical fact that the 1918 "Spanish Flu" epidemic, like many victims of the AIDS "epidemic," affected men in the prime of their lives, and at a 1/4th higher rate among new military recruits than civilians, but how could the virus "know?" In this context, The Pandemic of Influenza in 1918-1919 prepared by the US Department of Health, Education and Welfare Public Health Service National Office of Vital Statistics indicated that:

> "the extraordinary feature of 'the Great Spanish flu' was that it attacked young people in the prime of life unlike any other epidemics recorded." (Except AIDS)?
>
> "When appropriate adjustments are made for differences in the age and sex distribution of military and civilian populations, it appears that the death rate was about one-fourth higher in the Army than in the civilian population of the United States.
>
> "The relatively high mortality in young adults in 1918 and the 2 years immediately following seems to have been characteristic of that period and was not found in epidemics prior to or subsequent to this 3-year period."

Moreover, in these contexts, one might ask why there isn't a deeper sense of gratitude toward the scientific instincts and second great contribution of another one of Donald Rumsfeld's companies (a separate venture from Searle described earlier, Gilead Biosciences, who have made and promoted the drug Tamiflu to protect the world currently from "Bird Flu," which we have been told is a mutant from "The Great Spanish Flu pandemic," and who also now market the new AIDS drug atripola that outsold all other AIDS drugs last year-but more about that later).

"US Defense Secretary Donald Rumsfeld served as Gilead (Research)'s chairman from 1997 until he joined the Bush administration in 2001, and he still holds a Gilead stake valued at between $5 million and $25 million, according to federal financial disclosures filed by Rumsfeld. The forms do not reveal the exact number of shares Rumsfeld owns. Gilead made a loss in 2003, the year before concern about bird flu started. Then revenues from Tamiflu almost quadrupled, from $35 to $44.6m, helping put the company well into the black. Sales almost quadrupled again, to $161.6M in 2005. Mr Rumsfeld sold some of his Gilead shares in 2004 reaping – according to the financial disclosure report he is required to make each year – capital gains of > $5m (£2.9 m) ref. The report showed that he still had up to $25m-worth of shares at the end of 2004. Rumsfeld is not the only political heavyweight benefiting from demand for Tamiflu, which is manufactured and marketed by Swiss pharma giant Roche (Gilead receives a royalty from Roche equaling about 10% of sales). Former Secretary of State George Shultz, who is on Gilead's board, has sold more than $7 million worth of Gilead since the beginning of 2005. Another board member is the wife of former California Gov. Pete Wilson. In July, the Pentagon ordered $58 million worth of the treatment for U.S. troops around the world, and Congress is considering a multi-billion-dollar purchase. Rumsfeld recused himself from any decisions involving Gilead when he left Gilead and became Secretary of Defense in early 2001.

(**http://money.cnn.com/2005/10/31/news/newsmakers/fortune_rumsfeld/index.htm**).

HOW "ORIGINAL ANTIGENIC SIN" HAS COME ABOUT DURING THE ERA OF "HIV-AIDS" VACCINES

Toward the end of a Congressional document prepared by the Government Office of Technology Assessment, the term "**original antigenic sin**" was advanced to describe why by **1995**, 30 "HIV" vaccines had failed. Now in 2019 there have been 226 trials that have failed, because, according to AIDS INC:

A) When a vaccinated individual is exposed to a non-cross-reactive strain of HIV that induces the production of antibodies specific for the vaccine strain, that are unable to neutralize the newly encountered strain.
B) The fixing of an immune response in a "non-adaptive pattern."
C) When vaccinated individuals may be no worse off than unvaccinated individuals because non-vaccinated individuals also have a lag in generation of antibody to HIV, because their immune response has not been "primed" by vaccination.

The conclusions of The Office of Technology Assessment Book were presented to the 1995 Congress of the United States by the AIDS Research Advisory Committee (ARAC) of the National Institute of Allergy and Infectious Diseases (NIAID).

Toward the end of a Congressional document prepared by the Government Office of Technology Assessment, the term "original antigenic sin" was advanced to describe why by 1995, 30 "HIV" vaccines had failed:

A) When a vaccinated individual is exposed to a non-cross-reactive strain of HIV that induces the production of antibodies specific for the vaccine strain, that are unable to neutralize the newly encountered strain (in plain words, when an "HIV" vaccine does not work).
B) The fixing of an immune response in a "non-adaptive pattern."
C) When vaccinated individuals may be no worse off than unvaccinated individuals because non-vaccinated individuals also have a lag in generation of antibody to HIV, because their immune response has not been "primed" by vaccination.

The conclusions of The Office of Technology Assessment Book were presented to the 1995 Congress of the United States by the AIDS Research Advisory Committee (ARAC) of the National Institute of Allergy and Infectious Diseases (NIAID).

From these conclusions, it was recommended that Phase III clinical trials with enveloped vaccines should not proceed in the United States because of scientific, political, and ethical issues, and because of the significant level of scientific uncertainty about the wisdom of immediate trials" (1995 Congress of the United States: Office of Technology assessment. Adverse Reactions to HIV Vaccines: Medical, Ethical, and Legal Issues. Roger C. Herdman, Director).

More in-depth information about the importance of the "HIV'/AIDs era in the current context of COVID-19 testing and proposed treatments and vaccines will be presented later, but as a preliminary look, a list can convey the "certainty" with which this so-called epidemic, which officially began in 1984 has been such a failure, and why the current strategies of Fauci et all regarding vaccines will fail. For instance, one may ask why there were more than 100 failed "HIV" vaccines as of 2012, and why there are currently 230+ in the "HIV/AIDS" vaccine "pipeline." Emboldened words that appear throughout the following text and time-line are my emphasis-direct quotes usually are in italics.

1995 – SURVEY OF COMPETING THEORIES OF AIDS: A BRIEF HISTORY

Below is a list of **30 hypotheses** and a time-line of important events and publications that have been advanced about "HIV/AIDS" that have evolved during the past 3 decades. Following the hypotheses, I identify the source, institutions, and dates from which these hypotheses emerged in chronological sequence. Only a brief description as to the nature of the hypothesis is provided in the list below to demonstrate how the field of "HIV/AIDS" has evolved, and a more in-depth description and discussion entitled, "A brief history of AIDS" follows this survey section.

As you will hopefully discern, the field of "HIV/AIDS" and has departed from the "scientific and medical consensus" that had advanced the notion that Acquired Immune Deficiency Syndrome was caused by "HIV, " toward the recent 2009 documented claim made by Luc Montagnier, the Nobelist who is credited for the initial discovery of "HIV" and who now points to many co-factors, different causes than "HIV," and other hopeful news regarding "AIDS," such as his belief that:

> **"you can get rid of it in a few weeks."**

Some AIDS researchers and front-line AIDS doctors, following the lead of this Pasteur-Institute Nobelist credited for the discovery of "HIV" now recognize that AIDS is most likely caused by multi-factorial reasons that induce the set of at least 58 previously known syndromes that are collectively called Acquired Immune Deficiency Syndrome. You may be surprised to learn, in addition, that lymph node fibrosis, not the ill-termed and ill-conceived "viral load" readings (that never measured anything viral), or T-cell subset counts predict progression to fatal immune suppression, as researched and published by leading research institutions such as The Cleveland Clinic, or as seen in journals such as AIDS Clinical Care (see **Zugar A., 2009** in the list that follows below).

Here are 31 of the many most prominent hypotheses and theories of the men who now are calling the shots and whipping up the hysteria of COVID-19 during their last "run" during the era of AIDS, and the extent to which they encouraged academic freedom to question the growing IV drug epidemic and its consequences,

1. Cytomegalovirus causes AIDS because Dr. Michael Gottlieb found CMV (cytomegalovirus) in 100% of his first 5 patients at UCLA. (The CDC's Monthly Mortality Weekly Report, and, in the journal Nature, December **1981** issue).
2. Black slaves caused cancer because artwork evidence proved to Dr. Robert Gallo that the themes of these artworks depicted slaves who had caught a cancer virus in the 16th Century from monkeys during the slave trade. This logic in turn was used to explain the historical reasons as to how Japanese civilians in and near Nagasaki developed the high rate of leukemias from which they suffered after the atomic bombs were dropped on them. This hypothesis, in addition, was advanced to explain the origins of "HIV's" suspected "HTLV-1" origins by Robert Gallo in 1979-81, but this idea was rapidly dismissed by the scientific community, and abandoned by Gallo, and then "HTLV-II was imagined by Gallo to be the true "cancer virus" precursor, in order explained why 339 out of more than 600,000 Japanese acquired cancers in Southern Japan near Nagasaki.

   This is also why when the televised announcement was

made for the first time to the American public regarding "the probable cause of AIDS" had been found by Dr. Gallo in his sunglasses, and Health and Human Services Margaret Heckler standing at his side in 1984, that she was instructed by Gallo to use the phrase, "the probable cause of AIDS has been found…to be "HTLV-III…[which is] a known variant of a "cancer virus." "HTLV-III" was later renamed "HIV" by oncogene Nobelist Varmus's committee. (National Institute of Health: Gallo R.C., Sliski A., Wong-Staal F: Origin of T-cell leukemia-lymphoma virus. Lancet (ii): 962-963, **1983.**

3. The virus "LAV" (Lymphadenopathy-Associated Virus was associated with AIDS because Luc Montagnier's "Patient 1" had many diseases and was said to have pre-AIDS. Montagnier's so-called "LAV-BRU" or "LAV-LAI" "isolate's" association with pre-AIDS conditions was advanced despite the fact that Montagnier's "Patient One" had been treated **for syphilis, gonorrhea, cytomegalovirus, Epstein-Barr virus, and herpes viruses**. Yet, even though "Patient One's" lymphocytes were believed to harbor "LAV," (later also named "HIV" by Varmus's committee, **Montagnier later admitted they couldn't purify "HIV" despite "a Roman effort**," a required technical step in proving the association of any virus with disease (Pasteur Institute: Barre-Sinoussi, F,J.C. Chermann J.C., Rey F., Nugeyre MT., Chamaret, S., Gruest J., Dauguet C., Axler-Blin C., Vezinet-Brn F., Rouzioux, C., Rozenbaum R., & Montagnier L. Isolation of a T-lymphotropic retrovirus from a patient at risk for Acquired Immune Deficiency Syndrome. Science 230: 868-871, **1983**). Maybe this was not the best "Patient one" from which to launch The AIDS era?

Gallo's claim with Heckler in 1984 claimed that "HIV" was actually not a cancer virus but a cancer virus variant, and his claim that "HIV" causes AIDS, was based on the finding that 36% of 72 of his AIDS patients tested "HIV-positive," even though many were not sick. This claim was the basis of the first "HIV-test kits, and American-French patent for the kit. (It also was 64% less of an association that Gottlieb reported for CMV's association with his original AIDS patients). (National Institutes of Health: Popovic M, Sarngadharan MG, Read E, et al. Detection, Isolation,and Continuous Production of Cytopathic Retroviruses (HTLV-III) from Patients with AIDS and Pre-AIDS. Science, 224:497-500, **1984**; Gallo RC, Salahuddin SZ, Popovic M, et al. Frequent Detection and Isolation of Cytopathic Retroviruses (HTLV-III) from Patients with AIDS and at Risk for AIDS. Science 224:500-502, **1984**; Schupbach J, Popovic M, Gilden RV, et al. Serological analysis of a Subgroup of Human T-Lymphotrophic Retroviruses (HTLV-III) Associated with AIDS. Science, 224:503-505, **1984**; Sarngadharan MG, Popovic M,Bruch L, et al. Antibodies Reactive to Human TLymphotrophic Retroviruses (HTLV-III) in the Serum of Patients with AIDS. Science, 224:506-508, **1984**.

4. "HIV" emerged from barbaric African sexual practices to stimulate a man or a woman and induce them to intense sexual activity, monkey blood [for a man] or she-monkey blood [for a woman] was directly incubated in the pubic area and also the thighs and back. These magic practices would therefore unequivocally constitute an efficient experimental transmission model and could be responsible for the emergence of AIDS in man, as was published in The Lancet. (Noireau F. HIV transmission. From monkey to man-Lancet (i):1498-1499, **1987**).
5. "HIV" is a harmless passenger virus: "HIV" exists but does no harm and does not cause AIDS. (University of California, Berkeley: Peter H. Duesberg, "Retroviruses as Carcinogens and Pathogens: Expectations and Reality Cancer Research 47, 1199-1220, March 1, **1987**).
6. Smallpox vaccine campaigns in Africa caused AIDS as they woke up latent "HIV" harbored by blacks who were vaccinated. (The World Health Organization, published in Letters to The Lancet, and NEJM, London Times Edition 1 MON 11 MAY **1987**).

7. AIDS is actually a form of cryptic syphilis, "the great imitator," which presents with identical T—cell disturbances, profound immune suppression, and dementia (Washington's National Library of Medicine. Coulter HL. AIDS and Syphilis-The Hidden Link, CA, pps. 20, 21, **1987**).
8. AIDS is caused by Redox imbalances and by proteins and behaviors that oxidize cells and tissues (Royal Perth Hospital, Perth Australia, Papadopulos-Eleopulos E. Medical Hypotheses. 25: 151-162, **1988**).
9. Malnutrition, recreational and prescription drugs, and foreign proteins cause AIDS (University of California, Berkeley: Peter H. Duesberg, Proc. Natl. Acad. Sci. USA Vol.86, pp. 755-764, February **1989**).
10. Anti-HLA alloantigens cause AIDS (Michigan State University: Robert Root-Bernstein. Do we know the causes of AIDS? Perspectives in Biology and Medicine: Summer, 33:480-500, **1990**).
11. Mycoplasma incognitus causes AIDS: 22/34 patients with AIDS demonstrated high titres of M. incognitus in their tissues while 0 non-AIDS patients have the microbe (Armed Forces Institute of Pathology: Lo SC, Hayes MM, Wang RY, Pierce PF, Kotani H, Shih JW. Newly discovered mycoplasma isolated from patients infected with HIV. Lancet. Dec 7;338 (8780):1415-8, **1991**).
12. AIDS is caused by multiple –antigen-mediated-autoimmunity (MAMA) through idiotypic/anti-idiotypic immune reactions (Michigan State University: Robert Root-Bernstein, 'Rethinking AIDS; The tragic cost of premature consensus' The Free Press/ Macmillan USA, 527 pages, **1993**. ISBN 0-02-926905-9).
13. AIDS is caused by "HIV" hiding in lymph nodes and destroying them. (Pantaleo G, Graziosi C, Demarest JF, Butini L, et al. HIV infection is active and progressive in lymphoid tissue during the clinically latent stage of disease. Nature; 362(6418):355-8, **1993b**).
14. AIDS is caused by exposure to too many viruses, which is why

no vaccine is possible: AIDS is a chemical chain reaction because of all these virus infections. Kary Mullis, multiple institutions, Inventor of PCR-polymerase chain reaction used to detect COVID-19 and "HIV," Nobel Prize Recipient. (A hypothetical disease of the immune system that may bear some relation to the Acquired Immune Deficiency Syndrome. Genetica 95: 195-**1995**).

15. "HIV" is caused by oxidizing T-cell cultures with a plant lectin, phytohemagglutinin, and IL2. (Royal Perth Hospital, Perth Australia, Eleni Papadopulos-Eleopulos, Valendar F.Turner, John M. Papadimitriou, David Causer, Bruce Hedland-Thomas, Barry Page. a critical analysis of the HIV-T4-Cell-AIDS hypothesis. Genetica 95: 5-24, **1995**).
16. Influenza vaccines cause "HIV." (Simonsen L, Buffington J, Shapiro CN, et al. Multiple false reactions in viral antibody screening assays after influenza vaccination. Am J Epidemiol 141:1089-1096,**1995**).
17. "HIV" isn't sexually transmissible between 175 condom-using and condom avoiding serodiscordant sexual partners (where one sexual partner tests "HIV-positive" and the other sexual partner tests "HIV-negative) if folks receive expert counseling. Therefore, lack of expert counseling causes AIDS because transmission rate was reported in this experiment to have been 0% in victims who had received "expert counseling:" Padian, et al. Heterosexual Transmission of HIV in Northern California: Results from a Ten-Year Study." American Journal of Epidemiology. August, **1997**.
18. "HIV" does not exist because it has not been isolated by the minimum accepted standards of viral isolation, including purification, any animal model, no vaccine, its presence in patients that never express any symptoms of immune suppressive illness, that it never left risk groups initially linked to AIDS, etc. Eleni Papadopulos-Eleopulos, Valendar Turner, John Papadimitriou, Barry Page, David Causer, Helman Alfonso, Sam Mhlongo, Todd Miller, Andrew Maniotis, Christian Fiala.

A critique of the Montagnier evidence for the HIV/AIDS hypothesis. Med Hypotheses. 63(4):597-601, **2004.**

19. In a witty article published in Science in 2005, it was reported that "HIV"'s primary target of destruction is the gut, and specifically the Peyer's patches, which causes AIDS. (12th International conference on Retroviruses and Opportunistic infections Jon Cohen, Science Writer, Science, 4 March, Vol 307, p. 1395, **2005**).
20. Cigarette smoking causes "HIV" but cigarettes do not cause AIDS. (Dr Andrew Furber, of the South East Sheffield Primary Care Trust, London, Reuters, Thursday, Sep 21, **2006**).

    A Thy-1/Thy-2 lymphocyte imbalance caused by many stressors to the body causes AIDS and can be reversed. (German Federal HIV Study, Parliamentary HIV/AIDS Commission biostatistics unit of Wuppertal University, Raum & Zeit, **2006**).
21. Cross presentation of caspase-cleaved apoptotic self-antigens is induced by "HIV-infection" to cause AIDS. (University of Italy: Rawson et al., Cross presentation of caspase-cleaved apoptotic self-antigens in HIV infection. Nature Medicine Vol. 13, No 12, December **2007**).
22. "HIV" requires exactly 237 cellular proteins to cause AIDS. Harvard Medical School, Howard Hugues Medical Institute Stephen (J. Elledge, January 10, **2008**, in Science Express).
23. There is no AIDS because the world's AIDS epidemic is over, accept in Africa (WHO epidemiologist, Dr. Kevin de Cock, May 19, **2008**, Geneva AIDS conference).\
24. AIDS originated 125 years ago when the virus jumped from chimpanzees to blacks. (University of Arizona, Nature Commentary, October, **2008**).

In 2008, The Nobel Prize in Physiology or Medicine 2008 was divided, one half awarded to Harald zur Hausen "for his discovery of human papilloma viruses causing cervical cancer", the other half jointly to Françoise Barré-Sinoussi and Luc Montagnier "for their discovery of human immunodeficiency virus." Gallo received no credit.

25. MA new strain of "HIV" jumped from a gorilla to a black woman living in Cameroon as reported in 2008, proving unequivocally through phylogenetic analyses of "HIV" and "SIV" sequences that although the woman is not ill in any way, this new strain of virus rapidly mutated and adapted to her body, and now threatens to ignite a new deadly AIDS pandemic (University of Rouen, France, Jean-Christophe Plantier, reported in Nature, **2008**).
26. Viral loads or T-cell killing do not cause AIDS: fibrosis of the lymph nodes causes AIDS. (Evaluation of the pathogenesis of decreasing CD4+ T cell counts in human immunodeficiency virus type 1–infected patients receiving successfully suppressive antiretroviral therapy. **Nies-Kraske E. et al. J Infect Dis. Jun 1; 199:1648, 2009**). About this study, a commentary is presented by Abigal Zugar which reveals the true fibrotic condition of the classic "AIDS" patient and goes to painstaking lengths to point out that AIDS and "viral load" readings done with testing of supposed RNA sequences of "HIV" is a completely wrong approach to understanding the nature of AIDS. A little of this discussion may be useful to present here;
27. In a recent issue of AIDS Clinical Care (June 1, 2009), frontline workers on the AIDS issue published some statements that should concern every AIDS physician. An AIDS doctor, Dr. Abigail Zugar perhaps stated it in most clearly in the title of a recent summary she wrote, which, although slightly technical, the meaning is easy to understand, and the implications are clear:

    "The Puzzle of CD4-Cell Depletion Despite Good Viral Suppression In some patients, CD4-cell counts fail to rise as expected. Could extensive lymph node fibrosis be responsible?"

    In other words, AIDS is progressing without "HIV" being detected (suggesting an autoimmune etiology). This should be as alarming as waking up one morning, and despite the sun not shining, one gets sunburned.

    Even more concerning statements followed in Dr. Zugar's article:

"In a recent study, NIH researchers sought evidence to support any of several hypothetical explanations for the aberrant CD4-cell responses seen in four patients on combination ART whose CD4 counts had fallen from a median of 719 cells/mm3 to a median of 227 cells/mm3 despite persistently undetectable plasma viral loads."

In other words, these patients were taking a double AIDS-drug cocktail regimen, and yet their Tcells were plunging from relatively normal levels to the worrisome and CDC-defined level of when therapy should begin, at around 300 cells/mm3.

Drug resistance was "checked" and found not to be an issue. However, what is most troubling is that Dr. Zugar then recounts that "Residual replicating HIV did not seem to be the problem: Results of ultrasensitive PCR and assays for peripheral blood mononuclear cell–associated HIV RNA and proviral HIV DNA — and of assays for cell-associated HIV RNA and proviral DNA in mononuclear cells from inguinal lymph nodes — were similar to those obtained in other, successfully treated patients."

Translation: "Viral load" has nothing to do with any virus or T-cell levels in these AIDS patients (and never has been, as has been known by many doctors for a long, long time). The failure to correlate any "viral load" with disease progression has been a chief problem since the beginning of the AIDS era. And it is not the first time that fibrosis in the lymph nodes has been discussed as being a chief issue in "AIDS patients," as Dr. Zugar correctly states:

"The single unusual finding was a striking abnormality in inguinal lymph node architecture..."

Or: ...the unusual lymph node architecture documented in all four patients in this study may be related to (or even responsible for) the inadequate CD4-cell response — i.e., that CD4-cell depletion is independent of specific components of an antiretroviral regimen and is instead caused by lymph node fibrosis. They note that such architectural damage may well be "clinically irreversible with currently available interventions."

Interpretation: Fibrosis of the lymph nodes (and other organs such as the liver) are often linked drug toxicity (such as alcoholism) or toxic effects of many iatrogenically-prescribed drugs, or chronic autoimmune diseases, and not pathogens.

These observations regarding lymph node fibrosis, autoimmune disease, or iatrogenic or illicit drug or alcohol use, as mentioned, are not new: as these references suggest: Pantaleo G, Graziosi C, Demarest JF, Butini L, et al. HIV infection is active and progressive in lymphoid tissue during the clinically latent stage of disease. Nature 1993b;362 (6418):355-8]; Lymph node fibrosis impedes peripheral [CD4.sup.+] T-cell count; fibrosis could be better predictor of ability to recover after HAART. The Scientist | January 27, 2003 | Roberts, Josh P.; Jon Cohn. "It's the Gut, Stupid." 4 March Vol 307, p. 1395, 2005. These are only a few examples of discussions regarding this critically important, yet largely unnoticed or potentially life-ending "fibrous" condition in the lymph nodes.

The paper by Nies-Kraske E et al. [Evaluation of the pathogenesis of decreasing CD4+ T cell counts in human immunodeficiency virus type 1–infected patients receiving successfully suppressive antiretroviral therapy. J Infect Dis 2009 Jun 1; 199:1648] is just the latest warning that should be heeded, and implemented in Global AIDS policy, clinical trial evaluations, and medical appraisal with respect to so-called AIDS patients.

28. A defect in innate immunity causes AIDS that is mediated by the cellular protein tethering, because tethering inhibits the release of HIV-1, EBOLA, and Kaposi's associated herpesvirus 8, and probably all viruses from infected cells (University of California, San Diego, and the Veterans Affairs San Diego Healthcare System. 362:6 February 11, 2010. John Guatelli, M.D. 362:6 February 11, 2010).
29. Not enough smallpox vaccinations caused AIDS because

of the CCR5 receptor binds to both smallpox viruses, and "HIV," and Petri-dish experiments prove that a competition of smallpox virus with "HIV" for the CCR5 receptor inhibits "HIV. " George Mason University, Manassas, Virginia, from a team of researchers from George Washington University and UCLA (**Science Daily, May 18, 2010**).

30. "HIV" doesn't cause AIDS because if you have a good immune system, you can get rid of it in a few weeks, according to the Nobelist Montagnier, who first described "HIV." (Interview and documentary, House of Numbers: 2010. Brief clip: http://www.youtube.com/watch?v=WQoNW7lOnT4l, Entire documentary: http://www.facebook.com/l.php?u=http%3A%2F%2Fhiv-dissidents.taba.ru%2Fvideo%2Ff%2F26508_Dom_chisel.html&h=f6d5eYwjJV-GDsjmQI3gQp8u_Vg\).

These persons were then accused of harboring a virus, "HIV" by Robert Gallo and others, and condemned by some in the medical establishment to die in 3-10 years with no exceptions. The fact that 7 out of 11 out of the cohort of Gottlieb's first subjects eluded everyone and the focus was instead placed on the sexual preferences of the victims-a common oversight now well known among those who study addiction medicine. It should be emphasized also, because of the stigma associated with addictions to drugs and alcohol, including drugs which were endemic in the fast-track scene of this era of liberation, poppers which also are cancer-inductive chemicals were (and still are) sold in "head-shops" legally, and constituted an important part of the "fast-track" alternative scene of promiscuous and frequent sexual encounters. In other words, "HIV" and AIDS were instantly blamed on sexuality rather than the likely "first cause" identified by David Gottlieb, who may not have been aware of the use of poppers nor asked the question about popper use. Even if he had, 7 out of 11 of his subjects readily admitted "illicit" drug use.

Subsequently, Kaposi's sarcoma was Christened by the virologists as one of the first two deadly AIDS-indicator illnesses of this population of heavy drug-users, along with Pneumocystis carinii pneumonias (see **Duesberg, Inventing the AIDS Virus, Regnery Publishing, 1996**). However, it is most likely that Kaposi's sarcoma during the 1980's AIDS era was caused by exposure to the carcinogenic properties of AZT, which still is not banned, and is still sold over the counter as a room deodorizer, despite Professor and National Academy of Sciences member, Peter Duesberg's early warnings at the beginning of The AIDS era.

There also is evidence that a plethora of microbial infections, nutritional collapse, mycoplasmas, and other factors other than any virus can accompany the acquisition of AIDS and/or Kaposi's. Although Kaposi's sarcoma had been known previously to the AIDS era as an endemic, non-malignant and relatively harmless lesion mostly among men who lived in Africa or in the Mediterranean region, during the "HIV/AIDS" era of the 1980's and the use of AZT following the 1987 Fischl trial that was terminated at after 4 months because AZT "worked so well to cure "HIV infection(s) " thereafter, AIDS patients merely died from the anti-cancer drug AZT and were told they were dying of AIDS. Besides the recreational use of this known cancer-inducing carcinogenic drug AZT, it also became widely used to mindlessly treat both men, pregnant women, and with few exceptions (Ryan White-and a few others I had some contact with), mostly African American children who had been accused of having "HIV" infections. Yet although these drug-induced transitions to malignancy were believed to be caused by a new viral disease called "HIV/AIDS," and despite the fact that any evidence of T-cell defects could be identified in many who were studied and had the sarcoma, and despite many of its victims had normal T-cell sets according to a paper Robert Gallo and his colleagues wrote the following year in 1985, claiming that T-cell deficits were no longer needed to acquire full-blown AIDS, the madness accelerated (When David Gottleib it first described AIDS in 4 patients in 1981, he established that these men were profoundly anergic, which means they couldn't mount a normal immune response when soluble antigens were used to stimulate them in Petri dishes, or In Vivo (**Gottleib D., 1981**).

Fibrosis of the lung due to heavy crack cocaine or PCP use, opium uses or Ecstasy, also were also indifferently linked to other commonly seen AIDS-defining illnesses, by Anthony Fauci and others before and during the AIDS era. Moritz Kaposi, a dermatologist, described his lesion for the first time before the 1900's, and believed it to be endemic in Sub-Saharan African men, and probably the result of lack of sanitation. Yet later, because the virologists have at one time or another linked every disease known to man, and after inadequate viral isolations were performed, the cause of the African Koposi's was attributed to a herpesvirus HHV-8. Who could have predicted either the endemic African occurrence of Kaposi's, or the epidemic Kaposi's among predominantly intra-IV-drug-users?

Behavioral diseases are particularly clear examples in the way they show a relationship between endemic or epidemic syndromes and organic disease states, although their symptoms are difficult to understand. For example, addiction to drugs and alcohol has been endemic in human cultures forever, yet addiction was labeled as a disease as late as the 1950's by the medical establishment because it fulfilled the definitions of a disease in Western Medicine. This definition allows syndromes to enter the Western Medical Model's "disease club," if they can be shown to involve specific sub-organs or regions of the brain (the thalamus, nucleus accumbens, dorsal tegmentum, and part of the pre-frontal cortex), a defect in that organ or region (depleted dopamine and increasing cortisol levels typically associated with chronic stress), and the plethora of confusing symptoms (unpleasant survival behaviors characteristic of drug addicts and alcoholics who need their "fix," and who steal cars, commit thefts, engage in drug trafficking and all that goes with it, disruptions of marriages and families, and child neglect, etc.).

According to The National Institute on Drug Abuse, currently there is said to be an epidemic of opiate addiction in Florida and elsewhere in the US along with the predictable symptoms of addiction-associated criminal (survival) behaviors. As a now "doctor-OK'd real disease," addiction deaths now claim about 10 people/day who die in various counties from Fentanyl prescription abuse overdoses (prescriptions that are typically initiated by doctor), and other drugs also. In 2017, Florida providers wrote 60.9 opioid prescriptions for every 100 persons compared to the average U.S. rate of 58.7 prescriptions for every 100 persons. This is the lowest rate since 2006 when this data became available (CDC). In 2017, there were more than 70,200 opioid drug overdose deaths in the U.S.–an age-adjusted rate of 21.7 per 100,000 persons. Among these, 47,600 involved opioids. The sharpest increase occurred among deaths involving fentanyl and fentanyl analogs (other synthetic narcotics) with more than 28,400 overdose deaths in 2017. Therefore, addictions provide a clear example of epidemic and endemic (behavioral) disease.

Yet who could have predicted this opiate epidemic, or the British motives for the opium trade that went on during previous eras in China and throughout the world as best described in the Nancy Turner Banks, M.D.; AIDS, Opium, Diamonds, and Empire, The deadly virus of international greed, May. 2010, iUniverse.incorporated publishers).

DISEASE PROGRESSION DESPITE ANTIBODIES

It has been argued that HIV cannot cause AIDS because the body develops HIV-specific antibodies following primary infection (Duesberg, 1992). This reasoning ignores numerous examples of viruses other than HIV that can be pathogenic after evidence of immunity appears (Oldstone, 1989). Primary poliovirus infection is a classic example of a disease in which high titers of neutralizing antibodies develop in all infected individuals, yet a small percentage of individuals develop subsequent paralysis (Kurth, 1990). The entire AIDS era was a refutation of Jenner-a positive test meant you were going to die (unless you consumed life-ending cancer drugs like AZT.

It is believed that some viruses such as herpes virus and measles virus may persist for years in brain cells, eventually causing a chronic neurological disease despite the presence of antibodies (Gershon, 1990), IF the measles virus existed in the first place! Viruses such as cytomegalovirus, herpes simplex and varicella zoster may be activated after years of latency even in the presence of abundant antibodies (Weiss and Jaffe, 1990). “Lentiviruses” as “slow viruses” conjured up by “slow virologists with their imagined long and variable latency periods, such as visna virus in sheep, have been postulated to cause central nervous system damage even after the specific production of neutralizing antibodies (Haase, 1990). Furthermore, a litany is always chanted regarding how it is now so well-documented that HIV can mutate rapidly to circumvent all barriers to its replication and persistence.”

What this line of AIDS-company reasoning lacks is the ending of a sentence or two:

...high titers of neutralizing antibodies develop in all “infected” (naturally infected? vaccine infected?) individuals, yet a small percentage of individuals develop subsequent paralysis because that molecular marker or virus may have nothing to do with why paralysis (in this case) had occurred.

If you accept the premise that the universe is finite, or even if you do not, it has been said that the adaptive immune system since the appearance of the most primitive chordates some 800 million years ago (animals possessing a notochord) is capable of generating some 1016 possible different kinds of lymphocyte receptors (Laird et al., PNAS Vol. 97, No. 13, June 20, 2000). At present, synthetic antigens and antibodies are frequently used to “manufacture” immune responses made to order, because it is known that the immune system can generate responses even to molecules that have never existed in this universe. Or maybe this is not the way to think about how Nature has devised an immune system against non-self?

Amoebas will spit out microinjections of foreign amoebas because they can recognize molecules from other amoebas as non-self. Therefore, every cell might have the potential to recognize, and eliminate foreign molecules? Perhaps these other, simpler mechanisms can explain how the human immune system generates antibodies, or protection against disease. Antibody generation apparently is protective but is not protective in the case of “HIV,” and other suspected infectious molecular disease seroconversion profiles. With the understanding that evolution through natural selection has provided us with a mechanism for recognizing, and neutralizing (with neutralizing antibodies) a daunting number of different non-self-molecules. How can we reconcile the facts that "HIV" is recognized as foreign in 33 million "infected" carriers walking around at the moment, but these same molecules cannot induce the immune system to make an effective neutralizing antibody when the molecule is presented in the form of a vaccine? The AIDS era has run the gauntlet of lies demonstrating beyond any doubts, that vaccines do not work.

Given these concerns, what then should be done regarding all the healthy carriers of a particular molecular signature when universal testing programs are set into place and begin to record the inevitable high false-positive rates that will accumulate among "low risk" groups? Perhaps those of us who have tried to figure out or predict connections between molecular signatures and diseases should ask ourselves: if 1 out of 100, or 1 out of 1,000, or 1 out of 1,000,000 develop clinical illness although all may test positive for a particular molecular signature, while 99, 999, or 999,999 don't show clinical symptoms, are there any diseases or molecular signatures tied to certain disease states, like the ones discussed here, using any of the current paradigms, really caused by viruses? All of the molecular tests appear to be grievously non-predictive, and non-explanatory for any of these syndromes or their associated signatures or markers.

For example, those who harbor positive molecular signatures for "HIV" and are immunosuppressed, there is substantial evidence in the peer-reviewed scientific and medical literature to warrant changing the acronym "AIDS," which stands for Acquired Immune Deficiency Syndrome, to "AAIDS," which would represent Acquired Auto-Immune Deficiency Syndrome.

Such a change in nomenclature would represent and incorporate a major paradigm shift in our thinking about autoimmunity more generally, especially with respect to the way the immune system can target various tissues of the body, including itself, through such mechanisms as molecular mimicry, oxidation, serial infections, multiple-antigen-mediated-autoimmunity (MAMA), nutritional collapse, drug toxicity, and others.

If correct, this scenario, in turn, when examined in some depth, will hopefully lead to effective ways to reverse immune suppression in certain types of "AIDS" patients that are new and innovative approaches that have never been implemented in any large clinical trial that has focused on virus suppression.

Furthermore, the suggested change in "AIDS" nomenclature is not intended to be provocative. Such a change constitutes a necessary theoretical advance that is required in order to ask better questions. The state of our knowledge regarding the cell biology of the immune system, vaccines and vaccine adjuvants, cancer biology, epidemiology, test-kit development for viral pathogenesis, and many other areas which all point to huge gaps in current thinking regarding polio "virus," measles "virus," "AIDS" "virus(es)," "hepatitis B "viruses,"(HBV), "hepatitis C "viruses" (HCV), "human papilloma "virus" (HPV), "Human T-Cell Lymphotrophic "viruses" (HTLV-I,II, III) that all were shown to be fraudulent viruses before the AIDS era because Dr. Robert Gallo of the NIH didn't think the atomic bombs dropped on Japan in 1945 had anything to do with those populations in which he found HTLV-I and II, before claiming he found HTLV-III which became the AIDS virus, "HIV."

Other "molecular diseases" have advanced the same deceptions, and their "molecular signatures" are also in-frequently associated with any definable disease states. These gaps exist because it is not yet unknown how and under what circumstances the development of autoimmunity occurs in a wide spectrum of diseases.

1996 DTAP licensed; recommended for use instead of whole-cell DPT.

1996 Roche warns on its package insert that "The amplicor HIV-1 monitor test is not intended to be used as a screening test for HIV, nor as a diagnostic test to confirm the presence of HIV infection" (Roche's amplicor HIV-1 monitor test package insert, 1996) [a doctor is needed to determine if you are black, Hispanic, gay, OR even healthy enough for sexual activity, and would be an irresponsible physician if he doesn't ask who you slept with in the past].

1996 Hib-HepB combo licensed.

1996 De Serres, Gaston, MD, MPH, Boulianne N., MSC, Duval, B. MD, Déry, P. MD, Rodrigquez, A. M., MD, Massé, R., MD, and Halperin, S. MD, "[Ineffectiveness-emphasis mine] Effectiveness of whole cell pertussis vaccine in child-care centers and schools", The Pediatric Infectious Disease Journal, 1996;15:519-524

"Despite the high rate of pertussis vaccine coverage in children between the 2 and 9 years of age, pertussis was a common illness in these preschool and school age children. Although the whole cell vaccine was demonstrated to be effective, estimates of vaccine effectiveness were lower than the estimated in the United States and elsewhere. ... In those studies, a different whole cell vaccine manufactured by Connaught Laboratories Inc. (Swiftwater, PA) had an efficacy of 48% in Sweden and 36% in Italy."

1996 872 serious adverse events reported to VAERS in children under 14 years of age who had been injected with hepatitis B vaccine. 48 children were reported to have died after they were injected with hepatitis B vaccine that same year. By contrast, in 1996 only 279 cases of hepatitis B disease were reported in children under age 14.

HEPATITIS B VACCINE ACTUALLY CAUSED MORE ILLNESS THAN THE DISEASE BY A 20 TO 1 RATIO

1996 In 1996 only 54 cases of hepatitis B were reported in the 0-1 age group. There were 3.9 million births that year, so the observed incidence of hepatitis B in the 0-1 age group was just 0.001 %. VAERS received 1,080 total reports of adverse reactions from hepatitis B vaccine in 1996 in that same age group including 47 deaths. The hepatitis B vaccine actually caused more illness than the disease by a 20 to 1 ratio.

1996 – The 10 Stages of Genocide by Stanton

The Gregory Stanton paper was presented at the State Department in 1996, shortly after the Rwandan genocide, but it also analyzes the processes in the Holocaust, the Cambodian genocide, and other genocides. The preventive measures suggested are those that the United States, national governments, and United Nations could implement or influence other governments to implement.

#	Stage	Characteristics	Preventive measures
1	Classification	People are divided into "them and us".	"The main preventive measure at this early stage is to develop universalistic institutions that transcend… divisions."
2	Symbolization	"When combined with hatred, symbols may be forced upon unwilling members of pariah groups…"	"To combat symbolization, hate symbols can be legally forbidden as can hate speech".
3	Discrimination	"Law or cultural power excludes groups from full civil rights: segregation or apartheid laws, denial of voting rights".	"Pass and enforce laws prohibiting discrimination. Full citizenship and voting rights for all groups."
4	Dehumanization	"One group denies the humanity of the other group. Members of it are equated with animals, vermin, insects, or diseases."	"Local and international leaders should condemn the use of hate speech and make it culturally unacceptable. Leaders who incite genocide should be banned from international travel and have their foreign finances frozen."
5	Organization	"Genocide is always organized… Special army units or militias are often trained and armed…"	"The U.N. should impose arms embargoes on governments and citizens of countries involved in genocidal massacres, and create commissions to investigate violations"

6	Polarization	"Hate groups broadcast polarizing propaganda..."	"Prevention may mean security protection for moderate leaders or assistance to human rights groups...Coups d'état by extremists should be opposed by international sanctions."
7	Preparation	"Mass killing is planned. Victims are identified and separated out because of their ethnic or religious identity..."	"At this stage, a Genocide Emergency must be declared. Full diplomatic pressure by regional organizations must be invoked, including preparation to intervene to prevent genocide."
8	Persecution	"Expropriation, forced displacement, ghettos, concentration camps".	"Direct assistance to victim groups, targeted sanctions against persecutors, mobilization of humanitarian assistance or intervention, protection of refugees."
9	Extermination	"It is 'extermination' to the killers because they do not believe their victims to be fully human".	"At this stage, only rapid and overwhelming armed intervention can stop genocide. Real safe areas or refugee escape corridors should be established with heavily armed international protection."
10	Denial	"The perpetrators... deny that they committed any crimes..."	"The response to denial is punishment by an international tribunal or national courts"

1997 "Polio is not eradicated by vaccination, but likely lurks behind a disease redefinition and new diagnostic names like viral or aseptic meningitis.......According to one of the 1997 issues of the MMWR, there are some 30,000 to 50,000 cases of viral meningitis per year in the United States alone. That's where it is thought that 30,000 – 50,000 cases of polio disappeared after the introduction of mass vaccination."

"Today, various other forms of the word "polio" are still used to describe the effects of poisoning, though usually with regard to paralysis in animals. A search of Medline ("polio" and "poison") finds about 45 contemporary articles where poisoning causality is attributed to polio. The terminology found was: "polioencephalomalacia", "poliomyelomalacia", "polyradiculoneuritis", "neurological picture similar to that of poliomyelitis", "polioencephalomyelomalacia", "lumbal poliomyelomalacia", "cerebrocortical necrosis (polioencephalomalacia)", "Lead poisoning in grey-headed fruit bats (Pteropus poliocephalus)", "multifocal-poliomyelomalacia", "spinal poliomalacia", "Polio and high-sulfate diets", "atypical porcine enterovirus encephalomyelitis: possible interaction between enteroviruses and arsenicals", "polioencephalomalacia and photosensitization associated with kochia scoparia consumption in range cattle", "bovine polioencephalomalacia." Viral or aseptic meningitis, Guillaine Barre Syndrome (GBS), Chinese paralytic syndrome, chronic fatigue syndrome, epidemic cholera, cholera morbus, spinal meningitis, spinal apoplexy, inhibitory palsy, intermittent fever, famine fever, worm fever, bilious remittent fever, ergotism, ME, post-polio syndrome, acute flaccid paralysis (Jim West, Health and Research Publications).

1997 de Melker HE, et al. Pertussis in The Netherlands: an outbreak despite high levels of immunization with whole-cell vaccine. Emerg Infect Dis. 1997 Apr-Jun;3(2):175-8. PMID: 9204299; UI: 97348248.

BIRDS CATCH COLD FLUS TOO, BUT IT ISN'T PASSED FROM PERSON TO PERSON AND THE ENTIRE CHICKEN POPULATION OF HONG KONG IS SLAUGHTERED: THE BIRD INFLUENZA ERA BEGINS

1997 (April) Bird flu "virus" "H5N1" was isolated for the first time from a human patient in Hong Kong. "The virus" infected 18 patients who had had close contact with poultry, with six deaths. The virus did not spread from person to person. Within days of the press release, Hong Kong's entire chicken population was slaughtered to prevent further outbreak.

1997 Abbott labs warned that "ELISA testing alone could not be used to diagnose AIDS (Abbott Package HIV-I ELISA Test Kit insert, 1997) [because a doctor is needed to determine if you are black, hispanic, or gay, and to ask who you slept with in the past].

1997 It was reported that "no seroconversions" were observed among 175 HIV-discordant couples (where one partner tests positive, one negative), for a total of approximately 282 couple-years of follow up in a 10- year study (Padian, et al. Heterosexual Transmission of HIV in Northern California: Results from a Ten-Year Study." American Journal of Epidemiology. August, 1997).

1997 The biotech company Epitope warned on its package insert, "Do not use this kit as the sole basis for HIV infection" (Epitope HIV-I Western Blot Test Kit insert, 1997) [again, a doctor is needed to determine if you are black, hispanic, or gay, and to ask who you slept with in the past].

1997 News and Views Nature Medicine 3, 17 – 18 (1997) doi:10.1038/nm0197-17. **Live-attenuated HIV vaccines: How safe is safe enough?** Michael Murphey-Corb

Tulane Regional Primate Research Center, 18703 Three Rivers Road, Covington, Louisiana 70433, USA. "A live-attenuated SIV vaccine inducing protection in healthy adult monkeys appears both safe and effective but may be lethal when given in high doses to newborns.

THE BIRD FLU ERA STARTS CASHING OUT

1997 US Defense Secretary Donald Rumsfeld served as Gilead (Research)'s chairman from 1997 until he joined the Bush administration in 2001, and he held a Gilead stake valued at between $5 million and $25 million, according to federal financial disclosures filed by Rumsfeld. The forms did not reveal the exact number of shares Rumsfeld owned. Gilead made a loss in 2003, the year before concern about bird flu started. Then revenues from Tamiflu almost quadrupled, from $35 to $44.6 million, helping put the company well into the black. Sales almost quadrupled again, to $161.6 million in 2005. Mr Rumsfeld sold some of his Gilead shares in 2004 reaping – according to the financial disclosure report he is required to make each year – capital gains of > $5m (£2.9 million). The report showed that he still had up to $25m-worth of shares at the end of 2004.

Rumsfeld was not the only political heavyweight benefiting from demand for Tamiflu, which is manufactured and marketed by Swiss pharma giant Roche (Gilead receives a royalty from Roche equaling about 10% of sales). Former Secretary of State George Shultz, who was on Gilead's board, sold more than $7 million worth of Gilead since the beginning of 2005. Another board member was the wife of former California Gov. Pete Wilson.

The Pentagon ordered $58 million worth of the treatment for U.S. troops around the world, and Congress considered making a multi-billion-dollar purchase. Rumsfeld recused himself from any decisions involving Gilead when he left Gilead and became Secretary of Defense in early 2001.

(http://money.cnn.com/2005/10/31/news/newsmakers/fortune_rumsfeld/index.htm).

1997 Two teams of investigators, one consisting of a French-German collaboration [Gluschankof P, Mondor I, Gelderblom HR, Sattentau QJ. Virology. Mar 31;230(1):125-33, 1997], and another whose investigators were involved in the AIDS Vaccine Program, SAIC, National Cancer Institute-Frederick Cancer Research and Development Center, Maryland [Bess JW Jr, Gorelick RJ, Bosche WJ, Henderson LE, Arthur LO. Virology, Mar 31; 230(1):134-44, 1997]. The teams reported that:

PHA (phytohemagglutinin) and IL2 (interleukin-2) stimulated healthy cells to produce Human Immunodeficiency "viral like particles" and the molecular signatures of "HIV" only when stimulated with PHA and IL-2. They also claimed that: "macrovesicles were a source of contaminating cellular proteins found in purified HIV-1 preparations," as their titles of their papers suggest:

"Cell membrane vesicles are a major contaminant of gradient-enriched human immunodeficiency virus type-1 preparations" (Gluschankof et al.,1997).

"Microvesicles are a source of contaminating cellular proteins found in purified HIV-1 preparations" (Bess et al., 1997).

This work not only underscored the problem that there are no tissue or cell culture models of "HIV's pathogenic effect, but these facts raised issue regarding the basis of Gallo's and Montagnier's isolation and challenged National academy member Peter Duesberg's claims that the nucleic acids have been uniquely cloned, discrediting the hypothesis that the signature of "HIV" is due to ANY virus. Duesberg was vilified thereafter by the AIDS establishment.

In the Bess et al. paper, they also reported that "cellular debris was not distinguishable from other objects in the electron micrographs," and the Bess et al. authors specifically emphasized that:

"Identification and analysis of the virus are complicated by the presence of cellular membrane vesicles which COPURIFY (my emphasis) with the virus."

By another group it was reported that when certain proteolytic procedures are employed that effectively removed greater than 95% of proteins associated with membrane vesicles. This procedure also revealed that the cytoskeletal proteins, actin, ezrin, moesin, and cofilin were located in the interior of the "HIV" virions. (Ott et al., 1995b).

Such "advancements" in "HIV" isolation raised questions such as:

If the cell's cytoskeletal proteins, actin, exrin, and other proteins are located INSIDE the virions, how can one tell if p24, for instance, which is a faint band on most cellular gels that come from non-"HIV–infected" cells in most labs, if p24 and the other molecules thought to represent the specific molecules of "HIV" aren't also proteins of cellular origin?

Another important observation of Bess et al. Was that PHA activated human PBLs were also shown to produce micro vesicles that incorporated cellular proteins.

DIVISION OF AIDS (DAIDS) SAYS EVERYBODY'S GOT "HIV'S" CAPSID PROTEIN IN THEIR CELLS, BUT TO CONVICT ONLY THOSE WITH MORE THAN 30pg/ml P24 PROTEIN.

1997 The DAIDS official "HIV" culturing manual was published presenting a series of standard protocols for culturing "HIV." From the Reporting Results Section (section VII), a rationale was presented to unequivocally identify " HIV-infected" cells as truly "infected" by "HIV" cell culturing labs if:

Two consecutive HIV p24 antigen VQA CORRECTED values of > 30 pg/ml (from a healthy donor source), of which the second value is at least four times greater than the first value or out of range" (O.D.>2) or

Two consecutive HIV p24 antigen VQA CORRECTED values (from a healthy donor source) that are out of range" (Optical density.> 2); or

Three consecutive HIV p24 antigen VQA CORRECTED values of > 30 pg/ml (from a healthy donor source), where neither consecutive value is > four times the previous sample, but the third value is at least four times greater than the first.

1997 Poland, Gregory A., "Still more questions on pertussis vaccines", The Lancet, November 29, 1997, Vol. 350, pp. 1564-1565. "Despite sharply reducing severe pertussis and pertussis deaths, whole-cell vaccines have not stopped circulation of Bordetella in the population, do not induce sustained protective immunity, and are precluded from routine use as boosters in adolescents and adults because of their side-effects. In addition, questions about safety and efficacy remain."

1998 Hepatitis B Vaccine was linked to autoimmune rheumatoid diseases.

1998 15,000 French citizens filed a lawsuit against the French government for understating the risks and overstating the benefits associated with the hepatitis B vaccine. Hundreds of people were reported to have suffered from auto immune and neurological disorders, including multiple sclerosis, following hepatitis B vaccination. As a result, in October 1998, the French Minister of Health ended the mandatory hepatitis B vaccination program for all school children. "The French decision to continue hepatitis B immunization at birth while discontinuing immunization starting at school age suggests the French Ministry of Health may believe that they can decrease vaccine induced autoimmunity by giving vaccines starting in the first month of life. They appear to be accepting our findings" (Classen http://www.healing-arts.org/children/vaccines/vaccines-information.htm).

1998 Although infants and children are targeted by the hepatitis B vaccine, one of the initial target populations for the hepatitis B vaccine had been prostitutes and drug addicts, and although France had repealed the mandate because of high number of vaccine injuries, the CDC eventually admitted that the vaccine may not be effective after 7 yrs. for 30-50% of the infants vaccinated, so that when they grow up to become drug addicts and prostitutes, they are not protected,

1998 The hepatitis B Vaccine is mandated for school age children in first 46 and then 48 states in the US.

"HIV's" MOST IMPORTANT MOLECULE, REVERSE TRANSCRIPTASE IS FOUND IN CHICKEN VACCINES, AND IS DESTROYED WITH DNASE (reverse transcriptase is a protein, not a nucleic acid that would be sensitive to DNASE)

1998 The Center for Biologics Evaluation and Research Advisory Committee on Vaccines and Related Biological Products claimed in November in a chapter regarding the Update on Reverse Transcriptase Activity in Chicken Cell Derived Vaccines, by Dr. Arifa Khan (pages 13-15), that:

Initially Boni et al. (1996) published that low level reverse transcriptase activity was detected in ALL chicken cell derived vaccines using an overly sensitive PCR-based reverse transcriptase assay called PERT, which can detect one to ten virions which was reported to the WHO, and then additional studies were done by several laboratories in Europe, as well as the U.S., including the NIBSC, the CDC, as well as labs in the FDA to confirm this initial finding. However, after further work, it was discovered that this reverse transcriptase activity could be eliminated by treatment of extracts with DNAase, and that using Alu-based EAV sequence integration studies, that no integration of anything derived from the chicken cell supernatants was detected in Human PBMC cells.

1998 (November) Data from France released at the 62nd Annual Meeting of the American College of Rheumatology, held November 8-12, 1998, in San Diego, California links immunization against hepatitis B to the development of autoimmune rheumatoid diseases such as lupus and rheumatoid arthritis. The rise of autoimmunity following hepatitis B immunization in school children and adults has become a major public health concern. In October, the Ministry of Health in France suspended routine hepatitis B immunization of school children while continuing hepatitis B immunization at birth. The reason for this decision was reportedly the increased risk of autoimmune diseases that has been associated with the vaccine when it is given starting at school age or later. The data from France links hepatitis B immunization to both the development of newly diagnosed cases of autoimmune rheumatoid diseases as well as the exacerbation of previously diagnosed cases that were in remission. This finding is supported by data from Canada published in September which linked immunization against hepatitis B to the development of autoimmune rheumatoid diseases in firefighters.

"The data from humans and animals is noticeably clear, when you stimulate the immune system with vaccines you increase the risk of autoimmunity and exacerbate smoldering inflammatory conditions. Vaccine induced autoimmunity is a major public health problem because of the number of vaccine doses given and the large percentage of people with undiagnosed inflammatory conditions. We need to develop ways of giving vaccines without increasing the risk of autoimmune diseases" (Classen).

1998 Lyme vaccine (Lymerix) licensed.

1998 Paul Offit's rotavirus vaccine recommended by CDC for universal use in infants.

1998 The Cambridge Biotech HIV-1 Western Blot Kit insert warns: "The clinical implications of antibodies to HIV-1 in an asymptomatic person are not known." (The Cambridge Biotech HIV-1 Western Blot Kit, 1998).

1998 (August) Paul Offit's rotavirus vaccine licensed.

1998 (Sept). Johns Hopkins Newsletter Nov. 1998 stated Alzheimer's incidence would quadruple in coming years. According to Hugh Fudenberg, MD (the world's leading immunogeneticist, author of nearly 850 papers in peer-reviewed journals): "Individuals who have had five consecutive flu shots between 1970 and 1980 (years studied) have a ten times higher chance of getting Alzheimer's disease than if they had one, two or no shots... due to the mercury and aluminum in every flu shot. The gradual mercury and aluminum buildup in the brain causes cognitive dysfunction."

Also, in 1998, the head of the Swiss and European Blood Banks, the late Dr. Alfred Hassig (1921-1999) and his associates, including Dr. Hans Kremer (a specialist in drug addiction medicine), and a virologist (Stephan Lanka), made a series of claims suggesting that:

"The question of the specificity of the anti-HIV antibody test has to be re-evaluated as it was shown that the viral enrichment obtained from co-cultivations of patients lymphocytes with fetal cord blood by Barre-Sinouussi et al. and leukemia cells by Gallo et al., exclusively consisted of proteins of the cell types used in the cell culture. This precludes a clear separation of presumed retroviral and cellular proteins or extracellular matrix proteins. In this context it was shown that the anti-HIV antibody test detects autoimmune antibodies directed against cytoskeletal proteins e.g., the liver cells. Strongly augmented anti-actin autoantibodies is considered close to pathognomonic for chronically active hepatitis."

"The original assumption that reverse transcription from RNA to DNA is evidence for the existence of retroviruses was wrong. In fact, reverse transcription is a vital mechanism for the maintenance of the genome. The decrease in numbers of circulating lymphocytes can be explained by a stress-induced hyper-cortisolism. Up to date, direct HIV-mediated destruction of CD4 lymphocytes could not be proved. The same is true for the measuring of the "viral load." Shortcomings of the applied method to quantify the "viral load" do not permit definitive conclusions. Possibly, it may be taken as an expression of a stress induced weakening of the cellular immune reactions, in the course of which, nucleoside fragments resulting from the current cell turnover are inadequately eliminated. Furthermore, the treatment of patients with nucleoside analogs has a toxic effect on both the genome of the cell nucleus and the mitochondria. The latter, therefore, may produce insufficient amounts of ATP, causing organ failure and, eventually, death. The synthetic protease inhibitors used these days are associated with serious side-effects. Therefore, it seems worthwhile, in these patients, to bring back the catabolic situation of whole-body inflammation to homeostasis by administering anabolic phyto-polyenolic compounds."

In March, 1998, an "AIDS Alert" article on rapid tests appeared claiming:

Whether the tests will perform as well in the United States as they have abroad is still unknown, experts add. For one thing, using a single rapid test in a low-prevalence population will give a lower positive predictive value....That error rate will not matter much in areas with a high prevalence of HIV because in all probability the people testing false-positive will have the disease. But if the same test was performed on 1,000 white, affluent suburban housewives – a low-prevalence population – in all likelihood all positive results will be false, and positive predictive values plummet to zero. (Coming to your clinic: Candidates for Rapid Tests. Aids Alert, March 1998).

Translation: This is why the test kits cannot diagnose "HIV" infection: the physician has to observe with his own eyes if the person is black, hispanic, homosexual, and ask whom they slept with last night to diagnose "HIV/AIDS." There has never been one convincing demonstration that the so-called "AIDS virus," "HIV" has been isolated or even exists: at the level of electron microscopy, "HIV" was determined to be cellular garbage or debris. Gonda determined this when Gallo sent him the first so-called samples of "HIV."

This information has been suppressed to invent a world panic and justify the stigmatization of entire groups such as gay persons, Africans, African Americans, Hispanic peoples, and anyone else the Government deemed useless eaters.

HOW TO READ "AIDS" SCIENCE: DETERMINING SEROCONVERSION FROM VACCINES VERSUS TRUE "HIV" INFECTION DEPENDS ON WHAT SIZE YOUR CITY IS, COMMUNICATION, AND EMERGENCY PHONE NUMBERS

http://wwwn.cdc.gov/MLP/pdf/labhiv/TEvans.pdf.

1998 CONFERENCE ON THE LABORATORY SCIENCE OF HIV TESTING IN HIV-VACCINATED POPULATIONS. Thomas G. Evans, M.D., University of Rochester, Rochester, NY, Wednesday, September 16, 1998.

"Many problems arise in relation to vaccine testing and HIV 1 serology. Among the most complicated of these is the possibility of false HIV positive results appearing on serological tests. Such a result can have a number of possible consequences, including constraints on international travel, blood donation, military service, or health and life insurance. In addition, there can be discrimination from friends, employers and family."

"Such problems are only likely to become more magnified as increased testing of HIV 1 vaccine candidates moves into further Phase I, II, and III trials. At present there are six NIH-funded Phase I clinical trial sites of candidate HIV vaccines in the United

States. These include the University of Rochester, Vanderbilt University, University of Washington, the University of Alabama at Birmingham, St. Louis University, and Johns Hopkins University. These sites are primarily responsible for the Phase I and II trials that take place inside the AIDS Vaccine Evaluation Group (AVEG) of the NIH. These sites have been conducting trials of candidate HIV vaccines since 1998. There have been over 30 clinical trials which have used a variety of different vaccine approaches including subunit vaccines, peptide-based systems, canary pox vectors that encode most of the genes of HIV, Vaccinia vectors which also have encoded multiple genes, DNA vaccines, mucosal vaccines, Salmonella-based vaccines, and multiclade-based vaccines. To complicate matters further, these candidate vaccines have been given with over 10 different experimental adjuvants in these trials. The number of patients tested to date in these Phase I trials is not small. As of October 1998, over 2,600 seronegative volunteers had been enrolled in candidate HIV 1 vaccine trials. The majority of these volunteers have received vaccine and not placebo. Of these vaccines, approximately 2,000 were at low risk and approximately 500 at high risk. However, even low risk patients have some exposure risk. Evaluation in the AVEG reveals HIV 1 seroincidence in these Phase I trials ranging from 0.22% for low-risk individuals, up to 1.46% in the high-risk individuals. In these trials 32 individuals have become infected with HIV 1."

"This rate of infection potentially leads to a fairly major problem, that is, during vaccine trials, especially high-risk trials, there may be positive serology both from infection and from the vaccine itself. Distinguishing between these two conditions is obviously critically important."

"What percent of individuals that receive candidate HIV 1 vaccines will actually test positive?":

"The answer to this question lies in the serological tests used. (1)"

"When extremely specific serological tests are used which include reagents not included in the vaccine, the number of individuals testing positive is extremely low. However, when cell lysates or first- or second-generation ELISA tests are used, the rate can be fairly high. In initial trials of HIV 1 vaccines conducted in the early 1990's, approximately one half of all recipients of subunit gp160 and gp 120 vaccines tested positive by the Abbot HIV 1 second generation test at the time of their peak neutralization titer. However, now that these test kits are using synthetic peptides, the rate of testing positive has decreased. When tests are used based on the Sanofi kit which includes the immunodominant portions of gp41 and areas of pol, there is essentially little to no cross-reactivity with the gp120 vaccines."

"All gp160 vaccines that include the immunodominant epitopes of gp41 will tend to be problematic due to the fact that almost all commercially available testing is based on the that immunodominant sequence. In recent vaccine trials using canary pox vectors which encode multiple HIV genes and are boosted with gp120 subunits ("prime-boost"), the number of volunteers testing positive by the Abbot HIV 1/2 EIA is approximately 50% at the time of peak antibody titer. Persistence of these vaccine-induced antibody responses is quite variable. The antibody responses that are induced by subunit vaccines decline quickly over a three month to one year period. However, volunteers from AVEG trial 002, who received Vaccinia products which encoded gp160 and were boosted with subunit gp160 have had persistent antibody responses seen up to 10 years later."

"Are there any major implications for the numbers of individuals vaccinated?"

"In small cities such as Rochester and Nashville, the location of two of the AVEG units, it can be estimated that up to 100 people could have been positive due to vaccine trials rather than true infection when using blood bank screening methodologies that use an ELISA. In areas where only 2-3,000 individuals may be HIV positive, this could represent a significant number of the positive tests seen in the testing sites (vaccine-induced positives or "real positives-doesn't say)."

"Therefore, in cities that have vaccine units, close communication between health departments and the vaccine testing site is needed. Initially the number of such sites was relatively limited. They included the six AVEG sites mentioned above and the Phase II/III HIVNET sites in Chicago, San Francisco, New York, Denver, Philadelphia, Boston, Providence, and Seattle. However, with the initiation of the VaxGen Phase III efficacy trial of the bivalent gp120 subunit vaccine, the number of potentially affected individuals has markedly increased. This trial will enroll approximately 5,000 individuals in 50-60 centers across the United States. Two out of every three recipients will receive vaccine for a total vaccinated population of 3,333. Since the vaccine includes only the gp120 subunit, it would seem relatively simple to establish that a positive ELISA is not vaccine-[induced] by use of Western blot."

"However, in AVEG trials anywhere from 10-20% of individuals have a random falsely positive band at p24."

"If criteria are employed for interpreting Western blot which include one envelope band and a p24 band, then a large number of individuals that are vaccinated in this trial could eventually test positive if the Western Blot were interpreted by an inexperienced or uninformed interpreter. This trial will be further complicated by the fact that individuals will be receiving booster vaccines over three years and are likely to have high titer gp120 antibody responses during this entire vaccine period. The persistence of these vaccine responses after three years of immunization is not known at present."

"Do such false positive misinterpretations occur?"

"A number of these have occurred within the AVEG. One was published in the Lancet a year ago by Dr. David Schwartz from Johns Hopkins University.(2) In addition, a patient volunteer at another site who received a gp160 Vaccinia based vaccine with a gp160 boost had a Western blot interpreted as positive in a well-known research laboratory in the United States. He had an RNA PCR done which was also interpreted as positive. Follow-up at the site revealed his Western blot had not changed since vaccination. Two further RNA

PCRs, a DNA PCR, and a CD8+ co-culture revealed that this individual was not infected. However, he behaved as if he had been infected for over a six-month period. The cost of this workup was many thousands of dollars."

"It should be understood that this workup occurred approximately six years after initial vaccination. Thus, the potential problems from false positives are truly real. Basing tests on RNA PCR is also somewhat problematic. This is due to the fact that in some of the best surveys at present approximately 1-2% of sero-negative individuals may test falsely positive by RNA PCR. Although these false positives tend to have low absolute numbers (<10,000 copies), they can be problematic. For example, a physician may interpret an early ELISA or Western blot as potentially positive. An RNA PCR could be done which is also falsely positive. If that individual were quickly placed on very highly active antiretroviral therapy (HAART), as is now recommended, this could lead to a confusing situation. There may be no further seroconversion, negative follow-up PCR, and the physician or health care worker may inappropriately interpret the person as a transient infection and leave the patient on potentially toxic antiretroviral therapy. Such a scenario is not only somewhat likely but even probable with the number of individuals that will enter vaccine trials."

"What are the solutions to some of these problems?"

"The AVEG has used a photo identification card and an 800-telephone number. If a volunteer experiences social harm or problems, the number is called, and an intervention can occur. We have been successful at notifying insurance companies, employers, and other parties who have falsely interpreted vaccine-induced positive serology as being indicative of HIV 1 infection. The NIH has also stated that it will provide follow-up in NIH-sponsored vaccine trials as long as the individual tests seropositive by any conventional test used and licensed by the FDA. However, this may be more problematic because as individual pharmaceutical companies begin to undertake trials, the long-term follow-up of individuals in these company-based trials is not entirely clear. This situation is under consideration by the CDC, and appropriate guidelines will need to be developed. "It is also clear that as trials move forward, thought must be given to the methodology used to differentiate between seroconversion from the vaccine and from true infection. In the NIH-sponsored AVEG trials, an infection algorithm has been established, and can be accessed on the World Wide Web at http://www.emmes.com/avctn. This algorithm is then adapted specifically for each protocol depending upon the vaccine candidate that is tested. For some vaccines, a serological test can be a useful screen. There are a number of ELISA kits that are based merely on the gp41 subunit. Most of these are not presently licensed in the United States but can be used for research purposes. For example, if the Sanofi kit based on the gp41 and pol peptides is used, the number of serological false positives tend to be exceptionally low. Other kits made by other manufacturers that do not include pol are also quite useful."

"However, the use of full-length envelope vaccines that encode gp41, or the use of gp160 subunits can complicate the use of such serological testing. As previously stated, using the AVEG algorithms no identification of HIV 1 infection is ever made based on a single nucleic acid test. The belief is that the false positive rate is too high to take any chances on a single test. In addition, the FDA has not approved any nucleic acid-based test as a diagnostic test for HIV 1."

"Lastly, the AVEG and NIH are working in conjunction with CDC to test a number of rapid testing kits from different manufacturers around the world using sera from different vaccine trials. We hope to come up with specific algorithms that may work in the future."

"Dr. Robert Belshe and Robert Stein, Esq. of the AVEG have taken the lead in suggesting to the FDA language which is to be placed in the packaging of test kits. This exact language is now found in almost all test kits licensed in the United States. It is as follows: "A person who has antibodies to HIV 1 is assumed to be infected with the virus, except for a person who has participated in an HIV vaccine study may develop antibodies to the vaccine and may or may not be infected with HIV. Clinical correlation is indicated with appropriate counseling, medical evaluation, and additional testing to decide whether a diagnosis of HIV infection is accurate". This FDA language is included in the Sanufi kit, the Abbott kit, the Home Access kit, and the Murex SUDS kit. The use of multiple rapid testing mechanisms that are based on peptide-based sequences will also be extremely useful in algorithms for evaluating vaccine induced responses."

"It is also hoped that language similar to the above statement would be included in any algorithms adopted by the United States or the Association of Public Health Laboratories (APHL). Further information concerning the complex interaction between HIV candidate vaccines and serological testing can be found at the EMMES Corporation web site at http://www.emmes.com and at the NIH information number for serological testing, Ms. Mary Allen, 301-402-0846.In summary, when interpreting potential positive responses of HIV 1 serology, there is a need to remember the large number of vaccine recipients in the United States. The possibility for vaccine induced false positive responses will increase as further trials are undertaken in the United States."

1. Belshe RB, Clements ML, Keefer MC, Graham BS, Corey L, Sposto R, Wescott S, Lawrence D, NIAID AIDS Vaccine Clinical Trials Group. Interpreting HIV serodiagnostic test results in the late 990s: Social risks of HIV vaccine studies in uninfected volunteers. Ann Intern Med 1994:121:584-589.Schwartz DH, Laeyendeckar OB, Arango-Jaramillio S, Castillo RC, Reynolds MJ. Extensive evaluation of a seronegative participant in an HIV-1 vaccine trial as a result of false-positive PCR. Lancet 1997;350:25- 259.

1999 It was published in The Journal, AIDS, that children born to ZDV-treated mothers: "are more likely to have a rapid course of HIV-1 infection compared with children born to untreated mothers, as disease progression and immunological deterioration are significantly more rapid, and the risk of death is actually increased during the first 3 years of life." In 1999, it was also known that goat and cow proteins cause "HIV-positive" reactions.

On August 3, 1999, Dr. Howard Urnovitz testifies before The Committee on Government Reform that he does not want to vaccinate people against their own genes to cause adverse events with

"HIV subtype O." Here is the written testimony of Dr. Howard B. Urnovitz to the Committee on Government Reform and Oversight was presented claiming that:

House of Representatives I am grateful to this committee for allowing me to address the issue of vaccine safety. I am Dr. Howard B. Urnovitz. In 1979, I received my doctorate degree in Microbiology and Immunology from the University of Michigan, where I studied vaccines. I am testifying today as the Scientific Director of the Chronic Illness Research Foundation. For the record, I am also the chief science officer of a biotechnology corporation.

My testimony will describe the insights of recent scientific studies into the health consequences of exposing individuals to both toxic and foreign biologic materials, particularly multiple bacterial and live virus vaccines. The conventional wisdom concerning the use of vaccines needs to be reconsidered, considering the adverse medical effects that vaccines can have on the human body. Vaccine science must evaluate not only acute adverse side effects, but also possible associated chronic illnesses such as learning and behavior disorders, Autism Spectrum Disorders, intussusception, arthritis, cancer, diabetes, chronic fatigue syndrome, multiple sclerosis, autoimmune thyroiditis, and other chronic health problems. These chronic illnesses are increasingly costly to society in both human and financial terms.

By year's end, the Chronic Illness Research Foundation and its research colleagues will have published four peer-reviewed papers on the genetic basis of four different chronic diseases: vaccine associated human cancers, Gulf War Syndrome, multiple sclerosis, and AIDS. The implications of these findings for vaccine safety are:

...the human body retains a genetic memory of the foreign substances to which it has been exposed, including viral and bacterial vaccines; 2. each individual respond to foreign substances differently, based on his or her own unique genetic background;3. there appears to be a limit on how much foreign material to which the human body can be exposed before some level of genetic damage occurs and a chronic disease initiate.

It is known that our genetic blueprints for life, received from our mother and father, create new genetic material, allowing each individual to cope with toxic environmental exposures. Research needs to focus more intensely on precisely how the body handles the unprecedented level of gene-damaging substances in our air, water, food and even some medicines. These substances range from infectious agents, both natural and vaccine-related; pesticides, herbicides, petroleum by-products and other synthetic chemical hazards; and physical hazards such as radiation. Regarding vaccine safety, I suggest the initiation of serious inquiries into the following research areas:

How do genes change in response to vaccines, and what are the chronic consequences of these changes?

What are the acceptable limits of dose, age, timing, and combinations of vaccines that the body can handle? (Not only with respect to their ability to create an immune response to the infectious agent, but also with respect to their acute and chronic health effects).

How might we minimize vaccine adverse effects on our genome through lifestyle, diet, and pharmaceutical intervention?

How can we repair or minimize the effects of genetic damage?

Today, we are beginning to understand the indirect mechanisms that link toxic exposures and chronic disorders. Unfortunately, efforts by scientists to explore fully the possible negative effects of vaccines mandated by public policy has been met with stiff resistance by public health agencies.

Let me give you two examples of vaccine programs that are underway that lack a solid scientific foundation. First, several of my colleagues and I currently have a peer-reviewed paper in a major medical journal due out in September that contains the medical profile of a woman who died from a mysterious case of AIDS. Over several years, her laboratory tests showed a consistent pattern of negative or indeterminate HIV-1 blood antibody tests.

However, when an alternative fluid test was used, she was HIV-1 antibody positive in her urine. The virus was eventually isolated from this woman and sequenced. This HIV-1 variant came to be known as HIV-1 Group O. Analyses of the viral genetic material suggest that the virus originated, in part, from genetic reshuffling of human chromosomal material. HIV-1 could have serious consequences with respect to the initiation of autoimmune diseases. To put it simply, are we embarking on a course that will vaccinate people against their own genes?

The second example concerns the intensive effort to create a vaccine for the hepatitis C virus. If you read the literature very carefully, you will find that, while there is a strong marker for the disease, there is no hard scientific evidence to support the existence of a hepatitis C virus. Clearly, a non-A, non-B hepatitis disease exists, but the science behind an associated virus is weak at best. As a scientist I am compelled to ask, how can we vaccinate people against a disease-causing agent that has not been fully characterized?

Protecting the public against vaccine related chronic diseases is and will be a difficult task. Not only must researchers meet the scientific challenges, but increasingly they also must battle the politics of science. Research is showing that our understanding of chronic diseases, as illustrated by my two examples, often is seriously inadequate. Because the issue of vaccine safety involves both policy and science, the public needs to be better represented in the decisions made by public health agencies. In this realm, where science and politics collide, Congress should take a more active role in representing the public interest during the formulation of public health policies.

On the issue of informed consent: Had my mother and father known that the poliovirus vaccines of the 1950s were heavily contaminated with more than 26 monkey viruses, including the cancer virus SV40, I can say with certainty that they would not have allowed their children and themselves to take those vaccines. Both of my parents might not have developed cancers suspected of being vaccine-related and might even be alive today. Government, industry, and medicine should embrace the ethical principle of informed consent about possible adverse reactions associated with vaccines.

I appreciate the opportunity to discuss with you my research findings that span a quarter of a century. I will continue to work with my colleagues to unravel the links between toxic exposures and chronic illnesses. While others seek to map the human genome, our goal is to study the detours the human body's genes must take to survive in an increasingly toxic environment. I ask that the full text of my statement be submitted for inclusion in the record of this hearing. Thank you.

1999 Tomaszunas-Blaszczyk J Zaklad [Pertussis in 1997]. Epidemiologii Panstwowego, Zakladu Higieny, Warszawa. Przegl Epidemiol 1999;53(1-2):23-32 [Article in Polish] "In 1997 an epidemic increase of pertussis was observed in Poland. The incidence was 5.4/100,000 population and was more than six times higher than in the preceding year. No clear reason for a sudden increase in pertussis incidence was found, in particular the vaccination coverage rates have remained high. In December 1997, the DTP vaccine coverage rate for children below two with four doses of DTP was 97.5%. The distribution of cases according to age during the last 20 years was analyzed and it was shown that since the beginning of the '90 a growing proportion of cases occurs among fully vaccinated children and the average age of the cases has a steadily growing tendency."

1999 (October) Paul Offit's rotavirus vaccine pulled off the market due to significant adverse reactions such as perforation of the intestine.

1999 The Lancet Volume 353, Number 9150 30 January 1999. Risk of diphtheria among school children in the Russian Federation in relation to time since last vaccination.

Quote: In 1993, the Russian Federation reported 15,229 cases of diphtheria, a 25-fold increase over the 603 cases reported in 1989.1 The incidence rate among children 7-10 years of age (15·7 per 100000) was twice that of adults aged 18 years or over (7·9 per

100000).4 81% of the affected children aged 7-10 years had been vaccinated with at least a primary series of diphtheria toxoid, and most had received the first booster recommended to be given 12 months after completion of the primary series.

So, it is pretty hard to ascribe low immunization rates as a cause for the outbreak of Diptheria. A much more likely explanation is the social disruption that was going on at the time of great political upheaval. Breakdown of hygiene, poverty, etc.

1999 It is published that children who drink goats and cow's milk sometimes test "HIV-positive" (Willman et al., Heterophile Antibodies to Bovine and Caprine Proteins Causing False-Positive Human Immunodeficiency Virus Type 1 and Other. Enzyme-Linked Immunosorbent Assay Results. Clinical and Diagnostic Laboratory Immunology, p. 615-616, Vol. 6, No. 4, July 1999).

1999 (April) Journal of Infectious Diseases, vol. 179, 915-923. "Temporal trends in the population structure of Bordetella pertussis during 1949-1996 in a highly vaccinated population."

Despite the introduction of large-scale pertussis vaccination in 1953 and high vaccination coverage, pertussis is still an endemic disease in The Netherlands, with epidemic outbreaks occurring every 3-5 years." One factor that might contribute to this is the ability of pertussis strains to adapt to vaccine-induced immunity, causing new strains of pertussis to re-emerge in this well-vaccinated population.

1999 (Sept) "There are no data or evidence of any harm caused by the level of exposure that some children may have encountered in following the existing immunization schedule. Infants and children who have received thimerosal-containing vaccines do not need to be tested for mercury exposure." Joint Statement of the American Academy of Pediatrics (AAP) and JAMA.

1999 Bykowski, M., Pertussis in Adults", OB GYN News, November 1, 1999,Vol. 34, p. 29 "It was formerly believed that infection or immunization conferred lifetime immunity, but now appears that any resultant immunity is in fact short lived. Thus, there is a growing interest in the selective reimmunization of adults, he said. And while pertussis was once considered uncommon in adults and older adolescents, it is now believed that the disease is endemic in these populations, who actually serve as the primary reservoir for pertussis, explained Dr. Ogle, professor of pediatrics at the University of Colorado, Denver. Studies from throughout the developed world suggest a 25%-30% of persistent coughing illness in these age groups is pertussis, he added.

1999 In a review of the early polio era, Hans J. Eggers (Milestones in Early Poliomyelitis Research, 1840 to 1949, Journal of Virology, June 1999, p. 4533-4535, Vol. 73, No. 60) the following claims were made, although they were not entirely accurate especially with regards to Ender's group's contributions and conclusions, albeit the conclusions appeared in the Journal Virology:

The history of the etpiology of poliomyelitis is a history of errors. I mention only the "coccus era," when several investigators were prejudiced by a supposed parallelism between poliomyelitis and meningitis epidemic.

However, all in all, bacteriological findings were negative; likewise, attempts to transmit the disease to the usual laboratory animals, such as rabbits, guinea pigs, or mice, failed. Landsteiner and Popper (14) injected intraperitoneally into two Old World monkeys (Cynocephalus hamadryas and Macacus rhesus) a suspension of spinal cord from a 9-year-old boy who had succumbed to severe poliomyelitis after four days of illness. The two monkeys, in good condition, had been available from previous experiments with syphilis. The inoculated material, which was bacteriologically sterile, yielded negative results when injected into rabbits, guinea pigs, and mice. The two monkeys, however, exhibited lesions in the spinal cord, medulla, pons, and brain stem that were indistinguishable from those observed in cases of human poliomyelitis. One of the monkeys, the rhesus monkey, developed complete flaccid paralysis of both legs. Landsteiner and Popper were unable to passage the agent, but this was achieved soon afterward and independently in 1909 by Römer (22), Flexner and Lewis (8), Leiner and von Wiesner (15), and Landsteiner and Levaditi (13)

As early as 1910, Flexner and Lewis (9) had cautiously suggested that poliovirus gained access to the central nervous system via the nasal mucosa, a hypothesis supported by experiments with monkeys performed by Flexner's group and by Leiner and von Wiesner: swabs containing poliovirus were introduced into the nose and rubbed vigorously over the upper nasal mucous membrane, with ensuing clinical poliomyelitis. Flexner's views on the strict neurotropism of poliovirus and on its entry into the body by the nasal route (see above) dominated polio virology so that other experimental evidence was more or less neglected for about 25 years until the 1930s. In particular, the exciting results of a young Swedish team consisting of Carl Kling, Wilhelm Wernstedt, and Alfred Pettersson published in 1912 (11, 12) were disregarded: the authors had demonstrated poliovirus in fatal and nonfatal cases of poliomyelitis, not only as expected from the oropharynx and trachea but also from the small intestine. Certainly, one possible interpretation of the presence of virus in the intestines was that it had been swallowed. But the clue of poliovirus present in the intestines and its pathogenic significance was not seriously pursued. Revival of poliovirus infection as an intestinal disease came mainly from the work of Trask and Paul at Yale University (20) and the definite report by Albert Sabin and Robert Ward in 1941 (26) on the natural history of human poliomyelitis. By meticulous technique (the authors performed necropsies of fatal polio cases themselves), they proved that the virus is distributed predominantly in two systems: (i) certain regions of the nervous system and (ii) the alimentary tract.

The presence of virus in the walls of the alimentary tract appeared to be the primary localization and portal of entry. Virus was absent in the nasal mucosa, olfactory bulbs, and anterior perforated substance, which suggested that neither the upper respiratory tract nor the olfactory pathway is of significance in cases of natural human poliomyelitis.

Another highpoint of poliovirus research was the finding in 1931 by the Australians Frank M. Burnet and Jean Macnamara (4) that there existed antigenic differences between strains of poliovirus. So far, a complete similarity of the different strains had been assumed. The Australian authors compared the famous Rockefeller MV strain with a local strain isolated in Melbourne and found striking differences in cross-immunity experiments and neutralization tests in monkeys. The report was treated with skepticism, since it came from unknown investigators on a remote continent. But in light of the ill-fated vaccine trials of 1935, the significance of this finding was particularly realized by Hammon, Francis, and Rivers (2). Finally, the question was settled by the Committee on Typing of the National Foundation for Infantile Paralysis early in the 1950s (5).

A further highlight of poliovirus research was the adaption of the Lansing strain of poliovirus to mice by the persistent efforts of Charles Armstrong in 1939 (1). This meant that at least one strain of poliovirus was available for research purposes in an animal far less expensive than the monkey.

Some years earlier Maurice Brodie et al. (3) had already tried with ingenious techniques to reproduce poliovirus in mice for Brodie's vaccine trials, but with the vaccine failures this work was neglected. All the more must Armstrong's persistence be admired. In this context it should be mentioned that Max Theiler (quoted by Paul [20]) in analogy to his work on yellow fever formed more than 150 mouse passages of the Lansing strain and observed a dramatic attenuation-a term used first by John Kolmer of Philadelphia- in connection with poliomyelitis vaccines of the virus after intracerebral inoculation of monkeys with results of from 100 to 0% paralysis. In passing, I should like to mention that among all contemporary virologists, it was Max Theiler and likewise John Enders who were highly regarded by Albert Sabin.

There were attempts as early as 1913 by Constantin Levaditi (16) to replicate poliovirus in tissue culture. But as Sabin and Olitsky (25) stated in their famous paper of 1936, "there is no unequivocal evidence that the virus of poliomyelitis has as yet been successfully cultivated outside the body.

Sabin and Olitsky used various carefully dissected tissues of 3- to 4-month-old human embryos, e.g., brain and cord, lungs, kidney, liver, and spleen. The virus was the already mentioned MV (mixed virus) strain of the Rockefeller Institute, a virus mixture prepared by H. L. Amoss in 1914 and kept for decades through numerous intracerebral passages in monkeys (23). The authors found that the virus multiplied readily only in the presence of nervous tissue, as evidenced by experiments with monkeys, including neutralization tests. The experiment appeared interesting at the time but of no practical value.

Despite this depressing failure and in view of the mounting evidence of the extra neural multiplication of poliovirus (see above), John Enders and his young collaborators Thomas Weller and Frederick Robbins made further attempts to cultivate poliovirus in vitro, in particular after Weller's successful cultivation of mumps virus in vitro. Enders and coworkers (7) demonstrated the dramatic replication of Lansing virus (testable in mice) in human embryonic cultures composed chiefly of skin, muscle, and connective tissue from the arms and legs, in cultures of human embryonic intestine, and in those of nervous tissue. It was Robbins who first recognized differences in cell morphology between inoculated and uninoculated cultures (24a). Enders coined the term cytopathic effects (CPE).The implications of this famous paper, published in Science on 28 January 1949, were enormous and well recognized by the authors but surprisingly not by all colleagues in poliomyelitis research, at least initially. Enders et al. readily demonstrated the multiplication of all three poliovirus types in various primate tissues, in particular in non-nervous tissues, and showed that large amounts of virus could be propagated in vitro, that cultures most sensitive to the isolation of virus could be obtained in abundant amounts, and that precise quantitation of infectious virus could easily be achieved. Furthermore, besides Gilbert Dalldorf's and Grace Sickles' (6) isolation in newborn mice of coxsackieviruses, another major group of enteroviruses pathogenic for humans, the soon to be recognized potential of cell culture techniques led to the discovery of echoviruses, likewise important agents of human disease.

2000 (September) "UNINFECTED" WOMEN TEND TO TEST POSITIVE

In 2000, it was reported that pregnant women test positive for "HIV" at high frequency, and the appearance of the so-called specific and unique antigens of an "HIV's" molecular signature thus shares common molecular epitopes (molecular configurations) with those detected during pregnancy of certain women. In September, the study was published in The Archives of Family Medicine about false positive and indeterminate HIV test results in pregnant women: As the number of women being screened has increased, the proportion of false-positive and ambiguous (indeterminate) test results has increased....(Archives of Family Medicine, Sep/Oct 2000).

2000 (July) The first of many failures of genital lesion-causing microbicides on Africans was reported from a study of several microbicide trials funded by The Gates foundation, where it was claimed that spermicide does not actually reduce any risk of transmission of "HIV's" molecular profiles, but actually increased the rate of the appearance of its profiles. This finding ran contrary to what is known about how safe sex practices, including condoms and spermicide (Maggie Fox. Spermicide worsens HIV risk, study finds. Reuters 12 July 2000):

2000 (March 21) The Los Angeles Times (Paul Jacobs, Peter G. Gosselin, Times Staff Writers) reported that: "Scientists have uncovered what they believe are glaring errors in a patent issued last month to Human Genome Sciences Inc. for a human gene that plays a crucial role in AIDS. Errors Found in Patent for AIDS Gene Scientists Say; News comes amid concerns that genomics race could lead to shoddy science and profiteering. A few excerpts:

When we file a patent, we do not claim the sequence as the invention," said William A. Haseltine, chairman and chief executive of the Rockville, Md., company, which has filed about 7,500 gene patents. "The invention we claim is the gene we deposit with the ATCC. We know that our sequence and most sequences are not perfect." "Genomics companies such as Human Genome Sciences and its competitors Celera

Genomics and Incyte Pharmaceuticals are able to cast a broad net and haul in genes and gene fragments by the tens of thousands, using automated machines to spell out genetic code and sophisticated software to make reasonable guesses about their function.

In the months after the company filed its patent, however, other researchers at several academic centers, including the Aaron Diamond AIDS Research Center in New York and the NIH, made a remarkable series of discoveries about how HIV, the virus that causes AIDS, enters living cells, the first step in an infection.

Unaware of the company's patent application, these scientists found and isolated a protein that the virus requires for entry–the CCR5 receptor. And they isolated the gene that carries the instructions for building the receptor. A drug that can block the protein could be a new weapon against AIDS."…'The fight going on now is not a disinterested fight about who gets credit for it, but who gets money for it,' Haseltine said.

1999/2000 A Joint Statement by the U.S. Public Health Service, the AAFP, the AAP, and ACIP urging manufacturers to remove the preservative thimerosal (ethyl mercury) as soon as possible from vaccines routinely recommended for infants.

2000 Prevnar (pneumococcal conjugate vaccine) is licensed.

2000 CDC recommends use of IPV instead of OPV (polio vaccine).

2000 At a San Diego research meeting on autism, Dr. Stephanie Cave presented the following information:

By the age of two, American children have received 237 micrograms of mercury through vaccines alone, which far exceeds current EPA 'safe' levels of 0.1 mcg/kg. per day. That is one-tenth of a microgram, not one microgram. Three days in particular may be singled out as spectacularly toxic for infants:

Day of birth: hepatitis B—12 mcg mercury (30 times safe level).

At 4 months: DTaP and HiB on same day—50 mcg mercury (60 times safe level).

At 6 months: Hep B, Polio—62.5 mcg mercury (78 times safe level).

At 15 months the child received another 50 mcg (41 times safe level).

These figures are calculated for an infant's average weight in kilograms for each age. These one-day blasts of mercury are called 'bolus doses.' Although they far exceed 'safe' levels, there has never been any research conducted on the toxicity of such bolus doses of mercury given to infants all these years.

Autism and Mercury. [Testimony presented by Stephanie Cave, MD before the Committee on Government Reform, US House of Representatives, July 18, 2000. Also presented at the Defeat Autism Now! Conference, 15 Sep 2000, San Diego, CA].

2001 A DARK WINTER DESCENDS by Whitney Webb (full article here) https://unlimitedhangout.com/2020/04/investigative-series/all-roads-lead-to-dark-winter/

"In late June 2001, the U.S. military was preparing for a "Dark Winter." At Andrews Air Force Base in Camp Springs, Maryland, several Congressmen, a former CIA director, a former FBI director, government insiders and privileged members of the press met to conduct a biowarfare simulation that would precede both the September 11 attacks and the 2001 Anthrax attacks by a matter of months. It specifically simulated the deliberate introduction of smallpox to the American public by a hostile actor. The simulation was a collaborative effort led by the John Hopkins Center for Civilian Biodefense Strategies (part of the Johns Hopkins Center for Health Security) in collaboration with the Center for Strategic and International Studies (CSIS), the Analytic Services (ANSER) Institute for Homeland Security and the Oklahoma National Memorial Institute for the Prevention of Terrorism. The concept, design and script of the simulation were created by Tara O'Toole and Thomas Inglesby of the Johns Hopkins Center along with Randy Larsen and Mark DeMier of ANSER. The full script of the exercise can be read here. The name for the exercise derives from a statement made by Robert Kadlec, who participated in the script created for the exercise, when he states that the lack of smallpox vaccines for the U.S. populace means that "it could be a very dark winter for America." Kadlec, a veteran of the George W. Bush administration and a former lobbyist for military intelligence/intelligence contractors, is now leading HHS' Covid-19 response and led the Trump administration's 2019 "Crimson Contagion" exercises, which simulated a crippling pandemic influenza outbreak in the U.S. that had first originated in China. Kadlec's professional history, his decades-old obsession with apocalyptic bioweapon attack scenarios and the Crimson Contagion exercises themselves are the subject of Part III of this series."

2001 M.A. Fisher et al. publish that adverse events associated with hepatitis B vaccine in U.S. children less than six years of age, 1993 and 1994 and conclude: "Evidence from this study suggests that hepatitis B vaccine is positively associated with adverse health outcomes in the general population of US children." The hepatitis B vaccine is also associated with prevalent arthritis, acute ear infections, pharyngitis/nasopharyngitis (throat and nasal infections)." (Ann Epidemiol Jan; 11(1):13-21), 2001).

2001 (April) A number of studies have shown a link between the excessive mercury exposure due to vaccines and rising rates of autism in children (a report issued by the California Health and Human Services Agency revealed a 273 percent increase in California children diagnosed with autism in the past decade). One study noted: "A review of medical literature and US government data suggests that (i) many cases of idiopathic autism are induced by early mercury exposure from thimerosal; (ii) this type of autism represents an unrecognized mercurial syndrome; and (iii) genetic and non-genetic factors establish a predisposition whereby thimerosal's adverse effects occur only in some children." Bernard, S. et al., Autism: A novel form of mercury poisoning, Med Hypotheses 2001 Apr;56(4):462-71.

2001 (April) National Institutes of Health Statement: "Mercury is a potent neurotoxin ... Infants and young children are also very vulnerable to the impacts of mercury because it can affect their developing brains." National Institutes of Health April 26, 2001.

2001 (May) An article in the Sunday Times in London on May 27, 2001 observed, "Mercury in vaccines for babies and infants could be the cause of autism in children around the world, according to a growing number of scientists..."The National Autistic Society estimates that there are about 500,000 people with autism in Britain, 120,000 of them children. According to one recent study, there has been a tenfold increase [of autism] among children between 1984 and 1994."

2001 Once claimed by AIDS scientists to be a specific component required for "HIV" replication, and a surrogate marker for the presence of "HIV" in cultures, reverse transcriptase or RT is published in market magazines concerning biotechnology stocks having nothing to do with retroviruses (Pachez M. No need to be phased. Shares, 28-32, 2001).

2001 (APRIL) A press release about the National Institutes of Health (NIH) mercury-reduction program (April 26, 2001) noted: "Mercury is a potent neurotoxin... . Infants and young children are also very vulnerable to the impacts of mercury because it can affect their developing brains." And yet we continue to inject bolus doses of mercury directly into tiny infants with many childhood vaccines.

2001 The World Health Organization (WHO) outlines its new global laboratory proposal, aimed at improving the range, speed and quality of influenza virus surveillance (Science 293, 1729; 2001).

2001 FDA recalls Abbott Laboratories HIV p24 Antigen Test Kit lot 71843M101."The failure to deliver the Antibody to HIV-1 (Rabbit) component of the test kit to the reaction well could result in a false negative test. The recall notification instructs establishments that currently have in inventory the recalled product to discontinue use and discard the product" (but patients who were diagnosed positive with it are never informed).

2001 Vaccine Adverse Event Reporting System Tables published by the CDC in MMWR show adverse reactions from various vaccines, with the universally mandated hepatitis B vaccine by itself (9,022 cases) topping the list for adverse reactions between 1991-1995, followed by FLU vaccine (4,696 cases). Between 1996-2001, Vericel tops the lists with 9,820 cases, followed by hepatitis B (9,022 cases), followed by FLU vaccine (8,125 cases).

2001 The CDC's 2001 revised Isolation and Identification of Measles Virus in Culture protocol is analyzed and published by Janine Roberts, in her book 'Fear of the Invisible. "Monday, 18 August 2008. How 'Measles Virus' is isolated for a Vaccine (in 2001).

"In an online paper entitled 'Isolation and Identification of Measles Virus in Cell Culture,' the CDC, the central Health Research authority of the USA, lays out how isolation of this virus should be done so it can be used, say for a vaccine. It instructs, first obtain from the patient a small sample of urine or fluid from the nose or mouth."

"Next 'sacrifice' a marmoset monkey, take some of its cells, then make these cancerous, perhaps by exposing them to radiation, and then give them, on top of this, Epstein-Barr disease! Such extremely sick cells, the CDC informs us, are '10,000 times' more sensitive to the measles virus than are normal human cells."

"Now add to these cells a toxin called trypsin. The CDC tells us to expect some cells to fall off the sides of the vessel as if they have been poisoned. They have been. Now add nutrients and glucose and leave for two or three days so the cells can somewhat recover."

"Now add to the cells the sample gathered from the patient. After an hour, inspect the cells in the culture with a microscope to see if any of the cells are becoming distorted, or are floating free as they did when trypsin was added. If they are, the CDC says this is proof that measles virus is present and making the cells ill."

"This statement made me sit back and think. Why should this illness now be caused by a virus? They had poisoned the cells, made them cancerous.... and now the CDC was saying the cells must be ill because they had measles. Where was the logic in this?"

"The next stage involves the addition of two antibiotics, Penicillin and Streptomycin, to the culture and leaving it alone for a day. Again, the cells are inspected – and if small holes now appear between cells, it is now presumed that measles virus has caused these. If no sign of such damage, this process is repeated. If after this there are still no signs of damage, then the culture is discarded. However, if 50% or more of the cells are now seriously ill and distorted, the culture is set aside and kept in the fridge as 'isolated measles virus stock suitable for vaccines!' All this without actually detecting the virus itself!"

"This is the whole process as recommended by the CDC. There is no mention of the need to have a control culture, no mention of any need to isolate the measles virus or even to see it with an electron microscope. The cells are poisoned – and an unseen measles virus is blamed – even the disease the cells have is totally unlike measles. Where is the logic in this?"

2001 Carroll-Pankhurst et al., in her 2001 study published in the British Journal of Cancer report their thirty-five-year mortality study on people now in middle age following receipt of SV40-simian-(cancer) virus-contaminated and feces-derived polio vaccine. The study claimed that out of 1073 newborns that were vaccinated and carefully followed for 35 years, (which the authors cautiously claim is not really long enough to determine if the agent causes cancer in humans), and of those infants who were given this "cancer virus-contaminated vaccine " between 1959 and 1963, there has been no apparent increase in cancer above the expected background incidences in this carefully followed subgroup. Some scientists, however, such as Michele Carbone, and a group in Australia, that believe SV-40 has caused increases in mesothelioma, brain cancers, leukemias, and other cancers in Humans, but their cohorts have not been studied as long as Pankurst's (Carrol-Pankhurst et al. British Journal of Cancer, 85 (9), 1205-1207, 2001).

2001 The NucliSens(R) HIV-1 QT assay test kit package insert warns that NucliSens® HIV-1 QT assay "is not intended to be used as a screening test for HIV-1 nor is it to be used as a diagnostic test to confirm the presence of HIV-1 infection" (because a doctor is needed to determine if you are black, hispanic, or gay, and to ask who you slept with in the past).

2001 VAERS (Vaccine Adverse Event Reporting System of the US CDC) data from January 1, 1990 to November 1, 2001 show that: Following the DTP shot 807 children died. Following the DTaP shot 364 children died (acellular pertussis was adopted because of high reactions to live cell).

Following the hepatitis B shot 679 children died.

Following the haemophilus B shot 932 children died.

Following the poliovirus live oral vaccine 970 children died.

2001 (October 17), the law firm of Waters & Kraus revealed a confidential report by the Centers for Disease Control which studied autism as a neurological injury caused by mercury in vaccines. The CDC report stated: "We found increasing risks of neurological developmental disorder." Disorders noted were: Developmental Speech Disorder, Autism,...

The study found a 2.48 times increased risk of autism. Children with mercury exposure were more than twice as likely to develop autism as children not exposed. U.S. law states that: "In a vaccine injury case, a relative risk greater than 2.0 establishes that there is a greater than 50% chance that the injury was caused by the vaccine." New Yorkers for Vaccination Information and Choice press release by Waters & Kraus, Dallas, Texas.

Altered Report: A different version was made public and claimed results were inconclusive as to whether the mercury in vaccines has caused a nationwide epidemic of regressive autism and other neurological disorders in small children.

2001 The Infectious Diseases Society of America claimed that "HIV/AIDS" treatment is improving but more patients are dying who have undetectable "viral load" because of "treatment-related toxicities, and.......... end-organ failure in patients with HIV disease" [due to treatment-related toxicities:

Abstract: "We analyzed the deaths in an outpatient human immunodeficiency virus (HIV) care clinic at University Hospitals in Cleveland from January 1995 through December 1999. The number of annual deaths decreased progressively, from 112 in 1995 to 32 in 1999. The median final CD4+ cell count before death increased progressively from 10 cells/L in 1995 to 90 cells/L in 1999."

In the journal, Clinical Infectious Diseases (2001;32:492-497), this emerging clinical phenomenon was stated in the following way:

"End-stage liver disease is now the leading cause of death in our hospitalized HIV-seropositive population."

Translation: Treatments for AIDS are getting better as more patients are dying.

2001 (Feb) FDA recalls P24 antigen test kit (but patients who were diagnosed positive with it are never informed).

2001 ISIS Report (Institute for Science in Society)-July 19, 2001-GM AIDS Virus More Deadly:

Researchers have been creating one deadly virus after another in the laboratory, and the latest is 'SHIV', a hybrid between the human and monkey AIDS virus containing human interleukin genes that suppress immune response against viruses. At the same time, GM crops engineered with interleukin genes are being grown in open field trials.

2001. NucliSens(R) HIV-test kit package insert was published. 1The NucliSens(R) HIV-1 QT assay is not intended to be used as a screening test for HIV-1 nor is it to be used as a diagnostic test to confirm the presence of HIV-1 infection [a doctor is needed to determine if you are black, hispanic, or gay, and to ask who you slept with in the past].

2001 (November 9) The CDC publishes revised guidelines for "HIV" counseling, testing, and referral:

When a preliminary, positive rapid test is explained to clients, phrases like "a good chance of being infected" or "highly likely infected" can be used to indicate the likelihood of HIV infection and qualified based on the HIV prevalence in the setting and the client's individual risk." (CDC: "Revised Guidelines for HIV Counseling, Testing, and Referral" November 9, 2001).

2001 ISIS Report (Institute for Science in Society)-July 29, 2001-AIDS-Vaccine Trials Dangerous

The OECD Conference in Genoa announced a $1.2 billion package to help combat AIDS in the Third World. Vaccine developers and United Nation agencies are pushing for large-scale clinical trials of AIDS vaccines in vulnerable Third World populations "ravaged" by the AIDS pandemic. AIDS virologists point to evidence that the vaccines are not only ineffective but dangerous. Dr. Mae-Wan Ho reports.

"The intended vaccines all contain gp120, a glycoprotein (protein decorated with side-chains of carbohydrates) belonging to the envelope of the human AIDS virus, HIV-1. The candidates include recombinant HIV proteins and peptides (subunit vaccines), HIV-1 or SIV (the monkey AIDS virus), killed or 'attenuated', ie, rendered harmless by successive passage in cultured cells, and a wide range of recombinant viral, bacterial and plasmid vectors expressing HIV proteins. HIV researchers Dr. Veljko Veljkovic and his colleagues in Belgrade Yugoslavia, have shown that the gp120, is similar to the part of human immunoglobulin (antibody) proteins (Ig) involved in binding foreign antigens, a crucial step in the immune response. Thus, any AIDS vaccine containing the gp120 glycoprotein or the gene coding for it could strongly interfere with the immune system and make the host more vulnerable to the virus. And in the longer term, it could accelerate disease progression in HIV patients that do not yet have symptoms. But the gp120 gene has other properties that pose an even greater threat to the vaccinated population. It contains 'recombination hotspots' similar to those in bacteria and viruses such as Haemophilus influenzae, Mycobacterium tuberculosis, hepatitis B virus and herpes simplex virus, that often co-infect with the HIV, and also similar to recombination elements found in immunoglobulin genes and oncogenes (genes associated with cancer) in the human host. Recombination hotspots are breakpoints at which genetic exchange or recombination occurs much more frequently than usual. Recombination of HIV with bacteria and viruses would generate new pathogens. Within the human host, recombination with human genes would promote chromosomal rearrangements and formation of abnormal immunoglobulins, thus undermining immune responses. HIV-1 sequences integrated into the genome can act as retrotransposons (jumping genes) that can mutate genes by jumping into them, and some of the mutations may trigger cancer."

"Dr. Veljkovic's team, in collaboration with researchers in UK, Italy and US, already found evidence of recombination between gp120 and a gene from Haemophilus influenzae [2]. Recombination between an HIV gene and Mycoplasm fermentans has been implicated in 'Gulf war syndrome' [3] affecting a high proportion of soldiers from United States and the United Kingdom who served in the Gulf war. A new subtype of HIV-1 may also have resulted from recombination between HIV- 1 and SIV."

"The proponents of the AIDS vaccination trials argue that the desperate situation precipitated by the AIDS epidemic justifies acceptance of the 'small risks' involved. But Veljkovic and his colleagues have written a monograph documenting the lack of efficacy of the vaccines and the enormous risks involved [5]."

"Not effective and dangerous"

"In 1994, the AIDS Research Advisory Committee of the US National Institutes of Health (NIH) recommended that phase III clinical trials of gp120 vaccines should not be conducted 'at this time and in this country'. The reasons, according to Dr. A. Fauci, director of National Institute of Allergy and Infectious Diseases (NIAID), were that the vaccines were ineffective; and there was a remote chance that the vaccines would compromise the immune system and make the recipient more vulnerable to infection [6]. The possibility that a vaccinated individual runs a greater risk of developing an established infection, or of progressing to disease more rapidly once infected, was confirmed subsequently [7]. The recombinant gp120 subunit vaccine tested in HIV-negative individuals was ineffective in protecting them against infection. Those who became infected during or after vaccination actually had in their blood sera significant levels of antibodies against the vaccine before they became infected, but those antibodies failed to protect them from infection. On the contrary, the vaccine appeared to have acted as a decoy to fool the immune system into mounting an attack on it, while allowing the HIV itself to slip through the host defense to get established. This subunit vaccine is due to go on Phase III clinical trial in Thailand."

"Vaccine trials in breach of UNAIDS ethical, scientific and safety standards"

"According to the WHO report 2000, more than 90% of all AIDS cases are in developing countries. UNAIDS and NIH are the two most important organizations involved in developing AIDS vaccines. UNAIDS Executive Director Peter Piot has declared, 'It is our collective responsibility to ensure that all vaccine trials are conducted under the strictest possible ethical and scientific standards.' But Dr. Veljkovic has shown that current vaccines based on HIV-1 gp120 can harm the immune system of individuals and, on account of its recombinogenic tendencies, has the potential to generate deadly viruses and bacteria that can spread through the vaccinated populations and to wildlife.

"The intended vaccine trials are in serious breach of ethical, scientific and safety standards. "AIDS, more so than other diseases, cannot be addressed simply by vaccinations, even if efficacious and safe vaccines could be found."

"More than drugs and vaccines, we need to end poverty, malnutrition and environmental destruction, to reinstate social equity and free access to primary healthcare and education." (See Super viruses and Superbugs from AIDS vaccines, ISIS News 9/10 ISSN1474-1547(print), ISSN1474-1814 (online).

2002 (January 17) MANY CASES OF NO "HIV" TRANSMISSION AMONG SERODISCORDANT COUPLES, AND OTHER TEST KIT RECALLS.

The Journal of Infectious Disease featured an article about 17 women who remained "HIV" uninfected, despite a history of heavy exposure to HIV through repeated, unprotected sexual contact with an infected partner, and 12 of their regular, male HIV-positive partners.

2002 (February) "Merck Says Tens of Thousands May Need Another Hepatitis A Shot," Merck & Company said on Friday that an unknown number of people in as many as 27 nations, including 60 000 youngsters in Brazil, might need new shots to prevent infection with the hepatitis A virus because vaccines they received might have been defective.

2002 (February) Alarm bells are again sounded when the avian virus "H5N1" infects two people in Hong Kong, one fatal.

2002 The FDA recalled BioRad Genetic systems HIV Types 1 & 2 Synthetic Peptide containing test kits (but patients who were diagnosed positive with it are never informed).

2002 It was reported in The Journal of Virology, that saquinavir and other protease inhibitors are severely toxic to T-cells in the absence of "HIV" infection.

2002 (May 1) ISIS Report —Doubts Deepen over Safety of AIDS Vaccines

"Another key AIDS vaccine is abandoned before phase III trial. This latest setback comes at the end of a string of failures in developing vaccines that may be worse than useless." Dr. Mae-Wan Ho reports."

"The US government abandoned a controversial AIDS vaccine trial and announced it will combine the work of two federal institutions, the National Institutes of Health and the Department of Defense. Both institutions had proposed trials to test a combination of similar vaccines – a dose of canarypox virus engineered to carry HIV-1 proteins with a booster shot of the HIV protein gp120. The trial was designed to compare the types of immune responses the vaccine evoked with the protection it provided. That required the vaccine to produce an immune response in at least 30 per cent of volunteers. But analysis of the data suggests the response did not come up to scratch. "It didn't even come very close," said Anthony Fauci, director of the NIH's National Institute of Allergy and Infectious Diseases. The cancelled NIH trial, which would have involved 11,000 volunteers, was anticipated to cost $60 to $80 million dollars. The Department of Defense trial, which was designed to test only the efficacy of the vaccine, will still go ahead. But that may be a grave mistake."

"Some virologists have been warning for years that the entire class of AIDS vaccines based on the HIV gp120 gene or protein is not only ineffective, but also dangerous for the recipients and the human populations. There is evidence suggesting that gp120 can interfere with and undermine the immune system and can readily recombine with viruses and bacteria (used as vectors) to generate new pathogens."

"The envelope glycoprotein, gp120 of HIV-1, is similar to the region of human immunoglobulins that binds antigen, a crucial feature of the immune response. Thus, any AIDS vaccine containing the gp120 could interfere with the immune system and make people more vulnerable to the virus. And in the long term, it could accelerate disease progression in HIV patients that do not yet have symptoms."

"Recombinant viruses expressing gp120 could also be a source of potential new pathogens... Furthermore, HIV-1 sequences integrated into the genome have the potential to initiate a wide variety of diverse genetic effects caused by all mobile genetic elements, especially mutations of genes due to random insertion, some of which might trigger cancer."..."A recent theoretical study adds further fuel to their warning. Partially effective vaccines that inhibit the growth of the pathogen, such as the AIDS vaccines described here may leave death rates unchanged, or worse, increase deaths with the level of vaccination"... (see "Health warning over partially effective vaccines", this issue). "But a company in Texas, Prodigene, is putting gp120 into GM maize as a cheap, edible oral vaccine against HIV as announced in the internet journal, AIDScience. This will surely lead to widespread contamination of our food crops with disastrous consequences. Not only is this extremely hazardous for human beings. It will affect all organisms in the food chain and multiply the opportunities for this gene to recombine with bacteria and viruses in the environment, of which 99% cannot be cultured and are hence completely unknown. An edited version of our response was published on the internet journalhttp://www.aidscience.com".

2002 Pediarix (penta-valent DtaP/HepB/IPV) licensed (against diphtheria, tetanus, pertussis whooping cough, hepatitis B, and polio, all in 1 vaccine).

2002 Midwest Nurse Week, Vol. 3, No. 2; March/April 2002, p.27. "Nursing Home Residents Get Flu Despite Flu Shot. A flu outbreak in Nebraska's urban area killed one nursing home resident. Nearly all of the residents received flu shots. A similar outbreak at the Grand Island Veterans Home occurred although 98% of the residents were given flu shot."

2002 (May 16) FDA recalls Berna Biotech's Typhoid Vaccine Live Oral Ty21a lot numbers 16044.1a 16044.1b." The product may lose potency before the expiration date, even when kept at labeled refrigerated temperatures" (but patients who were diagnosed positive with it are never informed).

2002 (June) Mercury Horse Drug Recalled by the FDA. "Drug contains mercury: poisonous to horses and people. Purchasers should not use it. Contact local waste-management authorities to learn how to destroy it without endangering animals, people, or waterways." The Salt Lake Tribune, June 1, 2002

2002 Figures from the US Centers for Disease Control and Prevention showed there were 1,920 confirmed cases of polio reported by laboratories in 2002, up from 483 the previous year.

2002 (August) Shares crashed after the British drug maker PowderJect Pharmaceuticals said it was recalling its BCG tuberculosis vaccine in the UK. PowderJect said the move would reduce full-year pre-tax profits by about 5 million Pounds from previous estimates of about 25 million. The withdrawal followed the recent temporary suspension of its license in Ireland when the Irish Medicines Board found that some batches of the drug did not remain potent. Accusations of cronyism blew-up earlier this year after it emerged the company was awarded a 32 million government contract to supply smallpox vaccine, in case of a terrorist germ warfare attack.

2002 (August 7) FDA recalls Bio-Rad Laboratories Genetic Systems HIV1/HIV-2 Peptide EIA lot 105VP1. " The recalled test kits are qualitative enzyme immunoassays for the detection of antibodies to HIV-1 and/or HIV-2 in human serum and plasma, and also in cadaveric serum specimens. Microwell plates in this lot that are performing outside of expected performance ranges as indicated by invalid (low) HIV-1 and HIV-2 Positive Controls and elevated Negative Control values" (but patients who were diagnosed positive with it are never informed).

2002 British Medical Journal publishes article showing that: "Children vaccinated in infancy are at increased risk of hepatitis B virus infection in the late teens" (Hilton Whittle, Shabbar Jaffar, Michael Wansbrough, Maimuna Mendy, Uga Dumpis, Andrew Collison, Andrew Hall. Observational study of vaccine efficacy 14 years after trial of hepatitis B vaccination in Gambian children. (BMJ vol 325, 14 September, 2002).

2002 (Oct. 18) FDA recalls Aventis Pasteur's Meningococcal Polysaccharide Vaccine, Groups A, C, Y, W-135 Combined, single-dose vials (including single-dose in five dose packaging) lot numbers UB040AA, UB040AB, UB070AA, UB096AA.

2002 GSK pulled Lymerix (Lyme disease vaccine) off the market.

2002 The tuberculosis vaccine has been shown to have no efficacy against adult TB; the U.S. does not vaccinate and in 1999 had 6.4 tuberculosis cases per 100,000. Russia vaccinates for TB, but its rate of infection was 85 cases per 100,000. Today it is even higher, states the author of **Time Bomb: The Global Epidemic of Multi-Drug-Resistant Tuberculosis**. Lee B. Reichman, M.D., M.P.H., with Janice Hopkins Tanne, McGraw-Hill, 2002.

2003 HOW FAR FROM A HORMONE-BASED CONTRACEPTIVE VACCINE? By Peter Delves Journal Reproductive Immunology. 2004 Jun;62(1-2):69-78. doi: 10.1016/j.jri.2003.08.003.

Abstract

Antibodies of appropriate specificity are able to block the action of hormones which are obligatory for successful reproduction. Thus, if immunization using such hormones can provoke adequate titres of bioneutralizing antibodies in sexually mature individuals, **the vaccinee becomes infertile** ('immunocontraception') for as long as sufficient titres of the antibodies are maintained. **In the case of hormones that are required for the development of sexual maturity in the male, immunization of young animals can prevent sexual maturation ('immunocastration')**. The hormones which have been targeted are gonadotropin-releasing hormone (GnRH) for both immunocastration and immunocontraception, and follicle-stimulating hormone (FSH) and human chorionic gonadotropin (hCG) for immunocontraception.

2003 Inhaled flu vaccine (Flumist) being reviewed for approval by the FDA.

2003 (January 6) FDA recalls Abbott Laboratories HCV EIA 2.0 Test Kit lot 92527M101 (4/15/2003). "The manufacturer found an increase in frequency of Negative Control Out of Range High values, which results in an increased likelihood of invalid assay runs... Establishments that have the recalled product in inventory are instructed to discontinue use and destroy any remaining product," (but patients who were diagnosed positive with it are never informed).

2003 (February 17) FDA recalls antibody to Human Immunodeficiency Virus (Abbott HIVAG-1 Monoclonal EIA Test Kit lot numbers): 92677M200, 92677M201, 92677M202, 95132M100, 95132M101 (but patients who were diagnosed positive with it are never informed).

The manufacturer found an increase in the initial reactive rate when compared to historical performance expectations as shown in the package insert. This may result in an increased likelihood of invalid assay runs. Specificity, as defined by repeat reactive rate, and sensitivity continue to meet all performance requirements. Establishments that have the recalled product in inventory are instructed to discontinue use and destroy any remaining product.

2003 (February 28) Outbreaks of "chicken flu" occur in The Netherlands due to the "H7N7" avian flu virus. By April, the so-called virus has spread to nearly 800 poultry farms and resulted in the culling of almost 11 million chickens. The so-called imagined virus infects 83 people causing conjunctivitis and flu-like symptoms and kills one man. The drug Tamiflu is said to protect people against further spread of the virus.

2003 (March 19) FDA recalls Ortho-Clinical Diagnostics Ortho HCV (Hepatitis C virus) Version 3.0 ELISA Test System, lot number TXE358; Ortho Antibody to HBsAg ELISA Test System 2, lot number 2HB567;Ortho HBc ELISA Test System, lot numbers CHK423 and CHK424. " OPD Tablets that are packaged as components of Ortho ELISA Test Systems after receiving information that the OPD tablets may be discolored... if yellow or discolored OPD tablets are inadvertently used, the assay controls may be out of the acceptable range criteria as stated in the package insert resulting in an invalid plate." Patients who were diagnosed positive with these recalled tests are never informed.

2003 (May) Nature publishes statement that cows could foster flu pandemics. Vol 423, 5 (01 May 2003 doi:10.1038/423005b).

2003 Smallpox vaccine is mass produced for first-responders recommended following the events of 9/11, 2001 "terrorist attacks" during the second year of the G.W. Bush Administration.

2003 Cobra warns that "AmpliScreen HIV-1 Test is not intended for use as an aid in diagnosis" (COBAS AmpliScreen HIV-1 Test, version 1.5 Approval Date: 12/19/2003) [a doctor is needed to determine if you are black, hispanic, or gay, and to ask who you slept with in the past, or if you are healthy enough for sexual activity in the first place].

2003 Weeks after the announcement that the "HIV" vaccine, AIDSVAX, had failed, VaxGen (the makers of AIDSVAX) was hit with a shareholder lawsuit that accused the company's officials of continuing to make positive statements about their vaccine to artificially pump up the company's stock price, despite mounting evidence that it was not effective. The suit was dismissed last year and VaxGen, under new management, remade itself into a biodefense company, and is now supported with 887 million of our tax dollars.

BECAUSE THE U.S. VACCINE PROGRAMMES COULDN'T MAKE ANTHRAX VACCINE, GEORGE BUSH THREATENED CANADA NOT TO BUST BAYER'S PATENT RIGHTS ON CIPRO DURING THE EVENTS SURROUNDING 9/11

2003 "In the wake of anthrax being placed in the US mail following the events of 9/11, 2001 and "The Bush "terrorist attacks," the anthrax vaccine used in Desert Storm is found to be non-protective in animal experiments, and despite extensive domestic support for suspending Bayer's patent on Cipro, Tommy Thompson acting on behalf of the Bush Administration said it is "illegal" to suspend Bayer's patent on Cipro. Instead, he entered into negotiations with Bayer with the intention of lowering the price of Cipro. Facing an unprecedented public embarrassment, Bayer agreed to lower the price of Cipro for government purchase from $1.77 to $0.95. The Bush administration did not suspend the patent of Bayer largely because it was more concerned with the wider implications of such an action, particularly on the ongoing negotiations at the WTO. Realizing that scrapping Bayer's patent would set a precedent that could give legitimacy to the growing demands of the poor and developing world for more flexibility on patent issues, the US sent a clear message to the world that patents are more important than public health. Such a calculated move was not only meant to serve the corporate interests of drug manufacturers, but also to convey the message to the developing nations that the US administration would continue its discriminatory policy on the issue of patents."

2003 (December) South Korea has its first outbreak of avian flu in chickens, caused by "H5N1."

2003 (December 7) WHY YOU SHOULD AVOID TAKING VACCINES is published by Dr. James Howenstine, MD., former NIH fellow at UCSF, former Navy doctor, retired longtime assistant clinical professor of internal medicine from 1964 to 1991 at the University of California, San Francisco, and former Head of Internal Medicine at Thomas Davis Medical Center in Glendale, Arizona

"Dr. James R. Shannon, former director of the National institute of health declared, 'the only safe vaccine is one that is never used.' Cowpox vaccine was believed able to immunize people against smallpox. At the time this vaccine was introduced, there was already a decline in the number of cases of smallpox. Japan introduced compulsory vaccination in 1872. In 1892 there were 165,774 cases of smallpox with 29,979 deaths despite the vaccination program."

Much of the success attributed to vaccination programs may actually have been due to improvement in public health related to water quality and sanitation, less crowded living conditions, better nutrition, and higher standards of living. Typically, the incidence of a disease was clearly declining before the vaccine for that disease was introduced. In England, the incidence of polio had decreased by 82 % before the polio vaccine was introduced in 1956.

"In the early 1900s an astute Indiana physician, Dr. W.B. Clarke, stated "Cancer was practically unknown until compulsory vaccination with cowpox vaccine began to be introduced. I have had to deal with two hundred cases of cancer, and I never saw a case of cancer in a non-vaccinated [1] person."

"There is a widely held belief that vaccines should not be criticized because the public might refuse to take them. This is valid only if the benefits exceed the known risks of the vaccines."

Do Vaccines Actually Prevent Disease?

"This important question does not appear to have ever been adequately studied. Vaccines are enormously profitable for drug companies and recent legislation in the U.S. has exempted lawsuits against pharmaceutical firms in the event of adverse reactions to vaccines which are quite common. In 1975 Germany stopped requiring pertussis (whooping cough) vaccination. Today less than 10% of German children are vaccinated against pertussis. The number of cases of pertussis has steadily decreased[2] even though far fewer children are receiving pertussis vaccine."

"Measles outbreaks have occurred in schools with vaccination rates over 98% in all parts of the U.S. including areas that had reported no cases of measles for years. As measles immunization rates rise to high levels measles becomes a disease seen only in vaccinated persons. An outbreak of measles occurred in a school where 100% of the children had been vaccinated. Measles mortality rates had declined by 97 % in England before measles vaccination was instituted."

"In 1986 there were 1300 cases of pertussis in Kansas and 90% of these cases occurred in children who had been adequately vaccinated. Similar vaccine failures have been reported from Nova Scotia where pertussis continues to be occurring despite universal vaccination. Pertussis remains endemic[3] in the Netherlands where for more than 20 years 96% of children have received 3 pertussis shots by age 12 months."

"After institution of diphtheria vaccination in England and Wales in 1894 the number of deaths from diphtheria rose by 20% in the subsequent 15 years. Germany had compulsory vaccination in 1939. The rate of diphtheria spiraled to 150,000 cases that year whereas, Norway which did not have compulsory vaccination, had only 50 cases of diphtheria the same year."

"The continued presence of these infectious diseases in children who have received vaccines proves that lifelong immunity which follows natural infection does not occur in persons receiving vaccines. The injection process places the viral particles into the blood without providing any clear way to eliminate these foreign substances."

Why Do Vaccines Fail to Protect Against Diseases?

"Walene James, author of 'Immunization: The Reality Behind the Myth,' states that the full[4] inflammatory response is necessary to create real immunity. Prior to the introduction of measles and mumps vaccines children got measles and mumps and in the great majority of cases these diseases were benign. Vaccines "trick" the body so it does not mount a complete inflammatory response to the injected virus."

Vaccines and Sudden Infant Death Syndrome SIDS

"The incidence of Sudden Infant Death syndrome SIDS has grown from .55 per 1000 live births in 1953 to 12.8 per 1000 in 1992 in Olmstead County, Minnesota. The peak incidence for SIDS is age 2 to 4 months the exact time most vaccines are being given to children. 85 % of cases of SIDS occur in the first 6 months of infancy. The increase in SIDS as a percentage of total infant deaths has risen from 2.5 per 1000 in 1953 to 17.9 per 1000 in 1992. This rise in SIDS deaths has occurred during a period when nearly every childhood disease was declining due to improved sanitation and medical progress except SIDS. These deaths from SIDS did increase during a period when the number of vaccines given a child was steadily rising to 36 per child.

"Dr. W. Torch was able to document 12 deaths in infants which appeared within 3½ and 19 hours of a DPT immunization. He later reported 11 new cases of SIDS death and one near miss which had occurred within 24 hours of a DPT injection. When he studied 70 cases of SIDS two thirds of these victims[5] had been vaccinated from one half day to 3 weeks prior to their deaths. None of these deaths was attributed to vaccines. Vaccines are a sacred cow and nothing against them appears in the mass media because they are so profitable to pharmaceutical firms."

"There is valid reason to think that not only are vaccines worthless in preventing disease: they are counterproductive because they injure the immune system permitting cancer, auto-immune diseases and SIDS to cause much disability and death."

Are Vaccines Sterile?

"Dr. Robert Strecker claimed that the department of defense DOD was given $10,000,000 in 1969 to create the AIDS virus to be used as a population-reducing[6] weapon against blacks. By use of the Freedom of Information Act Dr. Strecker was able to learn that the DOD secured funds from Congress to perform studies on immune destroying agents for germ warfare."

"Once produced, the vaccine was given in two locations. Smallpox vaccine containing HIV was given to 100,000,000 Africans in 1977. Over 2000 young white homosexual males in New York City were given Hepatitis B vaccine that contained HIV virus in 1978. This vaccine was given at New York City Blood Center. The Hepatitis B vaccine containing the HIV virus was also administered to homosexual males in San Francisco, Los Angeles, St. Louis, Houston, and Chicago in 1978 and 1979. U.S. Public Health epidemiology studies have disclosed that these same 6 cities had the highest incidence of AIDS, Aids related Complex (ARC) and deaths rates from HIV, when compared to other U.S. cities."

"When a new virus is introduced into a community, it takes 20 years for the number of cases to double. If the fabricated story that green monkey bites of pygmies led to the HIV epidemic, the alleged monkey bites in the 1940s should have produced a peak in the incidence of HIV in the 1960s at which time HIV was nonexistent in Africa. The World Health Organization (WHO) began an African smallpox vaccination campaign in 1977 that targeted urban population centers and avoided pygmies. If the green monkey bites of pygmies truly caused the HIV epidemic the incidence of HIV in pygmies should have been higher than in urban citizens. However, the opposite was true."

"In 1954 Dr. Bernice Eddy (bacteriologist) discovered live monkey viruses in supposedly sterile inactivated polio vaccine[7] developed by Dr. Jonas Salk. This discovery was not well received at the NIH and Dr. Eddy was demoted. Later Dr. Eddy, working with Sarah Stewart, discovered SE polyoma virus. This virus was quite important because it caused cancer in every animal receiving it. Yellow fever vaccine had previously been found to contain avian (bird) leukemia virus. Later Dr. Hilleman isolated SV 40 virus from both the Salk and Sabin polio vaccines. There were 40 different viruses[8] in these polio vaccines they were trying to eradicate. They were never able to get rid of these viruses contaminating the polio vaccines. The SV 40 virus causes malignancies. It has now been identified in 43 % of cases of non-Hodgkin lymphoma[9], 36 % of brain tumors[10], 18 % of healthy blood samples, and 22 % of healthy semen samples, mesotheliomas, and other malignancies. By the time of this discovery SV 40 had already been injected into 10,000,000 people in Salk vaccine. Gastric digestion inactivates some of SV 40 in Sabin vaccine. However, the isolation of strains of Sabin polio vaccine from all 38 cases of Guillain Barre Syndrome[11] GBS in Brazil suggests that significant numbers of persons are able to be infected from this vaccine. All 38 of these patients had received Sabin polio vaccine months to years before the onset of GBS. The incidence of non-Hodgkin lymphoma has "mysteriously doubled since the 1970s."

"Dr. John Martin, Professor of Pathology at the Univ. of Southern California, was employed by the Viral Oncology Branch of the Bureau of Biologics (FDA) from 1976 to 1980. While employed there he identified foreign DNA in the live polio vaccine Orimune Lederle that suggested serious vaccine contamination. He warned his supervisors about this problem and was told to discontinue his work as it was outside the scope of testing required for polio vaccine."

"Later Dr. Martin learned that all eleven of the African green monkeys used to grow the Lederle polio virus Orimune had grown simian cytomegalovirus from kidney cell cultures. Lederle was aware of this viral contamination as their Cytomegaloviral Contamination Plan[12] clearly showed in 1972. The Bureau of Biologics decided not to pursue the matter, so production of infected polio vaccine continued."

"In 1955 Dr. Martin identified unique cell destroying viruses termed stealth viruses in patients with chronic fatigue syndrome. These viruses lacked genes that would enable the immune system to recognize them. Thus, they were protected by the body's failure to develop antiviral antibodies. In March of 1995, Dr. Martin learned that some of these stealth viruses had originated from African green monkey simian cytomegalovirus of a type known to infect man.'

"The Lederle vaccine experience suggests that the higher-ups are not concerned about sloppy and dangerous preparation of vaccines. Animal cross infection is a huge unsolved current problem for all vaccine manufacturing. If this vaccine production sounds like an unbelievable mess to you, you are right."

"The influential Club of Rome has a position paper in which they state that the world population is too large and needs to be reduced by 90 %. This means that 6 billion people must be reduced to 500 to 600 million. Obviously, creating famines and genocidal wars such as wreaked havoc in Africa, and loosing new laboratory-created diseases (HIV, Ebola, Marburg[13], and probably West Nile virus and SARS) can help reduce the population. Other elitist groups (Trilaterals, Bilderbergers) have expressed similar concerns about excess people on planet Earth."

"The company that was projected to produce the new smallpox vaccine in the U.S. was in serious trouble in England because of unsatisfactory quality of operations before setting up their facility in the U.S. Why would their performance here be any better than it was in England?"

"If there are important powerful groups of people that are determined to reduce the world population, what could be a more diabolically clever way to eliminate people than to inject them with a cancer-causing vaccine? The person receiving the injection would never suspect that the vaccine taken 10 to 15 years earlier had caused the cancer to appear."

Other Dangers from Vaccines

"The steady escalation in the number of vaccines administered has been followed by an identical rise in the incidence of auto-immune diseases (rheumatoid arthritis, subacute lupus erythematosus, psoriasis, multiple sclerosis, asthma) seen in children. While there is a genetic transmission of some of these diseases many are probably due to the injury from foreign protein particles, mercury, aluminum, formaldehyde and other toxic agents injected in vaccines."

"In 1999, the rotavirus vaccine was recommended by the Center for Disease Control for all infants. When this vaccine program was instituted several infants died and many had life endangering bowel obstructions. Obviously, there was no evidence that this vaccine would cause such serious problems before the vaccine was released for usage. Children's vaccines are not studied for toxicity possibly because such study might eliminate them from being used."

"A large study from Australia showed that the risk of developing encephalitis from the pertussis vaccine was 5 times greater than the risk of developing encephalitis by contacting pertussis by natural methods."

"Naturally acquired immunity by illness evolves by spread of a virus from the respiratory tract to the liver, thymus, spleen, and bone marrow. When symptoms begin, the entire immune response has been mobilized to repel the invading virus. This complex immune system response creates antibodies that confer lifelong immunity against that invading virus and prepares the child to respond promptly to an infection by the same virus in the future."

"Vaccination, in contrast, results in the persisting of live virus or other foreign antigens within the cells of the body, a situation that may provoke auto-immune reactions as the body attempts to destroy its own infected cells. There is no surprise that the incidence of autoimmune diseases (rheumatoid arthritis, subacute lupus erythematosus, multiple sclerosis, asthma, psoriasis) has risen sharply in this era of multiple vaccine immunization."

Vaccine Induced Type 1 Diabetes Mellitus

"Dr. John Classen has published 29 articles on vaccine-induced[14] diabetes. At least 8 of 10 children with Type 1 (insulin needing) diabetes have this disease as a result of vaccination. These children may have avoided measles, mumps, and whooping cough but they have received something far worse: an illness that shortens life expectancy by 10 to 15 years and results in a life requiring constant medical care." "Dr. Classen has shown in Finland, the introduction of Hemophilus type b vaccine caused three times as many cases of type 1 diabetes as the number of deaths and brain damage from Hemophilus influenza type b it might have prevented."

In New Zealand, the incidence of Type 1 diabetes in children rose by 61 % after an aggressive vaccine program against hepatitis B. This same program has been started in the U.S.A. so we can now look forward to many cases of Type 1 diabetes in children. Similar rises in Type 1 diabetes have been seen in England, Italy, Sweden, and Denmark after immunization programs against Hepatitis B."

Toxic Substances Are Needed to Make Vaccines

"Vaccines contain many toxic substances that are needed to prevent the vaccines from becoming infected or to improve the performance of the vaccine. Among these substances are mercury, formaldehyde and aluminum.[15]"

"In the past 10 years, the number of autistic children has risen from between 200 and 500 percent in every state in the U.S. This sharp rise in autism followed the introduction of measles, mumps and rubella vaccine in 1975."

"Representative Dan Burton's healthy grandson was given injections for 9 diseases in one day. These injections were instantly followed by autism. These injections contain a preservative of mercury called thimerosal. The boy received 41 times the amount of mercury which is capable of harm to the body. Mercury is a neurotoxin that can injure the brain and nervous system. And tragically, it did."

"In the United States the number of compulsory vaccine injections has increased from 10 to 36 in the last 25 years. During this period, there has been a simultaneous increase in the number of children suffering learning disabilities and attention deficit disorder. Some of these childhood disabilities are related to intrauterine cerebral damage from maternal cocaine use, but probably vaccines cause many of the others."

"Many vaccines contain aluminum. A new disease called macrophagic myofasciitis causes pain in muscles, bones, and joints. All persons with this disease have received aluminum containing vaccines. Deposits of aluminum are able to remain as an irritant in tissues and disturb the immune and nervous system for a lifetime."

"Nearly all vaccines contain aluminum and mercury. These

metals appear to play an important role in the etiology of Alzheimer's Disease. An expert at the 1997 International Vaccine Conference related that a person who takes 5 or more annual flu vaccine shots has increased the likelihood of developing Alzheimer's Disease by a factor of 10 over the person who has had 2 or fewer flu shots."

"When we take vaccines, we are playing a modern version of Russian Roulette. We not only get exposed to aluminum, mercury, formaldehyde, and foreign cell proteins but we may get simian virus 40 and other dangerous viruses which can cause cancer, leukemia, and other severe health problems because the vaccine pool is contaminated due to careless animal isolation techniques. Congress has protected the manufacturers from lawsuits, so dangerous vaccines simply increase profits at no risk to the drug companies."

"U.S. children aged 2 months began receiving hepatitis B vaccine in December 2000. No peer-reviewed studies of the safety of hepatitis B in this age bracket had been done. Over 36,000 adverse reactions with 440 deaths were soon reported but the true incidence is much higher as reporting is voluntary so only approximately 10 % of adverse reactions get reported. This means that about 5000 infants are dying annually from the hepatitis B vaccine. The CDC's Chief of Epidemiology admits that the frequency of serious reactions to hepatitis B vaccine is 10 times higher than other vaccines. Hepatitis B is transmitted sexually and by contaminated blood, so the incidence of this disease must be near zero in this age bracket. A vaccine expert, Dr. Philip Incao, states that "the conclusion is obvious that the risks [16] of hepatitis B vaccination far outweigh the benefits. Once a vaccine is mandated the vaccine manufacturer is no longer liable for adverse reactions."

"Dr. W.B. Clarke's important observation that cancer was not found in unvaccinated individuals demands an explanation and one now appear forthcoming. All vaccines given over a short period of time to an immature immune system deplete the thymus gland (the primary gland involved in immune reactions) of irreplaceable immature immune cells. Each of these cells could have multiplied and developed into an army of valuable cells to combat infection and growth of abnormal cells. When these immune cells have been used up, permanent immunity may not appear. The Arthur Research Foundation in Tucson, Arizona estimates that up to 60 % of our immune system may be exhausted[17] by multiple mass vaccines (36 are now required for children). Only 10 % of immune cells are permanently lost when a child is permitted to develop natural immunity from disease. There needs to be grave concern about these immune system injuring vaccinations! Could the persons who approve these mass vaccinations know that they are impairing the health of these children, many of whom are being doomed to requiring much medical care in the future?"

"Compelling evidence is available that the development of the immune system after contracting the usual childhood diseases matures and renders it capable to fight infection and malignant cells in the future."

"The use of multiple vaccines, which prevents natural immunity, promotes the development of allergies and asthma. A New Zealand study disclosed that 23 % of vaccinated children develop asthma, as compared to zero in unvaccinated children. "Cancer was an exceedingly rare illness in the 1890's. This evidence about immune system injury from vaccinating affords a plausible explanation for Dr. Clarke's finding that only vaccinated individuals got cancer. Some radical adverse change in health occurred in the early 1900s to permit cancer to explode and vaccinating appears to be the reason."

"Vaccines are an unnatural phenomenon. My guess is that if enough persons said no to immunizations there would be a striking improvement in general health with nature back in the immunizing business instead of man. Having a child vaccinated should be a choice not a requirement. Medical and religious exemptions are permitted by most states."

"When governmental policies require vaccinations before children enter schools coercion has overruled the lack of evidence of vaccine efficacy and safety. There is no proof that vaccines work, and they are never studied for safety before release. My opinion is that there is overwhelming evidence that vaccines are dangerous and the only reason for their existence is to increase profits of pharmaceutical firms."

"If you are forced to immunize your children so they can enter school, obtain a notarized statement from the director of the facility that they will accept full financial responsibility for any adverse reaction from the vaccine. Since there is at least a 2 percent risk of a serious adverse reaction they may be smart enough to permit your child to escape a dangerous procedure. Recent legislation passed by Congress gives the government the power to imprison persons refusing to take vaccines (smallpox, anthrax, etc.). This would be troublesome to enforce if large numbers of citizens declined to be vaccinated at the same time."

2003 (17th June) Professor Mye-Wan Ho, PHD Institute of Science in Society. AIDS Vaccines Worse Than Useless?

The US administration is offering AIDS-ravaged nations support for fighting AIDS tied to the purchase of GM products. The main anti-AIDS strategy is a class of vaccines that carries its own risks. Prominent AIDS researchers have called repeatedly for a moratorium as evidence of hazards accumulates. "Dr. Mae-Wan Ho reports.

George Bush has taken Europe to the World Trade Organization over Europe's de facto moratorium on GM imports. In the week of the G8 summit in Evian, France, Bush blasted Europe for perpetuating starvation in Africa by blocking US food aid with anti-GM policies and announced his pledge of $15bn to combat AIDS globally, especially in Africa.

The only AIDS vaccine to have progressed past phase 3 trial, made by VaxGen, took 5 years, and involved 5108 gay men and 309 women. Unfortunately, it proved ineffective, and may even be harmful.

A few days after Bush announced the AIDS package, US Congress was denounced for tying support for anti-AIDS research programmes in 50 countries to their acceptance of GM products. The gp120 protein is strongly immunogenic, which is why it is widely used in vaccines, in the hope that the body will produce antibodies against the protein and hence protect against the virus. But there have been many worrying signs that this may have just the opposite effect.

A recombinant gp120 vaccine tested in HIV-negative individuals in phaseI/II trails, was not effective in protecting against the disease. Not only that, but participants in the trials also had significant levels of circulating antibodies against the vaccine before they became infected and came down with AIDS disease. "The vaccine could also be dangerous. A vaccine based on the gp120 from the strain SF2, actually suppressed the production of antibodies that could neutralize the later infecting virus, while boosting the production of useless antibodies that were specific for the vaccine strain, SF2. In other words, gp120 acts as a molecular decoy to disarm the body's antiviral response, leaving it more vulnerable, and increasing the likelihood of rapid disease progression in those vaccinated that later became infected. This phenomenon is called "deceptive imprinting" of the immune system.

Veljkovic and his colleagues have repeated their call for an immediate moratorium on the current clinical trials of HIV-1 gp120/160 vaccines.

2003 (December) "At Kenyatta National Hospital [Kenya] ...out of 31 couples tested, 23 were discordant [one positive, one negative]. It was reported that some of them stayed in a sexual relationship with the infected partner for more than six years without the infected one passing the virus to the other. And when these discordant couples brought their children for testing, all of them were free of the virus... (Horizon Magazine, December 18, 2003).

2003 December 19 COBAS AmpliScreen HIV-1 Test package insert, version 1.5 was published (http://www.fda.gov/cber/label/hiv1roc121903LB.pdf): "This test is not intended for use as an aid in diagnosis." [a doctor is needed to determine if you are black, hispanic, or gay, and to ask who you slept with in the past, OR if you are healthy enough to have sex in the first place].

2004 FDA recalls bioMerieux NucliSens automated isolation reagent(s),DiaSoran's HIV-1 – HIV-2 Plus O EIA Testing Software, and Roche's Amplicor HIV Monitor test (but patients who were diagnosed positive with it are never informed).

2004 It was reported in The New England Journal of Medicine that vitamin supplements can ward off progression to AIDS in the absence of HAART (Highly Active Anti-Retroviral Therapy).

2004 Announcement of the failure of the 120-million-dollar AIDSVAX program: "A sound Rationale (is) needed for Phase III HIV vaccine trials."

The decision about whether or not to proceed with mounting a phase III HIV-1 vaccine trial needs to consider the likelihood of success and the consequences of failure, the value of what can realistically be learned, the human and financial costs involved. As a whole, the scientific community must do a better job of bringing truly promising vaccine candidates to this stage of development and beyond." (Gallo and others, Science, Vol 303 16 January, 2004).

2004 (January) Japan is claimed to have the first outbreak of avian influenza "H5N1" since 1925, but it isn't clear who sequenced the "H5N1" strain found in frozen snow samples from 1925.

2004 (January) WHO confirms "H5N1 infection" in 11 people, eight fatal, in Thailand and Vietnam, but no cases of person-to-person transmission. The virus has wreaked havoc among poultry in Thailand, Vietnam, Japan, and South Korea, and has also appeared in a duck farm in China. WHO is developing vaccine candidates using "H5N1" viruses isolated in 2003 and 2004, at laboratories in the U.S. and U.K. publishes that reverse genetics could offer forward-thinking flu vaccine (23 Jan 2004) doi:10.1038/news040119-15?

2004 (February) United Nations Food and Agriculture Organization advises governments in affected areas that mass culling of birds is failing to halt the disease and that vaccination of targeted poultry flocks is required as well.

2004 (February) West Africa polio campaign is boycotted by Nigerian states. A mass poliomyelitis vaccination campaign got under way to immunize 63 million children across west Africa but was boycotted by four predominantly Muslim states in Nigeria, where leaders claim the oral vaccine causes sterility and spreads AIDS (BMJ; 328:485 2004). The West African campaign was intended as a final push to stamp out the disease in the region and is part of the World Health Organization's 15-year drive to halt transmission of the poliomyelitis virus across the world by 2005. According to Dr Haruna Kaita, the head of the medical team that conducted the test in India, the vaccines contain "undeclared contaminants that can cause malfunctioning of the testes and cause infertility in women." The team also found "some toxic substances."

Polio controversy started long ago," said Dr Kaita. "If you find one batch defective, you should condemn all batches. What these people [proponents of the vaccine] are saying is unethical, illegal, and criminal, and they know that these things are contaminated, and they have the potential to cause human hazards. They should be banned rather than cause diseases in innocent children.

2004 (March) Avian "H5N1" flu "virus" is said to become more widespread among bird flocks in Asia, and is said to have caused 34 human cases, with 23 deaths. Nature reports that in a race to make a bird-flu vaccine, and that scientists are using "reverse genetics" to design new prototype vaccines against bird flu and establishing facilities for their mass production, including new cell culture as well as traditional egg-based methods. Biotechnology 22, 267 (01 Mar 2004) doi:10.1038/nbt0304-267a. Nature also reported that the race for pandemic flu vaccine rife with hurdles 432, 261 (18 Nov 2004) doi:10.1038/432261a.

2004 (April) Avian influenza virus "H7N3" confirmed in two poultry workers in British Columbia who developed flu-like symptoms.

2004 (June) Tests on chickens and mice show that avian flu "H5N1" virus isolated from ducks in 2004 is more virulent and harmful to mammals than in recent years.

2004 (July) Several countries, including Thailand, Vietnam, China, and Indonesia, report new infections in poultry with "H5N1."

2004 (August) "H5N1" virus is reported to have killed an additional three people in Vietnam.

2004 Nearly two dozen prominent AIDS researchers write an opinion piece in the journal Science in early 2004 calling Donald Francis's AIDSVAX vaccine completely incapable of preventing or ameliorating HIV infection and questioning the wisdom of the U.S. government's sponsoring the Thailand trial. "There are adverse consequences to conducting large-scale trials of inadequate [HIV] vaccines... . One price for repetitive failure could be crucial erosion of confidence by the public and politicians in our capability of developing an effective AIDS vaccine.

2004 (April 2) FDA recalls Aventis Pasteur's Imovax rabies vaccine lots:X0667-2, X0667-3, W1419-2, W1419-3. Precautionary measure stemming from the discovery through routine testing of a non-inactivated production strain of virus in a single product lot, which was not distributed.

2004 (May 13) FDA recalls DiaSorin's HIV-1 / HIV-2 Plus O EIA Testing Software. An error was contained on the ETI-LAB Applications disk for programming the BioRad HIV-1/HIV-2 Plus O assay. The error induced specimen and conjugate incubation temperatures for the assay to remain at ambient temperature rather than the required 37°C temperature;" (but patients who were diagnosed positive with it are never informed).

2004 (May 17) FDA recalls bioMerieux (Durham, NC) NucliSens HIV QT." Some irregularities have been observed with one lot's guanidine isothiocyanate (GuSCN) component, which may affect the sensitivity and accuracy of assays" (but patients who were diagnosed positive with it are never informed).

2004 (June 24) FDA recalls Roche's Amplicor HIV-1 Monitor Test, v 1.5." Roche has confirmed increased frequency of occurrence of "blue foci" with the Avidin-Horseradish Peroxidase (AV-HRP) Conjugate Lot E09659. Increased frequency of the occurrence of "blue foci" may lead to elevated and/or observed out of sequence optical density readings in the microwell plate assays that have used this particular lot of reagent." Patients who were diagnosed positive with it are never informed.

2004 The Institute of Medicine (IOM) of the U.S. National Academy of Sciences (NAS) retreats from the stated 1999 goal of the AAP and the PHS to remove thimerosal from U.S. vaccines ... "Despite its removal from many childhood vaccines, thimerosal is still routinely added to some formulations of influenza vaccine administered to U.S. infants, as well as to several other vaccines" (e.g., tetanus-diphtheria and monovalent tetanus) administered to older children and adults.

2004 (November) WHO warns that the "H5N1" bird flu virus might spark a flu pandemic that could kill "millions of people," and is concerned that "much of the world is unprepared for a pandemic" and needs to enhance preparedness to reduce its potential impact. WHO officials meet with vaccine makers, public-health experts, and government representatives in a bid to speed up the production of flu vaccines to avert a global pandemic.

2004 (December) WHO reports the first human case of "H5N1" in Vietnam since early September. Experts claim that sequencing of the chicken-genome (published in Nature 9 December 2004) may help provide insight into which genes prevent the spread of bird flu from person to person. Since the beginning of 2004, bird flu has caused the deaths of 32 people in Vietnam and Thailand, and millions of chickens across Asia due to culling and fear.

Normal flu is said to kill 30,000 Americans/year but the more conservative estimate is about 11,000/year U.S., as opposed to 32 in two other countries.

2004 "HIV" and "HBV" sequences found present in normal human genome analyses: McClure MA, Richardson HS, Clinton RA, Hepp CM, Crowther BA, Donaldson EF. Automated characterization of potentially active retroid agents in the human genome. Genomics. Apr;85(4):512-23, 2005).

2004 The American Red Cross reported that even after repeated "HIV" testing using different test kit types, that "low-risk" populations, such as blood donors (or military recruits or nuns) will typically yield 12 (PCR) positive or 2 (ELISA) positive results out of

37,000,000 million units of blood, which means that 10 out of 12 were false positives. In a follow-up analysis of this Red Cross study, it was then claimed that 6 of the 12 PCR-positive subjects tests seroconverted within several months, thereby obtaining a "HIV" molecular signature in 8/12 cases, out of 37 million negatives. Again, these numbers could represent statistical artifact, or the several who seroconverted may represent the detection of some kind of autoimmune condition in those who test positive, like psoriasis, arthritis, warts, or physiological stress, or a genetic polymorphism.

2005 (January 18) FDA recalls GEN-Probe Inc Procleix HIV-1/HCV Assay. " Procleix HIV-1 / HCV Assay, Master Lot 401254, was found to contain an elevated level of copper. The source of the elevated copper was the raw material, Trehalose, which is also a component of the Enzyme Reagent. The increase in copper may affect kit performance." Patients who were diagnosed positive with it are never informed.

2005 (January) Chinese authorities announce they have developed a new rapid test for bird flu that produces results in hours rather than days.

2005 Tetanus vaccine may be laced with anti-fertility drug. International / developing countries Vaccine Weekly.

1995 May 29 – Jun 5;9-10. https://pubmed.ncbi.nlm.nih.gov/12346214/

Abstract

PIP: A priest, president of Human Life International (HLI) based in Maryland, has asked Congress to investigate reports of women in some developing countries unknowingly receiving a tetanus vaccine laced with the anti-fertility drug human chorionic gonadotropin (hCG). If it is true, he wants Congress to publicly condemn the mass vaccinations and to cut off funding to UN agencies and other involved organizations. The natural hormone hCG is needed to maintain pregnancy. The hormone would produce antibodies against hCG to prevent pregnancy. In the fall of 1994, the Pro-Life

Committee of Mexico was suspicious of the protocols for the tetanus toxoid campaign because they excluded all males and children and called for multiple injections of the vaccine in only women of reproductive age. Yet, one injection provides protection for at least 10 years. The Committee had vials of the tetanus vaccine analyzed for hCG. It informed HLI about the tetanus toxoid vaccine. HLI then told its World Council members and HLI affiliates in more than 60 countries. Similar tetanus vaccines laced with hCG have been uncovered in the Philippines and in Nicaragua. In addition to the World Health Organization (WHO), other organizations involved in the development of an anti-fertility vaccine using hCG include the UN Population Fund, the UN Development Programme, the World Bank, the Population Council, the Rockefeller Foundation, the US National Institute of Child Health and Human Development, the All-India Institute of Medical Sciences, and Uppsala, Helsinki, and Ohio State universities. The priest objects that, if indeed the purpose of the mass vaccinations is to prevent pregnancies, women are uninformed, unsuspecting, and unconsenting victims.

2005 (February 4) FDA recalls Globus Media Inc. Rapid HIV Test Kits. "Rapid HIV Test Kits, marketed nationwide via the Internet, by Globus Media, were not reviewed for safety and effectiveness as required under U.S. law. Consequently, there is no assurance that the results from these kits are reliable. For example, one insert says: "DO NOT RELY ON ANY TEST RESULT FROM THESE RECALLED KITS. Consumers who have these products should not use them. Consumers who have used the RAPID HIV Test Kit, should consult a health care professional immediately to confirm any results." Patients who were diagnosed positive with them are never informed.

2005 (February 24) New bird flu symptoms reported, and the B.C. Centre for Disease Control is warning doctors to look out for new symptoms related to "the deadly" avian flu outbreak in Southeast Asia. At least two children in Vietnam who died of bird flu had diarrhea and seizures rather than classic respiratory symptoms. In the Feb. 17 issue of the New England Journal of Medicine, researchers from the Oxford University Clinical Research Unit in Ho Chi Minh City said two children died in February 2004 of acute encephalitis that was caused by the "H5N1" type of bird flu. Lab tests showed the "H5N1" virus in the children's feces, raising fears that the virus could be passed from person to person. Dr. Aleina Tweed, an epidemiologist, said doctors in British Columbia are being told to watch for gastrointestinal problems, especially in children, when they see sick people who have recently traveled in Southeast Asia. "We wanted to make sure that the medical health community was aware that there are different presentations of this, not to be looking only for respiratory illness among people who have recently traveled to this area," Tweed said. Late last year, doctors in B.C. were put on high alert to watch for signs of avian flu in people coming back from Southeast Asia. World Health Organization experts believe the "H5N1" flu strain poses the single greatest threat of a pandemic in humans. "What I'm questioning is this escalating rhetoric, led by the World Health Organization, that's trying to tell us that in fact we are on the verge of a pandemic," Dr. Richard Schabas told CBC Radio's the Current. "I don't think we really know what it is that triggers a pandemic, what it is that causes a particular virus to transform itself," added Schabas, Ontario's former chief medical officer of health. Tweed said while it is troubling to hear reports of new symptoms, a bird flu pandemic is not possible unless the virus spreads easily from one person to another. There is extraordinarily little information now about that risk. In Asia, it is more common to get "H5N1" directly from poultry, according to the UN Food and Agriculture Organization. "We certainly concur with the WHO that this is a profoundly serious threat. Whether it is a threat that will manifest itself, there is no way to know, until it actually happens," Tweed said." Whether it will happen this week, this month or never, we simply cannot predict," she said. "But we wouldn't want to take the chance, and not be as prepared as we can." The federal government acknowledged the threat in Wednesday's budget. A Vancouver-based company will receive about $20 million to develop a bird flu vaccine. "Symptoms of bird flu are said to consist of a fever, shortness of breath and a cough. Five patients there was a history of sputum production, and in three of these patients, the sputum was blood-stained. Two patients reported pleuritic pain. Diarrhea was reported in seven of the patients. Bleeding from the nose and gums was noted in one patient on the fourth day of illness. No patient had a sore throat, conjunctivitis, rash, or a runny nose. Physical examination in nine patients revealed fever, rapid respiratory rate (median 55 breaths per minute; range 28-70), respiratory distress, and crackles on examination of the chest. http://www.cbc.ca/health/story/2005/02/24/avian-flu050224.html

2005 Jan/Feb -13 additional cases of bird flu have occurred in Vietnam since December 2004, 12 fatal. [Typically, in the U.S. There are approximately 30 thousand influenza deaths during the same interval. Some Global pandemics!

2005 (February) First report of a bird flu case from Cambodia. A report of probable person to person transmission of bird flu in Vietnam is published (New Engl. J. Med, 352 333–340). WHO has made prototype "H5N1" vaccine strains available to a number of institutions and companies and several vaccines have been developed for clinical testing? 15 additional cases of "H5N1" infection in Vietnam, and one additional case in Cambodia, are reported. Bird flu has spread to 10 countries, including Democratic People's Republic of Korea, and killed around 50 million chickens.

2005 Evidence that vaccine adjuvants like squalene (MF-59), when they have been added to certain lots of anthrax (and perhaps "HIV") vaccines given to soldiers on threat of court martial if they do not roll up their shirt on command, have induced autoimmune syndromes in almost 100% of every sick Gulf-War I veteran tested, and have evoked antibodies to squalene in their blood (Gary Matsumoto. Vaccine A, Basic Books Publisher, 2005). Squalene and other adjuvants have been used by scientists for many years to induce rodents to develop arthritis, macrophagic myofasciitis, multiple-sclerosis (demyelinating syndromes), and lupus (Holmdahl et al. Arthritis induced in rats with nonimmunogenic adjuvants as models for rheumatoid arthritis

Immunol Rev. Dec;184:184-202, 2001; Gherardi NK. Lessons from macrophagic myofasciitis: towards definition of a vaccine adjuvant-related syndrome. Rev Neurol (Paris). Feb;159(2):162-4), 2003).

2005 An "encephalitis vaccine" mandated by the CDC for college-age (young adults) withdrawn for safety reasons (see FDA's 2005 recall list). Also see CDC's MMWR

http://www.cdc.gov/mmwr/preview/mmwrhtml/mm5541a2.htm

2005 Merck claims that its Human papilloma vaccine: "was 100 percent effective in preventing precancerous cervical disease, but only when given to women and girls who had never engaged in sex at the time of the shots," yet. "Documents prepared by the FDA suggest some women with persistent HPV infections could be at higher risk of cervical cancer after taking the vaccine."

Dr. Schiffman heads the HPV Troup in the Division of Cancer, Epidemiology, and Genetics at NCI and is a tenured senior investigator. In mid-March Dr. Mark Schiffman, MD, MPH, called CAP TODAY's editor to voice a troubling concern: that laboratories are failing to clinically validate their HPV tests" (September 2005 issue of Pathology/Laboratory Medicine/ and Laboratory Management article released monthly by The Collage of American Pathologists-CAP).

What surprises me is that this {the certainty with which these tests for HPV and cervical cancer} could in any way be controversial, he says. The issue is not so much controversial, of course, as it is loaded-with money and competitive claims, scientific complexity, and grave medical concerns (Dr. Schiffman).

In the same article, Even Attila Lorincz, PhD, chief scientific officer, and senior VP of research development at Digene (one of the HPV test-kit makers) says that "much of the confusion simply boils down to analytical and clinical accuracy is not well enough understood or described by people who write or talk about it," and that "the problem surfaces in the HPV literature with distressing regularity."

2005 (April) Vietnam has reported a total of 60 laboratory confirmed human cases of "H5N1" avian influenza since the outbreaks began, with 35 deaths; Thailand has confirmed a total of 17 infections of which 12 have been fatal, while Cambodia has confirmed two fatal cases. Same issue as stated above: 30,000/year with regular influenzas.

2005 (May) Rumor of human deaths in China from "H5N1" remain unconfirmed, while the virus has killed more than 1000 migratory birds. Indonesia's government confirms reports of "H5N1" infection in pigs.

2005 (May) WHO reports 97 cases and 53 deaths from bird flu in Vietnam, Cambodia, and Thailand since January 2004. news@nature.com publishes that heightened security after flu scare sparks biosafety debate (11 May 2005) doi:10.1038/435131a.

> Note: There are over 30,000 deaths reported in the U.S./year due to "influenza" (although the accurate number is thought to be around 2-4,000/yr). Yet 53 deaths from "bird flu," spread over 3 countries, is now considered a pandemic, if indeed these 53 cases were flu at all and not due to doctor-prescribed "remedies," such as pharmaceutical drugs like Tamiflu. The published case studies show this is indeed the case. These 53 deaths were due to doctors, not flu.

2005 (June) Indonesia confirms a man exposed to sick chickens has been infected with a deadly strain of avian flu virus. The farm laborer shows no symptoms, but his blood carries antibodies to the "H5N1" strain. Bird flu becomes resistant to the low-cost amantadine family of antiviral drugs. Chinese farmers' use of the compound in chickens is blamed, a claim formally denied by Chinese authorities who pledge to investigate the claim.

2005 (July) At the end of a three-day conference in Malaysia, World Health Organization officials announce that $150 million is needed to fight the spread of the disease in people and another $100 million to stop its spread in animals in Asia. The Philippines, so far, the only Asian country unaffected by bird flu, report their first case in a town north of the capital, Manila, but do not confirm whether it is the "H5N1" strain. On 29 July, the World Health Organization confirms that samples from an 8-year-old girl who died on the 14 July, two days after the death of her father, who was Indonesia's first confirmed human infection of influenza A ("H5N1").

2005 (August) The World Health Organization (WHO) confirms three new cases of "H5N1" in Vietnam. Of the three individuals infected, two died. Since mid-December 2004, 20 of the 63 cases of "H5N1" in Vietnam have been fatal. The Lancet publishes an article on 12 August 2005 saying the flu drug Relenza is at least as effective as Tamiflu but has fewer side effects and there is no evidence of resistance to Relenza, compared with resistance levels of up to 18% in those taking Tamiflu. The researchers recommend stockpiling both drugs. Vaccine manufacturer Maine Biological Labs is fined $500,000 for smuggling a chicken flu virus into the US. In 1998 the Maine biotechnology company illegally imported the virus from Saudi Arabia so that it could develop a vaccine for a disease-plagued poultry farm in that country. The company then used falsified documents to send 8000 bottles of the newly-created vaccine back to Saudi Arabia. WHO recommends that regional offices stockpile drugs against bird flu? The plan suggests that each office should stockpile drugs for a 5-day course of Oseltamivir (Tamiflu) for 30% of workers and their families. Both Russia and Kazakhstan report outbreaks of avian influenza in poultry in late July that are confirmed "H5N1" in early August. Outbreaks in both countries were attributed to contact between domestic birds and wild waterfowl via shared water sources. In early August, an outbreak of "H5N1" in poultry was detected in Tibet. Mongolia then issues an emergency report following the death of 89 migratory birds at two lakes in the northern part of the country.

2005 (August) Deception appears to be the name of the game when the facts reveal that current medical practices are doing major harm to America's children. The media is often deceived by medical "experts" whose agenda the reporters do not recognize. NBC's moderator, Tim Russert, appears to have been "had" when he accepted as Gospel what Dr. Feinberg's false claim that since 2003 there has been no Thimerosal preservative used in any vaccines given to infants (other than flu vaccine).

FDA's current table of vaccine contents calls the lie.

(See: http://www.FDA.gov/cber/vaccine/thimerosal.htm). "The latest table still lists Multiple dose DT by Aventis Pasteur ltd as fully preserved; TT vaccine is preserved with Thimerosal; Japanese encephalitis vaccine JE-VAC is thimerosal preserved; Meningococcal vaccine (Menomune) in multidose vials is preserved with Thimerosal. Tim Russert's effort to reassure parents that there is no longer any thimerosal in any vaccines was inappropriate–as it helps perpetrate deceptions."

"21CFR610.15(A) is part of the Code of Federal regulations. It is a law, and it is legally binding. It states that a manufacturer must prove that the component is "safe" before putting it into a vaccine as a preservative. This SAFETY test has never been done. And FDA has never been taken to task for allowing preservatives that are known to cause neurological damage to be used in vaccines. According to our testing results from January of this year, there are vaccines that contained from .019 micrograms up to 66 micrograms per mL that either expired in 2005 or will not expire until 2006. The flu vaccine we tested that expired in June 2005 contained 48 micrograms per mL, or 24 micrograms per adult dose (and I assume 12 micrograms per adolescent dose) and that it is being used as a preservative." Dawn Winkler, Executive Director, Health Advocacy in the Public Interest (HAPI) http://www.hapihealth.com.

2005 BIODEFENSE AND PANDEMIC AND VACCINE AND DRUG DEVELOPMENT ACT IS PASSED BY GEORGE BUSH'S ADMINISTRATION, FACILITATED BY DR. BILL FRIST CHANGING SENTENCES BURIED IN THOUSAND-PAGE-LONG DOCUMENTS HOURS BEFORE THE HUGE DOCUMENTS ARE PRESENTED TO OFFICIALS IN CONGRESS FOR A VOTE

The Biodefense and Pandemic and Vaccine and Drug Development bill was written as a bill to amend the Public Health Service Act to enhance biodefense and pandemic preparedness activities, to use untested vaccines, drugs, medical products, or "security countermeasures." without any liability for claims for loss of property, personal injury, or death arising out of, reasonably relating to, or resulting from the design, development, clinical testing and investigation, manufacture, labeling, distribution, sale, purchase, donation, dispensing, prescribing, administration, or use of a security countermeasure or qualified pandemic or epidemic product distributed, sold, purchased, donated, dispensed, prescribed, administered, or used in anticipation of and preparation for, in defense against, or in response to, or recovery from an actual or potential public health emergency that is a designated security countermeasure or a qualified pandemic or epidemic product..." (http://thomas.loc.gov/ Search Bill Title or Number – S.1873RS click 'enter bill number).'

2005 Newsweek reports that VaxGen, a little-known California biotechnology company, will start its first delivery of its anthrax vaccine to the government six months later than originally slated. The company was awarded an $877.5 million contract to produce and manufacture the vaccine, which was developed by the U.S. Army Medical Research Institute of Infectious Diseases (USAMRIID). Seventy-five million doses of VaxGen's vaccine are to be procured for the Strategic National Stockpile under Project Bioshield, a joint Department of Homeland Security (DHS) and Department of Health and Human Services (HHS) initiative to stimulate the creation of a domestic biodefense industry. Five million doses of Vaxgen competitor Bioport's vaccine were procured earlier this year in response to Bioport's aggressive lobbying and anti-VaxGen campaign. VaxGen's vaccine has not been approved by the Food and Drug Administration. Bioport's vaccine, which has been used by the Defense Department, has been controversial because of its side effects and its FDA approval has been disputed (Project on Government Oversight, Vera Hassner Sharav).

2005 (September) Three more laboratory-confirmed cases of "H5N1" strike Indonesia. A 37-year-old woman dies on 10th September and is the fourth fatality associated with "H5N1" to hit the country. Indonesia's third laboratory-confirmed case of "H5N1" since July 2005 involves an 8-year-old boy who survives. Later, a 27-year-old woman from Jakarta, who developed symptoms after direct contact with diseased and dying chickens in her household, dies on 26 September. Viet Nam officials retrospectively confirm an additional fatal case of "H5N1" infection, bringing the total in Viet Nam since mid-December 2004 to 64 cases, a third of which (21) were fatalities. Two independent studies, each reaching different conclusions, suggest it would be possible to contain an emerging pandemic if the virus were detected quickly, if it did not spread too fast, if sufficient antiviral drugs were deployed around the outbreak's epicenter, and if strict quarantine and other measures were also used employed. President George W. Bush calls for an international partnership that would require countries facing an influenza outbreak to share information and samples with the WHO. But experts say research would speed up if the US Centers for Disease Control and Prevention's (CDC) influenza branch threw open its databases of virus sequences and immunological and epidemiological data and complain that too few of the flu data collected by the CDC are made generally available.

2005 (October) Greece becomes the first EU country with a bird flu infection as the country's Centre for Veterinary Institutes detects bird flu in one turkey on the eastern Aegean island of Chios. Officials confirm the virus is a member of the "H5 strain," but not yet identified as "H5N1." The WHO reiterates that the level of pandemic alert remains unchanged at phase 3: a virus new to humans is causing infections but does not spread easily from one person to another. On 13 October WHO states that tests conducted by the World Organization for Animal Health (OIE) confirm the presence of "H5N1" avian influenza in samples taken from domestic birds in Turkey. Days later, the presence of the virus is confirmed in

Romania. A fifth laboratory-confirmed case of "H5N1" is reported from Indonesia on 10 October 2005. The 21-year-old Sumatran man had contact with diseased chickens shortly before he became ill. The case brings the total number of human infections with influenza A ("H5N1") since December 2003 to 117.http://www.nature.com/nature/focus/avianflu/timeline.html

2005 (November) Chinese scientists report "H5N1" avian flu infection in pigs, raising concerns that the virus could exchange genes with human flu strains in this 'mixing vessel'. None of these pigs was ill, according to National Geographic article, Nov. 2005. "H5N1" virus has spread throughout most of SE Asia, resulting in the culling of over 100 million chickens. In Vietnam and Thailand, the pandemic has infected at least 37 people, with 26 deaths.

2005 THE ILLINOIS PARENT TEACHERS ASSOCIATION VERSUS THE ILLINOIS DEPARTMENT OF PUBLIC HEALTH

A small group of physicians and scientists, including author of this book Dr. Andrew Maniotis and his then wife Rita Maniotis, gained the support of the Illinois PTA in a unanimous decision to support a current halt to the current mandated hepatitis B vaccine. Another way of saying this is that every school representative present at the convention, when shown the data we had obtained, had agreed with our concerns, and immediately held a brief session to advance a motion to direct PTA funding to disseminate literature so that parents would be informed. This group of perhaps a thousand parents (mostly women), appeared to have only one concern: the total welfare, protection, and education of the school children of Illinois. It should be stated emphatically, that the current hepatitis B mandate threatens not only our children's health, but also serves to threaten our children's education and admission to all kinds of institutions (day care and school admission), with the bluff that "if you don't get your kid vaccinated against this STD, that is detected only in subpopulations of injection drug users and perhaps highly promiscuous persons, healthy black Australian aboriginal men, Micronesians, Vietnamese, Taiwanese, Native Americans, patients with Down syndrome, leukemia and transfusion recipients, he or she cannot enter school to learn how to read and write." This is not overstating it. Children cannot gain admission into day-care, Kindergarten, elementary schools, junior highs, high schools, and now even colleges, without showing evidence of a mandated (federally-recommended), and dangerous vaccine (hepatitis B). Pursuing these issues, we presented the current head of the IDPH (Illinois Department of Public Health Director Whitaker and his staff), with the same publicly available data from Medline, the vaccine manufacturer's package inserts warnings, data from the Vaccine Adverse Events reporting System, the CDC, Vaccine-link, and other databases, that we had presented to the Illinois PTA convention. After visits with numerous Senators, and public officials during the past several years, over a year later, in June of 2005, we finally were granted a brief meeting with the IDPH, after they could put us off no longer. As a response to our pleas to institute informed consent regarding the dangers of the hepatitis B vaccine's side effects and safety record as it appears on the Federal government's VAERS database, and after many weeks of deliberation, Dr. Whitaker and his staff emailed us a one paragraph letter stating: "Parents are currently given enough informed consent."

2006 (March) Article appears in the New England Journal of Medicine confirming that "HIV" tests show positive results after recent flu vaccination. (Christian, P. Erickson, Todd McNiff, Jeffrey D. Klausner. Influenza Vaccination and False Positive HIV Results New England Journal of Medicine, Number 13, Volume 354:1422-1423, March 30, 2006).

2006 (March) An article in the March 10, 2006 issue of the Journal of American Physicians and Surgeons (JPandS.org) shows that since mercury was removed from childhood vaccines, the alarming increase in reported rates of autism and other neurological disorders (NDs) in children not only stopped, but actually dropped sharply – by as much as 35%.

Using the government's own databases, David A. Geier, B.A. and

Mark R. Geier, M.D., Ph.D. analyzed reports of childhood NDs, including autism, before and after removal of mercury-based preservatives. The authors analyzed data from the CDC's Vaccine Adverse Event Reporting System (VAERS) and the California Department of Developmental Services (CDDS) in "Early Downward Trends in Neurodevelopmental Disorders Following Removal of Thimerosal-Containing Vaccines."

The numbers from California show that reported autism rates hit a high of 800 in May 2003. If that trend had continued, the reports would have skyrocketed to more than 1000 by the beginning of 2006. But in fact, the Geier's report that the number went down to only 620, a real decrease of 22%, and a decrease from the projections of 35%. This analysis directly contradicts 2004 recommendations of the Institute of Medicine which examined vaccine safety data from the National Immunization Program (NIP) of the CDC. While not willing to either rule out or to corroborate a relationship between mercury and autism, the IOM soft-pedaled its findings, and decided no more studies were needed. The authors write: "The IOM stated that the evidence favored rejection of a causal relationship between thimerosal and autism, that such a relationship was not biologically plausible, and that no further studies should be conducted to evaluate it.

2006 EDITORIAL-WHY IS THE HEPATITIS B VACCINE STILL MANDATED?

Andrew Maniotis, PhD a Program Director in the Cell and Developmental Biology of Cancer Department of Pathology, Anatomy and Cell Biology, and Bioengineering, College of Medicine Research Building 909 South Wolcott Ave. University of Illinois at Chicago

Evidence from many sources show the hepatitis B vaccine is not safe or effective and is linked to many autoimmune syndromes. Hepatitis B syndrome is rare (0.00024%-hovering near zero percent for both adults and children), while over 10.4% of hepatitis B vaccine recipients experience adverse vaccine reactions. According to package inserts, 1% of these are serious enough for emergency room admission. France discontinued its vaccination of school-aged children because of the types and high rate of catastrophic illnesses linked to the vaccine. Molecular markers (HBsAg, anti-HBsAg, HbeAg, anti-HbeAg, or HBV-DNA) are not diagnostic or predictive of liver disease, and Down syndrome, leukemia, and genetic polymorphisms related to differences in disease susceptibility were central to the discovery of HBV. Cell culture, animal models, and human studies have failed to show cytopathic effects in liver consistent with the hypothesized pathogenicity of HBV infection. In regions where the HBV markers are endemic, long-term study has shown that the vaccine increased the rate of hepatitis B syndrome in teens. The claim that seropositivity for HBV markers is linked to liver cancer decades later may be a form of molecular mimicry, and it is unsupported by evidence: it is like claiming that a freckle on an infant signal that melanoma will develop decades later. To date, and despite congressional investigations and numerous studies questioning the safety of the hepatitis B vaccine, informed consent and the original trial safety data has not been provided by the public health service.

2006 (March) Chiron Recalls Nearly 5.5 Million Vaccine Doses. California-based biotechnology company Chiron Corp. announced Thursday that it is recalling and withdrawing almost 5.5 million doses of a measles, mumps and rubella vaccine distributed to developing countries and in Italy. The move was made because the vaccine caused a higher rate of such adverse effects such as fever, allergic reactions, and glandular swelling than other similar vaccines, the Associated Press reported. The reactions occurred just after inoculation and do not indicate any long-term risk, according to Chiron, which described the recall and withdrawal as a precaution. About five million doses of the vaccine were distributed to developing countries and about 450,000 doses were distributed in Italy. Other Chiron vaccines are not affected by the recall, the AP reported. In 2004, Chiron failure to deliver half the United States' expected 100 million flu shots triggered widespread public health concern. The company could not fill the order because contaminated vaccine was discovered at its plant in Liverpool, England. Last fall, Chiron said problems at the same plant meant the company would not ship out as many flu shots as initially planned.

2006 (April) Associated press releases article claiming that Bangladesh will vaccinate about 18 million children aged 5 and under to combat polio, which recently re-emerged after authorities believed it had been eradicated five years ago, the country's health minister said Saturday. Bangladesh carried out extensive vaccination programs in 1995-2004, with the last polio case reported in August 2000, according to the government and WHO.

2006 During National Infant Immunization week, statistics are released that show to date, the National Vaccine Injury Compensation Program (VICP) has paid $1.2 billion to families who have proven that their children suffer permanent disabilities or have died from a vaccine reaction. Less than 25 percent of families who apply through VICP ever get compensated. Many more families never apply for compensation since they do not recognize the symptoms of vaccine damage. In 2019 this sum rose to 4 Billion according to The National Vaccine Information Center and CDC.

2006 (June) Press Release for Immediate Release June 29, 2006. Contact: CDC Media Relations. Phone: (404) 639-3286 CDC's Advisory Committee Recommends Changes in Varicella Vaccinations. A Second dose of varicella vaccine is being suggested to offer more protection for children, adolescents, and adults.

The Advisory Committee on Immunization Practices (ACIP) to the Centers for Disease Control and Prevention (CDC), in its meeting in Atlanta today, voted to recommend a second dose of varicella (chickenpox) vaccine for children four to six years old to further improve protection against the disease. The first dose of varicella vaccine is recommended at 12 to 15 months old.

Fifteen to 20 percent of children who have received one dose of the vaccine are not fully protected and may develop chickenpox after coming in contact with varicella zoster virus. Additionally, one dose of the vaccine may not continue to provide protection into adulthood when chickenpox is more severe. A second dose of varicella vaccine provides increased protection against varicella disease compared to one-dose. The ACIP also recommended that children, adolescents and adults who previously received one dose should receive a second dose."

We have made great progress in reducing chickenpox during the past ten years," said Dr. Anne Schuchat, director of CDC's National Center for Immunization and Respiratory Diseases. "This recommendation will further reduce outbreaks of chickenpox and provide better individual protection.

Before licensure of the varicella vaccine in 1995, each year there were about four million cases of varicella, 13,500 hospitalizations and 150 deaths (yet in NY State alone, the register claims 64 potential deaths and 54 actual deaths for that state alone). Cases of varicella have steadily declined 80 to 85 percent in surveillance sites since the licensure. From 1995 to 2001, varicella hospitalizations declined by 72 percent and deaths, among those 50 years old and younger, decreased by 75% or more.

However, in recent years varicella outbreaks have continued to occur among vaccinated school children. During these chickenpox outbreaks, between 11 and 17 percent of vaccinated children developed varicella. Varicella in vaccinated children is usually mild, but the children are contagious and can transmit the virus to others including their parents who are at higher risk of severe disease.

The ACIP, consisting of 15 members appointed by the Secretary of the Department of Health and Human Services (HHS), advises the director of CDC and Secretary of HHS on control of vaccine-preventable disease and vaccine usage. Recommendations of the ACIP become CDC policy when they are accepted by the director of CDC and are published in CDC's Morbidity and Mortality Weekly Report (MMWR). There are no federal laws requiring the immunization of children. All school and daycare entry laws are state laws and vary from state to state.

2006 (Sept 1) Polio reported on the rise in Nigeria Lagos, Nigeria despite near-universal vaccination. Nigerian authorities on Friday reported a sharp rise in the number of polio cases in Africa's most populous country over recent months, despite a government immunization drive.

"A total of 784 cases of the disease were registered in 17 states at the end of July, the National Programme on Immunization said. In June, the figures were 501 cases in 15 states, compared to 244 cases in 18 states for the same period in 2005, it said in a statement."

"From June 29 to July 3, Nigerian health officials in collaboration with United Nations health agencies launched an ambitious five-day Polio Plus immunization campaign of 10-million children in northern Nigeria aimed at eradicating the deadly disease from the country by the end of 2006."

2006 One of the chief dissenters of AIDSVAX, the failed program now funded to make an anthrax vaccine for 887 million of taxpayer money following announcement of that failure, Robert C. Gallo, scoffs at the notion that the trial will be successful.

"I thought we'd learn more if we had extract of maple leaf in the vaccine," he said derisively.

2006 Toronto International AIDS Conference. Barre-Sinoussi (one of Montagnier's original group who thought "HIV" was associated with AIDS and who received the Nobel with Montagnier in 2009) "came out of the closet" http://www.aids2006.org/PAG/PSession.aspx?s=653):

It is not clear if therapeutic vaccines might be useful, since 15 trials to date have not demonstrated definitive evidence of improved outcomes.

2006 (October 6) FDA recalls Home Access Health Corporation (Hoffman Illinois) Home Access and Home Access Express HIV-1 Test System lots 042108, 042109, 042110, 042111, 042113, 052101, 042010, 042011, 042012, 042013, 042014, 042015, 042016, 042017, 052001. "The lancets may not be sterile as of the printed "Use By" date. These lots should have been labeled with a "Use By" date of October 2006. HAHC recommends that these lots be removed from distribution and they will not be able to provide results for any blood specimen collected after October 31, 2006." It is not clear how aseptically-sealed blood-letting lancets lose their sterility over time.

2006 December Senate approves Burr's bioterrorism bill-a bill to establish the Biomedical Advanced Research and Development Authority, commonly referred to as BARDA, which passed by unanimous consent. The bill describes how forced vaccines and quarantines should be signed into law as the 'debate' regarding Bush's wars in Iraq and Afghanistan and "rooting out terrorism" continues.

2006 FDA recalls Vironostika HIV-1 test kit lots: 259606, 121566, 1008926, 259606, 121567, 1008926, 259606,121568, 1008926, 259605, 259717, 160342, 1011220, 259605, 259717,160339, 1011021."These HIV-1 finished kit lots in the field have been reported to contain EnzAbody reagent that appears noticeably cloudy and/or flocculent, instead of clear and non-turbid as expected 30 minutes after reconstitution. Use of cloudy EnzAbody could possibly increase your risk of inaccurate HIV test results in patients and therefore should be avoided." Patients who were diagnosed positive with them are never informed.

2006 A nationwide team of AIDS researchers led by doctors Benigno Rodriguez and Michael Lederman of Case Western Reserve University in Cleveland dispute the value of viral load tests-a standard used since 1996 to assess health, predict progression to disease, and grant approval to new AIDS drugs after their study of 2,800 HIV positives concluded viral load measures failed in more than 90% of cases to predict or explain immune status..."Viral load is only able to predict progression to disease in 4% to 6% of HIV-positives studied, challenging much of the basis for current AIDS science and treatment policy" (Rodriquez B, Sethi AK, Cheruvu VK, et al. Predictive value of plasma HIV RNA level on rate of CD4 T-cell decline in untreated HIV infection. JAMA 296(12):1498-506, 2006).

2006 (November) Cervical cancer vaccination funding for Australian girls rejected. CSL Limited, Australia's leading biopharmaceutical company, announced that the Pharmaceutical Benefits

Advisory Committee (PBAC) rejected CSL's funding application for its cervical cancer vaccine GARDASIL(r). CSL applied to the PBAC for National Immunization Program funding for the vaccine for three groups of women, based on the use approved by the Therapeutic Goods Administration (TGA). An ongoing cohort of 11–12-year-old girls delivered through a schools-based program at the end of primary school, a catch-up program for high-school girls (aged 13-18) delivered through secondary schools and a general practice-based program for women aged 19-26. Although disappointed, CSL remains committed to securing Government funding for GARDASIL in Australia and will continue to work closely with the Government and PBAC until this is achieved.

Last week, the Centers for Disease Control and Prevention issued new immunization schedules, including the first separate ones for adolescents. The recommendations cover two new vaccines for teenagers: one for the virus that causes cervical cancer and the other for a bacterium that causes meningitis and other diseases.

The agency has updated its recommended list of vaccines several times over the past 15 years, always after lengthy debate. Each state, rather than the C.D.C., decides which vaccines to make compulsory for entry into school. And some new vaccines are recommended rather than required because their prices are so high.

The timing of injections is complex and must be overseen by a doctor. But in general, these are the recommendations:

By age 6: Polio, Measles, Mumps, Rubella, Chickenpox, Diphtheria, Tetanus, Whooping cough, Hib (meningitis), PCV (pneumonia), Rotavirus (diarrhea), Hepatitis A and B, Flu (annually).

By age 18: Cervical cancer* (Incorrectly said to be caused by "human papillomaviruses")Meningococcus (bacterial infection).

From 18-65: Between ages 18-65, the vaccination you should get depends on risk factors: Flu (annually when available, always after age 50)Tetanus and diphtheria (every 10 years)Measles, mumps, rubella, chicken-pox (for everyone not previously infected).

Some high-risk categories include:

MULTIPLE DISEASES: Military recruits, health care workers, emergency responders, sewer workers

HEPATITIS: Gay men, sex workers, drug injectors

PLAGUE, RABIES: Veterinarians, animal handlers

ANTHRAX: Hide handlers

BY REGION: Travelers and immigrants may need vaccination, depending on their location. People with compromised immune systems should not take some vaccines.

By age 65:Pneumococcal pneumonia flu (annually).

*Girls only; an HPV vaccine for boys is being developed." (Source by Centers for Disease Control and Prevention).

2006 (December) Despite the 2004-5 west African polio eradication campaign intended as a final push to stamp out the disease in the region and is part of the World Health Organization's 15-year drive to halt transmission of the poliomyelitis virus across the world by 2005, the CDC, and WHO report that Nigeria now leads the world in new polio cases http://www.who.int/vaccines/immunizationmonitoring/en/diseases/poliomyelitis/afpextract.cfm.

"Country: Nigeria-Year: 2006-AFP cases (acute flaccid paralysis) reported: 4937-Non-polio AFP rate: 6.7%-AFP rate with adequate specimens: 88-Total confirmed polio cases: 1044-Wild-virus confirmed polio cases: 1043-Polio cases attributed to vaccine.

2007 – While working fully time at the University of Illinois as a cancer researcher, in his free time **Dr. Andrew Maniotis published "Sacrifice of the Virgins, and the Other First Anti-Cancer Vaccine" e-book about the HPV vaccine dangers** and fake science proclamations by Merck and public health agencies about its proven efficacy in preventing cervical cancer in the mainstream media. https://andrewmaniotis.wordpress.com/cancer-2/sacrifice-of-the-virgins-and-the-other-first-anti-cancer-vaccine/

1) **HPV vaccine prevents cervical cancer—no evidence.**
2) **HPV causes cervical cancer—no evidence.**

3) **HPV is the first cancer vaccine–what about hepatitis B and hepatocellular carcinoma? Merck told us 20 years ago that that the hepatitis B vaccine was the first cancer-preventative vaccine, and Taiwan, and Korean studies are often provided to support that the vaccine reduced cancer in these countries. Can't these folks remember the history of their own vaccinology for 20 years prior to the present?**
4) **"The unanimous recommendation inspired cheers from the medical community, which said the vaccine could help save the lives of tens of thousands of women worldwide."**

   But you do not hear the parents of vaccine damaged children cheering (as many as 10% are severely damaged by the hepatitis B vaccine according to Merck's own package insert-which in many cases is being co-administered along with GARDASIL-see VAERS reports toward the end of this article). Many of our colleagues who have worked directly with "HPV" diagnosis and treatment also aren't cheering, because they diagnose and treat cervical cancers and they know that the molecular HPV tests have not been validated, nor have the cell based smears been elucidated (why would the ASCUS test mean Atypical Squamous Cell Carcinoma of UNDETERMINED SIGNIFICANCE if this were not the case)?Certainly, the US's chief and most respected workers in HPV research aren't cheering because they stated in a CAP Today article (College of American Pathologists Today) there are grave medical concerns even regarding the validity of HPV test kits. Moreover, we worked with HPV in my laboratory, and we were horrified at such a dangerous suggestion-the implementation of this vaccine will place the lives of millions of our daughters at risk. Where are the long-term safety data? Will they be conveniently lost like the hepatitis B data that we asked the CDC to show us several years ago?
5) **"...this is a watershed event ... that we hope will help usher in a new era of cancer prevention,"**

It is a "watershed event" designed to reap untold profits at almost $900 dollars for the series at the expense of our daughter's (and possibly son's health).

6) **"Haupt doesn't expect women to be tested routinely for HPV before being inoculated, in part because commercial tests can't pinpoint which HPV strain a woman has."**

   How can any scientific study on vaccine efficacy be conducted without an accurate test to "pinpoint" the presence of a suspected pathogen?

7) **Documents prepared by the FDA suggest some women with persistent HPV infections could be at higher risk of cervical cancer after taking the vaccine.**

How could this be science based upon the immunology that we learned in school, or anything resembling science? Why should some women be at greater risk if they receive the vaccine? Is the HPV vaccine, GARDASIL, like the SV40-contaminated polio vaccines that increased the polio rate 3-fold in California, and 15-fold in Idaho, and hundreds of folds in certain outbreaks over normal summer background incidences of polio in the US weeks after the first vaccine wave was given? Does it increase disease like MMR and pertussis vaccines have, or is it due to the possibility that the HPV vaccine contains poisons, toxins, other viruses, or non-disclosed immune-disease-stimulating adjuvants (such as squalene) that cause autoimmune disease such as lupus, demyelinating syndromes, arthritis, or even cancer in animals?

What leading pathologists are saying about the molecular HPV kits and their validation as cancer diagnostics?

Both of these Chicago Tribune articles differ considerably from a front-page statement and 5-page article published in the September 2005 issue of Pathology/Laboratory Medicine/ and Laboratory Management article released monthly by The College of American Pathologists (CAP). Instead of asking Merck, The Public Health Service, or Moms and their children what they think about the merits of the new Gardasil "HPV" vaccine, a highly pointed and critical

5-page article was advanced regarding the uncertainties of "HPV" testing. A few examples from the article make the point:

"Dr. Schiffman heads the HPV Troup in the Division of Cancer, Epidemiology, and Genetics at NCI and is a tenured senior investigator. In mid-March, Dr. Mark Schiffman, MD, MPH, called CAP TODAY's editor to voice a troubling concern: that laboratories are failing to clinically validate their HPV tests."

In two subsequent interviews with CAP TODAY, Dr. Schiffman says labs are stumbling badly. His case is straightforward. Laboratories that use HPV tests need to make sure those tests are clinically validated. "It's amazing to me that someone would sell a product that's influencing a patient's life in terms of treatment for cervical cancer without being sure, based on data, that they can do it again and again and again with reliability."

Mark Stoler, M.D., professor of pathology and clinical gynecology and associate director of surgical pathology and cytopathology, University of Virginia Health System, Charlottesville, says the problem is a major concern, not 'some' concern. It's beyond anecdotal."

"I certainly see-in the chat areas of the different organizations, at conferences, on the Internet-advertisements and statements that are troubling, because they're indicating an excessive faith in poorly validated assays."

In the CAP TODAY article, Dr. Stoler also pointedly asks, "The essential question for ASCUS triage (atypical squamous cells of <u>undetermined</u> significance), is what is the sensitivity of the HPV test, and therefore its negative predictive value, in patients who have equivocal cytology for high-grade lesions? Many physicians, however, focus instead on the positive predictive value of the test, that is, the likelihood of finding high-grade lesions with colposcopy."

"The problem," he says, "is colposcopy is a terrible gold standard, missing anywhere from one-third to one-half of high-grade disease." "Lots and lots of labs say, 'We think the PCR test is more sensitive because we can pick up fewer DNA copies.' That has nothing to do with what we are talking about," says Dr. Stoler. "If you're going to bring forward a test, you've got to do a clinical validation trial that establishes its performance relative to these other benchmarks," he continues. "And the standard is not analytical molecules of DNA. It is not the analytic validation that matters, it is the clinical validation-how does the test perform in the real world? How sensitive are you with finding high-grade disease in a population of minimally abnormal cytology patients?"

2007 (January) "Virological failure" is a technical term among "HIV/AIDS" shills that simply means a lethal and toxic liver-destroying drug has failed to suppress "virus" because it doesn't work, and patients tend to die taking the drugs anyway. On January 11, 2007 in the New England Journal of Medicine, it was reported by Max Essex's Harvard group that nevirapine (withdrawn because of its toxicity in the U.S. and instead given to pregnant African women in order to experiment on them) increases the failure of the drug cocktail by 41.7% compared to controls:

"Nevirapine remains central to the prevention of mother-to-child transmission of human immunodeficiency virus type 1 (HIV-1) and to combination antiretroviral treatment throughout much of the developing world. Nevirapine administered as one dose to the mother and one to the newborn reduces mother-to-child transmission of HIV-1 by 41 to 47%, and well over 875,000 women and infants have received a single dose of nevirapine. A single dose of nevirapine is the cornerstone of the regimen recommended by the World Health Organization (WHO) to prevent mother-to-child transmission among women without access to antiretroviral treatment and among those not meeting treatment criteria. However, nevirapine resistance is detected (with the use of standard genotyping techniques) in 20 to 69% of women and 33 to 87% of infants after exposure to a single, peripartum dose of nevirapine. Among 60 women starting antiretroviral treatment within 6 months after receiving placebo or a single dose of nevirapine, no women in the placebo group and 41.7% in the nevirapine group had virologic failure."

2007 (March) ALLIANCE FOR HUMAN RESEARCH PROTECTION (AHRP) PROMOTING OPENNESS, FULL DISCLOSURE, AND ACCOUNTABILITY http://www.ahrp.org

"Two weeks ago, the controversial anthrax vaccine which has not been fully tested for safety, became mandatory for the military. Since then, Meryl Nass, MD, (AHRP board member) has received numerous requests for help and information from military personnel who refuse to be vaccinated with this controversial vaccine."

"The military has issued an unsigned, anonymous "informational brochure" filled with misinformation about the anthrax vaccine. The very fact that no one in the military wants "credit" for this document should raise red flags about its veracity!"

"Dr. Nass has appended the DOD "informational brochure" with relevant facts, additional information, comments and copious references about the Surveillance Program for Short-term Health Effects of AVA and Surveillance Program for Long-term Health Effects of AVA. She demonstrates how the DOD misrepresents the findings of several vaccine safety studies."

"For example, Dr. Nass writes: Military medical providers have been loath to file anthrax vaccine adverse event reports due to perceived adverse effects on their careers if they do so. This probably stems from the instruction to medical providers NOT to report adverse events unless the patient missed more than 24 hours of work, was hospitalized, or contamination of an entire lot of vaccine was suspected."

"Therefore, after changing this guidance in response to Congressional testimony about the failures to file, repeated instructions to file these reports by top military leaders have been issued to providers in 1999, 2000 and 2004. This would suggest that military medical providers continued to fail to file the reports." See complete annotated document at:

http://www.anthraxvaccine.org/NassDOD.htm;

http://www.anthraxvaccine.org/NassDOD.htm

2007 (March) Varicella Vaccine Waning -Waning Immunity with the Varicella Vaccine. A population-based study shows declining immunity over time in individuals who receive only a single dose of varicella vaccine.

"Although varicella incidence has decreased dramatically in the U.S. since the introduction of universal varicella immunization in 1995, disease outbreaks have continued to occur in highly vaccinated populations. Might vaccine-induced immunity diminish with time? To find out, researchers from the CDC and the Los Angeles County Department of Health Services examined varicella surveillance data from Antelope Valley, California (population, 350,000)."

"From 1995 through 2004, 11,356 cases of varicella were reported in this population, including 1080 cases (9.5%) with onset >42 days after vaccination. During the decade of observation, annual varicella incidence decreased by 85%, and the proportion of cases in immunized children increased from 1% to 60%. Among vaccinated children, the incidence of moderate-to-severe disease increased from 18% in 1995–1998 to 31% in 2001–2004. Moderate-to-severe disease was significantly more likely in 8- to 12-year-olds who had been vaccinated? 5 years previously than in those vaccinated within the previous 5 years (odds ratio, 2.6; 95% confidence interval, 1.2–5.8). The rate of varicella disease following vaccination increased significantly each year after vaccination, ranging from 1.6 per 1000 person-years in year 1 to 58.2 per 1000 person-years in year 9 which isn't bad because it is only increased 36 times in the disease frequency among the vaccinated compared to the non-vaccinated!"

Comment: These findings were part of the evidence underlying the June 2006 recommendation from the Advisory Committee on Immunization Practices to provide a second dose of varicella vaccine to children aged 4 to 6 years, despite the fact that disease incidence is increasing among the vaccinated. "Exogenous re-exposure to varicella virus has probably helped in maintaining immunity to this pathogen. Given the ongoing decline in varicella incidence, and thus in opportunities for community exposure to the virus, a second dose of vaccine may also be needed for high-risk populations such as healthcare workers."— Richard T. Ellison III, MD Journal Watch Infectious Diseases March 14, 2007. Citation(s): Chaves SS et al. Loss of vaccine-induced immunity to varicella over time. N Engl J Med 2007 Mar 15; 356:1121-9.

2007 Fri Mar 30, 1:45pm EDT By Anne Harding

NEW YORK (Reuters Health) – "Rules that allow parents to exempt their children from immunization requirements for "philosophical" reasons are putting all kids at risk of outbreaks of vaccine-preventable disease, Arkansas researchers warn. Since 2003, when the state began allowing these exemptions from school vaccine rules, rising numbers of children have been going without immunization, Dr. Joseph W. Thompson of the Arkansas Center for Health Improvement in Little Rock and colleagues found. Arkansas had previously allowed exemption from vaccine requirements for religious or medical reasons, but parents had to belong to a "recognized religion that included tenets against immunization" for the exemption to be allowed, Thompson and colleagues explain in the American Journal of Preventive Medicine. Parents challenged the law, and a federal court ruled that requiring a religion to be "recognized" was not constitutional. Arkansas now allows religious, philosophical, and medical exemptions, which must be renewed annually. Since the change, Thompson and his team found, the number of exemptions requested by parents has steadily risen, while the percentage of exemptions that are non-medical has made up an increasingly large portion of the total.

For example, in 2001 (when the philosophical exemption was not available) there were 419 religious exemptions and 110 medical exemptions statewide. In 2004-2005, there were 721 philosophical exemptions, 362 religious exemptions, and 62 medical exemptions.

And in the 10 districts with the highest exemption rates, none were medical. In order for vaccines to be effective, Thompson noted, they must provide an individual with immunity, and they must also provide "herd" immunity by covering a certain percentage of people in the community, estimated to be at least 93 percent for measles, for example.

"Concentrations of children who are not immunized could result in a loss of community-level immunity and ultimately erode public health protection against vaccine-preventable illness," the researchers warn "Nationwide we're seeing parents increasingly undervalue the protection that vaccines give because the diseases they have never seen," Thompson said. "When polio affected a child in every school, the polio vaccine was rapidly adopted." According to Thompson, policymakers and medical professionals need to do a better job of informing parents about the risks and benefits of vaccines. "Just throwing information at them without putting it in the context of what their concerns are probably is not going to be very valuable." SOURCE: American Journal of Preventive Medicine, March 2007.

2007 April. FDA recall of Combivir/Ziagen (lamivudine and zidovudine) Tablets because counterfeit labels are discovered.

2007 June. HIV infection theory challenged:

"T cells are lost at a slow rate. A longstanding theory of how HIV slowly depletes the body's capacity to fight infection is wrong, scientists say. The researchers used a mathematical model of the processes by which T cells are produced and eliminated. Using this they showed that the current theory of an uncontrolled cycle of T cell activation, infection, HIV production and cell destruction – dubbed the "runaway" hypothesis – was flawed. They concluded that it could not explain the terribly slow pace of depletion that occurs in HIV infection. If the theory were correct, then T helper cell numbers would fall to exceptionally low levels over a number of months, not years."

2007 (July) The clout of the immense pharmaceutical giants is used to persuade and coerce state and National government officials to embrace massive, expensive vaccination programs. For example, over the last seven years, the industry has contributed more than $800 million in federal and state lobbying and campaign donations. No other industry has spent more money to sway public policy to use their products: drugs and vaccines. (REF: **"Drug Lobby Second to None." Center for Public Integrity. July 7, 2007).**

2007 July. Six health care workers that were to be placed before a firing squad in Libya for "infecting 426 children" are released because black health care workers from sub-Saharan Africa are blamed instead by Luc Montagnier for spreading "the infection."

EPILOGUE IN LIBYA: A SPREADING AIDS EPIDEMIC by Elisabeth Rosenthal Thursday, July 26, 2007

ROME: Five Bulgarian nurses and a Palestinian doctor landed in Sofia this week, freed of a death sentence after eight years in Libyan prisons, an apparent victory of diplomacy at long last.

Officially, two visits to Libya by Cécilia Sarkozy, the French president's wife, precipitated the release of the six medics who had been found guilty – not once, but twice – of infecting more than 400 children with HIV as part of a plot by the Israeli secret service.

Sarkozy's visit was only the latest in countless pilgrimages by diplomats and scientists to the Libyan leader, Muammar el-Qaddafi, to plead the medics' cause. Recent visitors included the U.S. secretary of state, Condoleezza Rice, the European Union's external relations commissioner, Benita Ferrero-Waldner, and Richard Roberts, a Nobel laureate, who represented more than 100 Nobel Prize winners.

He and another expert, Dr. Luc Montagnier, the French virologist whose team discovered HIV, concluded that the AIDS virus was present in the hospital before the nurses arrived, probably brought to Libya by guest workers from countries in sub-Saharan Africa. (In other words, it the fault of the blacks, if this quote from Montagnier is accurate).

Comment: In other words, Montagnier claims that the "epidemic" of more than 400 "HIV/AIDS" cases in hospitalized children in Libya "treated" by the 5 nurses and one doctor was instead really caused by Black people coming up to work in (and around?) the Libyan hospital from "Sub-Saharan" Africa, somehow.

2007 On Monday, July 23, 2007, in Nkange, Botswana, it was reported that (Craig Timberg Washington Post Foreign Service) in Botswana, step to cut AIDS proves a formula for disaster:

Doctors noticed two troubling things about the limp, sunken-eyed children who flooded pediatric wards across Botswana during the rainy season in early 2006: They were dying from diarrhea, a malady that is rarely fatal here. And few of their mothers were breast-feeding, a practice once all but universal. After the outbreak was over and at least 532 children had died — 20 times the usual toll for diarrhea — a team of U.S. investigators solved the terrible riddle. A decade-long, global push to provide infant formula to mothers with the AIDS virus had backfired in Botswana, leaving children more vulnerable to other, more immediately lethal diseases, the U.S. team found after investigating the outbreak at the request of Botswana's government.

2007 July – A total recall of an important AIDS drug widely used in developing countries has disrupted treatment for tens of thousands of the world's poorest patients, with no clear word from the manufacturer on when shipments will resume.

The recall of the drug, Viracept, by Roche Pharmaceuticals of Switzerland, went largely unnoticed in the developed world when it was announced in early June, after the company had discovered that some batches made at its Swiss plant contained a dangerous chemical. But the recall has caused growing concern among global health officials and in AIDS programs in many poor nations. They say the company did an inadequate job of informing patients and officials about the potential risks and helping them find affordable access to newer alternative drugs.

2007 "September AIDS Effort Suffers Big Blow as Merck Vaccine Fails to evoke seroconversion or protection from "HIV," by Marilyn Chase and Mark Schoofs:

"In a major setback, one of the leading experimental AIDS vaccines not only failed to prevent test subjects from becoming infected with HIV, but it didn't offer any indication it might delay the onset of full-blown AIDS, which had been a key hope."

The collapse of the trial leaves Merck & Co., which had spent a decade developing the vaccine, with no remaining prospects in the global hunt for an AIDS immunization. The vaccine was tested in a network funded by the National Institutes of Health."

"We've been kicked in the teeth," said Bruce Walker, a veteran AIDS researcher at Harvard University who was not involved in the study. Lawrence Corey, a leader of the NIH-funded HIV Vaccine Trials Network, said he was 'mourning. "The vaccine's failure to protect recipients from acquiring "HIV" was also a big disappointment to the recipients of the anti-"HIV" vaccine. The "HIV" vaccine recipients tested positive for "HIV" slightly more frequently than the non-"HIV"-vaccinated, but the differences between the groups were not significant in any arms of the STEP trial, or in any other "HIV" vaccine trial. All of these men who now test "HIV-positive" will be regarded and treated now as AIDS patients."

MORE SUCCESS WITH ANIMAL MODELS OF "HIV/AIDS"

Although SIV has always been a better model of "HIV" than "HIV," because the chimps that were injected with "HIV" or AIDS patient blood more than 20 years ago never became ill, as they were built new retirement homes, at least one group of investigators recently challenged this long-standing belief: Sodora's paper provides evidence, using the sooty mangabey SIV natural host, that virally induced CD4 T-cell depletion, by itself, is not sufficient to induce AIDS in a natural host. "When we first observed the dramatic CD4 depletion in all the tissues we examined in these monkeys, we were concerned that they might begin to exhibit clinical signs of AIDS," said Jeffrey Milush, Ph.D., lead author on the paper. "But after more than six years, we are sure that CD4 depletion by itself does not necessarily result in progression to AIDS".

"Sodora contributed to a second paper, with senior author Guido Silvestri, M.D., of the University of Pennsylvania. In a study of disease free SIV–infected sooty mangabeys, Silvestri proposed that these African monkeys preserve immune function despite a major loss of mucosal CD4 T-cells as a result of an evolutionary adaptation to reduce immune activation in response to virus replication."

"The third of the three papers published this week in The Journal of Immunology, with Ivona Pandrea, M.D., Ph.D., and Cristian Apetrei, M.D., Ph.D., from Tulane University as lead authors, shows that a severe loss of intestinal CD4 T-cells in another natural host, the African green monkey, is also not predictive of SIV virulence."

2007 ONE-HUNDRED-THIRTEEN VACCINE ANTIGENS FROM AT LEAST 10 DIFFERENT VACCINES HAD BEEN ADDED AS SCHOOL REQUIREMENTS

"... Many parents are asking: How many more vaccines are going to be forced on children in order to obtain tax-funded, public education? Now, more than ever, parents are starting to say no. Many parents blame the health problems of their children on the sheer number of vaccines and additives they receive. Tens of thousands of parents have watched their children regress into poor health after vaccinations. They believe their children are at high risk and may suffer reactions from further doses. Parents who barely questioned their doctors' decisions in the past are now becoming informed and challenging vaccination recommendations. Many are choosing the risk of the infection over the risk of the vaccine. Legitimate concerns have been met by steely resistance from the medical profession and public health officials. A flurry of articles, closed-door meetings, congressional hearings, and position papers from the Institutes of Medicine defend the national vaccination program as widely accepted, an economic necessity and a small personal sacrifice for the good of the community. Resisters are marginalized as "wackos who believe in conspiracy theories." This tactic is not new. As far back as 1894, those who opposed vaccination were blasted in the New York Times as engaging "in a futile attempt to head off human progress and to reopen a question about which pretty much all of the world has made up its mind." REF: Cited in Brooklyn Medical Journal. 8(1894):576 and reference in Colgrove, p.14.

October 25, 2007; Thursday Warning Is Sent to AIDS Vaccine Volunteers: South Africans Among Recipients Who May Be at Higher Risk of Contracting Virus. Page A20, By Craig Timberg. JOHANNESBURG, Oct. 24 — "South African AIDS researchers have begun warning hundreds of volunteers that a highly touted experimental vaccine they received in recent months might make them more, not less, likely to contract HIV in the midst of one of the world's most rampant epidemics."

"The move stems from the discovery last month that an AIDS vaccine developed by Merck & Co. might have led to more infections than it averted among study subjects in the United States and other countries. Among those who received at least two doses of the vaccine, 19 contracted HIV compared with 11 of those given placebos."

2007, December 13 Audrey Serrano wins first-ever lawsuit including $2.5 M award overturning her AIDS diagnosis based on faulty virus tests. Dr Andrew Maniotis, author of this book, acts as chief scientific advisor https://www.cbsnews.com/news/woman-misdiagnosed-with-hiv-awarded-25m/.

2008 January. Prince George's County, Upper Marlboro, Maryland (CNN). A crowd of frustrated parents gathered on a chilly Saturday morning outside Prince George's County Circuit Court to comply with an order from the school system to have their children vaccinated — or else.

"Prince George's County State's Attorney Glenn Ivey, whose office began the effort, was at the courthouse to answer questions. Judge C. Philip Nichols, who signed the letters threatening parents with jail or fines, said he felt the tactic worked."

"We got a thousand kids back in school just by sending one letter," he said.

"Nichols ordered parents to come to court Saturday to either immunize the children on the spot, or to provide proof that they already had their shots," according to The Associated Press.

"Families who failed to comply could face 10 to 30 days in jail."

"The schools started out with phone calls, even home visits, and this became a last resort for parents who wouldn't comply one way or another," Ivey said.

All states require school-age children to be immunized against diseases such as mumps, measles, and polio. But the parents said they objected to the heavy-handed way Ivey has handled it. Families could opt out of the required shots by providing medical or religious waivers. Citing cases of serious adverse reactions, some parents worry about the safety of vaccines. The patient should have a choice. I just don't think Big Brother should have that much power," said Donna Hurlock, a physician and activist concerned about parental rights and privacy issues. Jim Moody was among the parents protesting the policy.

There are serious considerations for safety that need to be addressed before compelling people to get vaccines," he said. Public health officials said the benefits of vaccinations against child-hood diseases outweigh the risks. It was the school's mistake. [My daughter] did not have documentation. This is the second or third time we had to redo her again because her shot records got misplaced," Ron Brooking told CNN. Authorities said they will decide in the next few days what to do with families who refused to obey the vaccination order. Ivey was still mulling whether to prosecute parents not in compliance. "We have to sit down with school and health services," he told the AP. "We haven't ruled anything out. We need to figure out where we stand." The parents of about 1,700 children received letters from Ivey reminding them of the consequences for not complying, said John White, spokesman for Prince George's County Public Schools." That number was down to 1,111 by Thursday, and was reduced to 939 children by Saturday evening, he said. White said that number was the lowest since a law requiring additional vaccinations went into effect January 1. But "obviously, we still have some more work to do," he told the AP. 101 vaccinations were administered at the courthouse and 71 records were updated," he said.

2008 (January 1) 18 states as of this date allow an exemption to the procedure based on philosophical opposition to vaccination: Arizona, Arkansas, California, Colorado, Idaho, Louisiana, Maine, Michigan, Minnesota, New Mexico, North Dakota, Ohio, Oklahoma, Texas, Utah, Vermont, Washington, and Wisconsin. Mississippi, which has only a medical exemption for the public school system, allows an automatic exemption for home-schooled students. REF: Home School Legal Defense Association. http://www.hslda.org/Legislation/State/wv/2007/WVSB91/default.asp

2008 January 3, NEJM Volume 358:93-94, Number 1. Early Thimerosal Exposure and Neuropsychological Outcomes by Thompson, W. W.

To the Editor: "Thompson et al. (Sept. 27 issue) reports about the results of a study investigating the neuropsychological outcomes of early exposure to thimerosal. As a dissenting member of the panel of external consultants for this study, I object to the authors' conclusion that there is no causal association between thimerosal and children's brain function. The sample comprised children who were least likely to exhibit neuropsychological impairments. Specifically, children with congenital problems, those from multiple births, those of low birth weight, and those not living with their biological mother were excluded. The sample was skewed toward higher socioeconomic status and maternal education — factors that are associated with lower rates of neurobehavioral problems and higher intervention rates and that were not measured. The sampling frame included only children enrolled from birth in the health maintenance organization (HMO) and still enrolled after 7 to 10 years, excluding children in higher-mobility families, who tend to have lower academic and behavioral function.2 Children with neurobehavioral problems may have been less likely to remain with the HMO. Only 30% of families selected for recruitment participated, a low rate for scientific research. Among the families selected for recruitment, 26% refused to participate. Another 28% "could not be located," which included families that did not respond to multiple recruitment attempts (internal documentation from the study contractor, Abt Associates) — another form of refusal."

2008, June. HPV Vaccination: Is It Cost-Effective? Immunizing preteens before sexual exposure makes economic sense; cost-effectiveness of vaccinating older teens and young-adult females is less clear. By Ann J.

"In June, 2008, the reported death toll linked to Gardasil vaccine rises. Complications include foaming at mouth, convulsions, coma, anaphylactic shock, grand mal convulsion, "coma, and paralysis are a few of the startling descriptions included in a new federal report describing the complications from Merck & Co.'s Gardasil medication for sexually transmitted human papillomavirus – which has been proposed as mandatory for all schoolgirls."

The document was obtained from the U.S. Food and Drug Administration by Judicial Watch, a Washington group that investigates and prosecutes government corruption, and it has details of 10 deaths just since September.

"Given all the questions about Gardasil, the best public health policy would be to re-evaluate its safety and to prohibit its distribution to minors. In the least, governments should rethink any efforts to mandate or promote this vaccine for children," said Judicial Watch President Tom Fitton.

"The organization's work uncovered reports of about one death each month since last fall, bringing the total death toll from the drug to at least 18 and as many as 20. There also were 140 "serious" reports of complications including about three dozen classified as life- threatening, 10 spontaneous abortions and half a dozen cases of Guillain-Barre Syndrome."

"The document reveals the case of an 18-year-old woman who got the Gardasil vaccine, was found unconscious that evening, and died. Another woman, age 19, got the drug and the next morning was found dead in her bed. The new documents also reveal a total of 8,864 Vaccine Adverse Event Reporting System records, up from a total of 3,461 that had been reported in a document just last fall."

2008 July 10, 12 Babies Die During Vaccine Trials in Argentina. (Trading Markets). "At least 12 infants who were part of a clinical study to test a pneumonia vaccine have died in Argentina over the course of the past year. The study was sponsored by GlaxoSmithKline and uses children from poor families. According to the Argentine Federation of Health Professionals, the families are "pressured and forced into signing consent forms." The vaccine trial is still ongoing despite the denunciations."

2008 (August) Austrian Baxter scientist involved in H1N1 vaccine patent also advises WHO.

Baxter's Vaccine Patent Application US 2009/0060950 A1 gives "Kistner et al" as the applicant for the patent for the H1N1 vaccine that was provisionally filed on August 28, 2008. Baxter Files Swine Flu Vaccine Patent A Year Ahead of Outbreak US 20090060950A1 to Baxter International filed 28th August 2008. See Baxter Vaccine Patent Application...

"Baxter are nothing if not prepared for this 'swine flu' outbreak if the wording in this 2008 US patent application is anything to go by: In particular preferred embodiments the composition or vaccine comprises more than one antigen.....such as influenza A and influenza B in particular selected from of one or more of the human *H1N1*, H2N2, H3N2, H5N1, H7N7, H1N2, H9N2, H7N2, H7N3, H10N7 subtypes, of the pig flu *H1N1,* H1N2, H3N1 and H3N2 subtypes, of the dog or horse flu H7N7, H3N8 subtypes or of the avian H5N1, H7N2, H1N7, H7N3, H13N6, H5N9, H11N6, H3N8, H9N2, H5N2, H4N8, H10N7, H2N2, H8N4, H14N5, H6N5, H12N5 subtypes."

"Suitable adjuvants can be selected from mineral gels, aluminum hydroxide, surface active substances, lysolecithin, Pluronic polyols, polyanions or oil emulsions such as water in oil or oil in water, or a combination thereof. Of course, the selection of the adjuvant depends on the intended use. E.g., toxicity may depend on the destined subject organism and can vary from no toxicity to high toxicity."

"Three different influenza strains, two A-strains Hiroshima (HR, H3N2), a New Calcdonia (NC, H1N1) and a B-strain, Malaysia (MA), were produced in Vero cell cultures. After virus propagation the infectious virus harvest is inactivated prior to purification...."

2008 RELIGIOUS TERMINOLOGY, FOOTBALL STRATEGIES, AIDS RESEARCH, AND ORIGINAL ANTIGENIC SIN

The term, "Hail Mary," has been used after numerous failures of the "HIV equals AIDS hypothesis" to describe the 100-billion-dollar failures of AIDS research (HIV vaccine may never be found, warns leading scientist Mark Henderson, Science Editor, in Boston. From Times Online, February 14, 2008):

"Professor David Baltimore, a Nobel laureate who is President of the American Association for the Advancement of Science, told its annual conference in Boston that the failure of every promising approach to an HIV vaccine had led many scientists to wonder whether it would ever be possible to create one."

"While Professor Baltimore has a major grant from the Bill and Melinda Gates Foundation to research a new approach to HIV therapy and treatment, he said it was a last-ditch effort with only a slim hope of success. He compared it to a "Hail Mary" play in American football – a desperate attempt at a long pass, in which the quarterback throws the ball up and prays it will be caught by a teammate.

Specialized proteins that are not found in nature that can attack "HIV?"

Hail Mary indeed!

These kinds of strategies based upon football, and faith-based science and medicine have been employed since the first decade of "HIV" vaccine research. As shown a book obtained from The Office of Technology Assessment of "HIV" vaccine development, up until 1995, the recommendations of The Office of Technology presented to the 1995 Congress by the AIDS Research Advisory Committee (ARAC) of the National Institute of Allergy and Infectious Diseases (NIAID) were no more promising than those statements about the failed STEP trial we hear about from Dr. Baltimore and others today (1995 Congress of the United States: Office of Technology assessment. Adverse Reactions to HIV Vaccines: Medical, Ethical, and Legal Issues. Roger C. Herdman, Director).

The conclusions of this 1995 assessment recommended that Phase III clinical trials with enveloped vaccines should not proceed in the United States because of scientific, political, and ethical issues, and because of the significant level of scientific uncertainty about the wisdom of immediate trials. Not only were warnings presented about the danger of giving an "HIV" vaccine to already immunocompromised individuals (such as ARC or AIDS patients).

Such violations of biological principles and facts also may be the reason why the FDA and other agencies so frequently recall "HIV" test kit as shown even recently on the following dates (and these are only a few listed here to make the point, and only the ones that have made the Wall Street Journal: In 2001- FDA recalled 24 antigen test kit; in 2002, the FDA recalled BioRad Genetic systems HIV Types 1 &2 Synthetic Peptide containing test kits; in 2004, the FDA recalled bioMerieux NucliSens automated isolation reagent(s), DiaSoran's HIV-1 – HIV-2 Plus O EIA Testing Software, and Roche's Amplicor HIV Monitor test; in 2005, the FDA also recalled Globus Media Rapid HIV test kits; in 2006, the FDA recalled BioMerieux, in 2006 FDA recalled Vironostika HIV-1 test kit, and Abbott's Home access HIVAG-1 Monoclonal EIA Test Kit. It is a shame that "HIV" test kits are being recalled a full decade after unfortunate individuals who were caught in the "AIDS trap" may have tested positive in 2006, and their lives thereafter ruined. And as I have emphasized throughout this timeline, patients who were diagnosed positive with these phony diagnostic tests are never informed, and frequently, their lives are ruined. It is as certain as these facts or occurrences represent human rights violations of the darkest kind, it is certain also that those who tested positive on such recalled or fraudulent tests, or any others, are never informed that their lives have been ruined by fraudulent tests that cannot detect any virus in the first place.

With respect to the Military-Thailand trial, some highly creative "book-keeping" should be examined briefly. The vaccine track record of "HIV" vaccines, with their 64 failed trials, and the 172 duds currently in the NIH "HIV" vaccine pipeline are the best evidence we have that no such virus exists as an exogenous entity, and this most recent trial, said not to achieve statistical significance unless the data were manipulated, proves this view once more. Not only is it irrational to expect that seroconversion to gp120, which happens to about 98% of the multiple booster injections with the so-called env protein, indicates vaccine-acquired immunity, as it does with hepatitis C antibody which is believed to protect those who recover from that disease for life, and yet still an "HIV" partial positive test indicates active infection in the minds of the medical establishment, contrary to the fundamental laws and track record of vaccination seroepidemiology.

In fact, the track record and intensity of "HIV" vaccine research is the best evidence in the history of vaccination that the Jennerian paradigm, expanded by Pasteur, is even tenable. The results of the latest Military-Thailand trial, that used the past failed AIDSVAX vaccine was simply re-used and boosted with aluminum in multiple injections, among 16,000 unsuspecting Thailand people.

When control-vaccinated groups seroconvert more frequently than "HIV" vaccinated groups even after repeated booster vaccinations as they did in THE STEP trial, and they invariably stop these trials early because of what they call "futility" and potential adverse harm to the recipients is tragic. Using modern techniques and isolation(s) of so-called "HIV," rather than continuing to site or analyze the dusty old papers written by Montagnier, we can begin to appreciate how much of a scam "HIV/AIDS" science has become. As mentioned, even the co-Nobelist and co-discoverer of the molecular signature of "HIV" now claims, "we can catch it many times, no problem if you have a good immune system you can get rid of it,": etc. Who knows what went on at the Pasteur 30 years ago?

2008 GARDASIL LINKED TO SEVENTY-EIGHT OUTBREAKS OF GENITAL WARTS

"The Gardasil vaccine has been linked to 78 outbreaks of genital warts, according to an article in The Fiji Times entitled "Are our girls guinea pigs?" by Matelita Ragogo.

That is right. In addition to all of the other adverse reactions to this controversial vaccine, children who receive it are subject to outbreaks of genital warts. Unfortunately, not too many doctors take the time to educate parents about some of these possible reactions prior to giving little girls this expensive jab."

Deaths, Miscarriages and Other Adverse Events

"While genital warts are certainly disgusting, parents who think that genital warts are the worst possible adverse reaction to the vaccine should think again. According to Ragogo, as of August 14th, including the 78 outbreaks of genital warts, there have been 9,748 adverse events reported as per Judicial Watch, a non-profit watchdog group. Judicial Watch also reports that there have been 21 deaths, not including the deaths (by miscarriage) of 10 unborn babies."

https://www.lifesitenews.com/news/gardasil-vaccination-results-in-three-outbreaks-of-genital-warts-in-fiji-sc

MOST PATIENTS SHOULD BE SCREENED FOR H.I.V., PHYSICIANS GROUP SAYS: New York Times, December 2, 2009. By Roni Caryn Rabin

By the end of 2009 in December, and whether or not they had engaged in "risky behaviors, the American College of Physicians urged doctors to screen all patients for "HIV" routinely beginning at the age of 13.

These guidelines differed slightly from those of the federal Centers for Disease Control and Prevention, which recommended routine screening of patients until age 64, unless the prevalence of "HIV" was known to be less than 0.1 percent in the patient population in a specific geographical area or among a certain demographic. The recommendations also differed from those put forth by the U.S. Preventive Services Task Force, which urged routine screening only of patients at "increased risk for infection."

"But most patients don't tell their doctors about their risky behaviors," said Dr. Amir Qaseem, senior medical associate with the American College of Physicians, a professional group that represents internists. Moreover, "it is almost impossible for a physician to know what the "HIV" prevalence rate is among certain patients, Dr. Qaseem added.

In 2009 it was estimated that "1 million to 1.2 million Americans had "HIV," but 24 to 27 percent were undiagnosed or unaware of their infection," Dr. Qaseem said. Dr. Qaseem added: "We're recommending clinicians just adopt routine screening in their patients."

"The American College of Physicians had set no upper age limit on testing at that time because it was believed that 20 percent of people with "HIV" were over 50 years of age," Dr. Qaseem said. He also said, "clinicians should decide whether repeat screening is required on a case-by-case basis."

Even though the CDC had recommended routine testing two years previously, hospitals and clinics were slow to incorporate "HIV" screening into daily care. At that time only 50 to 100 of the nation's 5,000 emergency rooms routinely tested for "HIV," said Dr. Richard Rothman, who was an associate professor of emergency medicine at Johns Hopkins School of Medicine, and the rationale for this policy was justified in part because of a lack of funding.

"The CDC's view was that you would get an "HIV test just like you would have a complete blood count or any other test as part of your care," Dr. Rothman said... "But in many states, there was no mechanism for reimbursement, so emergency rooms that try to do it have to foot the bill themselves or find creative ways of paying for it."

The American College of Obstetricians and Gynecologists also recommended routine screening of all women ages 19 to 64, regardless of their risk factors for "HIV" infection. It was believed that early diagnosis maximized the "benefit" from antiretroviral therapy and also helped contain the spread of the disease by decreasing inadvertent transmissions.

2008 TOURIST VISA FROM INDIA: Declaration to be made by applicants seeking to stay in India for more than one year:

"I hereby undertake that I shall subject myself to a medical test, including for AIDS within one month of arrival in India. In case I am found positive for AIDS, I will leave India."

VACCINES CAUSE MICRO-VASCULAR STROKES: Dr. Andrew Moulden, Canadian Doctor (September 27, 2008) http://newsblaze.com/story/20080927170755tsop.nb/topstory.html

How long does it take a medical breakthrough to be acted upon? A Canadian doctor, Dr. Andrew Moulden says he conclusively proved seven years ago that vaccines cause micro-vascular strokes. Dr Moulden has a 21-year record of award-winning medical study and practice starting at Nipissing University, but he has been unable to get the attention of the College of Physicians or politicians to investigate his findings, which have been corroborated by other doctors. How vaccines cause micro-vascular strokes – Dr. Moulden says the shots cause our body's own immune systems to hyper-react as large white blood cells naturally rush to attack the foreign particles injected into our bloodstream. The white blood cells are too big to enter, so they surround tiny capillaries where the foreign particles land, clog and collapse the capillaries. This cuts off pathways for the smaller red blood cells to carry oxygen to the organs near those capillaries that contain the foreign particles. When the particles float near the brain, this lack of blood supply can lead to autism, SIDS and many other diagnosed illnesses in both children and adults. Our immune systems will continue fighting the particles leading to long-term or chronic illness. Different organs are affected depending on where the particles are, which leads to different symptoms and 'disease' names, but the basic causes are the same and before this discovery were unknown. The main cause of the problem is the additives in the vaccines. The purpose of the additives is to generate a faster response from white blood cells. This works perfectly – white blood cells rush to the site of the introduced foreign matter – and that is the source of the problem. The white blood cells block the capillaries and also collapse them, trying to destroy the foreign matter. Much more on this through http://brainguardmd.com/

2008 TUCSON, Arizona, October 2, (ENS) – New research indicates that the most pervasive global strain of HIV began spreading among humans as early as 1884, suggesting that growing urbanization in colonial Africa through the early 1900s set the stage for the current HIV/AIDS pandemic...The virus responsible for HIV/AIDS jumped from chimpanzees to humans...

2008 BARRE-SINOUSSI, LUC MONTAGNIER, HAROLD ZUR HAUSEN RECIEVE NOBEL PRIZE FOR "HIV" AND HPV: GALLO SAYS THEY DESERVE IT

The 2008 award went to Harald zur Hausen in recognition of his discovery that human papillomavirus (HPV) can cause cervical cancer, and to Françoise Barré-Sinoussi and Luc Montagnier for discovering the human immunodeficiency virus (HIV).[1] Whether Robert Gallo or Luc Montagnier deserved more credit for the discovery of the virus that causes AIDS has been a matter of considerable controversy. As it was, Gallo was left out and not awarded a prize. [2, 3]

Additionally, there was scandal when it was learned that Harald zur Hausen was being investigated for having a financial interest in vaccines for the cervical cancer that HPV can cause. AstraZeneca, who with a stake in two lucrative HPV vaccines could benefit financially from the prize, had agreed to sponsor Nobel Media and Nobel Web. According to Times Online, two senior figures in the selection process that chose zur Hausen also had strong links with AstraZeneca. Http://www.webcitation.org/5qpa5pF7G

References for Zur Hausen and Montagnier's Prize

"The Nobel Prize in Physiology or Medicine. Nobelprize.org. Retrieved 20 June 2010.

Jump up Cohen J, Enserink M (October 2008). "Nobel Prize in Physiology or Medicine. HIV, HPV researchers honored, but one scientist is left out". Science. 322 (5899): 174 5.doi:10.1126/science.322.5899.174. PMID 18845715.

Jump up Enserink, Martin; Jon Cohen (6 October 2008). "Nobel Prize Surprise". Science Now. AAAS. 2008 Harald zur Hausen, Françoise Barré-Sinoussi, Luc Montagnier

Charter, David (19 December 2008). "AstraZeneca row as corruption claims engulf Nobel prize" The Sunday Times. timesonline.co.uk. Retrieved 22 June 2010.

2008 October 6. Montagnier, Barre-Sinoussi and zur Hausen Share Nobel Physiology or medicine prize recognizes work on HIV and human papillomavirus (HPV) linked to cervical cancer–but leaves out Robert Gallo By Jordan Lite in Scientific American

A pair of French scientists who isolated the AIDS-causing human immunodeficiency virus (HIV) and a German scientist who determined that human papillomavirus (HPV) causes cervical cancer were awarded the Nobel Prize in Physiology or Medicine today.

The Nobel committee's decision to give the prize to Luc

Montagnier and Francoise Barre-Sinoussi, who isolated HIV in 1983, caps a long, bitter dispute between the Pasteur Institute in Paris, where they made their discovery, and American scientist Robert Gallo, who linked HIV to AIDS separately but was snubbed by the Nobel committee.

Gallo, then a division chief at the National Cancer Institute, made the connection between HIV and AIDS in research published in 1984 in the journal Science. A year later, the Pasteur Institute sued him for allegedly using one of its samples of HIV to draw his conclusion. In 1992 a review panel of the National Academy of Sciences determined that the sample Gallo used was contaminated with material from the Pasteur Institute, and accused him of "intellectual recklessness of a high degree." That same year, Gallo was found guilty of scientific misconduct by the Office of Research Integrity of the U.S. Public Health Sericeous determinations were overturned on appeal. Gallo and Montagnier, 76, co-authored at least two papers, one for Scientific American in 1988, and another in Science in 2002 in which they credited each other with aspects of the discovery. Today, members of the Nobel committee said the award was given to the right scientists....

Against the prevailing view during the 1970s, Harald zur Hausen postulated a role for human papilloma virus (HPV) in cervical cancer. He assumed that the tumor cells, if they contained an oncogenic virus, should harbor viral DNA integrated into their genomes. The HPV genes promoting cell proliferation should therefore be detectable by specifically searching tumor cells for such viral DNA. Harald zur Hausen pursued this idea for over 10 years by searching for different HPV types, a search made difficult by the fact that only parts of the viral DNA were integrated into the host genome. He found novel HPV-DNA in cervix cancer biopsies, and thus discovered the new, tumorigenic HPV16 type in 1983.However, a few opponents led by P. Duesberg argued and are still arguing that there is no real demonstration that the virus does exist and is the cause of AIDS according to Koch's postulates.

This violates all the seroepidemiological rules of vaccination-where the presence of antibodies is indicative of immunity. Either the rules of vaccinology are wrong, "HIV" does not exist as an exogenous retrovirus, or the epitopes tested for in either situation are not reactive. This single fact strongly suggests that the AIDS era was necessary in order to realize that vaccines cannot possibly benefit mankind. This theme will be fully supported in the "HIV/AIDS" section of this website.

2009 THE PUZZLE OF CD4-CELL DEPLETION DESPITE GOOD VIRAL SUPPRESSION: "HIV" "VIRAL LOAD" OR CD4-DEPLETION NO LONGER CAUSES AIDS. LYMPH NODE FIBROSIS CAUSES AIDS Published in AIDS Clinical Care June 1, 2009 in some patients, CD4-cell counts fail to rise as expected. Could extensive lymph node fibrosis be responsible?

"We expect that when combination antiretroviral therapy (ART) suppresses a patient's HIV viremia [dampens retroid production], a steady increase in CD4-cell count will ensue. In some patients, however, such increases are minimal or fail to occur, and in others, CD4-cell counts plummet after an initial rise, even though viral load [retroid expression] remains undetectable. The combination of ddI and tenofovir has been associated with these aberrant CD4-cell responses, but the underlying mechanism is unclear, and the phenomenon is also seen in patients taking other drugs. In a recent study, NIH researchers sought evidence to support any of several hypothetical explanations for the aberrant CD4-cell responses seen in four patients on combination ART whose CD4 counts had fallen from a median of 719 cells/mm3 to a median of 227 cells/mm3 despite persistently undetectable plasma viral loads [retroids]. Three of the four patients were receiving a regimen containing tenofovir and ddI.

Residual replicating HIV did not seem to be the problem: Results of ultrasensitive PCR and assays for peripheral blood mononuclear cell–associated HIV RNA and proviral HIV DNA — and of assays for cell-associated HIV RNA and proviral DNA in mononuclear cells from inguinal lymph nodes — were similar to those obtained in other, successfully treated patients. No evidence of occult drug resistance sabotaging treatment was found. Changing ART regimens to avoid the tenofovir/ddI combination had little effect on CD4-cell counts during the follow-up period (median duration, 10 months).

The single unusual finding was a striking abnormality in inguinal lymph node architecture in the four patients: From 24% to 34% of the T-cell zone was replaced by collagen. In contrast, collagen levels in six successfully treated patients have been reported to range from 2% to 12% (J Clin Invest 2002; 110:1133).

Comment: We do not know the exact pathogenesis of CD4-cell depletion in untreated HIV infection, so creating logical hypotheses to explain aberrant CD4 responses is especially challenging. These authors offer the intriguing suggestion that the unusual lymph node architecture documented in all four patients in this study may be related to (or even responsible for) the inadequate CD4-cell response — i.e., that CD4-cell depletion is independent of specific components of an antiretroviral regimen and is instead caused by lymph node fibrosis. They note that such architectural damage may well be "clinically irreversible with currently available interventions."

Citation(s):Nies-Kraske E et al. Evaluation of the pathogenesis of decreasing CD4+ T cell counts in human immunodeficiency virus type 1–infected patients receiving successfully suppressive antiretroviral therapy. J Infect Dis 2009 Jun 1; 199:1648.

2009 American Thoracic Society (2009, May 20)

http://www.sciencedaily.com/releases/2009/05/090519172045.htmScienceDaily.

CHILDREN WHO GET FLU VACCINE HAVE THREE TIMES RISK OF HOSPITALIZATION FOR FLU, STUDY SUGGESTS

"The inactivated flu vaccine does not appear to be effective in preventing influenza-related hospitalizations in children, especially the ones with asthma. In fact, children who get the flu vaccine are more at risk for hospitalization than their peers who do not get the vaccine, according to new research that will be presented on May 19, at the 105th International Conference of the American Thoracic Society in San Diego."

"Flu vaccine (trivalent inactivated flu vaccine-TIV) has unknown effects on asthmatics."

"The concerns that vaccination maybe associated with asthma exacerbations have been disproved with multiple studies in the past, but the vaccine's effectiveness has not been well-established," said Avni Joshi, M.D., of the Mayo Clinic in Rochester, MN. "This study was aimed at evaluating the effectiveness of the TIV in children overall, as well as the children with asthma, to prevent influenza-related hospitalization."

"The CDC's Advisory Committee on Immunization Practices (ACIP) and the American Academy of Pediatrics (AAP) recommend annual influenza vaccination for all children aged six months to 18 years. The National Asthma Education and Prevention Program (3rd revision) also recommends annual flu vaccination of asthmatic children older than six months."

"In order to determine whether the vaccine was effective in reducing the number of hospitalizations that all children, and especially the ones with asthma, faced over eight consecutive flu seasons, the researchers conducted a cohort study of 263 children who were evaluated at the Mayo Clinic in Minnesota from six months to 18 years of age, each of whom had had laboratory-confirmed influenza between 1996 to 2006.

The investigators determined who had and had not received the flu vaccine, their asthma status and who did and did not require hospitalization. Records were reviewed for each subject with influenza-related illness for flu vaccination preceding the illness and hospitalization during that illness."

They found that children who had received the flu vaccine had three times the risk of hospitalization, as compared to children who had not received the vaccine. In asthmatic children, there was a significantly higher risk of hospitalization in subjects who received the TIV, as compared to those who did not (p= 0.006). But no other measured factors-such as insurance plans or severity of asthma-appeared to affect risk of hospitalization."

"While these findings do raise questions about the efficacy of the vaccine, they do not in fact implicate it as a cause of hospitalizations," said Dr. Joshi. "More studies are needed to assess not only the immunogenicity, but also the efficacy of different influenza vaccines in asthmatic subjects." Adapted from materials provided by American Thoracic Society, via EurekAlert! a service of AAAS.

2009 (June) By Navy Lt. Jennifer Cragg. U.S. Army scientists are studying a new DNA vaccine-delivery method that is needle-free and painless, said a senior Army research scientist at Fort Detrick, Md.

One of the newest DNA vaccine-delivery methods relies on technology known as the "gene gun," which is capable of delivering the vaccine directly into cells. This needle-free vaccination method is more cost-effective, and it is less painful for the recipient.

"DNA offers a number of advantages over conventional vaccine approaches, especially with regard to biodefense vaccines. This is important when rapid vaccine development is needed for a newly emerging disease threat or possibly for a genetically engineered biological warfare pathogen," Dr. Connie Schmaljohn, senior research scientist at the U.S. Army Medical Research Institute of Infectious Diseases (USAMRIID) told "Armed with Science: Research and Applications for the Modern Military" listeners during a live audio webcast on May 27.

USAMRIID is currently conducting a human study of DNA vaccines using this delivery method. Schmaljohn's research team has isolated small amounts of DNA from the Hantaan and Puumala viruses to develop the vaccines. These particular viruses are known health threats to U.S. troops stationed in Europe and Asia. Both vaccines are now in Phase I clinical testing, the first step toward licensure by the U.S. Food and Drug Administration.

"The DNA is first coated onto very, very tiny gold beads, and those gold beads with the DNA are then put inside of a plastic device that's about the size of a small flashlight. Inside that device is also a little canister of compressed helium gas," Schmaljohn explained. "When the trigger of the gene gun device is pushed, the gas is released, and it propels the gold [bead] coated with the DNA out of the device [and] into the skin of the vaccine recipient."

USAMRIID is producing a DNA vaccine for the Asian and European hantaviruses that can cause hemorrhagic fever with renal syndrome. This disease was first recognized as a threat during the Korean War.

"The hantaviruses, once they infect humans, can cause one of two serious human illnesses – hemorrhagic fever with renal syndrome, which occurs in Asia and Europe — or hantavirus pulmonary syndrome, which occurs in the Americas," Schmaljohn said. "Today there's more than 100,000 cases of hemorrhagic fever with renal syndrome each year, with the highest number occurring in China, Russia...Scandinavia and other parts of Europe."

These viruses are found in many types of rodents, including rats, field mice, and meadow voles.

HOW DID MY DAUGHTER, 10, GET HIV IN 2009?

ASIAONE / HEALTH / NEWS / STORY Sun, Aug 23, 2009 The New Straits Times

JOHOR BARU, Malaysia: A 39-year-old single mother is puzzled how her daughter was born with the human immuno-deficiency virus (HIV) although the rest of her family have tested negative for the virus.

The girl, who is now 10, had been in and out of hospitals for the past eight years due to frequent bouts of lethargy and difficulty in swallowing food. Blood tests had been regularly done on her daughter. "But it was only late last year that a doctor told me that she was HIV-positive.

"This came as a shock to me," the mother said at her home in Bukit Mutiara yesterday.

Worse, she was told that her daughter, the second of three children, had only six months to live.

"Although I am heartbroken knowing that she is suffering, I have vowed to make this Ramadan and Hari Raya Aidilfitri something for her to remember and be proud of," said the woman tearfully.

But how did her daughter contract the virus in the first place? The woman said blood tests had been carried out among her two other children and her former husband.

"The blood tests were all negative. "So where did my daughter get the virus from?"

"Moreover, she is suspected to have contracted the virus from the time she was born. Even the doctors could not give proper answers to my queries," she said.

Recounting the events that led to the diagnosis of her daughter's condition, the woman said she had first taken her daughter to a specialist hospital to find out why she was always lethargic and had trouble eating.

"But the hospital could not determine my daughter's ailment," she said.

"It was only after going for another treatment at another private hospital that I was told the bad news.

"I am terribly upset to know that after eight years of frequenting hospitals, it was only last year that my daughter's actual condition was diagnosed.

"The doctors carried out tests for other diseases such as chikungunya and dengue, but the tests were all found to be negative.

"If I remember correctly, no blood transfusion took place during my delivery. So how could she have been infected at birth?"

Puteri Wangsa state assemblyman Datuk Abdul Halim Suleiman visited the family and handed over some cash assistance for Ramadan.

The woman, who is a clerk, said her daughter still attended morning school regularly but had quit religious school in the evening since she was too tired.

"I hope there is someone out there who can help me find out the cause of my daughter's infection," she said. The girl is now on free medication supplied by a government hospital.

2009 (June 11) NEW REPORT FORECASTS MORE THAN DOUBLING OF VACCINE SALES BY 2013

NEW YORK, NY, Jun 11, 2009 (MARKETWIRE via COMTEX) — 2008 was another stellar year for the world vaccine market. Sales grew 21.5% since 2007 to reach $19.2 billion. Few areas of pharmaceuticals have seen the fast-moving developments in the marketplace that the vaccine market has. A new report from leading life science market research publisher Kalorama Information, "Vaccines 2009: World Market Analysis, Key Players, and Critical Trends in a Fast-Changing Industry," forecasts the market to more than double by 2013 due to a strong pipeline of new products and rising usage of current products around the world.

New products and better-than-expected profits, as well as merger activity, have transformed the vaccine marketplace," says Bruce Carlson, publisher of Kalorama Information. "Continued sales of influenza and cervical cancer vaccines have provided a foundation for growth in the adult market. Meanwhile, the pediatric market was fueled by several major products including Wyeth's pneumococcal vaccines Prevnar and Merck's new rotavirus vaccine TotaTeq. "Though vaccination programs typically focus on children, adults in industrialized countries are more likely than children to die as a result of vaccine-preventable diseases. For example, vaccines can prevent about 50% of deaths from pneumococcal disease and 80% of deaths from influenza-related complications in the elderly.

Immunization rates for these diseases continue to be low in at-risk populations, but increased educational efforts aiming to promote the benefits of immunization should contribute to continued growth.

Growth is also being fueled by vaccines that have recently been introduced or are in the approval process that address meningitis, swine flu, malaria, and Japanese encephalitis, as well as a growing number of combination vaccines which are enjoying one of the highest growth rates of any vaccine segment. Both Sanofi Pasteur's Penacel, which protects against pertussis, diphtheria, tetanus, polio and Haemophilus influenzae type B, and GlaxoSmithKline's Kimrix, which protects against pertussis, diphtheria, tetanus, and polio, were approved by the FDA in mid-2008.

Kalorama Information's new report, "Vaccines 2009: World Market Analysis, Key Players, and Critical Trends in a Fast-Changing Industry," covers all the latest trends and issues for both pediatric and adult vaccines. Market data is broken down by type of vaccine, and includes market size and forecasts, product reviews and pipelines, and competitive analyses of leading providers.

(Note: It should not escape the notice of the reader that Kawasaki disease has been added to rotavirus package inserts (Kawasaki's disease does not have a diagnosis: it is akin to vascular inflammation or what is termed "vasculitis," causes heart attacks, rheumatic fever, vascular diseases of all kinds, and profound morbidity. It is consistent with inflammation and desquamation of endothelial cells along the vasculature, and it is fatal in many cases. It is significant that it does appear on the vaccine damage part of rotavirus package inserts as of 2009 at least)

2009 In times of crisis, Big Pharma turns to vaccines Novavax shares skyrocket on new vax pact By John Carroll.

Shares of Rockville, MA-based Novavax shot up more than 30 percent on Tuesday afternoon after the developer announced a licensing deal covering its use of virus-like particles in new vaccines. Spain's Rovi Pharmaceuticals Laboratories plans to use Novavax's technology to develop exclusive new seasonal and pandemic vaccines for Spain and Portugal. Rovi also gets a non-exclusive license for Europe, Latin America, and Africa. And Rovi is making a $3 million equity investment in Novavax in the partnership deal.

A non-profit foundation, jointly sponsored by ROVI and the Spanish authorities, will be formed and funded with a 25-million-euro credit line from the Spanish government to support Phase III clinical development and other studies necessary to achieve marketing authorization of the VLP influenza vaccines in the European Union in 2012.

The deal represents a coup for Novavax, which has been looking to partner up as a way to gain new capital. "We continue to discuss opportunities with other pharmaceutical companies and governments to implement this compelling influenza vaccine technology around the globe," CEO Rahul Singhvi says.

2009 (June 5) Novavax shares soar on NIH swine flu agreement. By Calisha Myers

Novavax saw its stock soar 75 percent to a high of $3.26 yesterday after the Rockville, MD-based company announced it will be working with the National Institutes of Health to evaluate its first batch of H1N1 vaccine. The vaccine developer says it completed its first batch of H1N1 virus-like particles back in May, just three weeks after the CDC released the genetic sequence of the H1N1 virus. The VLP–nearly identical to the swine flu virus–was developed from a strain of H1N1 isolated from an infected person in California. The particles are not infectious and cannot replicate but are designed to produce an immune response.

Novavax says it also already manufactured the master seed stock necessary to produce the vaccine in larger quantities. The National Institute of Allergy and Infectious Diseases' Division of Microbiology and Infectious Diseases unit has agreed to work with Novavax to evaluate the VLP vaccine.

2009 Vical surges on successful swine flu vaccine tests Associated Press, 06.30.09, 01:25 PM EDT NEW YORK

Biopharmaceuticals company Vical Inc. said Tuesday that animal tests of a potential swine flu vaccine were successful.

In the preclinical tests, Vical said all mice and rabbits who were injected with the vaccine were protected from the flu virus. It said 75 percent of the animals reached or surpassed the protection threshold after one dose. Vical said it is ready to move on to large scale manufacturing for testing on humans once it gets the necessary funding.

The San Diego company's shares climbed on the news, rising 45 cents, or 20 percent, to $2.65 in heavy afternoon trading.

Rodman & Renshaw analyst Reni Benjamin noted the speed of the vaccine's development, as Vical received a sample of swine flu from the Centers for Disease Control and Prevention on April 30, shortly after the H1N1 strain emerged. "These results provide additional validation for Vical's technology platform, demonstrating not only efficacy and but also speed in generating a vaccine to an influenza strain that emerged in April 2009," he wrote. Vical is developing its vaccine under an agreement with the U.S. Navy.

2009 Inovio forms collaboration for development of influenza vaccine. Tue. June 30, 2009; Posted: 09:36 AM Jun 30, 2009 (Datamonitor via COMTEX)

Inovio Biomedical, a late-stage biomedical company, has established a new collaboration with the National Microbiology Laboratory of the Public Health Agency of Canada and the University of Pennsylvania to further evaluate the company's DNA vaccine candidates against swine influenza A virus. As a part of its universal influenza vaccine program, Inovio has designed and manufactured consensus DNA vaccines for H1N1 influenza strains. These consensus vaccines, delivered using Inovio's proprietary electroporation technology, have the potential to provide protection against a broad scope of existing as well as currently unknown, unmatched influenza strains that could emerge – one of the perpetual challenges in trying to protect against influenza, the company said. The purpose of this collaboration is to test these vaccine candidates against pandemic and seasonal influenza strains in animal models and will include testing against a recently identified swine H1N1 strain. Inovio's influenza vaccine constructs were designed using the company's novel SynCon technology, which facilitates the design of DNA-based vaccines capable of protecting against unmatched sub-types and strains of pathogens.

"Joseph Kim, Inovio's CEO, said: "The current swine flu outbreak highlights the fact that the world cannot rely solely on the 'catch-up' strategy of influenza vaccine design. We need vaccines that provide at least some broad protective capability against evolving seasonal influenza strains and those with pandemic potential. We have already achieved significant validating data in large animal models regarding the ability of Inovio's consensus vaccines to protect against unmatched strains of different influenza sub-types and look forward to the data resulting from this collaboration of vaccine experts."

July 2009 Scottish government reports that it "is unable to legislate on this issue (of annual vaccination) since legislation on veterinary medicines and veterinary surgeons is a reserved matter." 2009 (July) WHO – Vaccinate Health Care Workers, Pregnant Women, School Aged Children First

BAXTER WORLDWIDE, BIG GOVERNMENT, BIG PHARMA, PANDEMIC, VACCINES TRANSCRIPT OF VIRTUAL PRESS CONFERENCE WITH GREGORY HARTL, WHO SPOKESPERSON FOR GLOBAL ALERT AND RESPONSE, AND DR. MARIE-PAULE KIENY, DIRECTOR OF THE INITIATIVE FOR VACCINE RESEARCH, WORLD HEALTH ORGANIZATION JULY 4, 2009

Mr Gregory Hartl: This is WHO Headquarters in Geneva. We welcome you all to this virtual press briefing today. My name is Gregory Hartl and with us today is Dr Marie-Paule Kieny, the Director of the Initiative for Vaccine Research at WHO Headquarters who will make a few opening remarks about the results of the SAGE Committee meeting of last week and their recommendations and then we will open the floor to questions. As always, please, if you have a question to ask please dial 01 to get into the queue to ask the question and state your name and organization. Dr Kieny over to you:

Dr Marie-Paule Kieny: Thank you very much Gregory. It is a pleasure to be with you again to give you this update on the recommendation of the SAGE on H1N1 vaccine and vaccination. The SAGE is the Strategy Advisory Group of Experts, that is the highest level of advisory body in WHO on immunization matters and they met last week on 7 July to be updated about the epidemiological status and the clinical status of H1N1 as well as being provided with an update on expected vaccine availability. They also reviewed the status of production of the current seasonal epidemic vaccine.

As you know we are coming to the end of the production

campaign for the vaccine which is meant to be used to fight seasonal epidemic of influenza in the northern hemisphere starting this fall and they also met to review various vaccine options that would be available both for seasonal immunization and for H1N1, and to make recommendations to the Director-General. The SAGE, which was helped by a number of experts and also by another committee that we have established in May, which is more specific about the expertise in the area of influenza, so the group together came together with recommendations that were endorsed by the Director-General on Friday. In general, these recommendations take into consideration as I said the epidemiology, the severity of the disease, the expected availability of H1N1 vaccine and have come up with a number of recommendations. I will be incredibly happy to detail them following questions but just to give you an idea of how they go.

First, the Committee recognized that the H1N1 pandemic is unstoppable and therefore that all countries will need to have access to vaccines. Second, the Committee also recognized, really acknowledged the fact that different countries have different epidemiological and other situations and therefore that the countries themselves will have to take decisions that are best adapted to their own national situation but in terms of giving indicative consideration and guidance to countries, SAGE recommended first that healthcare workers should be immunized in all countries in order to maintain functional health systems as the pandemic evolves. So, there are several reasons to protect health workers when they put themselves at risk, when they care for patients; the other one is because they need to remain in good health condition to care for pandemic influenza sick people and the third is because during the time of a pandemic people will continue to be ill with other diseases and these diseases will also need to be taken care of. Second the SAGE considered the of the disease in various groups and considered that countries gravity may have different strategies when they implement immunization campaigns. So, the first one would be to try to stop transmission and if you want to stop transmission as much as you can, and this may still be possible, in certain settings at least to mitigate transmission, you target different population groups, and if you just want to have other objectives: So, the first objective is to reduce transmission as much as possible. Another objective might be to reduce morbidity and mortality and the third objective, but there is no priority in order, would be as I said, to protect the health care system.

In view of these three objectives countries might have, and depending on their own decision, they may consider immunization of several different groups – one of them being pregnant women e.g., as I am sure you have followed in the news, pregnant women are at elevated risk of severe diseases and death; other groups would be anybody over 6 months of age with chronic health conditions and these induced variety of conditions which are putting more people more at risk from having severe illness. This could be chronic respiratory disease – it could be obesity which has been now shown as being a risk factor. Another group to be considered would be healthy adults of over 15 years of age and less than 49 which have been shown also to be surprisingly, although were healthy, at risk of death. Yet another group would be healthy children, and this is mainly to reduce transmission as we discussed because children are amplifiers of infection because they meet in groups. Yet another group would be healthy elderly adults and all country conditions need to be taken into consideration when countries make decisions.

The SAGE also then, to further go into decision and in going out with recommendation for target groups, considered the safety of adjuvant vaccines and they noted that there was, so far, no concern of the safety of vaccine adjuvanted with the new oil-in-water adjuvants but that it was urgent to collect safety data in groups for which safety data is not available in numbers for the time being. They also noted that because these vaccines are novel, use for some of them, a particularly good post marketing surveillance and pharmaco- vigilance has to be implemented when the vaccine is deployed and that international cooperation is requested to have results of any signal that some vaccine might not be safe, which we do not expect but you never know, be shared with the international community as soon as possible.

Finally, they considered recommendations on seasonal influenza vaccination. They were informed that the campaign for preparation of seasonal vaccine for the northern hemisphere were close to completion with more than 90% of production being finalized by end of July and therefore considered that there was no need to recommend a switch from seasonal to H1N1 vaccine. They also considered that at the current time there would be no change in recommendation of WHO for the seasonal vaccine for the next season for the northern hemisphere, that preparations should continue for this immunization as if there would not have been a pandemic. So, these are the main messages, and I will be most happy to answer your questions.

Mr Gregory Hartl: Dr Kieny, thank you very much. Before we go to questions can I remind journalists that the audio file and transcript will be available shortly afterwards as usual on the WHO website. In addition, a web update outlining in summary, the conclusions of the SAGE meeting will be posted shortly. Once again, journalists who want to ask questions please press 1 on their keypad.

Fergus Walsh, BBC: Regarding the southern hemisphere can you tell me were there any decision made to ask companies like CSL and Sanofi Pasteur who will, in the general run of things, make seasonal flu vaccine for the southern hemisphere, they would normally expect in the autumn, to get the strain from you and do that. Whether or not you are planning to allow next winter's southern hemisphere seasonal flu vaccine to go ahead or whether you consider the pandemic is serious enough and that they should just concentrate on the pandemic vaccine and secondly, when would you expect the first doses of pandemic vaccine from cell culture to arrive?

Dr Marie-Paule Kieny: In terms of southern hemisphere, this was of course discussed, and SAGE considered that it was too early to make recommendations on the upcoming production of the southern hemisphere vaccine. Indeed, the southern hemisphere seasonal epidemic has started and now we are in the middle of it. It seems that there is still significant proportion or number of cases which are caused notably by H3N2, one of the seasonal strains. There really needs to be more data accumulated on what is circulating in terms of the new virus or the traditional H1, H3 and B strains.

So, we expect that all these data, much more data and evidence will be available in September when traditionally WHO will hold its meeting to determine which strain should be put into the seasonal vaccine and by that time, we hope that we will be able to be more explicit in giving recommendations in one direction or another. I still need to note that seasonal influenza is a severe disease in certain population groups, like the elderly or the very the young and nobody would want to have an epidemic of severe and preventable seasonal epidemic in nursing homes when winter comes in the southern hemisphere. So, this is something which is watched very carefully but it is too early to give any recommendations.

On when the first doses of pandemic vaccine made from cell culture would be available, there are already vaccine doses available. They are produced but they are by no means ready to be licensed yet. So, both the doses are available for clinical trials, from both manufacturers who have been making vaccines from cell cultures but also coming very soon or are already there, as you may know, from manufacturers who are making vaccines from egg products. Notably, CSL in the southern hemisphere has really been rushing to prepare for clinical trials. So, when we hear that vaccine is available already, certainly, yes, vaccine has been produced but it is still an experimental vaccine awaiting results of both pharmaceutical characterizations to be licensed as well as upon request of regulatory authority clinical trials.

Helen Branswell, Canadian Press: If I could ask 2 questions. The first is a clarification. Dr Kieny you talked about a variety of different groups who might be vaccinated – am I correct in thinking that what you are saying is that the SAGE did not say these people should be first, these people should be second, these people should be third, but that it put a strong priority on health-care workers but after that its somehow left in the hands of individual countries? And I would have a follow-up question.

Dr Marie-Paule Kieny: So, you are right: the SAGE identified the health- care workers as a main priority group for the three reasons that I already have given. In terms of the other group, it really depends on the strategy that each country wants to follow. In certain cases, as I mentioned countries may want to try to mitigate transmission and therefore, children would be an obvious target. In some other cases, they want to rather concentrate on reducing morbidity and mortality and then some other groups may be more the target. But there is identification on various options, but no ranking and no priority are given to these options.

Helen Branswell, Canadian Press: The follow-up I wanted to ask in your presentation to that made in last week, you refer to the fact WHO has done a survey of vaccine manufacturers asking them about their plans and if I read the slides correctly, only 12 of the proposed pandemic vaccines are planned to have adjuvants in them. Is WHO getting a sense that a number of manufacturers are not planning of using adjuvants? And do you have a position on whether or not that is appropriate under the circumstances?

Dr Marie-Paule Kieny: Indeed, it is exceedingly difficult in a situation like in a pandemic when you want to have a vaccine which can be distributed safely to the population in the shortest possible time, it is very difficult to say that you take the adjuvant of one company and you mix it with antigens of another company when they have never been tested together. So, we know for example that clinical trials financed by the US Government have looked at some of these combinations, but these are very specific combinations. So it is very difficult to imagine because as you have seen in the slides, manufacturers are actually, although the vast majority of vaccine doses is coming from companies in certain areas of the world, there are actually vaccines manufacturers in other parts of the world, and these are producing less vaccines in terms of output in number of doses, but it would be very difficult to say let us just for the sake of taking an example that you take vaccines from country X in Asia which has never been a mix of any of this new adjuvant and then you just make the mix and you say that this is my vaccine and it will be safe because the safety of adjuvant is not only depending on the adjuvant itself, it is quite often combined fact between the purity of the antigen of a certain characteristics of the antigen and the adjuvant. So, this is why a number of manufacturers who currently have never made any other vaccines than non-adjuvanted vaccines are still planning to go with non-adjuvanted vaccines. I may also add a comment on that for the time being there is still the question to know whether the immunogenicity of the A(H1N1) vaccine will be more like that we are used to for seasonal vaccine where no problem with 15 micrograms not adjuvanted, just one dose is fine or will it be more like H5N1 where all the trials have shown that you either need to have a very potent adjuvant or you need to increase the dose quite significantly, so in the absence of these responses, yes a number of manufacturers are planning to go ahead with 50 microgram without adjuvant.

Martin Enserink, Science Magazine: Helen Branswell reported this morning or late last night from those presentations that the virus is not growing very well. I wonder if you can comment on that, and whether that will cause any delay? Secondly, has SAGE made any recommendations with regard to international solidarity? Is there any talk of any recommendations to create equity between countries, for instance you mentioned that countries can have different strategies, but would it not be recommendable that they use only the vaccine for those high-risk groups and save vaccines for other countries?

Dr Marie-Paule Kieny: First, in terms of yields, maybe there is some confusion between the reality that is in the slides, that is now recognized by the manufacturers and the regulatory authorities and the WHO Network that we have a strain which are currently available to make inactivated vaccine, the manufacturers only get moderately affected yields. This is not to say that the viruses grow poorly, it is that for a reason or another the hemagglutinin they can produce is either not stable or exceptionally low. It is not known what is exactly happening but in terms of output that they have of hemagglutinin at the end when they grow a virus, they have poor yields, poor as between 25 and 50 percent of the normal yields that they have with good yielders. What is the reason for this is difficult to know, that it is well known that some strains are good yielders, and some are bad yielders, it happens that for the first series of strains which were generated and unfortunately, we did not come up with a good yielder?

So that in order to remedy to that the WHO laboratory network is again trying to generate new vaccines viruses from wild type virus isolated from patients, and these will be tested again by the manufacturers and we hope that at least one of them or more than that we hope will be giving higher yields that would be comparable to the ones obtained with seasonal vaccines. So, for the time being, these are strains which are available and are still giving of course enough production yields in order to make clinical batches into test immunogenicity of new vaccines. We understand that the regulatory authorities have said that when better yielders are available there will not be a need to have bridging studies between the results obtained with the strains available now and the new strains because actually there will be difference in yields and not in antigenicity or immunogenicity. So, we hope that as soon as possible the situation can be improved upon but for the time being there is no reason to be really anxious about that.

In terms of equity, yes of course, SAGE has also made a note that WHO should try to help with as much equity as is there in the distribution of vaccines. We are all committed to that, we have several strategies, we are discussing with the industry and we have already, this was announced in the press, we have already secured a number of donations from industry, we have also secured access to real time production during the pandemic. WHO at the highest level is discussing with Governments to see how much they can help to either help negotiate some doses with industry but also help finance these vaccines and finally, but very importantly, we are also discussing with new manufacturers who have started to acquire the technology to make influenza vaccines in the past three years with technical and financial support from us, to help them accelerate their preparation and be able to produce some vaccines for their own country? So, this is the situation in terms of trying to ensure equity for vaccines.

Richard Knox, National Public Radio: Dr Kieny, you said earlier that you do not expect safety issues to arise with the pandemic vaccine and tests, but do you think that there is less risk of Guillain-Barre syndrome with this new swine flu vaccine than there was in 1976 and why? And secondly, I wonder with the accelerated safety tests that will be necessary, how many subjects will you expect to have tested and how can experts draw conclusions about safety from these tests when the vaccine has put into a hundred of millions of people.

Dr Marie-Paule Kieny: It is not completely known why the vaccine which was distributed against the swine flu in 1976 induced higher risk of Guillain-Barre syndrome. There are a number of hypotheses and one of the hypotheses is that the vaccine was contaminated by a component coming from a bacterial infection that was inducing antibodies that cross reacted with self-protein and therefore, caused Guillain-Barre syndrome. The vaccines which are produced now are much better purified than the way they were in 1976, so we really do not think that it is likely that we will have these side effects again, but to be absolutely honest, of course it is only when you have a large-scale distribution of vaccines that you know with certainty the safety profile of the vaccine.

Modern vaccines such as those which are used to immunize children and adults currently in all countries of the world are very safe products. Nevertheless, in an exceedingly small number of people they do induce adverse reactions, and this can be the case as well for adjuvanted vaccines and non-adjuvanted vaccines. So, what needs to be put in place and everyone is working towards this direction is a very good surveillance system and monitoring adverse effects so that as soon as a signal pops up it can immediately be followed-up, investigated and adequate public health measures be taken to respond to that.

Now, in terms of these new vaccines, new adjuvants there is one manufacturer who has had an oil-in-water adjuvanted influenza vaccine in use for many years for seasonal vaccination and the safety database for this particular antigen is exceptionally large although mainly in elderly people and there does not seem to be any signal for any unexpected severe event like Guillain-Barre. But as I said, all must be put in place to detect any signal as early as possible.

Journalist, Sky Television: Your referred previously that the obese people should probably be among those that the national government should consider vaccinating. On what scientific basis are made these recommendations and if you could elaborate more on the body mass index? And the second question is, if we have the vaccine later than October in the Northern Hemisphere, don't you think it would be too late to protect the people from the second pandemic wave?

Dr Marie-Paule Kieny: In terms of obesity, obesity has been observed as being one of the risk factors for more severe diseases other than H1N1 influenza. This is an observation. We still do not know exactly if it is obesity itself which is a risk factor, or if it is other health conditions which arise because of obesity. For the time being it is an observation, and a lot of investigations are conducted to try and understand this better.

It has been observed in several countries that people with a body mass index over 30, and even more, over 40, have a higher chance of having a severe disease than noon obese people. This is why one of the groups that was mentioned, that was listed by SAGE, and that was worth considering for pandemic influenza vaccination contains all populations over 6 months of age with risk factors, and one of the risk factors listed is obesity. It is not the only one of course, you have asthma, chronic lung disease. All these are considered as being risk factors based on observation so far. About availability of vaccines, all the manufacturers and the regulatory authorities are working to have vaccine available as soon as possible. Vaccines will be available starting from September or October. If the situation remains as it is, of course the regulatory authorities will certainly want to have a better handle at the safety in clinical trials and dosing in clinical trials and these clinical trials will take some time, and therefore, to have a full license of this new vaccine may take until the end of the year. This being said, many countries have provision in their law, so if there is an emergency, they can invoke an emergency situation to use vaccine for which you would have already good characterization in terms of pharmaceutical data but not yet, all the data on clinical trials. We certainly look towards seeing how the epidemic evolves and when it unfolds, to see what the situation in countries and we are will take our own decisions on whether or not to use vaccine under an emergency provision as compared to waiting for full registration of these vaccines.

Maggie Fox, Reuters: If WHO wants to reassess its best-case scenario for how many vaccine doses might be available – I think the last number for the best-case scenario was 4.9 billion.

And I am also wondering about this issue with the virus strain not producing good results. Was this also the same for the live vaccine or only for the killed vaccine?

Dr Marie-Paule Kieny: In terms of updating the figures that we have published for likely vaccine supply over the next 12 months, we will update these figures, but we want to wait to have some further information to update these with some meaningful changes. First as we have to have a definite idea of what yield manufacturers are getting with inactivated vaccines is it the same as seasonal, which was the assumption that we took when we made the first calculation, or is it 50%, and these of course as you may imagine will change the total output. The other information which is still lacking as what is a dose of inactivated H1N1 vaccine. Is it, without adjuvant, is it 50 micrograms, is it 30 micrograms, we do not know? And we will know as soon as the result of the first clinical trial will come out, although the result will certainly be very adapted or relevant only to the vaccine which will be tested, it will still give a flavor of what kind of results we will have with the other inactivated vaccines. You asked a question about the live-attenuated vaccine, the response, and the way this vaccine induces an immune response is quite different because these are replicative organisms, so they induce antibodies and also anti-cell response.

So, for the time being, the results that we have from the manufacturers who make live-attenuated vaccines, is that in terms of yields, and this is yields in terms of growth this time – how these vaccine strains grow – there does not seem to be any surprise and they grow with the same titres as the seasonal vaccine that they have obtained in normal production for a seasonal vaccine. Still there need to be clinical trials to know what titres of these live-attenuated vaccines will have to be used in a dose to make an effective dose. So, the quick response is that we don't know, but in terms of growth they seem to be behaving normally.

Journalist, Scrip Pharmaceutical News: When the new pandemic vaccine becomes available later this year, will WHO or Member States have any new pharmaco-vigilance initiative to pick up ADRs (ADVERSE REACTIONS) to this new vaccine. For example, in some countries, they allow patients to report ADRs as other do not. Is WHO thinking about this or are you quite happy with existing pharmaco-vigilance systems?

Dr Marie-Paule Kieny: Although in some countries the pharmaco-vigilance system is working very well and we will pick up signals (ADVERSE REACTIONS) very easily, in other countries there need to be an increased attention to the pharmaco-vigilance system, notably in the developing countries and WHO is already working with countries to try and use systems in place, like the system that the Polio Initiative uses to detect cases of acute flaccid paralysis to try and help detect any signs of Guillain- Barre for example. We are both strengthening the network as well as working on new guidelines that will be more adapted to the detection of adverse events following vaccination with pandemic influenza vaccine.

Helen Branswell, Canadian Press: I would like to get some information about adjuvants and children. Obviously, young people are among the people hardest hit by this strain so far, but I don't think that there is much evidence at all about safety of adjuvants in that group. I was looking at a document yesterday that shows that with MS59 for instance, it has been given to 6 or 700 children which is not a long safety record. Are there any other vaccines – not influenza vaccines –but marketed vaccines with these kinds of adjuvants that children receive now and that might give us a sense of whether or not they are safe to use in children?

Dr Marie-Paule Kieny: You are absolutely right that safety data, at least in terms of numbers are lacking in certain population groups. You mentioned the children, certainly there are no data in children more than 6 months old and less than 3 years, there are no data in pregnant women, there are no data in asthmatics, so there are quite a number of populations for which there are no data. SAGE has also made the point that as quickly as possible data should be obtained on these populations groups if they are to be vaccinated with these new vaccines. In terms of use of this new novel adjuvant in children, there is no vaccine for incredibly young children that is using the formulation. The closest being the vaccine, which is currently developed as the malaria vaccine, which has been tested in a few thousand children and is being tested now in Africa with this indication for malaria in a few thousand children, but apart from that, these data are still lacking.

Journalist, German Television: If I understand correctly, talking about the doses for the next winter, do we have to go for a mid- seasonal vaccine and then also to go for two other doses for the new pandemic vaccination, will there be enough vaccine for all the countries then?

Dr Marie-Paule Kieny: The vaccine against seasonal influenza for the Northern Hemisphere is finishing production. We expect to have more than 90% of doses which were planned to be produced, so this is awfully close to the number of doses that were produced in 2008. We do not envisage changes in the recommendation for seasonal vaccination, so vaccination will still target the same persons and as in the previous national recommendations mainly in most countries these people will be the elderly, over 60 or 65 years of age, also in some countries children as well, so yes, certain of these groups may receive during the upcoming fall three shots which could be one of seasonal vaccine and two for the pandemic vaccine.

Mr Gregory Hartl: Dr Kieny, thank you very much. That closes our virtual press conference for today, 13 July, from WHO headquarters in Geneva. And just before we say goodbye, one last reminder that there will be 3 things posted on the WHO website shortly: the normal audio file and transcript and in addition, a web update which outlines recommendations from the SAGE meeting will also be shortly available.

2009 July. Swiss army stockpiles "swine flu" vaccines in preparation for mass vaccination. The army in Switzerland is starting to stockpile "swine flu" vaccines as it gears up for a mass vaccination of the Swiss population in autumn, according to a report in Basler Zeitung. http://bazonline.ch/schweiz/standard/Erste-Impfspritzen-in-der-Schweiz eingetroffen/story/22051646

The Swiss army today received the first shipment of a total of 16 million doses of vaccines as well as needles in readiness for mass forced vaccination of the entire population using two doses.

Thomas Meister, the head of pharmacy products and technology of the army pharmacy department, told Swiss TV that the vaccines came from USA, Germany, and Spain, but it is not clear which pharmaceutical companies delivered them and whether Baxter was one of them.

It is not clear either whether the vaccines have passed clinical trials or whether they have been subjected to any safety tests.

The Swiss Ministry of Health ordered the army to buy the vaccines on the basis of the country's pandemic plan – and WHO's instructions to all 194 member states to mass vaccinate their populations by use of force.

The Cantons of Switzerland are reported to have plans already in place to force every single person living in each Canton to appear at a "vaccine center" at a specified time to take the vaccine or face prison.*

The local police have been instructed to go through the register and ring every single person to get them to go to their vaccine center during the pandemic "emergency" predicted by "WHO" to occur from September onwards*. No exceptions to the vaccine will be allowed.

2009 July. The Norwegian health authorities will this fall begin a program of mass vaccination against the A H1N1 flu, also called the swine flu. A total of 9.4 million doses have been ordered from the suppliers. All will be given two inoculations, two weeks apart, Bergens Tidende reports. The total cost will be NOK 650 million. So far, only 23 cases of the flu have been diagnosed in Norway, but the authorities expect that the number will increase.

2009. GREECE TO VACCINATE 12 MILLION AGAINST H1N1 SWINE FLU PANDEMIC

Filed Under Pandemic, Vaccines, Greece will vaccinate its entire population of 12 million against the H1N1 swine flu pandemic which has swept around the world in weeks, killing hundreds of people, the country's health minister said on Friday.

The Mediterranean country, which receives about 15 million tourists every year, has confirmed more than 700 swine flu cases and no deaths, but world health experts say the true number of cases globally is far higher as only a few patients get tested. "We decided that the entire population, all citizens and residents, without any exception, will be vaccinated against the flu," Health Minister Dimitris Avramopoulos said after a ministerial meeting.

Greece has already earmarked 40 million euros for vaccines and has placed orders with Novartis, Glaxo, and Sanofi for 8 million vaccine doses, to be received gradually by January. Vaccine experts say people will likely need two doses of vaccine to be protected from H1N1 swine flu, so Greece would need a total of 24 million doses to vaccinate its entire population. Other countries are taking similar steps.

"Greece will order 16 million more doses from the same companies in the future," a health ministry official who declined to be named told Reuters.

"We are only waiting for the European Union's approval to start vaccinating everyone."

The European Medicines Agency has begun reviewing pandemic flu vaccines under development, aiming to get them approved before the flu season starts, sometime in September.

The health ministry official said children, the elderly and ailing would be the first to be vaccinated.

About 800 people have died worldwide since the outbreak of the flu in April! And from heath attacks, stokes, murders? Car accidents?

http://tvnz.co.nz/health-news/greece-vaccinate-population-swine-flu-2881876

2009-10. ONE WOMAN IN CAMAROON CATCHES "HIV" FROM A GORILLA AND LIKE THE ANDROMEDA STRAIN, IT MUTATES IMMEDIATELY TO FORM A NEW, RAPIDLY GROWING, PROBABLY WIDESPREAD, DEADLY PANDEMIC AIDS VIRUS...

New HIV strain discovered in woman from Cameroon, Randolph Schmidt Ap Science Writer

A new strain of the virus that causes AIDS has been discovered in a [black] woman from the African nation of Cameroon. It differs from the three known strains of human immunodeficiency virus and appears to be closely related to a form of simian virus recently discovered in wild gorillas, researchers report in Monday's edition of the journal Nature Medicine.

The finding "highlights the continuing need to watch closely for the emergence for new HIV variants, said the researchers, led by Jean-Christophe Plantier of the University of Rouen, France.

The three previously known HIV strains are related to the simian virus that occurs in chimpanzees. The most likely explanation for the new find is gorilla-to-human transmission, Plantier's team said. But they added they cannot rule out the possibility that the new strain started in chimpanzees and moved into gorillas and then humans or moved directly from chimpanzees to both gorillas and humans. The 62-year-old patient tested positive for HIV in 2004, shortly after moving to

Paris from Cameroon, according to the researchers. She had lived near Yaounde, the capital of Cameroon, but said she had no contact with apes or bush meat, a name often given to meat from wild animals in tropical countries. The woman currently shows no signs of AIDS and remains untreated, though she still carries the virus, the researchers said. How widespread this strain is remains to be determined? Researchers said it could be circulating unnoticed in Cameroon or elsewhere. The virus' rapid replication indicates that it is adapted to human cells, the researchers reported. Their research was supported by the French Health Watch Institute, the French National Agency for Research on AIDS and Viral Hepatitis and Rouen University Hospital.

September 2009 by Christine England, American Chronicle: Fourteen-year-old Natalie Morton, walked into school yesterday a happy, healthy little girl. Sadly, today she did not and tragically she will never walk through her school gates again. Yesterday Natalie was given one dose of the Cervarix HPV vaccine, the vaccine that the UK Government has portrayed as safe, a vaccine that Glaxo Smith Kline has said over and over is safe. For this little girl Cervarix was not because she died just a few hours later.

If Natalie were an isolated incident it could be seen to be a tragic but extremely rare allergic reaction. It is a recognized fact that all vaccines and medications carry risks but Cervarix has been in use for just under a year and although this is the first death associated with the vaccine, it is far from being the first adverse event. The adverse events are mounting up at an alarming rate.

These are recent figure taken from the MHRA or the Yellow Card reporting system.

"This report summarizes the adverse reactions suspected to have been caused by Cervarix human papillomavirus (HPV) vaccine in the UK. This includes reports received between 14 April 2008 and 23 September 2009. These reports have been voluntarily submitted to the MHRA by healthcare professionals and members of the public via the Yellow Card Scheme.

SUMMARY OF UK SAFETY EXPERIENCE

Total number of reports received: 2,137.

Total number of suspected reactions: 4,657

Estimated number of doses administered across the UK: at least 1.4 million doses."

These are the number reported so far as of 24th September 2009.

409 0f these reports are of anaphylactic shock which can if left untreated lead to death, so is a severe reaction more common than we are led to believe?

As yet it is not known conclusively that Natalie died from the Cervarix vaccine but given that classmates also suffered reactions albeit mild in comparison, it is definitely time to get worried. A full investigation is under way and the batch of vaccines that all the girls were vaccinated with has been quarantined as a precaution. A possible faulty batch is being blamed.

August 24, 2009. Christina England, American Chronicle

This week has shown that a large number of reports stating that Gardasil is proving unsafe. News stations around the world have reported that Gardasil the HPV vaccine has been found to cause adverse reactions. The adverse reactions range from mild, such as headaches, nausea, and fainting, to the more severe such as seizures, blood clots, Guillain Barre Syndrome and even death. This information has come to light since the publication of the JAMA papers on the 19th of August 2009, showing the results of the VAERS Vaccine Adverse Event Reporting System. The Gardasil data published was collected from June 1, 2006 through December 31, 2008.

Merck has only recently changed packaging showing acknowledgement that this vaccine causes fainting and seizures in some children.

Information Pertaining to Labeling Revision for Gardasil

"On June 9, 2009, the Food and Drug Administration (FDA) approved a revised label for Gardasil, a vaccine to protect against cervical, vulvar and vaginal cancers caused by Human Papillomavirus (HPV) types 16 and 18 and genital warts caused by HPV types 6 and

11. In the new label, information pertaining to syncope (fainting) is now also included in the Warnings and Precautions section, and this section has new information noting that individuals who faint sometimes have tonic-clonic (jerking) movements and seizure-like activity. The addition of syncope to the Warnings and Precautions section emphasizes that healthcare providers and consumers should be alert that fainting may occur following vaccination with Gardasil, sometimes resulting in falling and injuries. To prevent falls and injuries all vaccine recipients should remain seated or lying down and be closely observed for 15 minutes following vaccination."

Cynthia Janak a USA journalist has been writing and proving this vaccine is unsafe for the last few years. Her website Only the Truth gives tribute to the many girls who have lost their life after taking Gardasil shots. This site points out and lists the adverse reactions, showing pictures of beautiful young woman now no longer with us, other pages have stories of girls suffering every day from the adverse reactions to this vaccine. There is up to date news and views on Gardasil.

News stories have been hitting America for three years about the dangers of this vaccine. Stories like this one 2007 Did Gardasil Vaccine Cause a 12-yr-old Girl's Paralysis and Girl Dies after HPV Jab – CDC Blame Birth Control Pill

Merck says however, Merck Says FDA And CDC Reaffirm Safety Profile of Gardasil – Update

"Based on the review of available information by FDA and CDC, Gardasil continues to be safe and effective, and its benefits continue to outweigh its risks." Confusing that because if Merck were so convinced that their vaccine was safe why have they recently changed the labelling? Diane Harper who worked on the Gardasil trials has reservations. Harper told CNN she has concerns about the safety of the HPV vaccine for pre-adolescents, noting that a small number of girls have died or suffered neurological damage after receiving the shot. However, despite the controversy surrounding this vaccine, with much information proving it to be unsafe, it appears not only is still being offered to teenage girls across the USA and the world today but is a mandatory vaccine for immigrants wanting to come into the USA. In a sickening story in a letter passed to me – a grandmother who has been raising her grandchild and was trying to escape to the USA from domestic violence was refused entry because she refused to vaccinate her grandchild after researching the Gardasil vaccine. The letter also shows 140 immigration rights, women´s rights, public health, medical, and reproductive justice organizations including an attorney have joined a coalition in NYS. The letter to the CDC was written as the author felt the vaccine activists might want to know the names of political organizations opposing the US immigration regulation that requires immigrants receive the Gardasil shot.

So why is it that USA citizens in many states have the option to choose whether they or their children have the HPV vaccine, but immigrants cannot? In order to become a permanent, legal resident of the U.S, immigrants now must receive a vaccine that is not required of U.S. citizens. This is like saying these people are less important or more likely to be infected. This surely is wrong.

One comment on the subject on the Age of Autism in 2008 from a concerned professional said:-

"Thirty-six death reports with Gardasil, VAERS database now has 13,667 adverse events reports. Merck knew that boric acid causes convulsions in 1945. Your FDA and CDC and Merck still denies the problems with this aluminum vaccine.

"DO NOT TREAT THESE IMMIGRANTS LIKE LAB RATS. THEY HAVE SUFFERED ENOUGH, DO NOT DESTROY THEIR HEALTH AND THEIR FUTURE OFFSPRING AND HEALTH WITH THIS TOXIC VACCINE. IT IS THE POLYSORBATE 80 AND THE BORIC ACID THAT IS IN THE VACCINE THAT WILL CAUSE CANCER. PLEASE DO NOT USE THE IMMIGRANTS AS GUINEA PIGS. THIS IS AN EXPERIMENTAL VACCINE, PLEASE, DO NOT EXPERIMENT ON THE IMMIGRANTS."

The letter outlines that 140 organizations oppose the Gardasil Mandate: Clearly this shows massive opposition and anger that this vaccine is being forced on all 11 – 26 female immigrants wishing to enter the USA. This shows a degree of possible discrimination against immigrants, not only by the CDC but by the American Government. To force a vaccine that is essentially against the HPV virus which is being advertised as being a STD on any children is wrong. All parents should have the rights to refuse a vaccine, especially in the light of what is in the JAMA papers. Is this the first step to vaccines becoming mandatory throughout the whole of the USA? Maybe the CDC needs to rethink this decision, especially in the light of the recent evidence showing that this vaccine is proving to be unsafe. Immigrants should have the same rights as anyone else to the freedom of choice, as the concerned professional said many have suffered enough.

2009 PERHAPS THE LARGEST FAILURE OF THE AIDS ERA WAS PUBLISHED IN 2009 IN THE NEJM, WITH ANTHONY FAUCI AND OTHERS CLAIMING FOR THE FIRST TIME, A 3% RATE OF PROTECTION (OVER BACKGROUND LEVELS WITHOUT THE VACCINE

However, if you look at the numbers published regarding the trial involving 16,000 recipients, 8,000 controls injected with aluminum, and 8,000 injected with aluminum and gp120, and a difference a in "true seroconversion" between the two groups was 0.6% (of 8,000) aluminum "HIV": versus 0.8% with aluminum only.

However, the CIA website (of all places-you will see later how Bill Clinton and these agencies deemed "HIV" a National Security Issue in the information presented about A History of AIDS on this website) and find that the rate of seroconversion in Thailand at background levels is 1.3 percent without any vaccination, one only can conclude that the cheapest way to "immunize" those promiscuous barbarians is to inject them with aluminum (its cheap)!

Here are the numbers more visibly:

Aluminum boosted Aluminum without Background "HIV" detection:

gp120 "background"	gp120 Military	-Thailand trial aluminum
1.3%	0.6%	0.8%

The numbers would make it appear that it is a good idea to inject everybody with aluminum only because it is cheap-and will reduce the levels of "HIV" detection by 0.5% in the absence of co-injected and expensive to acquire and manufacture gp120 (1.3 is the background levels) -0.8=0.5%). This trial cost 101 + million? But that is not all we got for that expenditure combined with the 500 million a year spent for the 172 vaccines currently in "the pipeline."

Look at the numbers for the largest trial ever conducted, which Fauci says had a 31% success rate and had no statistical significance that involved no more than 50 people in the experimental versus 7 1 in the control-who went on to acquire "REAL" HIV." If background level of detection of "REAL" "HIV" is 1.3%, then you go like Fauci did and eliminate two types of statistical analyses (the "intent to treat group and per protocol group), and only count the "modified intent to treat analysis" as statistically significant when 30% of the folks not analyzed in the "modified intent to treat group" are dropped from that analysis, and yes, you achieve statistical significance) !!!. Such creative figure juggling provides Fauci with his 31%, and, according to my reading of this interesting paper, we have both an end to the fraudulence of the AIDS era, or vaccination: take your pick. And somehow, according to Fauci, the efficacy shoots up to a staggering 50% success rate, by dropping only 1/3 of the recipients by counting only those in the first of 3 years following the first vaccination of the series and eliminating the rest.

Translation: But this is cheating using numbers and fancy words. It is not science. It is highly premeditated lying?

This is not to mention the 7 patients that "seroconverted" during "the window period" to a "true" "HIV-positive result" that were dropped from the modified intent to treat analysis, changing the numbers to 57 versus 71, or conversely, 79 versus 51, depending on which of the two groups these excluded groups belonged to in the initial recruitment, which would completely change the 0.6% versus 0.8% groups, with only these few individuals dropped from that analysis. Then you add the deaths due to the experimental or control vaccines laced with the toxic metal aluminum that number somewhere between 5-10 (it is not clear), and the statistics change again. Or try counting in the NEMJ analysis the poor Thailand folks that developed potentially lifelong health issue(s) (defined as unable to work on the NEMJ supplement document) due to the either the experimental or placebo vaccine. These damaged individuals due to both the experimental (and placebo) aluminum-laced vaccines also were not counted, or they were excluded from the analysis published in the "supplement" in The New England Journal of Medicine but not in the main article. The numbers according to my estimation amount to about 340 "HIV/Aluminum" vaccinated, versus about 71 controls (aluminum only) that would have had adverse reactions and missed work because of disability due to the control or experimental vaccines.

2009, December 3

THE MILITARY-THAILAND TRIAL THAT DIDN'T ACHIEVE STATISTICAL SIGNIFICANCE WITH MORE THAN 16 THOUSAND PARTICIPANTS UNLESS YOU FUDGE THE DATA AND CHEAT AND EXCLUDE 1/3 OF THE FOLKS

Donald Stablein, Ph.D., Deborah L. Birx, M.D., Supamit Chunsuttiwat, M.D., Chirasak Khamboonruang, M.D., Prasert Thongcharoen, M.D., Ph.D., Merlin L. Robb, M.D., Nelson L. Michael, M.D., Ph.D., Prayura Kunasol, M.D., and Jerome H. Kim, M.D. for the MOPH–TAVEG InvestigatorsDonald Stablein, Ph.D., Deborah L. Birx, M.D., Supamit Chunsuttiwat, M.D., Chirasak Khamboonruang, M.D., Prasert Thongcharoen, M.D., Ph.D., Merlin L. Robb, M.D., Nelson L. Michael, M.D., Ph.D., Prayura Kunasol, M.D., and Jerome H. Kim, M.D. for the MOPH–TAVEG Investigators N Engl J Med 2009; 361:2209-2220l, December 3, 2009 (December 3, 2009).

"A total of 26,676 volunteers were screened and 16,402 were enrolled (intention-to-treat group). The 12,542 subjects who completed all (6) vaccination visits on schedule and were not found to have HIV-1 infection after receiving the full vaccination regimen were included in the per-protocol analysis. Seven volunteers who were found to be seropositive for HIV-1 on the first test after vaccination were determined by RNA testing to have been infected at enrollment and were not included in the modified intention-to-treat analysis, leaving 16,395 volunteers: 8197 in the vaccine group and 8198 in the placebo group. This group consisted of 10,064 men (61.4% of the subjects) and 6331 women (38.6%). Baseline characteristics were similar for selected variables, and there was no imbalance between the two groups in self-described risk behavior. Baseline Characteristics of the Subjects (Modified Intention-to-Treat Population)."

"There were no substantive changes in serial self-reports of risk behavior during the trial. No data were collected on the status of male circumcision or on serologic analyses for adenovirus type 5 or herpes simplex virus type 2."

There were 52,985 person-years of follow-up (15% more than planned). At 42 months, 14,672 of the volunteers (89.5%) had completed the trial and were HIV-seronegative.

Adverse Events

"Most local and systemic reactions to the vaccine were mild to moderate and reflected the findings of studies on the safety of these products that have been reported previously. Most reactions were mild to moderate and resolved within 3 days after vaccination (but some killed recipients and prevented them from returning to work for an undisclosed period of time). At least one adverse event was reported in 69.4% of subjects in the two study groups. The number of deaths and the frequency and severity of adverse events and serious adverse events were similar in the two groups."

Primary End Points: "HIV-1 Infection"

"HIV-1 infection was diagnosed in 132 subjects (56 in the vaccine group and 76 in the placebo group) during 52,985 person-years of follow-up in the intention-to-treat analysis, in 86 subjects (36 in the vaccine group and 50 in the placebo group) during 36,720 person-years of follow-up in the per-protocol analysis, and in 125 subjects (51 in the vaccine group and 74 in the placebo group) during 52,985 person-years of follow-up in the modified intention-to-treat analysis.

One subject in the placebo group who was identified by hospital record as being seropositive for HIV after dying from Pneumocystis jirovecii pneumonia was included in the analysis before the unblinding of the study. This diagnosis of HIV-1 infection was the only one that occurred outside planned procedures.

— **INTENTION-TO-TREAT ANALYSIS:** 132 SUBJECTS INFECTED (56/8197 VACCINATED AND 76/8198 PLACEBO—PER PROTOCOL ANALYSIS: 86 SUBJECTS INFECTED (36 VACCINATED, 50 PLACEBO):

— **MODIFIED INTENTION-TO-TREAT ANALYSIS** (the analysis Fauci frequently cites claiming a 31%$ success rate regarding a "protective effect" of this vaccine): and the ONLY "HIV" trial ever carried out that has exhibits STATISTICAL SIGNIFICANCE. The numbers reported where obtained after 1/3 of the patients were dropped from the analysis-which is cheating. Yet it remains as the only trial reported as being the first "HIV" vaccine trial to show promise since 1983, as it appears in the NEJM. Here are how the numbers look:

Out of 16,395, 125 experimentally-vaccinated subjects, 8197 subjects became "infected, 51 that were fully vaccinated: out of 8198 subjects vaccinated with placebo, 70 were "infected" that were fully vaccinated (with placebo).

There were 86 HIV-1 infections in the per-protocol population and 125 infections in the modified intention-to-treat population. There were three categories into which the 39 subjects with HIV-1 infection who were excluded from the per-protocol population could be organized: 10 subjects: 3 in the vaccine group and 7 in the placebo group were infected during the vaccination phase and received all vaccinations on schedule; but one or more vaccinations were not administered during the pre-specified window; and 19 subjects in the vaccine group and 10 in the placebo group were infected after the vaccination but did not receive all vaccinations.

"In this clinical trial, we evaluated the efficacy of ALVAC-HIV priming and AIDSVAX B/E boosting for the prevention of HIV-1 infection in more than 16,000 young Thai adults at community risk for such infection. In the intention-to-treat group (which included seven subjects who were found to have had HIV-1 infection at baseline), there was a trend toward prevention of infection with the vaccine regimen. In the per-protocol analysis, which excluded 30% of the end points and person-years of follow-up, the results were not significant. However, after the exclusion of the subjects who were infected with HIV-1 before vaccination, the modified intention-to-treat analysis showed a significant, though modest, reduction in the rate of HIV-1 infection, as compared with placebo. "Although there were increased env responses in the vaccinated, and increased gag responses in placebo, neither is statistically significant. (Env 165 and LAI gag (120?) peptides were used)?The trial demonstrated that the vaccine regimen was safe and modestly effective in preventing HIV infection. The results show that the prime-boost combination lowered the rate of HIV infection by 31.2 percent compared to placebo based on the modified intent-to-treat (mITT) population (n=51 vs. n=74, respectively; p=0.04). NO infections" ("VIRAL LOAD MEASUREMENTS).Vaccination with ALVAC and AIDSVAX to Prevent HIV-1 Infection in Thailand

http://www.nejm.org/doi/full/10.1056/NEJMoa0908492#t=article

For the number of deaths due to vaccine which outnumber the quantity excluded from the analysis (10 deaths here and there due to vaccine), see:

http://www.nejm.org/doi/suppl/10.1056/NEJMoa0908492/suppl_file/nejm_rerks-ngarm_2209sa1.pdf

To determine the viral load in samples tested in Thailand, the scientists used AMPLICOR'S 1.5 TEST. But 1996 and in 2004, Roche warned on its package insert that "The amplicor HIV-1 monitor test is not intended to be used as a screening test for HIV, nor as a diagnostic test to confirm the presence of HIV infection" (Roche's amplicor HIV-1 monitor test package insert, 1996).

To determine viral load in samples sent to the states, a recalled test was used called Procelix: In January of 2005, the FDA recalled Procleix HIV-1 – HCV Assay.

The official narrative and official Faucitopian conclusions about the largest "HIV" vaccine trial in history from these numbers, which are available for all to see and analyze, continues to be:

"We do not understand the immune mechanisms mediating the results that we observed. The ALVAC-HIV and AIDSVAX B/E prime–boost regimen induces a broad constellation of immune responses against HIV-1, including T-cell–line adapted neutralizing antibody (71% with response), antibody-directed, cell-mediated cytotoxicity, CD4+ lymphoproliferation (61% with response to gp20 MN, 63% with response to gp120 CM244), and CD8+ T cells (24% with response to 51Cr-release cytotoxic T-cell assay; 17% with positive response on ELISPOT),17,33,43 but these may not be the relevant responses."

2010 THE ROCKEFELLER FOUNDATION PUBLISHES SCENERIOS FOR THE FUTURE OF TECHNOLOGY AND INTERNATIONAL DEVELOPMENT which presciently predicts a global pandemic causing a global shutdown of the world economy and new authoritarian measures against civilian populations where China will be seen as a role model of successful pandemic authoritarianism.

China's government was not the only one that took extreme measures to protect its citizens from risk and exposure. During the pandemic, national leaders around the world flexed their authority and imposed airtight rules and restrictions, from the mandatory wearing of face masks to body-temperature checks at the entries to communal spaces like train stations and supermarkets. Even after the pandemic faded, this more authoritarian control and oversight of citizens and their activities stuck and even intensified. In order to protect themselves from the spread of increasingly global problems — from pandemics and transnational terrorism to environmental crises and rising poverty — leaders around the world took a firmer grip on power.

At first, the notion of a more controlled world gained wide acceptance and approval. Citizens willingly gave up some of their sovereignty — and their privacy — to more paternalistic states in exchange for greater safety and stability. Citizens were more tolerant, and even eager, for top-down direction and oversight, and national leaders had more latitude to impose order in the ways they saw fit. In developed countries, this heightened oversight took many forms: biometric IDs for all citizens, for example, and tighter regulation of key industries whose stability was deemed vital to national interests. In many developed countries, enforced cooperation with a suite of new regulations and agreements slowly but steadily restored both order and, importantly, economic growth.

2010 – SCIENTISTS DISCOVER A NEW VIRUS CAUSING AIDS. January 2010 News: World by Nikolai Terziev

Chinese scientists have discovered a previously unknown virus that can cause a syndrome of acquired immune deficiency (AIDS). Until now it was believed that a person may develop AIDS only after infected with HIV. But Chinese scholars argue that there is another virus that has yet to be studied and led to the development of the disease. "Thousands of patients who have AIDS have tested negative for HIV test," said one of the doctors. Experts explain that this hypothetical mutation of HIV is more aggressive and dangerous when transmitted through sex [as opposed to sharing a hamburger with someone—my observation]. Studies of the new virus began on Monday and still no clear date when results will be announced.

2010 (March) DANISH SCIENTIST POUL THORSEN WHO ALLEGEDLY "PROVED" VACCINES DON'T CAUSE AUTISM DISAPPEARED WITH $ 2 MILLION AND IS A FUGITIVE FROM AMERICAN JUSTICE SYSTEM FOR FRAUD

See the Copenhagen Post Online article at: http://www.cph-post.dk/news/international/89-international/48229-researcher-accused-of-cheating-uni-out-of-millions.html.

A Danish scientist who was a key researcher in two studies that purport to show that mercury used in vaccines and the measles mumps-rubella (MMR) vaccine do not cause autism. Thorsen is believed to have used forged documents to steal $2 million from Aarhus University in Denmark according to reports in the Copenhagen Post Online and a statement from Aarhus University. Paul Thorsen, MD PhD, headed up a research unit at Aarhus University that was hired by the Centers for Disease Control and Prevention to prepare a series of studies that would exonerate thimerosal, a mercury-based preservative and adjuvant used in vaccines, and the MMR vaccine from any role in causing autism. The veracity of the three studies he co-authored is now in doubt. These studies formed the foundation for the conclusions of several Institute of Medicine reports that claimed that it was highly unlikely that thimerosal or MMR were implicated in autism.

In a statement Aarhus University official said that believe Poulsen forged documents supposedly from the CDC to obtain the release of $2 million from the University. Poulsen resigned abruptly in March 2009 and left Denmark. Since then, Thorsen has held several jobs in the US, first at Emory University in Atlanta and then at Drexel University in Philadelphia. Documents show that as late as January 22, 2009. Thorsen was employed at Drexel. Any reference to Poulsen has now been deleted from the Drexel website.

Investigations also revealed that while employed full-time for the University of Aarhus in Denmark, Poulsen simultaneously held a fulltime position at Emory University in Atlanta and drew salaries from both Universities despite a contract with Aarhus forbidding outside employment. According to the statement from Aarhus University.

Autism advocacy groups have published extensive analyses on

Thorsen's studies and found many problems in methods, assumptions and conclusions that are supported by the data. And Thorsen is the lynchpin in the series of studies used to dismiss concerns about thimerosal and MMR causing autism.

See the statement from Aarhus University: http://www.rescuepost.com/files/thorsen-aarhus.pdf

The two studies now in doubt include:

Thimerosal and the occurrence of autism: negative ecological evidence from Danish population-based data. Madsen KM, Lauritsen MB, Pedersen CB, Thorsen P, Plesner AM, Andersen PH, Mortensen PB, Pediatrics. 2003 Sep;112(3 Pt 1):604-6.

A population-based study of measles, mumps, and rubella vaccination and autism. Madsen KM, Hviid A, Vestergaard M, Schendel D, Wohlfahrt J, Thorsen P, Olsen J, Melbye M.,N Engl J Med. 2002 Nov 7;347(19):1477-82.

EXPERTS SUGGEST THAT SMALLPOX VACCINE WOULD PROTECT AGAINST HIV (instead of cause it as they said before)

2010 (June). Instead of triggering the era of AIDS as was chronicled earlier in this book, The Church of Modern Medicine now claims the smallpox vaccine could protect people against HIV infection, as it was said an article released in the journal BMC Immunology. According to the publication, researchers from George Mason University, George Washington and UCLA in Los Angeles, USA, showed that in the laboratory the vaccinia virus, the basis of the vaccine, reduced the replication of HIV. It appears that the compound blocks a receptor, called CCR5, on the surface of white blood cells, the same as the HIV virus uses to infect cells. However, more studies are needed before recommending the general use of the immunogen in the fight against AIDS. After the disappearance of the disease in 1977 (first eradicated throughout the world), the World Health Organization recommended removing the vaccine, something that happened in the same period of time when HIV and AIDS was discovered. Hence, one researcher suggested that the removal may have been the cause of the rapid spread of HIV in Africa. Several explanations were given on how HIV spread in the black continent, including wars, use of unsterilized needles and the contamination of polio vaccines, said Raymond Weinstein, author of the work. But no theory has been able to determine the behavior of the pandemic, he said. "Our finding that previous immunization with vaccinia virus can give a person some protection against subsequent HIV infection suggests that the withdrawal of this vaccine may have been the explanation for the rapid spread of HIV in Africa" Weinstein concluded.

Did the End of Smallpox Vaccination Cause the Explosive Spread of HIV? ScienceDaily (May 18, 2010) — Vaccinia immunization, as given to prevent the spread of smallpox, produces a five-fold reduction in HIV replication in the laboratory. Researchers writing in the open access journal BMC Immunology suggest that the end of smallpox vaccination in the mid-20th century may have caused a loss of protection that contributed to the rapid contemporary spread of HIV. See Also: Health & Medicine – HIV and AIDS Infectious Diseases Viruses Plants & Animals Virology Biology Genetics Reference Vaccination Flu vaccine HPV vaccine MMR vaccine.

Raymond Weinstein, a family doctor turned laboratory scientist at George Mason University, Manassas, Virginia, worked with a team of researchers from George Washington University and UCLA. The researchers looked at the ability of white blood cells taken from people recently immunized with vaccinia to support HIV replication compared to unvaccinated controls. They found significantly lower viral replication in blood cells from vaccinated individuals. Weinstein said, "There have been several proposed explanations for the rapid spread of HIV in Africa, including wars, the reuse of unsterilized needles and the contamination of early batches of polio vaccine. However, all of these have been either disproved or do not sufficiently explain the behavior of the

HIV pandemic. Our finding that prior immunization with vaccinia virus may provide an individual with some degree of protection to subsequent HIV infection suggests that the withdrawal of such vaccination may be a partial explanation. "Smallpox immunization was gradually withdrawn from the 1950s to the 1970s following the worldwide eradication of the disease, and HIV has been spreading exponentially since approximately the same time period. Weinstein and his colleagues propose that vaccination may confer protection against HIV by producing long term alterations in the immune system, possibly including the expression of a certain receptor, CCR5, on the surface of a person's white blood cells which is exploited by both viruses. Speaking about the results, Weinstein said, "While these results are very interesting and hopefully may lead to a new weapon against the HIV pandemic, they are very preliminary, and it is far too soon to recommend the general use of vaccinia immunization for fighting HIV." Source: Adapted from materials provided by BioMed Central, Journal Reference: Raymond S Weinstein, Michael M Weinstein, Kenneth Alibek, Michael I Bukrinsky and Brichacek Beda. Significantly Reduced CCR5-tropic HIV-1 Replication in vitro in Cells from Subjects Previously Immunized with Vaccinia Virus. BMC Immunology, 2010; (in press)

Flashback to 1987: Despite these claims that the end of smallpox vaccination of Africans caused the AIDS epidemic, can you remember what was written at the beginning of the AIDS era? In case you are unaware of this information, I have provided it here (and not in 1987 where it would go along the timeline):

"1987 SMALLPOX VACCINE 'TRIGGERED AIDS VIRUS" By Pearce Wright, Science editor, London Times edition, Monday, May 11, 1987.

The Aids epidemic may have been triggered by the mass vaccination campaign which eradicated smallpox. The World Health Organization, which masterminded the 13-year campaign, is studying new scientific evidence suggesting that immunization with the smallpox vaccine Vaccinia awakened the unsuspected, dormant human immuno defense virus infection (HIV).(Article presented in its entirety before-see 1987). (Look at the 1987 entry on the timeline in its entirety (in the year 1987).

2011 Newsflash: Feds urge churches to peddle flu shots to members, partner with drugstores to sponsor flu clinics.

In 2011, while she served as deputy director for the laboratory science policy and practice program office, and as a graduate of serving as former senior health preparedness and response, an office that oversaw the allocation process for $1.5 billion in terrorism preparedness, and which led the sham 2009 H1N1 flu vaccine debacle, Dr, Kimberly Quinlan Lindsey and her CDC security guard boyfriend were arrested and charged with two counts of alleged child molestation and one count of bestiality. She also oversaw the dangerous Pandemrix vaccine program that increased the risk of narcolepsy by 900% in children and adolescents below the age of 19, and which was linked with abnormally high rates of miscarriage and stillbirths, during a time when her involvement with the CDC's AIDS program. After President Barack Obama declared 2009 H1N1 swine flu a national emergency, the U.S. Centers for Disease Control released reports that the flu has become widespread in 46 of the 50 U.S. states at a level comparable to the peak of ordinary flu seasons but far earlier and with more waves of infection.

https://www.reuters.com/article/us-flu-usa-obama-id USTRE59N19E20091024

It took time, but eventually it was revealed that the 2009 H1N1 Influenza vaccine increased the risk for narcolepsy-an exceedingly rare and devastating sleeping disorder in a cohort of Swedish children and adolescents by 660% following Pandemrix influenza vaccination in Europe.

https://www.cdc.gov/vaccinesafety/concerns/history/narcolepsy-flu.html

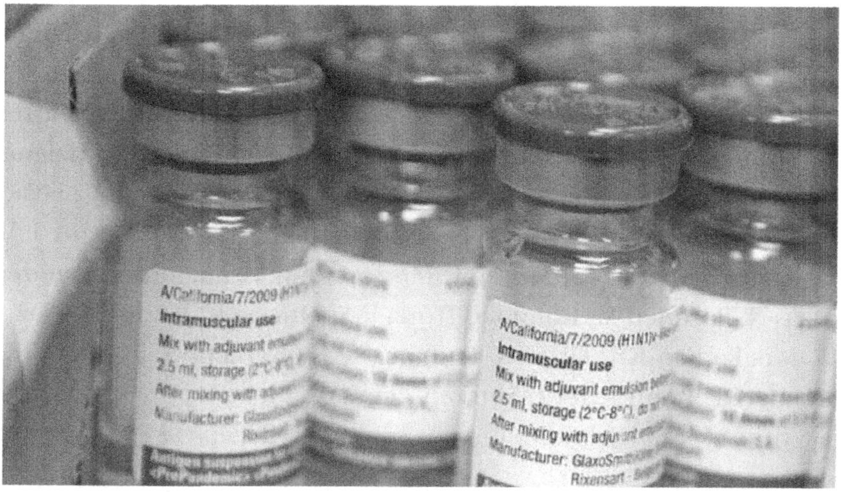

IN 2011, some countries reported that "PANDEMRIX" H1N1 vaccine increased the risk of narcolepsy by 900 percent in children and adolescents below the age of 19. In the US, the H1N1 flu vaccine was statistically linked with abnormally high rates of miscarriage and stillbirths.

"An increased risk of narcolepsy was found following vaccination with Pandemrix, a monovalent 2009 H1N1 influenza vaccine that was used in several European countries during the H1N1 influenza pandemic. Narcolepsy is a chronic neurological disorder caused by the brain's inability to regulate sleep-wake cycles normally. This risk was initially found in Finland, and then some other European countries also detected an association. Scientists at the United Kingdom's (UK) Health Protection Agency (HPA) found evidence of an association between Pandemrix and narcolepsy in children in England. The findings were consistent with studies from Finland and other countries. Pandemrix was manufactured by GlaxoSmithKline in Europe and was specifically produced for pandemic 2009 H1N1 influenza. It was not used before 2009 and has not been used since the influenza pandemic season (2009-2010). It contained an oil-in-water emulsion adjuvant called ASO3. Adjuvants are substances added to a vaccine to increase the body's immune response to that vaccine."

Vaccine. 2013 Feb 6;31(8):1246-54. doi: 10.1016/j.vaccine.2012.12.015. Epub 2012 Dec 16.

The incidence of narcolepsy in Europe: before, during, and after the influenza A (H1N1)pdm09 pandemic and vaccination campaigns.

Wijnans L1, Lecomte C, de Vries C, Weibel D, Sammon C, Hviid A, Svanström H, Mølgaard-Nielsen D, Heijbel H, Dahlström LA, Hallgren J, Sparen P, Jennum P, Mosseveld M, Schuemie M, van der Maas N, Partinen M, Romio S, Trotta F, Santuccio C, Menna A, Plazzi G, Moghadam KK, Ferro S, Lammers GJ, Overeem S, Johansen K, Kramarz P, Bonhoeffer J, Sturkenboom MC.

https://www.ncbi.nlm.nih.gov/pubmed/23246544

Abstract

BACKGROUND:

In August 2010 reports of a possible association between exposure to AS03 adjuvanted pandemic A(H1N1)pdm09 vaccine and occurrence of narcolepsy in children and adolescents emerged in Sweden and Finland. In response to this signal, the background rates of narcolepsy in Europe were assessed to rapidly provide information for signal verification.

CONCLUSIONS:

The results of this incidence study provided useful information for signal verification on a population level. The safety signal of increased narcolepsy diagnoses following the start of the pandemic vaccination campaign as observed in Sweden and Finland could be observed with this approach. An increase in narcolepsy diagnoses was not observed in other countries, where vaccination coverage was low in the affected age group or did not follow influenza A(H1N1) pdm09 vaccination. Patient level analyses in these countries are being conducted to verify the signal in more detail.

https://www.ncbi.nlm.nih.gov/pubmed/31130313

Biologicals. 2019 Jul;60:1-7. doi: 10.1016/j.biologicals.2019.05.005. Epub 2019 May 23.

Meeting report narcolepsy and pandemic influenza vaccination: What we know and what we need to know before the next pandemic? A report from the 2nd IABS meeting.

Edwards K1, Hanquet G2, Black S3, Mignot E4, Jankosky C5, Shimabukuro T6, Miller E7, Nohynek H8, Neels P9.

Abstract

A group of scientific and public health experts and key stakeholders convened to discuss the state of knowledge on the relationship between adjuvanted monovalent inactivated 2009 influenza A H1N1 vaccines used during the 2009 influenza pandemic and narcolepsy. There was consensus that an increased risk of narcolepsy was consistently observed after Pandemrix (AS03-adjuvanted) vaccine, but similar associations following Arepanrix (AS03-adjuvanted) or Focetria (MF59-adjuvanted) vaccines were not observed. Whether the differences are due to vaccine composition or other factors such as the timing of large-scale vaccination programs relative to H1N1pdm09 wild-type virus circulation in different geographic regions is not clear. The limitations of retrospective observational methodologies could also be contributing to some of the differences across studies. More basic and epidemiologic research is needed to further elucidate the association between adjuvanted influenza vaccine and narcolepsy and its mechanism and to inform planning and preparation for vaccination programs in advance of the next influenza pandemic.

September 2010 https://www.eurosurveillance.org/content/10.2807/ese.15.35.19652-en

Virus excretion in vaccinees has been reported before [8-10], but to our knowledge, this is documented for the first time for the Schwarz vaccine strain. Interestingly, although the blood for serology testing was obtained 14 and 32 days after vaccination, the child still had no antibodies to rubella virus in either serum sample. It is

unclear why there was no seroconversion to rubella 32 days after vaccination, although this is not an unusual finding. The dynamics of measles and mumps antibodies were as expected for someone who had either been vaccinated or had natural infection, indicating that the child did not have impaired antibody production kinetics in general.

We demonstrated excretion of the Schwarz measles vaccine virus in a child with a vaccine-associated febrile rash illness in urine and in pharyngeal excretions.

2011 – Harvard Professor Charles Lieber invents nano-technology transistors that are so tiny they can penetrate human cells and organs https://www.harvardmagazine.com/2011/01/virus-sized-transistors

"Digital electronics are so powerful that they dominate our daily lives," Lieber points out. "When scaled down, the difference between digital and living systems blurs, so that you have an opportunity to do things that sound like science fiction—things that people have only dreamed about." Imagine being able to signal an immune cell to generate antibodies that would fight bacteria or even cancer. That fictional possibility is now a step closer to reality with the development of a bio-compatible transistor the size of a virus. Hyman professor of chemistry Charles Lieber and his colleagues used nanowires to create a transistor so small that it can be used to enter and probe cells without disrupting the intracellular machinery. These nanoscale semiconductor switches could even be used to enable two-way communication with individual cells. Lieber has worked for the past decade on the design and synthesis of nanoscale parts that will enable him to build tiny electronic devices (see "Liquid Computing,)" Devising a biological interface, in which a nanoscale device can actually communicate with a living organism, has been an explicit goal from the beginning, but has proven tricky."

2012 POLIO VACCINES NOW THE # 1 CAUSE OF POLIO PARALYSIS. Sayer Ji, Contributing Writer, GreenMedInfo.

The Polio Global Eradication Initiative (PGEI), founded in 1988 by the World Health Organization, Rotary International, UNICEF, and the U.S. Centers for Disease Control and Prevention, holds up India as a prime example of its success at eradicating polio, stating on its website (Jan. 11 2012) that "India has made unprecedented progress against polio in the last two years and on 13 January, 2012, India will reach a major milestone — a 12-month period without any case of polio being recorded."

This report, however, is highly misleading, as an estimated 100-180 Indian children are diagnosed with vaccine-associated polio paralysis (VAPP) each year. In fact, the clinical presentation of the disease, including paralysis, caused by VAPP is indistinguishable from that caused by wild polioviruses, making the PGEI's pronouncements all the more suspect.

According to the Polio Global Eradication Initiative's own statistics there were 42 cases of wild-type polio (WPV) reported in India in 2010, indicating that vaccine-induced cases of polio paralysis (100-180 annually) outnumber wild-type cases by a factor of 3-4. Even if we put aside the important question of whether or not the PGEI is accurately differentiating between wild and vaccine-associated polio cases in their statistics, we still must ask ourselves: should not the real-world effects of immunization, both good and bad, be included in PGEI's measurement of success? For the dozens of Indian children who develop vaccine-induced paralysis every year, the PGEI's recent declaration of India as nearing "polio free" status, is not only disingenuous, but could be considered an attempt to minimize their obvious liability in having transformed polio from a natural disease vector into a man-made (iatrogenic) one.

VAPP is, in fact, the predominant form of the disease in developed countries like the US since 1973.3 The problem of vaccine-induced polio paralysis was so severe that the United States moved to the inactivated poliovirus vaccine (IPV) in 2000, after the Advisory Committee on Immunization Practices (ACIP) recommended altogether eliminating the live-virus oral polio vaccine

(OPV), which is still used throughout the third world, despite the known risks.

Polio underscores the need for a change in the way we look at so-called "vaccine preventable" diseases as a whole. In most people with a healthy immune system, a poliovirus infection does not even generate symptoms. Only rarely does the infection produce minor symptoms, e.g., sore throat, fever, gastrointestinal disturbances, and influenza-like illness. In only 3% of infections does virus gain entry to the central nervous system, and then, in only 1-5 in 1000 cases does the infection progress to paralytic disease. Due to the fact that polio spreads through the fecal-oral route (i.e., the virus is transmitted from the stool of an infected person to the mouth of another person through a contaminated object, e.g., utensil) focusing on hygiene, sanitation and proper nutrition (to support innate immunity) is a logical way to prevent transmission in the first place, as well as reducing morbidity associated with an infection when it does occur.

Instead, a large portion of the world's vaccines are given to the Third World as "charity," when the underlying conditions of economic impoverishment, poor nutrition, chemical exposures, and socio-political unrest are never addressed. You simply cannot vaccinate people out of these conditions, and as India's new epidemic of vaccine-induced polio cases clearly demonstrates, the "cure" may be far worse than the disease itself.

1 Cono J, Alexander LN (2002). "Chapter 10: Poliomyelitis" (PDF). Vaccine-Preventable Disease Surveillance Manual.2 http://www.polioeradication.org/Dataandmonitoring/Poliothisweek.aspx3 Strebel PM, Sutter RW, Cochi SL, et al. Epidemiology of poliomyelitis in the United States one decade after the last reported case of indigenous wild virus-associated disease. Clin Infect Dis 1992;14:568-79.

2012 January 25 PREMATURE BABIES USED AS LAB RATS IN MANIPULATED VACCINE TRIALS http://sanevax.org/premature-babies-used-as-lab-rats-in-manipulated-vaccine-trials/ By Christina England

While reading the results of a vaccination trial on premature babies funded by GlaxoSmithKline, I noticed something was not quite right.

The trial, whilst sickening in itself, was testing out the rotavirus vaccine on a group of 988 premature babies ranging between 27 weeks and 36 weeks.

The paper reporting the trial was published on the 'Pediatric SuperSite' and was entitled 'Human rotavirus immunogenic, well-tolerated for preterm infants' by Felix Omenaca MD. PhD, and colleagues (1) The paper stated the following:

"The researchers grouped preterm infants by ages—infants born at gestational ages 27 to 30 weeks and those born at 30 to 36 weeks. They administered rotavirus vaccine (RIX4414, GlaxoSmithKline) in two doses to 658 preterm infants, and 330 received a placebo along with routine vaccinations, including diphtheria, tetanus, pertussis, hepatitis B, Haemophilus influenzae type B and poliovirus. Infants from France and Spain also received Streptococcus pneumoniae concomitantly; infants from Portugal and Spain also received Neisseria meningitides...

The researchers then asked parents/guardians to report adverse effects, and they noted no statistically significant difference in the reporting of severe adverse reactions in the vaccine or placebo group (5.1% and 6.2%, respectively). Unsolicited adverse effects, which included fever of more than 39.5·C, six or more bouts of diarrhea per day, three or more episodes of vomiting per day, appetite loss and irritability, were reported in 29.3% of preterm infants in the vaccine group and 40.7% in the placebo group. (own emphasis)

The problems I see are as follows:

All the infants were given multiple vaccinations, therefore, there was no control group.

Of a group of 988 children, approximately 2/3 were given the vaccine for rotavirus and 1/3 were given the placebo, then the researchers compared the results like for like. This cannot be done because one group is significantly larger than the other. Because all of the infants received multiple vaccinations it is impossible to tell which vaccine if any caused the side effects.

Here is the abstract and some related articles:

Felix Omenaca, Jean Sarlangue, Leszek Szenborn, Marta Nogueira Pemmaraju, V. Suryakiran, Igor V. Smalenov, Htay H Han, Rota-054 Study Group. **Safety, reactogenicity and immunogenicity of the human rotavirus vaccine in preterm European Infants: a randomized phase IIIb study.**

Abstract

Background: Rotavirus disease is more severe in preterm infants than in full-term infants. This study assessed the safety, reactogenicity and immunogenicity of a human rotavirus vaccine, RIX4414, in European preterm infants.

Methods: A total of 1009 preterm infants were randomized (2:1, vaccine:placebo) and stratified into 2 groups: 20% of early (27-30 weeks, group 1) and 80% of late (31-36 weeks, group 2) gestational age preterm infants in each group. Two doses of RIX4414/placebo were administered to these preterm infants according to the recommended chronologic age for full-term infants with an interval of 30-83 days between doses. Serious adverse events were recorded throughout the study period. Solicited and unsolicited adverse events were recorded for 15 and 31 days post-each dose. Antirotavirus IgA concentrations (enzyme-linked immunosorbent assay cutoff = 20 U/mL) and geometric mean concentration were determined predose 1- and 30-83-days post-dose 2 in a subset of 300 infants. This study is registered with ClinicalTrials.gov, number NCT00420745 (eTrack106481).

Results: Serious adverse events were reported at a similar frequency in both groups (P = 0.266). Fifty-seven infants reported at least 1 serious adverse event (5.1% [3.5-7.0] in the RIX4414 group and 6.8% [4.3-10.0] in the placebo group). During the 15-day post-vaccination follow-up period, diarrhea, vomiting, and fever occurred at a similar frequency in both groups; fever could have been due to concomitant vaccines. Five cases (RIX4414 = 3, Placebo = 2) of rotavirus gastroenteritis were reported. The onset of rotavirus gastroenteritis in the RIX4414 group was 1-5 days after vaccination (vaccine strain identified in all cases) and in the placebo group it was 3-4 days after receiving placebo (wild-type rotavirus identified from both cases). Antirotavirus IgA seroconversion rates at 30-83 days post-dose 2 were 85.7% (79.0-90.9) in the RIX4414 group and 16.0% (8.8-25.9) in the placebo group. Geometric mean concentrations were 202.2 U/mL (153.1-267.1) in the RIX4414 group and <20 U/mL in the placebo group. Seroconversion rate in groups 1 and 2 in RIX4414 recipients were 75.9% (95% confidence interval [CI]: 56.5-89.7%) and 88.1% (95% CI: 80.9-93.4%), respectively; the geometric mean concentrations in the respective groups were 110.2 U/mL (95% CI: 56.1-216.5) and 234.8 U/mL (95% CI: 173.4-318.0; exploratory analysis).

Conclusions: Two doses of RIX4414 were immunogenic and well-tolerated in European preterm infants.

2013 Murti M, Krajden M, Petric M et al. **Case of Vaccine Associated Measles Five Weeks Post-Immunization,** British Columbia, Canada, October 2013. Eurosurveillance Dec. 5, 2013; 18(49).

2014 'A mass sterilization exercise': Kenyan doctors find anti-fertility agent in UN tetanus vaccine was registered with ClinicalTrials.gov, number NCT00420745 (eTrack106481).

'This WHO campaign is not about eradicating neonatal tetanus but a well-coordinated forceful population control mass sterilization exercise using a proven fertility regulating vaccine.'

https://www.lifesitenews.com/news/a-mass-sterilization-exercise-kenyan-doctors-find-anti-fertility-agent-in-u

UPDATE (Nov. 12): Kenya's government has launched an investigation into the Catholic Church's allegations.

Kenya's Catholic bishops are charging two United Nations organizations with sterilizing millions of girls and women under cover of an anti-tetanus inoculation program sponsored by the Kenyan government.

According to a statement released Tuesday by the Kenya Catholic Doctors Association, the organization has found an antigen that causes miscarriages in a vaccine being administered to 2.3 million girls and women by the World Health Organization and UNICEF. Priests throughout Kenya reportedly are advising their congregations to refuse the vaccine.

"We sent six samples from around Kenya to laboratories in South Africa. They tested positive for the HCG antigen," Dr. Muhame Ngare of the Mercy Medical Centre in Nairobi told LifeSiteNews. "They were all laced with HCG."

Dr. Ngare, spokesman for the Kenya Catholic Doctors Association, stated in a bulletin released November 4, "This proved right our worst fears; that this WHO campaign is not about eradicating neonatal tetanus but a well-coordinated forceful population control mass sterilization exercise using a proven fertility regulating vaccine. This evidence was presented to the Ministry of Health before the third round of immunization but was ignored."

Several things alerted doctors in the Church's far-flung medical system of 54 hospitals, 83 health centers, and 17 medical and nursing schools to the possibility the anti-tetanus campaign was secretly an anti-fertility campaign.

Why, they ask does it involve an unprecedented five shots (or "jabs" as they are known, in Kenya) over more than two years and why is it applied only to women of child-bearing years, and why is it not being conducted without the usual fanfare of government publicity?

"Usually, we give a series three shots over two to three years, we give it anyone who comes into the clinic with an open wound, men, women or children." said Dr. Ngare. "If this is intended to inoculate children in the womb, why give it to girls starting at 15 years? You cannot get married till you are 18." The usual way to vaccinate children is to wait till they are six weeks old."

But it is the five-vaccination regime that is most alarming. "The only time tetanus vaccine has been given in five doses is when it is used as a carrier in fertility regulating vaccines laced with the pregnancy hormone, Human Chorionic Gonadotropin (HCG) developed by WHO in 1992."

It is HCG that has been found in all six samples sent to the University of Nairobi medical laboratory and another in South Africa. The bishops and doctors warn that injecting women with HCG, which mimics a natural hormone produced by pregnant women, causes them to develop antibodies against it. When they do get pregnant, and produce their own version of HCG, it triggers the production of antibodies that cause a miscarriage.

"We knew that the last time this vaccination with five injections has been used was in Mexico in 1993 and Nicaragua and the Philippines in 1994," said Dr. Ngare. "It didn't cause miscarriages till three years later," which is why, he added, the counterclaims that women who got the vaccination recently and then got pregnant are meaningless.

Ngare said WHO tried to bring the same anti-fertility program into Kenya in the 1990s. "We alerted the government, and it stopped the vaccination. But this time they haven't done so."

Ngare also contrasted the secrecy of this campaign with the usual fanfare accompanying national vaccination efforts. "They usually bring all the stakeholders together three months before the campaign, like they did with polio a little while ago. And they use staff in all the centers to give out the vaccine." But with this anti-tetanus campaign, "only a few operatives from the government are allowed to give it out. They come with a police escort. They take it away with them when they are finished. Why not leave it with the local medical staff to administer?"

In the previous cases, said Clowes, the vaccinators insisted their product was pure until it was shown not to be. Then they claimed the positive tests for HCG were isolated, accidental contaminations in the manufacturing process.

LifeSiteNews has obtained a UN report on an August 1992 meeting at its world headquarters in Geneva of 10 scientists from

"Australia, Europe, India and the U.S.A" and 10 "women's health advocates" from around the world, to discuss the use of "fertility regulating vaccines." It describes the "anti-Human Chorionic Gonadotropin vaccine" as the most advanced.

One million Kenyan women and girls have been vaccinated so far with another 1.3 million to go. The vaccination is targeting women, according to the government, in order to inoculate their children in the womb against tetanus as well. The government says 550 children die of tetanus yearly.

In covering the contest of words, the pro-government Nation found plenty of women who had been vaccinated and were now pregnant, even one who was the wife of a former Catholic priest who left the Church to marry. The paper ignored Kenya's reliance on the Catholic medical system, while setting the bishops' stand in a questionable historical context of irrational responses "largely based on religious beliefs," the more recent murder of vaccination teams in Nigeria, and even of CIA conspiracy theories.

Why would the UN want to suppress the population in developing countries? "Racism," is Brian Clowes' first explanation. "Also, the developed countries want to get hold of their natural resources. And lately, there is the whole bogus global warming thing."

Dr. Ngare said it was the Catholic Church's hope that the government could have resolved the matter quietly by testing the vaccine. "But the government has chosen to be combative," forcing Kenya's bishops and Catholic doctors to go public.

WHO's Kenyan office and several WHO media contacts in Washington; D.C. failed to respond to LifeSiteNews enquiries over a 24-hour period.

June 10, 2014 Daily Beast -Irish Care Home Scandal Grows as Children Revealed to Be Used As Vaccine Guinea Pigs, by Tom Sykes

https://www.thedailybeast.com/irish-care-home-scandal-grows-as-children-revealed-to-be-used-as-vaccine-guinea-pigs

The Irish mother-and-baby home scandal has continued to grow, with shocking allegations that children in homes for 'fallen women'—as unmarried mothers, who often were put by their families into institutions, were known—were used as guinea pigs in vaccine trials by pharmaceutical companies.

The revelations came as the Irish government today bowed to pressure and announced a full enquiry into the homes.

Last week, it was revealed that almost 800 children and babies were buried in unmarked graves in the grounds of a home run by the Bon Secours sisters in Tuam, County Galway. Reports that the bodies of the children had been 'dumped' in a septic tank have, however, proved to be wide of the mark.

However, the Irish radio station Newstalk has now claimed in an exclusive report that 80 children in a care home became ill after they were given an experimental bovine vaccine.

The children allegedly became unwell after they were given a vaccine intended for cattle in a trial at five care homes and orphanages in Dublin in the mid-'70s.They were among 298 children experimented on in drug trials.

The information is contained in a report from the Chief Medical Officer of the Department of Health's report to the Oireachtas in the year 2000, obtained by Newstalk.

One man who was adopted from one of the homes—Bessborough House, in County Cork—and who gave his name only as Christy, said: "My arms and legs were very badly scarred. But when I asked my (adopted) Mum why, she basically said, 'When you arrived your arms were very sore, and they were bandaged'… I did not know anything about vaccination trials. I've since been to a few doctors and they said they had never seen anything like it, so many injections… I had eight injections between my two arms and two on my legs… I have been to a few doctors and they said they can't understand it."

2015 Disney Measles Outbreak https://www.cbsnews.com/news/disney-measles-outbreak-may-have-originated-in-the-philippines/

In the month and a half since public health officials in California confirmed the first case of measles linked to Disneyland, the measles outbreak has grown to at least 182 cases in 18 states and the District of Columbia, according to the latest count by CBS News. But state and federal health officials are still uncertain of the exact source of the outbreak.

February 20 2015 https://www.cdc.gov/mmwr/preview/mmwrhtml/mm6406a5.htm

The California Department of Public Health (CDPH) was notified about a suspected measles case. The patient was a hospitalized, unvaccinated child, aged 11 years with rash onset on December 28. The only notable travel history during the exposure period was a visit to one of two adjacent Disney theme parks located in Orange County, California. On the same day, CDPH received reports of four additional suspected measles cases in California residents and two in Utah residents, all of whom reported visiting one or both Disney theme parks during December 17–20. By January 7, seven California measles cases had been confirmed, and CDPH issued a press release and an Epidemic Information Exchange (Epi-X) notification to other states regarding this outbreak. Measles transmission is ongoing.

As of February 11, a total of 125 measles cases with rash occurring during December 28, 2014–February 8, 2015, had been confirmed in U.S. residents connected with this outbreak. Of these, 110 patients were California residents.28 intentionally unvaccinated patients, 18 were children (aged <18 years), and 10 were adults.

2016, June 6 – mRNA Vaccine Delivery Using Lipid Nanoparticles https://pubmed.ncbi.nlm.nih.gov/27075952/

Abstract

mRNA vaccines elicit a potent immune response including antibodies and cytotoxic T cells. mRNA vaccines are currently evaluated in clinical trials for cancer immunotherapy applications, but also have great potential as prophylactic vaccines. Efficient delivery of mRNA vaccines will be key for their success and translation to the clinic. Among potential nonviral vectors, lipid nanoparticles are particularly promising. Indeed, lipid nanoparticles can be synthesized with

relative ease in a scalable manner, protect the mRNA against degradation, facilitate endosomal escape, can be targeted to the desired cell type by surface decoration with ligands, and as needed, can be codelivered with adjuvants.

September 2016 – Future leader of the World Health Organization Tedros Adhanom accused in Jerusalem Post editorial of executing hundreds of innocent civilian protesters and accused of being a war criminal and guilty of accepting bribes and stealing wealth from the Ethiopian public https://www.jpost.com/Opinion/Ethiopia-lacks-a-model-of-leadership-467052

The current Ethiopian government is widely recognized as a criminally organized group with high rates of human rights abuses. According to The New York Times and Human Rights Watch, tens of thousands of peaceful protesters against the government have been incarcerated, and over 700 have been killed, in recent months. The Ethiopian athlete Feyisa Lilesa made a powerful public gesture in solidarity with his oppressed countrymen at the Summer Olympics in Rio last month and was warned not to return home afterward. The International Committee to Protect Journalists reports that Ethiopia is among Africa's leading jailers of journalists and has destroyed its own independent civil society. The UN Commissioner for Human Rights has requested an independent evaluation of the deaths of hundreds of peaceful civilian protesters in recent months at the hands of the Ethiopian army. However, Foreign Minister Adhanom and his government have refused external evaluation of human rights abuses complained of by large numbers of citizens.

2017 Communist Ethiopian Accused War Criminal Tedros Adhanom nominated to head World Health Organization https://globalvoices.org/2017/05/21/ethiopias-cholera-denying-candidate-to-lead-the-worlds-top-health-body-is-taking-a-battering-online/

Dr Frank Ashall, an Oxford trained Ethiopian Medical School Professor stated in June of 2017 "Your words are mixed up – you should have said that Dr Tedros Adhanom was "exceptionally unethical" as MoH in Ethiopia. He deliberately neglected cholera epidemics, and there are published scientific investigations that show this. He neglected tobacco deals, he supported ungodly human rights abuse of poor Ethiopians by involving health extension workers in government oppression, denying people of food aid and proper care. Worse still, he was key politburo official of a group that was listed as a terrorist organization- Tigray People's Liberation Front (TPLF), which continues to this day to oppress, torture, jail and kill anyone who dare criticize its evil deeds. Shame for WHO and shame for humanity!"

2017 Study prompts call to examine flu vaccine and miscarriage. CBS News- https://www.cbsnews.com/news/study-prompts-call-to-examine-flu-vaccine-and-miscarriage

NEW YORK — A puzzling study of U.S. pregnancies found that women who had miscarriages between 2010 and 2012 were more likely to have had back-to-back annual flu shots that included protection against swine flu.

2018 A lowered probability of pregnancy in females in the USA aged 25-29 who received a human papillomavirus (HPV) vaccine injection by Professor Gayle Delong J Toxicol Environ Health 2018;81(14):661-674. doi: 10.1080/15287394.2018.1477640. Epub 2018 Jun 11.

This study analyzed information gathered in National Health and Nutrition Examination Survey, which represented 8 million 25-to-29-year-old women residing in the United States between 2007 and 2014. Approximately 60% of women who did not receive the HPV vaccine had been pregnant at least once, whereas only 35% of women who were exposed to the vaccine had conceived. For married women, 75% who did not receive the shot were found to conceive, while only 50% who received the vaccine had ever been pregnant. Using logistic regression to analyze the data, the probability of having been pregnant was estimated for females who received an HPV vaccine compared with females who did not receive the shot. Results suggest that females who received the HPV shot were less likely to have ever been pregnant than women in the same age group who did not receive the shot. If 100% of females in this study had received the HPV vaccine, data suggest the number of women having ever conceived would have fallen by 2 million. Further study into the influence of HPV vaccine on fertility is thus warranted.

CHAPTER III

THE TIMELINE OF THE SARS-COVID 19 GREAT RESET

JANUARY 2019: CRIMSON CONTAGION VIRUS FROM CHINA EXERCISE SCENARIO OVERVIEW – US federal government agencies including Department of Health & FEMA and DHS and City of Chicago, Illinois and New York and other local cities and states run a "pandemic exercise" where a novel respiratory virus comes from China via travelers and causes a shutdown of the United States and school closures.

The Crimson Contagion 2019 Functional Exercise scenario was based on a novel influenza A (H7N9) virus that originates in China and is antigenically distinct (not matched) from stockpiled vaccines. The scenario starts off with tourists becoming ill in China with non-severe acute respiratory illness and then departing the Lhasa airport to other cities in China before flying back to their respective countries. During their flights home, additional tour group members, who were not ill when they embarked on their return flights from China,begin to experience the onset of respiratory symptoms and some develop fever. Figure 3 below shows how the virus begins to spread around the world, as the ill tourists fly back to their countries of origin. Figure1. Map of III Tourists Flying Back to Their Countries of Origin COUNTRIES OF ORIGIN OF ILL TOURISTS INITIAL ORIGIN POINTS The virus rapidly spreads via human -to -human transmission around the world and to the continental U. S., where the virus is first detected in Chicago, Illinois. The virus continues to spread to other metropolitan areas across the U. S. Figure 4 below shows the extent of the outbreak across the U. S. at the start of the exercise. Conduct of the Crimson Contagion 2019 Functional Exercise began 47 days after the identification of the first case of H7N9 in the U. S. By this point in the scenario, the HHS Secretary has declared a national public health emergency and the World Health Organization has declared an influenza pandemic – the 2019 Influenza Pandemic. The federal government has decided to use stockpiled H7N9 vaccines as a FOR OFFICIAL USE ONLY COORDINATING DRAFT DO NOT DISTRIBUTE priming dose for selected persons at high risk of complications from influenza and designated critical work force groups, but vaccination has not yet been implemented.

July 5, 2019 BREAKING NEWS: **NYC MAYOR BILL de BLASIO ORDERS FORCED VACCINATIONS IN BROOKLYN, NYC,** sends "Disease Detectives" in Jewish Neighborhoods Looking for Unvaccinated-Attorneys Prepare Lawsuits. Comments by Brian Shilhavy Editor, Health Impact News

Just days after the New York Supreme Court struck down a ban on unvaccinated children in Rockland County, New York, after declaring a state of emergency over a measles outbreak, New York City Mayor Bill de Blasio has taken even more drastic actions in certain Jewish populated neighborhoods in Brooklyn, ordering forced vaccinations for measles. "There's no question that vaccines are safe, effective and life-saving," de Blasio said. "I urge everyone, especially those in affected areas, to get their MMR vaccines to protect their children, families and communities." There have been no reported deaths due to measles anywhere in the United States this year. The Mayor's order goes beyond what Rockland County Supervisor Ed Day ordered, and includes EVERYONE who is unvaccinated within zip codes 11205, 11206, 11221 and 11249 which are part of Williamsburg, Brooklyn, to be vaccinated within 48 hours. From the order: IT IS HEREBY ORDERED that any person who lives, works or resides within the 11205, 11206, 11221 and/or 11249 zip codes and who has not received the MMR vaccine within forty-eight (48) hours of this Order being signed by me shall be vaccinated against measles unless such person can demonstrate immunity to the disease or document to the satisfaction of the Department that he or she should be medically exempt from this requirement. IT IS FURTHER ORDERED that the parent or guardian of any child older than six months of age who lives, works or resides within the 11205, 11206, 11221 and/or 11249 zip codes and who has not received the MMR vaccine within forty eight (48) hours of this order being signed by me shall cause such child to be vaccinated against measles unless such parent or guardian can demonstrate that the child has immunity to the disease or document that he or she should be medically exempt from this requirement. According to WCBS radio in New York: Members of the city's Health Department will check the vaccination records of any individual who may have been in contact with infected patients. Those who have not received the vaccine or do not have evidence of immunity may be given a violation and **could be fined $1,000**.

2019 October Crimson Contagion Report published on US preparedness for a "Novel Chinese respiratory virus" https://archive.org/details/crimson-contagion-2019/page/19/mode/2up

2019 October – Oral Polio Vaccine Causing Paralysis in Indian Kids Study https://www.newindianexpress.com/nation/2019/oct/23/oral-polio-vaccine-causing-paralysis-in-kids-study-2051670.html

Expert calls for review of India's oral polio vaccination programme, but health ministry officials say OPV benefits far outweigh the risks.

NEW DELHI:

At least 400 children in India would have developed polio after receiving the oral polio vaccine (OPV) over the past five years, a top Indian pediatrician has revealed in a just published scientific paper that questions the ethics of the continued use of OPV.

T Jacob John, who has earlier advised the World Health Organization and the Indian government on polio eradication policies, has described the continued use of OPV as an "ethical anomaly" that is causing avoidable polio to children.

November 7, 2019 "THE NEXT PANDEMIC RELEASED BY NETFLIX" FEATURING BILL GATES…

2019 November 25 – The Associated Press More polio cases now caused by vaccine than by wild virus.

More polio cases now caused by vaccine than by wild virus as 4 African countries report them.

LONDON — Four African countries have reported new cases of polio linked to the oral vaccine, as global health numbers show there are now more children being paralyzed by viruses originating in vaccines than in the wild.

In a report late last week, the World Health Organization and partners noted nine new polio cases caused by the vaccine in Nigeria, Congo, Central African Republic, and Angola. Seven countries elsewhere in Africa have similar outbreaks and cases have been reported in Asia. Of the two countries where polio remains endemic, Afghanistan and Pakistan, vaccine-linked cases have been identified in Pakistan.

2019 October 18 – Event 201 Tabletop Exercise by the Bill & Melinda Gates Foundation, World Economic Forum, Johns Hopkins – A Preparation for a Hyped Pandemic?

The Event 201 scenario http://www.centerforhealthsecurity.org/event201/scenario.html Event 201 simulates an outbreak of a novel zoonotic coronavirus transmitted from bats to pigs to people that eventually becomes efficiently transmissible from person to person, leading to a severe pandemic.

The pathogen and the disease it cause are modeled largely on SARS, but it is more transmissible in the community setting by people with mild symptoms. The disease starts in pig farms in Brazil, quietly and slowly at first, but then it starts to spread more rapidly in healthcare settings. When it starts to spread efficiently from person to person in the low-income, densely packed neighborhoods of some of the megacities in South America, the epidemic explodes. It is first exported by air travel to Portugal, the United States, and China and then to many other countries. Although at first some countries are able to control it, it continues to spread and be reintroduced, and eventually no country can maintain control.

There is no possibility of a vaccine being available in the first year. There is a fictional antiviral drug that can help the sick but not significantly limit spread of the disease. Since the whole human population is susceptible, during the initial months of the pandemic, the cumulative number of cases increases exponentially, doubling every week. And as the cases and deaths accumulate, the economic and societal consequences become increasingly severe.

The scenario ends at the 18-month point, with 65 million deaths. The pandemic is beginning to slow due to the decreasing number of susceptible people. The pandemic will continue at some rate until there is an effective vaccine or until 80-90 % of the global population has been exposed. From that point on, it is likely to be an endemic childhood disease.

Event 201 was funded by the **Bloomberg School of Public Health**, which is named in honor of Michael Bloomberg, who has contributed close to $3 billion to Johns Hopkins, in partnership with the World Economic Forum and the Bill and Melinda Gates Foundation.

November 17 2019 First Covid-19 Patient Zero in Wuhan China https://www.msn.com/en-ca/news/world/the-first-covid-19-case-originated-on-november-17-according-to-chinese-officials-searching-for-patient-zero/ar-BB119YOI#image=BBZaM5o|2

- The original case of the novel coronavirus emerged on November 17, according to data from the Chinese government reviewed by South China Morning Post.
- The identity of the person has not been confirmed, but it appears to be a 55-year-old from the Hubei province.

- It was not until December that Chinese authorities realized they had a new type of virus on their hands.

December 1, 2019 Alleged patient zero in Wuhan, China started to experience alleged SARS-COVID-19 symptoms. He was never at the Huanan Seafood Wholesale Market.

December 21, 2019 Chinese Center for Disease Control and Prevention (CCDC) published an article on January 20, 2020, stating that the first cluster of patients with "pneumonia of an unknown cause" had been identified on December 21, 2019.

January 12, 2020 CCTV of China reported on January 12, 2020, that Wuhan virus started around December 12, 2019.

January 28, 2020 Harvard Professor Charles Lieber federally indicted. Charles Lieber, the Harvard Professor & inventor of biological nano-transistors, indicted for lying about being on the payroll of the Chinese Wuhan University of Technology.

https://www.cnn.com/2020/01/28/politics/harvard-professor-chinese-nationals-arrest-espionage/index.html.

"The complaint alleges that Lieber had lied about his affiliation with the Wuhan University of Technology (WUT) in China and a contract he had with a Chinese talent recruitment plan to attract high-level scientists to the country. He was being paid $50,000 per month by the Chinese university and given $1.5 million to establish a nanoscience research lab at WUT, the complaint said."

"CNN has reached out to an attorney for Lieber. In a statement, Harvard called the charges 'extremely serious.' Harvard is cooperating with federal authorities, including the National Institutes of Health, and is conducting its own review of the alleged misconduct, the university said in a statement. Professor Lieber has been placed on indefinite administrative leave."

March 2020 New epidemiological study shows death rate in Wuhan of 0.04% to 0.12% and thus rather lower than seasonal flu.

https://www.medrxiv.org/content/10.1101/2020.02.12.20022434v2.

March 17 2020 A fiasco in the making? As the coronavirus pandemic takes hold, we are making decisions without reliable data By JOHN P.A. IOANNIDIS https://www.statnews.com/2020/03/17/a-fiasco-in-the-making-as-the-coronavirus-pandemic-takes-hold-we-are-making-decisions-without-reliable-data/.

The current coronavirus disease, Covid-19, has been called a once-in-a-century pandemic. But it may also be a once-in-a-century evidence fiasco. At a time when everyone needs better information, from disease modelers and governments to people quarantined or just social distancing, we lack reliable evidence on how many people have been infected with SARS-CoV-2 or who continue to become infected. Better information is needed to guide decisions and actions of monumental significance and to monitor their impact.

Draconian countermeasures have been adopted in many countries. If the pandemic dissipates — either on its own or because of these measures — short-term extreme social distancing and lockdowns may be bearable. How long, though, should measures like these be continued if the pandemic churns across the globe unabated? How can policymakers tell if they are doing better than harm? Vaccines or affordable treatments take many months (or even years) to develop and test properly. Given such timelines, the consequences of long-term lockdowns are entirely unknown.

March 5 2020 Preliminary study shows 50% false positives from coronavirus tests https://pubmed.ncbi.nlm.nih.gov/32133832/?fbclid=IwAR1hTB9NNkfFqK3837ktl5HIj8_MN6Ipdetk1_we9lBlTv4OLIQeTa1-FiQ.

March 11, 2020 World Health Director General & accused war-crimes perpetrator Ethiopian communist party leader Tedros Adhanom declares SARS-CoV-2 a global pandemic https://www.who.int/dg/speeches/detail/who-director-general-s-opening-remarks-at-the-media-briefing-on-covid-19–11-march-2020

March 11, 2020 World Health Organization and World Economic Forum announce partnership on Covid-19 https://www.

businessinsider.com/wef-and-who-launch-covid-action-platform-for-business-2020-3?op=1

The World Health Organization and The World Economic Forum are launching an emergency task force in response to the global outbreak of coronavirus, the organizations announced Wednesday. The task force, called the COVID Action Platform, was created following a World Economic Forum conference call of more than 200 corporate leaders from around the globe concerned about the outbreak. Members include companies like Alphabet, Nasdaq Inc, KPMG, HP, Volkswagen, Bank of America, and Deloitte.

The group's main goals are to ensure global supply chains of key commodities remain intact, facilitate business donations to public health needs, develop vaccines and diagnostics, and pursue collaborations to address business and economic disruptions.

March 17 2020 Coronavirus / Covid-19 Italian National Health Institute ISS has published a new report on test-positive deaths:

https://www.epicentro.iss.it/coronavirus/bollettino/Report-COVID-2019_17_marzo-v2.pdf

The median age is **80.5** years (79.5 for men, **83.7** for women). 10% of the deceased was over 90 years old; **90% of the deceased was over 70 years old**. At most 0.8% of the deceased had no pre-existing chronic illnesses.

March 21 2020 Politico Coronavirus by BETSY WOODRUFF SWAN. The DOJ seeks new emergency powers amid coronaviruses pandemic.

One of the requests to Congress would allow the department to petition a judge to indefinitely detain someone during an emergency. 195 The Justice Department has quietly asked Congress for the ability to ask chief judges to detain people indefinitely without trial during emergencies — part of a push for new powers that comes as the coronavirus spreads through the United States. In one of the documents, the department proposed that Congress grant the attorney general power to ask the chief judge of any district court to pause court proceedings "whenever the district court is fully or partially closed by virtue of any natural disaster, civil disobedience, or other emergency situation." The proposal would also grant those top judges broad authority to pause court proceedings during emergencies. It would apply to "any statutes or rules of procedure otherwise affecting pre-arrest, post-arrest, pre-trial, trial, and post-trial procedures in criminal and juvenile proceedings and all civil process and proceedings," according to draft legislative language the department shared with Congress. In making the case for the change, the DOJ document wrote that individual judges can currently pause proceedings during emergencies, but that their proposal would make sure all judges in any particular district could handle emergencies "in a consistent manner."

The request raised eyebrows because of its potential implications for habeas corpus — the constitutional right to appear before a judge after arrest and seek release. "Not only would it be a violation of that, but it says, 'affecting pre-arrest,'" said Norman L. Reimer, the executive director of the National Association of Criminal Defense Lawyers. "So that means you could be arrested and never brought before a judge until they decide that the emergency or the civil disobedience is over. I find it absolutely terrifying. Especially in a time of emergency, we should be incredibly careful about granting new powers to the government." Reimer said the possibility of chief judges suspending all court rules during an emergency without a clear end in sight was deeply disturbing. "That is something that should not happen in a democracy," he said.

March 24 2020 – 12 experts questioning the coronavirus panic.

https://off-guardian.org/2020/03/24/12-experts-questioning-the-coronavirus-panic/

March 24 2020 – https://hitchensblog.mailonsunday.co.uk/2020/03/an-expert-says-the-current-response-to-the-corona-virus-is-grotesque-absurd-and-very-dangerous.html

An Expert says the Current response to the Coronavirus is 'Grotesque, Absurd and Very Dangerous.'

A recent interview with Professor Dr Sucharit Bhakdi, an

infectious medicine specialist. The Professor is one of the most highly cited medical research scientists in Germany. He was head of the Institute for Medical Microbiology at the Johannes Gutenberg University of Mainz, one of Germany's most distinguished seats of learning.

March 24 2020 – Is the Coronavirus as Deadly as They Say?

https://www.wsj.com/articles/is-the-coronavirus-as-deadly-as-they-say-11585088464

March 24, 2020 Current estimates about the Covid-19 fatality rate may be too high by orders of magnitude.

By Eran Bendavid and Jay Bhattacharya

If it is true that the novel coronavirus would kill millions without shelter-in-place orders and quarantines, then the extraordinary measures being carried out in cities and states around the country are surely justified. But there's little evidence to confirm that premise—and projections of the death toll could plausibly be orders of magnitude too high.

March 30 2020 Coronavirus testing effort hampered by kits contaminated with Covid-19

Traces of the virus were detected in parts due for delivery from overseas in the coming days By Bill Gardner and Harry Yorke, POLITICAL CORRESPONDENT30 March 2020 • 9:00pm

https://www.telegraph.co.uk/news/2020/03/30/uks-attempt-ramp-coronavirus-testing-hindered-key-components/

April 1st 2020 Coronavirus Test Kits Meant for the UK found to be contaminated with Covid-19

https://www.cbs17.com/community/health/coronavirus/coronavirus-test-kits-meant-for-the-uk-found-to-be-contaminated-with-covid-19/

April 1 2020 – All Roads Lead to Dark Winter by Whitney Webb
https://unlimitedhangout.com/2020/04/investigative-series/all-roads-lead-to-dark-winter/

The leaders of two controversial pandemic simulations that took place just months before the Coronavirus crisis – Event 201 and

Crimson Contagion – share a common history, the 2001 biowarfare simulation Dark Winter. Dark Winter not only predicted the 2001 anthrax attacks, but some of its participants had clear foreknowledge of those attacks.

April 3, 2020 –Foreign Policy magazine published "How WHO Became China's Coronavirus Accomplice." https://foreignpolicy.com/2020/04/02/china-coronavirus-who-health-soft-power/

April 15, 2020 from Swiss Policy Research: https://swprs.org/facts-about-covid19-archive/

"In Germany, a medical lawyer who filed a complaint against the corona measures with the Federal Constitutional Court and called for demonstrations, was arrested and sent to a prison psychiatric ward for two days. The public prosecutor is investigating for "public provocation to commit crimes". Another lawyer asks in an open letter to the German Federal Chamber of Lawyers: "Lawyers sent to psychiatric hospital for protest? Is it that time again in Germany?"

April 15, 2020 – from Swiss Policy Research: https://swprs.org/facts-about-covid19-archive/ "In Switzerland, a "corona critical" doctor was arrested by a special police unit for alleged "threats against relatives and authorities" and sent to a psychiatric clinic. See here: https://www.srf.ch/news/regional/aargau-solothurn/festnahme-von-corona-kritiker-verschwoerung-oder-normale-intervention-der-aargauer-behoerden

The family has since declared that there were no threats against relatives. The doctor also stated that he was not accused of "threats against authorities" during the interrogation. The police justified the deployment of the special unit by assuming that the doctor was in possession of a weapon – but this was the usual Swiss medical army pistol without ammunition. The transfer of the doctor to a psychiatric clinic was justified on the grounds of an alleged "incapacity to serve in prison" (as is the case of nursing patients) – this, too, may be seen as a pretext. Based on the current state of knowledge, it is therefore possible that the measure was indeed politically motivated.

Former US Congresswoman Cynthia McKinney has already drawn attention to the Swiss case."

April 20 2020 CDCs Failed Coronavirus Tests were Tainted with Coronavirus Feds Confirm

https://arstechnica.com/science/2020/04/cdcs-failed-coronavirus-tests-were-tainted-with-coronavirus-feds-confirm/?fbclid=IwAR2ZaEgzi32_7K4g0I5UZk0QoeEBWj8Vj54JdiV8xyaXeXA5hSPBjtaAxEI

April 21 2020 How One Model Simulated 2.2 Million U.S. Deaths from COVID-19 by Alan Reynolds

https://www.cato.org/blog/how-one-model-simulated-22-million-us-deaths-covid-19

When it came to dealing with an unexpected surge in infections and deaths from SARS-CoV-2 (the virus causing COVID-19 symptoms), federal and state policymakers understandably sought guidance from competing epidemiological computer models.

On March 16, a 20-page report from Neil Ferguson's team at Imperial College London quickly gathered enormous attention by producing enormous death estimates.

Dr. Ferguson had previously publicized almost equally sensational death estimates from mad cow disease, bird flu and swine flu. All of them proved to be grossly in error, over-estimating deaths in some cases by 100 times or more the actual number who did die. But he is the modeler who became "the world's authority" of prediction and Bill Gates man, despite his previous track record of failures and over-estimates.

As described by John Rappaport, author of AIDS INC.

Neil Ferguson: the ghost in the machine

Why do governments salute when he predicts a pandemic and tells them to lockdown their countries? Does anyone care about his past? Why does he still have a prestigious job? Who is he connected to? Neil Ferguson, through his institute at London's Imperial College, can call the shots on a major percentage of the global population. He's Mr. Genius, when it comes to projecting computer models of epidemics. Fellow experts puff up his reputation. According to the Business Insider

(4/25, 2020), "Ferguson's team warned Boris Johnson that the quest for 'herd immunity' [letting people live their lives out in the open in the UK] could cost 510,000 lives, prompting an abrupt U-turn [massive national lockdown in the UK]...His simulations have been influential in other countries as well, cited by authorities in the US, Germany, and France. Not only cited, not only influential, but swallowed whole. Business insider continues: "On March 23, the UK scrapped 'herd immunity' in favor of a suppression strategy, and the country prepared for weeks of lockdown. Ferguson's study was responsible."

Same BI article: "Dr **Deborah Birx**, coronavirus response coordinator to the Trump administration, told journalists at a March 16, 2020 press briefing that the Imperial paper [Ferguson's computer projection] prompted the CDC's new advice to work from home and avoid gatherings of 10 or more."

Ferguson, instigator of LOCKDOWN. Stripping away of basic liberties. Economic devastation. So, let's look at Ferguson's track record, spelled out in the BI piece. "Ferguson co-founded the MRC Centre for Global Infectious Disease Analysis, based at Imperial, in 2008. It is the leading body advising national governments on pathogen outbreaks." "It gets tens of millions of dollars in annual funding from the Bill & Melinda Gates Foundation, and works with the UK National Health Service, the US Centers for Disease Prevention and Control (CDC), and is tasked with supplying the World Health Organization with 'rapid analysis of urgent infectious disease problems'."

Gates money goes to Ferguson.

Ferguson predicts dire threat from COVID, necessitating lockdowns–thus preparing people to accept a vaccine. The vaccine Gates wants. Ferguson supplies a frightening computer projection of COVID deaths–to the CDC and WHO. Ferguson thus communicates a rationale for the Gates vaccine plan. National governments surrender to WHO and CDC. LOCKDOWNS.

Business Insider: "Michael Thrusfield, a professor of veterinary epidemiology at Edinburgh University, told the paper he had "déjà vu' after reading the [Ferguson] Imperial paper [on COVID], saying Ferguson was responsible for excessive animal culling during the 2001 Foot and Mouth [mad cow] outbreak."

"Ferguson warned the government that 150,000 people could die. Six million animals were slaughtered as a precaution, costing the country billions in farming revenue. In the end, 200 people died."

"Similarly, he [Ferguson] was accused of creating panic by overestimating the potential death toll during the 2005 Bird Flu outbreak. Ferguson estimated 200 million could die. The real number was in the low hundreds. In 2009, one of Ferguson's models predicted 65,000 people could die from the Swine Flu outbreak in the UK — the final figure was below 500." So, you have to ask yourself, why would anyone believe what Ferguson has been predicting in this COVID hustle? Are his fellow experts that stupid? Are presidents and prime ministers that stupid? And the answer is: This is a monumental covert op; some people are that stupid; some are caught up in the op and are afraid to say the emperor has no clothes; some are aware of what is going on, and they want to destroy national economies and lead us into, yes, a new world order. Gates knows he has his man: Ferguson. As the recipient of tens of millions of dollars, a year from the Gates Foundation, Ferguson isn't about to issue a model that states: COVID is nothing to worry about, let people live their lives and we'll be all right. The chance of that happening is on a par with researchers admitting they never properly identified a new virus as the cause of illness in 2019, in Wuhan. In order to justify injecting every man, woman, and child in the world with heavy metals, synthetic genes that alter genetic makeup, a host of germs, and who knows what else, Gates needs A STORY ABOUT A DEADLY VIRUS THAT NECESSITATES SHUTTING DOWN AND IMPRISONING THE PLANET, ACHIEVING A CAPTIVE AUDIENCE. He has got the story, all dressed up in a computer model, composed by a man with a past record of abject and devastating failures.

April 26 2020 Stanford Hospital Lays Off Employees Because of Lack of Patients?

https://www.sfchronicle.com/bayarea/article/Stanford-hospital-system-to-cut-pay-20-furlough-15227591.php

At the height of the SARS-CoV-2 global pandemic in April, 2020, the April 26 San Francisco Chronicle printed a story claiming that:

Stanford hospital system to cut pay 20%, furlough workers during coronavirus pandemic.

Spokeswoman Lia Kim said emergency room visits at Stanford Hospital are down about 40% since the region's shelter-in-place order March 16. Hospitals have also shut down revenue-generating elective surgeries, and Stanford did not see the expected surge of patients during the pandemic — all of which is provoking the employees' cuts.

The pay reductions will apply to all employees at Stanford Hospital, Lucile Packard Children's Hospital and Stanford-ValleyCare, according to Palo Alto Weekly, which was first to report the story. Hospital leadership and a health care workers union said the cuts will be "across the board" among the roughly 14,000 employees.

April 19 2020 No Vaccine for Coronavirus a Possibility https://www.news.com.au/lifestyle/health/health-problems/no-vaccine-for-coronavirus-a-possibility/news-story/34e678ae205b50ea983cc64ab2943608

One of Australia's most eminent vaccine developers says there may never be a vaccine against COVID-19 for some particularly good reasons. Professor Ian Frazer, the immunologist who co-invented the human papilloma virus (HPV) vaccine which prevents cervical cancer, said a coronavirus vaccine was "tricky". He told news.com.au that although 100 different teams around the world were testing for vaccines, medical scientists did not have a model of how to attack the virus. The professor of medicine at Queensland University, which is testing for its own COVID-19 vaccine, said immunization against coronavirus was similar to immunizing against the common cold. "It is tricky, vaccines for upper respiratory tract diseases, because the virus lands on the outside of you," Prof Frazer said.

May 2020 CDC Mask Study – Nonpharmaceutical Measures for Pandemic Influenza in Nonhealthcare Settings—Personal Protective and Environmental Measures

https://www.cdc.gov/eid/article/26/5/19-0994_article

*In this review, we did not find evidence to support a protective effect of personal protective measures or environmental measures in reducing influenza transmission. Although these measures have mechanistic support based on our knowledge of how influenza is transmitted from person to person, randomized trials of hand hygiene and face masks have not demonstrated protection against laboratory-confirmed influenza, with 1 exception (*18*). We identified only 2 RCTs on environmental cleaning and no RCTs on cough etiquette.*

*Hand hygiene is a widely used intervention and has been shown to effectively reduce the transmission of gastrointestinal infections and respiratory infections (*26*). However, in our systematic review, updating the findings of Wong et al. (*8*), we did not find evidence of a major effect of hand hygiene on laboratory-confirmed influenza virus transmission (Figure 1). Nevertheless, hand hygiene might be included in influenza pandemic plans as part of general hygiene and infection prevention.*

We did not find evidence that surgical-type face masks are effective in reducing laboratory-confirmed influenza transmission, either when worn by infected persons (source control) or by persons in the general community to reduce their susceptibility (Figure 2). However, as with hand hygiene, face masks might be able to reduce the transmission of other infections and therefore have value in an influenza pandemic when healthcare resources are stretched.

May 14 2020 Targets of T-Cell Responses to SARS-CoV-2 Coronavirus in Humans with Covid-19 Disease and Unexposed

https://www.cell.com/cell/fulltext/S0092-8674(20)30610-3

There is a critical need for foundational knowledge about T cell responses to SARS-CoV-2. Here, we report functional validation of predicted epitopes when arranged in epitope MPs, utilizing PBMCs derived from convalescing COVID-19 cases. The experiments also used protein-specific peptide pools to determine which SARS-CoV-2 proteins are the predominant targets of human SARS-CoV-2-specific $CD4^+$ and $CD8^+$ T cells generated during COVID-19 disease.

Importantly, we utilized the exact same series of experimental techniques with blood samples from healthy control donors (PBMCs collected in the 2015–2018-time frame), and substantial cross-reactive coronavirus T cell memory was observed. **This important Cell study shows that many people with T cells from past common cold viruses (coronaviruses) may be already have immunity to COVID-19.**

May 17, 2020 The Head of the Hydra the Rise of Robert Kadlec-A powerful network of political operatives, a global vaccine mafia and their man in Washington by Whitney Webb

https://unlimitedhangout.com/2020/05/investigative-series/head-of-the-hydra-the-rise-of-robert-kadlec/

"Thanks to a long and deliberate process to introduce biodefense policy, driven by Robert Kadlec and his sponsors, $7 billion dollars-worth of federally-owned vaccines, antidotes and medicines – held in strategically arranged repositories across the country in case of a health emergency – are now in the hands of one single individual. Those repositories, which compose the Strategic National Stockpile (SNS), are the exclusive domain of HHS' ASPR, a post created under Kadlec's watchful eye and tailored over the years to meet his awfully specific requirements. From this perch, Robert Kadlec has final say on where the stockpile's contents are sourced, as well as how, when and where they are deployed. He is the sole source procurer of medical material and pharmaceuticals, making him the best friend of Big Pharma and other healthcare industry giants who have been in his ear every step of the way.

May 2020 "Neil Ferguson's Imperial model could be the most devastating software mistake of all time."

https://analyticsindiamag.com/the-most-devastating-software-mistake-of-all-time-why-is-the-imperial-model-under-criticism/

Neil Ferguson, a popular epidemiologist from the Imperial College, London, whose model forecasted the possible deaths due to COVID-19 with and without lockdown, has turned to be inaccurate and the events followed has even led to his resignation.

Ferguson's forecasts have been around for a while. He has been doing this for over a decade — during swine flu, mad cow disease and other outbreaks. One thing that is common in all of his models was, the results were nowhere near to the reality.

But why should we talk about only Ferguson's forecasting model and its flaws when there have been many over the years?

June 2020 – Predicted Covid-19 Fatality Rate Based on Age, Sex, Comorbidities, and Health System Capacity – Stockholm University Ghisolfi,1,2 Ingvild Almås,1 Justin C Sandefur, 3 Tillman von Carnap,1 Jesse Heitner,4 Tessa Bold1

https://gh.bmj.com/content/bmjgh/5/9/e003094.full.pdf

Here is another way of expressing the above chart in the Swedish study on Covid-19:

Figure 1 cIFRs, adjusted for health system capacity, by country income group (log scale). cIFRs, infection fatality rates conditional on age, sex and comorbidity; HICs, high-income countries; LICs, low-income countries; LMICs, lower middle-income countries; UMICs, upper middle-incomecountries.

Table 1 cIFRs, adjusted for health system capacity, by income group (percentage points)

	LIC				LMIC			
	Females		Males		Females		Males	
Comorbidity	0	>0	0	>0	0	>0	0	>0
Age, years								
0–19	0.0003	0.2583	0.0003	0.2807	0.0002	0.1670	0.0002	0.1825
20–29	0.0016	0.3727	0.0025	0.6551	0.0010	0.2435	0.0016	0.4324
30–39	0.0066	0.9167	0.0098	1.3538	0.0043	0.6080	0.0063	0.9127
40–49	0.0142	1.1632	0.0249	1.8018	0.0092	0.7912	0.0161	1.2563
50–59	0.0783	3.4838	0.1263	3.8523	0.0511	2.4923	0.0832	2.8623
60–69	0.2917	5.4639	0.7042	7.4230	0.1941	4.1954	0.4768	5.9842
70–79	1.0952	8.3357	2.7756	12.1281	0.7466	6.8290	1.9421	10.4667
80+	6.7997	19.3879	19.9064	42.2803	4.7666	16.7857	14.4353	38.4637

cIFRs, infection fatality rates conditional on age, sex and comorbidity; LIC, low-income country; LMIC, lower middle-income country.

	UMIC				HIC			
	Females		Males		Females		Males	
Comorbidities	0	>0	0	>0	0	>0	0	>0
Age, years								
0–19	0.0001	0.1001	0.0001	0.1098	0.00004	0.0361	0.00004	0.0397
20–29	0.00060	0.1470	0.00095	0.2631	0.00021	0.0534	0.00034	0.0963
30–39	0.0025	0.3713	0.0038	0.5645	0.0009	0.1364	0.0014	0.2100
40–49	0.0055	0.4928	0.0097	0.7985	0.0020	0.1847	0.0035	0.3057
50–59	0.0308	1.6196	0.0505	1.9255	0.0112	0.6353	0.0185	0.7865
60–69	0.1188	2.9143	0.2959	4.3776	0.0438	1.2395	0.1105	2.0008
70–79	0.4659	5.0878	1.2381	8.3111	0.1749	2.3906	0.4755	4.3483
80+	3.0436	13.3843	9.4946	32.8492	1.1708	7.0568	3.7759	19.9581

Table reports the health-system adjusted cIFR derived in Section Predicting the cIFR and online supplementary appendix A1.
HIC, high-income country; UMIC, upper middle-income country.

Ghisolfi S, *et al. BMJ Global Health* 2020;**5**:e003094. doi:10.1136/bmjgh-2020-003094 3

Chance of Surviving Covid-19 By Age and Se

AGE	FEMALE No Underlying Conditions	FEMALE One or Greater Underlying Conditions	MALE No Underlying Conditions	MALE One or Greate Underlying Conditions
0-9	99.99996	99.9639	99.99996	99.9603
10-19	99.99996	99.9639	99.99996	99.9603
20-29	99.9998	99.9466	99.9997	99.9037
30-39	99.9991	99.8636	99.9986	99.79
40-49	99.998	99.8153	99.9965	99.6943
50-59	99.9888	99.3647	99.9815	99.2135
60-69	99.9562	98.7605	99.8895	97.9992
70-79	99.8251	97.6094	99.5245	95.6517
80+	98.9087	92.8152	96.3318	79.9154

***"Predicted COVID-19 Fatality Rates Based on Age, Sex, Comorbidities, and Health System Capacity, Stockholm University"*, June 2020**

July 2020 – Lockdowns are Killing More People than Would Have Died Without Lockdowns says University Researchers in the United Kingdom

https://www.lboro.ac.uk/news-events/news/2020/july/new-approach-to-recording-covid-deaths/#.XyhDhoJ56Pg.twitter

The new study, co-authored by **Karligash Glass**, Professor of Financial Economics and a respected economic data scientist within Loughborough University's **School of Business and Economics**, Professor Anthony Glass (Professor of Managerial Economics, the University of Sheffield), Sam Williams (founder and Director of Economic Insight) and Alasdair Crookes (Consultant at Economic Insight) proposes an enhanced approach to crunching the COVID numbers.

The authors have used statistical techniques to better identify deaths due to COVID, applying the excess death framework more robustly and controlling for other factors that affect mortality. The key findings are as follows:

- Actual deaths due to COVID are some 54% or 63% lower than implied by the standard excess deaths measure, and reported excess deaths likely include a significant number of non-COVID deaths.
- While it is well known that COVID deaths are concentrated in the elderly, the study finds them to be particularly acute in the very elderly (75-84 and 85+ years old).
- Over the lockdown period as a whole Government policy has increased mortality rather than reduced it.

July 2020 – How Sweden Faced COVID19 Without Lockdowns The real reasons New York failed to "attenuate the curve" and Sweden succeeded https://catalyst.independent.org/2020/07/17/lockdowns-sweden-beat-covid-19/

Coronavirus deaths have slowed to a crawl in Sweden. With the exception of a single death on July 13, no deaths in this nation of 10 million have been reported since July 10.

But the debate over Sweden's approach to the COVID-19 pandemic, which relied on individual responsibility instead of government coercion to maintain social distancing, is far from over.

Last week, The New York Times labeled Sweden's approach to the pandemic a "cautionary tale" for the rest of the world, claiming it "yielded a surge of deaths without sparing its economy from damage."

To be accurate, Sweden has outperformed many nations around the world with its "lighter touch" approach and was one of the few nations in Europe to see its economy grow in the first quarter of 2020.

Meanwhile, Anders Tegnell, Sweden's top infectious disease expert, continues to defend his nation's approach to the pandemic.

"I'm looking forward to a more serious evaluation of our work than has been made so far," Tegnell said in a recent podcast published by Swedish public radio before taking a scheduled vacation. "There is no way of knowing how this end."

July 29 2020 – Moderna's Mysterious Coronavirus Vaccine Delivery System by Nathan Vardi

https://www.forbes.com/sites/nathanvardi/2020/07/29/modernas-mysterious-coronavirus-vaccine-delivery-system/?sh=65c9620e62d9

For a decade, Moderna has been working to develop mRNA technology that could turn the body's cells into drug factories. In order for the approach to work, Moderna needs to safely deliver the mRNA to the body's cells without the payload breaking down in the bloodstream. As a result, any mRNA vaccine or therapeutic consists of two components, the actual sequence mRNA, and the delivery mechanism. Moderna has clearly engineered the first component, but there remain questions about the second. No mRNA vaccine or medicine has ever been approved by U.S. or European regulators .... The preprint of the study that tested the vaccine in mice described the mRNA for mRNA-1273 as being encapsulated into LNP "at molar ratio of 50:10:38.5:1.5 (ionizable lipid:DSPC:cholesterol:PEG-lipid)."

The first claim of the upheld Arbutus patent describes "a cationic lipid comprising from 50 mol % to 65 mol % of the total lipid present in the particle;" a non-cationic lipid comprising a mixture of phospholipid and cholesterol, where the "phospholipid comprises from 4 mol % to 10 mol %" and the cholesterol comprises "30 mol % to 40 mol %;" and a conjugated lipid "comprising from 0.5 mol % to 2 mol %."

August 2020 – CDC Director Acknowledges Hospitals Have a Monetary Incentive to Overcount Coronavirus Deaths

https://www.washingtonexaminer.com/news/cdc-director-acknowledges-hospitals-have-a-monetary-incentive-to-overcount-coronavirus-deaths

U.S. Centers for Disease Control and Prevention Director Robert Redfield agreed that some hospitals have a monetary incentive to overcount coronavirus deaths as they do deaths for other diseases.

"I think you're correct in that we've seen this in other disease processes, too. Really, in the HIV epidemic, somebody may have a heart attack but also have HIV — the hospital would prefer the [classification] for HIV because there's greater reimbursement," Redfield said during a House panel hearing Friday when asked by Rep. Blaine Luetkemeyer about potential "perverse incentives."

Redfield continued: "So, I do think there's some reality to that. When it comes to death reporting, though, ultimately, it is how the physician defines it in the death certificate, and … we review all of those death certificates. So, I think, probably it is less operable in the cause of death, although I will not say there are not some cases. I do think though [that] when it comes to hospital reimbursement issues or individuals that get discharged, there could be some play in that for sure. "Questions have been raised about coronavirus counting in hospitals across the country, and conflicting conclusions have been raised about whether or not deaths are being accurately counted.

August 29 2020 – NY Times: **Your Coronavirus Test Is Positive. Maybe It Should Not Be.**

The usual diagnostic tests may simply be too sensitive and too slow to contain the spread of the virus.

https://www.nytimes.com/2020/08/29/health/coronavirus-testing.html

Some of the nation's leading public health experts are raising a new concern in the endless debate over coronavirus testing in the United States: The standard tests are diagnosing huge numbers of people who may be carrying relatively insignificant amounts of the virus.

Most of these people are not likely to be contagious and identifying them may contribute to bottlenecks that prevent those who are contagious from being found in time.

September 9 2020 Bloomberg News: AstraZeneca Must Explain Spinal Ailment to Resume Vaccine Trial by Robert Langreth and Riley Griffin

A day after pausing its Covid-19 vaccine trials due to a possible serious neurological problem in one patient, AstraZeneca Plc faced numerous questions about what exactly caused the issue and whether it could be related to the vaccine.

On Tuesday, AstraZeneca and its partner, the University of Oxford, confirmed it had stopped giving patients the experimental shot after a person in the U.K. who was participating in one of their studies got sick, triggering a review of safety data.

U.S. National Institutes of Health Director Francis Collins told a Senate committee Wednesday the trial had been halted due to a "spinal cord problem." AstraZeneca is one of several drug companies taking part in the U.S. government's Operation Warp Speed program to accelerate the development of a coronavirus vaccine.

October 4 2020 – Great Barrington Declaration released and signed by thousands of academic medical scientists and medical doctors around the world calling for focused protection for the elderly and an end to Covid lockdowns of the young and healthy https://gbdeclaration.org/

"The Great Barrington Declaration – As infectious disease epidemiologists and public health scientists we have grave concerns about the damaging physical and mental health impacts of the prevailing COVID-19 policies and recommend an approach we call Focused Protection."

First signers of the Great Barrington Declaration are Dr. Martin Kulldorff, professor of medicine at Harvard University, a biostatistician, and epidemiologist with expertise in detecting and monitoring infectious disease outbreaks and vaccine safety evaluations. **Dr. Sunetra Gupta**, professor at Oxford University, an epidemiologist with expertise in immunology, vaccine development, and mathematical modeling of infectious diseases. **Dr. Jay Bhattacharya**, professor at Stanford University Medical School, a physician, epidemiologist, health economist, and public health policy expert focusing on infectious diseases and vulnerable populations.

October 12 2020 – Dr David Nabarro of the World Health Organization who leads WHO strategy on Covid-19 says in an interview that lockdowns are devastating to poor people and need to stop. "Lockdowns just have one consequence that you must never ever belittle, and that is making poor people an awful lot poorer," he said.

He agrees with some of the key points of the Great Barrington Declaration Covid lockdowns are the wrong strategy and begs nations to stop locking their countries down as a primary method of stopping Covid-19. Dr. David Nabarro is a medical doctor who has made his career in the international civil service, working for either the Secretary-General of the United Nations or the Director-General of the World Health Organization. Most recently from February 2020 he has helped the DGWHO deal with the COVID-19 pandemic. He also claimed that the only thing lockdowns achieved was poverty – with no mention of the potential lives saved.

https://www.news.com.au/world/coronavirus/global/coronavirus-who-backflips-on-virus-stance-by-condemning-lockdowns/news-story/f2188f2aebff1b7b291b297731c3da74

October 13, 2020 Facemask against viral respiratory infections among Hajj pilgrims: A challenging cluster-randomized trial https://journals.plos.org/plosone/article?id=10.1371/journal.pone.0240287

Abstract

Background

In this large-scale cluster-randomized controlled trial (cRCT) we sought to assess the effectiveness of facemasks against viral respiratory infections.

Methods and results

Over three consecutive Hajj seasons (2013, 2014, 2015) pilgrims' tents in Makkah were allocated to 'facemask' or 'no facemask' group. Fifty facemasks were offered to participants in intervention tents, to be worn over four days, and none were offered to participants in control tents. All participants recorded facemask use and respiratory symptoms in health diaries. Nasal swabs were collected from the symptomatic for virus detection by reverse transcription polymerase chain reaction. Clinical symptoms and laboratory results were analyzed by 'intention- to-treat' and 'per-protocol'. A total of 7687 adult participants from 318 tents were randomized: 3864 from 149 tents to the intervention group, and 3823 from 169 tents to the control group. Participants were aged 18 to 95 (median 34, mean 37) years, with a male to female ratio of 1:1.2. Overall, respiratory viruses were detected in 277 of 650 (43%) nasal/pharyngeal swabs collected from symptomatic pilgrims. Common viruses were rhinovirus (35.1%), influenza (4.5%) and parainfluenza (1.7%). In the intervention arm, respectively 954 (24.7%) and 1842 (47.7%) participants used facemasks daily and intermittently, while in the control arm, respectively 546 (14.3%) and 1334 (34.9%) used facemasks daily and intermittently. By intention-to-treat analysis, facemask use did not seem to be effective against laboratory-confirmed viral respiratory infections (odds ratio [OR], 1.4; 95% confidence interval [CI], 0.9 to 2.1, p = 0.18) nor against clinical respiratory infection (OR, 1.1; 95% CI, 0.9 to 1.4, p = 0.40). Similarly, in a per-protocol analysis, facemask use did not seem to be effective against laboratory-confirmed viral respiratory infections (OR 1.2, 95% CI 0.9–1.7, p = 0.26) nor against clinical respiratory infection (OR 1.3, 95% CI 1.0–1.8, p = 0.06).

Conclusion

This trial was unable to provide conclusive evidence on facemask efficacy against viral respiratory infections most likely due to poor adherence to protocol.

October 16 2020 – Flu cases decline dramatically in 2020. World Health Organization chart comparing global influenza cases so far in 2020 against global influenza cases in 2019.

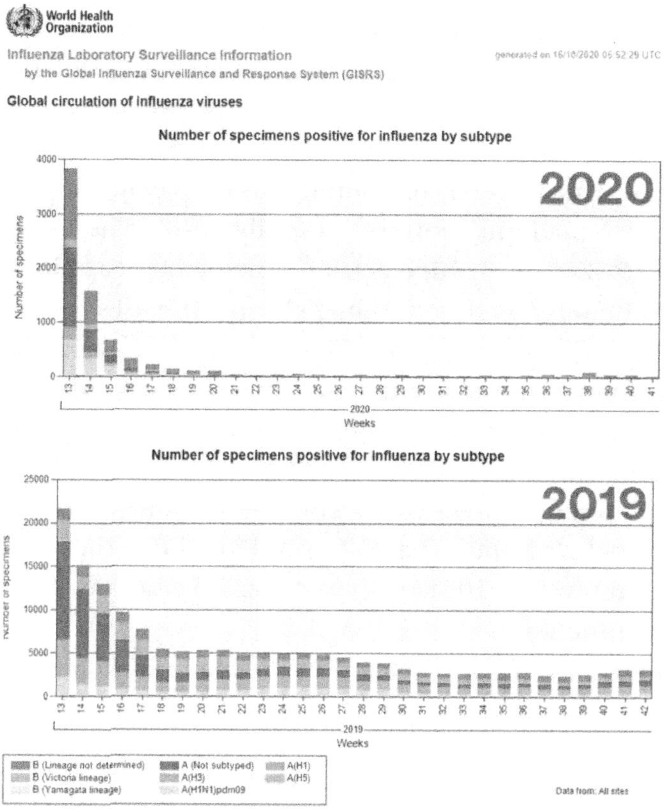

October 17 2020 Twitter censors White House Covid advisor Dr. Scott Atlas, a critic of lockdowns and mandatory masks, by deleting his post and locking him out of his Twitter account for publishing scientific evidence that face masks are worthless.

October 22 2020 The Head of Operation Warp Speed & The Gates Foundation Are Pushing BioElectronics & Vaccine Patches by Derrick Broze

https://www.thelastamericanvagabond.com/the-head-of-operation-warp-speed-and-the-gates-foundation-are-pushing-bioelectronics-and-vaccine-patches/

"To understand the goals of Operation Warp Speed we

must understand Dr. Moncef Slaoui and his connections to Big Pharma and the Gates Foundation… In mid-May, Donald Trump announced he was appointing Dr. Moncef Slaoui, a former executive with vaccine manufacturer GlaxoSmithKline, to lead Operation Warp Speed, the public-private partnership launched by the Trump administration to rapidly develop and distribute a COVID-19 vaccine … Bioelectronic medicine is a relatively new research field focused on tackling chronic diseases by **using "miniaturised, implantable devices that can modify electrical signals that pass along nerves in the body, including irregular or altered impulses that occur in many illnesses" …** Galvani's plan to use miniature implantable devices within the body was described by MIT Technology Review as "hacking the nervous system." In 2016, Slaoui said, "We hope to have approval and be in the marketplace in the next seven to 10 years. It is not science fiction. And it's progressing quite well."

October 29, 2020 France Says Second Lockdown Will Cut Economic Output by 15% By Rudy Ruitenberg https://www.bloomberg.com/news/articles/2020-10-29/france-says-second-lockdown-will-cut-economic-output-by-15

France is aiming to limit the drop-in economic activity to 15% during the country's second coronavirus lockdown starting on Friday, Finance Minister Bruno Le Maire said in a government briefing on Thursday. That would be half of the 30% drop-in activity during the country's first lockdown that started in March, which was caused in particular by a halt of construction work, Le Maire said.

October 29, 2020 A Useful Pandemic: Davos Launches New 'Reset,' this Time on the Back of COVID by Andrew Stuttaford, Editor of National Review's Capital Markets

COVID-19 is a bad disease that has been used to breathe new life into bad ideas. And so it comes as no surprise that the World Economic Forum ("Davos") is deploying the pandemic as an argument for what it labels, with characteristic modesty, The Great Reset" initiative.

There is an urgent need for global stakeholders to cooperate in simultaneously managing the direct consequences of the COVID-19 crisis. To improve the state of the world, the World Economic Forum is starting The Great Reset initiative. Even if we pass over the presumption of the reset's name, this is a small classic of the prose of soft authoritarianism. There is an "urgent need" that must be met. There is to be cooperation and management, the world is to be "improved," and all of this is to be put in place by "global stakeholders," — a conveniently vague phrase, with more than a suggestion of democracy bypassed about it.

https://www.nationalreview.com/2020/10/a-useful-pandemic-davos-launches-new-reset-this-time-on-the-back-of-covid/

October 30 2020 Recent Vatican ambassador to the US government, Archbishop Carlo Viganò, warns Trump about "Great Reset' plot to "subdue humanity,' destroy freedom using Covid pandemic as tool to bring totalitarian health dictatorship and forced vaccinations https://www.docdroid.com/Mz92diV/open-letter-to-potus-pdf

"A global plan called the Great Reset is underway. Its architect is a global élite that wants to subdue all of humanity, imposing coercive measures with which to drastically limit individual freedoms and those of entire populations. In several nations this plan has already been approved and financed; in others it is still in an early stage. Behind the world leaders who are the accomplices and executors of this infernal project, there are unscrupulous characters who finance the World Economic Forum and Event 201, promoting their agenda. The purpose of the Great Reset is the imposition of a health dictatorship aiming at the imposition of liberticidal measures, hidden behind tempting promises of ensuring a universal income and cancelling individual debt. The price of these concessions from the International Monetary Fund will be the renunciation of private property and adherence to a program of vaccination against Covid-19 and Covid-21 promoted by Bill Gates with the collaboration of the main pharmaceutical groups. Beyond the enormous economic interests that motivate the promoters of the Great Reset, the imposition of the vaccination will be accompanied by the requirement of a health passport and a digital ID, with the consequent contact tracing of the population of the entire world. Those who do not accept these measures will be confined in detention camps or placed under house arrest, and all their assets will be confiscated" https://www.lifesitenews.com/news/abp-vigano-warns-trump-about-great-reset-plot-to-subdue-humanity-destroy-freedom

October 31, 2020 England goes into 2nd lockdown: UK Prime Minister Boris Johnson announces month-long national lockdown of England – The lockdown will last five weeks, ending on December 2 https://www.foxnews.com/world/johnson-month-long-lockdown-england

November 5, 2020 – German doctors write letter to German Chancellor Angela Merkel declaring Covid as an over-hyped illness that has not been as deadly as the press and politicians have said. Call for investigation https://www.globalresearch.ca/german-doctors-write-letter-chancellor-merkel/5728843

German Doctors Letter to Chancellor Merkel, Put an End to the Covid "Fear Machine" by Dr. Robert Kluger, Dr. Bruno Weil, et al…

Dear Chancellor Dr. Merkel,

We, the signatories, are doctors from all areas of healthcare, who have been serving people in practices and clinics for decades. During this time, we have witnessed more than one seasonal infection in Germany, most of them with far more severe conditions and significantly more deaths than since January 2020 from COVID infectious diseases. Together we serve approx. 70.000 people.

The circumstances of the coronavirus wave in the FRG have been perceived differently than the media and the ongoing warnings of politics, which were unjustified in fact, presented to the public for months. Predictions of individual advisory virologists with millions of seriously ill and hundreds of thousands of deaths in Germany have not been true in any way.

November 9, 2020 Dr. Fauci Told the Truth About COVID-19 Tests in July and Has Been Misleading the Public Ever Since

https://pjmedia.com/news-and-politics/stacey-lennox/2020/11/09/dr-fauci-told-the-truth-about-covid-19-tests-in-july-and-has-been-misleading-the-public-ever-since-n1131938

Joining the hosts of This Week in Virology in July, Fauci directly responded to a question about COVID-19 testing, specifically how patients with positive tests might determine whether or not they are actually infectious and need to quarantine.

"What is now sort of evolving into a bit of a standard," Fauci said, is that "if you get a cycle threshold of 35 or more … the chances of it being replication-[competent] are minuscule."

"It's very frustrating for the patients as well as for the physicians," he continued, when "somebody comes in, and they repeat their PCR, and it's like [a] 37 cycle thresholds, but you almost never can culture virus from a 37-threshold cycle."

So, I think if somebody does come in with 37, 38, even 36, you got to say, you know, it is just dead nucleotides, period."

March 1 2021 3 Dozen Cases of Spontaneous Miscarriages, Stillbirths Occurring After COVID-19 Vaccination

BY MEILING LEE, EPOCH TIMES

https://www.theepochtimes.com/3-dozen-cases-of-spontaneous-miscarriages-stillbirths-occurring-after-covid-19-vaccination_3716385.html

Thirty-four cases of pregnant women experiencing spontaneous miscarriages or stillbirths after receiving a COVID-19 vaccine have been submitted to the Vaccine Adverse Event Reporting System (VAERS).

VAERS is a passive reporting system that allows people to submit a report of an adverse event after vaccination and is run by the Food and Drug Administration (FDA) and the Centers for Disease Control and Prevention (CDC). Research funded by the CDC has shown that fewer than 1 percent of reactions from vaccinations are being reported on VAERS.

In one case, a physician in Tennessee, at five weeks pregnant, suffered a miscarriage 13 days after being immunized with a Pfizer vaccine. The 31-year-old woman had no known allergies or medical history.

While a 33-year-old Indiana nurse in her third week of pregnancy had

a miscarriage five days after receiving her second Pfizer vaccine. She also reported that the adverse event caused a birth defect.

And a 32-year-old woman in Virginia who was eight weeks pregnant reported having a miscarriage five days after being injected with the first dose of a Moderna vaccine in January. She had consulted with two obstetrics and gynecologists (OB-GYN) prior to receiving the vaccine on Jan. 14. She experienced abdominal cramping and vaginal bleeding two days later and had a miscarriage on Jan. 19. She had only been taking prenatal vitamins.

In Michigan, a 35-year-old woman who was 28 weeks and five days pregnant said that the baby's movements decreased two days after her first Pfizer vaccine in December 2020. The woman delivered a stillborn baby weighing two pounds and seven ounces at 29 weeks. She was being closely monitored for an umbilical cord abnormality called velamentous cord insertion.

Both Pfizer and Moderna did not respond to a request by The Epoch Times for comment.

In addition, the FDA did not reply to The Epoch Times' inquiry on whether the regulatory agency will be looking into the VAERS report. An FDA spokesperson told The Epoch Times in an email that their subject matter experts working with vaccines are "quite busy" at the moment.

Dr. Shelley Cole, MD, an OB-GYN and a member of America's Frontline Doctors, says it's concerning that a vaccine still in an experimental phase is being recommended to pregnant and lactating women and that science is no longer protecting them.

"As an obstetrician-gynecologist, it is a concern," Cole told The Epoch Times. "We're [now] throwing science and the scientific medicine method out the window and jeopardizing pregnancies and future pregnancies."

"It concerns me that the CDC says that there are no studies, but it's okay to get it and you don't even need to discuss it with your doctor," Cole added. "I mean this is the opposite of everything that the scientific models and methods, and standard of care has been for a century."

March 2021 Effectiveness of Adding a Mask Recommendation to Other Public Health Measures to Prevent SARS-CoV-2 Infection in Danish Mask Wearers Henning Bundgaard, DMSc Johan Skov Bundgaard, BSc

https://www.acpjournals.org/doi/10.7326/M20-6817
A Randomized Controlled Trial

Results:
A total of 3030 participants were randomly assigned to the recommendation to wear masks, and 2994 were assigned to control; 4862 completed the study. Infection with SARS-CoV-2 occurred in 42 participants recommended masks (1.8%) and 53 control participants (2.1%). The between-group difference was −0.3 percentage point (95% CI, −1.2 to 0.4 percentage point; P = 0.38) (odds ratio, 0.82 [CI, 0.54 to 1.23]; P = 0.33). Multiple imputation accounting for loss to follow-up yielded similar results. Although the difference observed was not statistically significant, the 95% CIs are compatible with a 46% reduction to a 23% increase in infection.

Limitation:
Inconclusive results, missing data, variable adherence, patient-reported findings on home tests, no blinding, and no assessment of whether masks could decrease disease transmission from mask wearers to others.

Conclusion:
The recommendation to wear surgical masks to supplement other public health measures did not reduce the SARS-CoV-2 infection rate among wearers by more than 50% in a community with modest infection rates, some degree of social distancing, and uncommon general mask use. The data were compatible with lesser degrees of self-protection.

March 9 2021 – Scotland Freedom of Information Act Request on Deaths within 28 days of a Covid Vaccine

Public Health Scotland

Date 9 March 2021
Our Ref 2021-000426
Enquiries to phs.foi@phs.scot

[redacted]

Freedom of Information Reference: [redacted]

Thank you for your information request of 20th February 2021.

"Could you please provide the total number of deaths for any reason within 28 days of having a covid vaccine from the start of the vaccination roll out to date."

I confirm that Public Health Scotland holds the information you have requested and that this can be provided to you.

Using the latest mortality data available (up to 26th February), 2,207 people have died within 28 days of vaccination (number of days between vaccine and death is 0-27 where 0 is the day of vaccination). Please note that these deaths are due to any cause.

PHS is not currently aware of any deaths in Scotland that are considered conclusively linked to vaccination.

The Medicines and Healthcare Products Regulatory Agency (MHRA) is the UK's regulator of medicines, medical devices and blood components for transfusion, responsible for ensuring their safety, quality and effectiveness. Part of the MHRA's continuous analysis includes an evaluation of natural death rates over time, to determine if any specific trends or patterns are occurring that might indicate a vaccine safety concern. To date (period 9 December 2020 to 21 February 2021), the MHRA has received 212 UK reports of suspected adverse reactions to the Pfizer/BioNTech vaccine in which the patient died shortly after vaccination, 244 reports for the Oxford University/AstraZeneca vaccine and 4 where the brand of vaccine was unspecified. Review of individual reports and patterns of reporting does not suggest the vaccines played a role in the deaths. For more information on deaths following vaccination, please refer to the MHRA weekly adverse events report (https://www.gov.uk/government/publications/coronavirus-covid-19-vaccine-adverse-reactions/coronavirus-vaccine-summary-of-yellow-card-reporting, see under 'Events with a fatal outcome' section).

If you are unhappy with our response to your request, you have the right to request a review. Your request should be made within 40 working days of receipt of this correspondence, and we will reply within 20 working days of receipt. The review will be undertaken by a reviewer who was not involved in the original decision-making process.

The reviewer can be contacted as follows:

5 Cadogan Street, Glasgow G2 6QE

March 2021 – Despite avoiding lockdowns, 2020 all cause mortality rates in Sweden below or comparable to its Nordic peers.

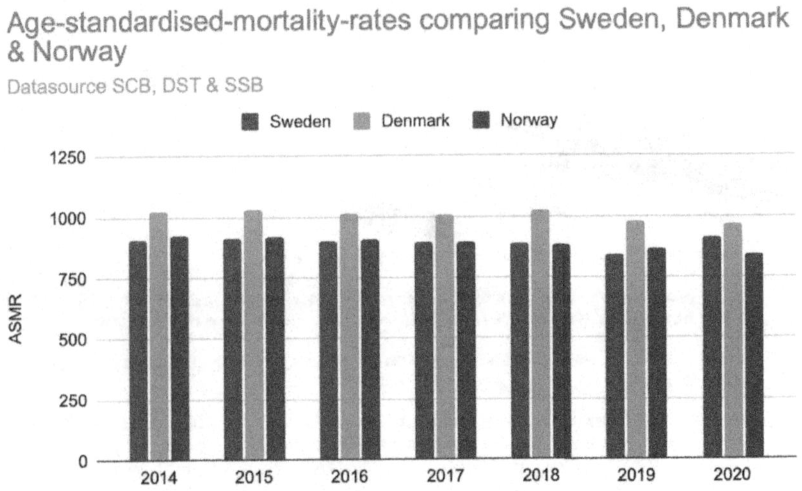

March 3 2021 Preprint: Age-dependent immune response to the Biontech/Pfizer BNT162b2 COVID-19 vaccination by Lisa Müller, Marcel Andrée, Wiebke Moskorz, Ingo Drexler, Lara Walotka, Ramona Grothmann, Johannes Ptok, Jonas Hillebrandt, Anastasia Ritchie, Denise Rabl, PhilipNiklas Ostermann, Rebekka Robitzsch, Sandra Hauka, Andreas Walker, Christopher Menne, Ralf Grutza, Jörg Timm, Ortwin Adams, Heiner Schaal

doi: https://doi.org/10.1101/2021.03.03.21251066

https://www.medrxiv.org/content/10.1101/2021.03.03.21251066v1

Results – While the majority of participants in both groups produced specific IgG antibody titers against SARS-CoV-2 spike protein, titers were significantly lower in elderly participants. Although the increment of antibody levels after the second immunization was higher in elderly participants, the absolute mean titer of this group remained lower than the <60 group.

After the second vaccination, 31.3 % of the elderly had no detectable neutralizing antibodies in contrast to the younger group, in which only 2.2% had no detectable neutralizing antibodies.

March 16 2021 Sweden joins Germany, France, and 15 other countries in suspending AstraZeneca's vaccine over possible side effects

https://www.businessinsider.com/astrazeneca-covid-vaccine-countries-suspend-denmark-thailand-batch-blood-clots-2021-3

Multiple countries have paused the use of AstraZeneca's COVID-19 vaccine as a precaution while investigators look into cases of blood clots among vaccinated people.

Austrian authorities said March 7 that a 49-year-old woman had died as a result of severe coagulation disorder after taking the shot, and that a 35-year-old had developed blood clots in the lungs, but was recovering. Both had received vaccines from the same batch, the authorities said.

March 18 2021 Norwegian experts say deadly blood clots were caused by the AstraZeneca covid vaccine https://sciencenorway.no/covid19/norwegian-experts-say-deadly-blood-clots-were-caused-by-the-astrazeneca-covid-vaccine/1830510

"Our theory that this is a powerful immune response most likely triggered by the vaccine, has been confirmed", says professor and chief physician Pål Andre Holme. Three Norwegian health workers under the age of 50 have been hospitalized. One is dead.

March 17, 2021 UK mulling vaccine passport options for at home and abroad, minister says

https://www.reuters.com/article/uk-health-coronavirus-britain-vaccine-pa-idUSKBN2B90WN

LONDON (Reuters) – Britain is reviewing the idea of vaccine certificates to allow access to travel, hospitality and entertainment and discussing the best way to proceed in terms of fairness, said business minister Kwarsi Kwarteng. P&O Cruises said on Tuesday that it would only accept as passengers those who have had both doses of the vaccine for its trips around the UK this summer, sparking a fresh debate on the issue.

When asked about the fairness of companies requiring proof of vaccination to grant entry and what the government's stance was on the matter, Kwarteng said it was under review.

"We are discussing what the best way to proceed is," Kwarteng told the BBC. More than half of Britain's adult population will have received the first shot of a COVID-19 vaccine by the end of the week.

Kwarteng said there were two separate issues, that of vaccine certification or so-called vaccine passports for access to theatres, restaurants and venues within Britain, and that of vaccine certification to allow travel abroad.

March 18 2021 Pensioner given Covid breach warning over socially-distanced cup of tea https://www.itv.com/news/westcountry/2021-03-18/pensioner-given-covid-breach-warning-over-socially-distanced-cup-of-tea

A pensioner has been given a Covid breach warning by police after having a socially-distanced cup of tea in her communal garden.

The 82-year-old was visited by police after she had been reported for drinking tea outside with neighbours from her sheltered housing complex.

The woman, from Charlton Kings, was watching television in bed when there was a knock at the door at 9.45pm.

The pensioner's daughter Lesley Magovern, 56, from Cheltenham said: "My mother heard a knock at the door and it was very late and she wondered really who it could be.

Police visited the pensioner and warned her about a potential Covid breach.

'She was quite frightened'

"My mother is quite deaf and she asked who it was and she thought the voice said 'It's me'. Then mother assumed it was in fact me and she then opened the door.

"There were two officers stood there, a man and a woman with masks on and they asked if they could come in and speak to her.

"They did not show her any identification so she just trusted the uniform and she was quite frightened. My mother has never been in trouble with the police in her life."

The residents all share a communal garden and her mother moved in just before lockdown.

They told mother if it were to happen again she would be fined.

Lesley

March 19, 2021 VAERS (Vaccine Adverse Event Reporting System United States) https://www.openvaers.com/covid-data

2050 deaths from Covid vaccines reported in the USAs

4450 hospitalizations from vaccine side effects reported in the USA

7485 urgent care visits due to Covid vaccine side effects

6759 office visits due to Covid vaccine side effects

354 Anaphylaxis reports following Covid vaccines

421 reports of Bells Palsy following Covid vaccines

434 Heart Attacks reported due to Covid vaccines

76 Miscarriages reported following Covid vaccines

2550 Allergic Reactions reported from Covid vaccines

March 20 2021 Covid Vaccines: Post-Vaccination Deaths https://swprs.org/covid-rna-vaccines-deaths/

Data from vaccine adverse event reporting systems in the US (VAERS), the EU (EUDRA) and the UK (MHRA) indicates that covid vaccinations have already been associated with about ***5000 deaths*** *and several thousand* *non-trivial 'adverse events', including anaphylactic (allergic) shocks, temporary facial paralysis, cardiovascular disorders, and, in some cases, miscarriages. These figures may be an underestimate, as vaccine reporting systems typically cover only a fraction of adverse events. Post-vaccination deaths may be unrelated to the vaccination. However, in the US, 47% of post-vaccination deaths occurred in people who became ill within 48 hours of being vaccinated and 31% of deaths occurred within 48 hours of vaccination. 20% of deaths were related to cardiac disorder.*

In the US, the average age of those who died after covid vaccination was 78 years. The youngest death confirmed was a 23-year-old. Some young and healthy doctors were affected, too. Furthermore, in the UK, by mid-March about 50 cases of blindness, about 60 cases of deafness, and about 30 cases of spontaneous abortions were reported shortly after covid vaccinations.

March 24 2021 Outbreaks continue in some Oregon senior care homes after vaccination clinics. Why?

https://www.oregonlive.com/coronavirus/2021/03/outbreaks-continue-in-some-oregon-senior-care-homes-after-vaccination-clinics-why.html

*By **Fedor Zarkhin | The Oregonian/OregonLive***

More than a dozen Oregon senior care homes have reported coronavirus outbreaks even after staff and residents were offered vaccines, The Oregonian/OregonLive has found, pointing to the reality that vaccine access, while extraordinarily important, has not been a panacea for completely ending some outbreaks.

At one facility, a resident got sick and died with COVID-19 more than two weeks after getting both shots of the vaccine, a facility director said. In a third facility, seven people tested positive after they should have reached full immunity – triggering reports to the state and federal government in search of potential variants of the disease.

In all, at least 15 nursing, assisted living and memory care homes in Oregon have seen coronavirus outbreaks weeks after residents and staff were offered shots, three of them exceeding 30 cases. New cases continue to emerge.

March 28, 2021

The Washington Po

'Vaccine passports' are on the way, but developing them won't be easy

Dan Diamond, Lena H. Sun, Isaac Stanley-Becker 3 hrs ago

https://www.msn.com/en-us/news/politics/vaccine-passports-are-on-the-way-but-developing-them-wont-be-easy/ar-BB1f39Cc

The Centers for Disease Control and Prevention, which is participating in the WHO's effort to create "digital vaccination certificates," also is preparing to help advise on the passport rollout. The health agency says it is expecting to play a role in determining which organizations will credential and issue the certificates, in addition to informing the public, according to CDC documents reviewed by The Post.

Donald Rucker, who led the health IT office during the Trump administration, said myriad technical issues await the rollout of vaccine credentials, including how they are tracked, whether they are enforced and who pulls together the initial records of which Americans have gotten shots. Rucker said keeping vaccine credentials could help officials better understand coronavirus vaccination, including possible long-term side effects, if the data is connected with the health information exchanges that states maintain. "The tracking of vaccinations is not just simply for vaccine passports," Rucker said. "The tracking of vaccinations is a broader issue of 'we're giving a novel biologic agent to the entire country,' more or less."

March 29, 2021 –Covid-19: US cases rise while vaccinations increase **British Medical Journal by** *Janice Hopkins Tanne*

The US reported more than 61 000 cases of covid-19 per day in the past week, an increase of 12% over the average two weeks ago, even as vaccinations were increasing to about 2.5 million a day, according to the New York Times.[1]

Cases are high and rising in 26 states and are increasing in three other states that had a low number of cases. As of 28 March, there have been more than 30.2 million cases of covid-19 and 548 000 deaths in the US.

March 31, 2021 SARS-CoV-2 Spike Protein Impairs Endothelial Function via Downregulation of ACE 2

https://www.ahajournals.org/doi/10.1161/CIRCRESAHA.121.318902

April 13, 2021 – Johnson and Johnson Vaccine Paused by the FDA in the USA due to blood clots

https://www.fda.gov/news-events/press-announcements/joint-cdc-and-fda-statement-johnson-johnson-covid-19-vaccine

As of April 12, more than 6.8 million doses of the Johnson & Johnson (Janssen) vaccine have been administered in the U.S. CDC and FDA are reviewing data involving six reported U.S. cases of a rare and severe type of blood clot in individuals after receiving the J&J vaccine. In these cases, a type of blood clot called cerebral venous sinus thrombosis (CVST) was seen in combination with low levels of blood platelets (thrombocytopenia). All six cases occurred among women between the ages of 18 and 48, and symptoms occurred 6 to 13 days after vaccination. Treatment of this specific type of blood clot is different from the treatment that might typically be administered. Usually, an anticoagulant drug called heparin is used to treat blood clots. In this setting, administration of heparin may be dangerous, and alternative treatments need to be given.

April 15, 2021 – The Norwegian Institute of Public Health has recommended stopping further use of the AstraZeneca vaccine (Vaxzevria) in the Coronavirus Immunization Programme in Norway. https://www.fhi.no/en/news/2021/astrazeneca-vaccine-removed-from-coronavirus-immunisation-programme-in-norw/

Since use of the AstraZeneca vaccine was put on hold on 11th March, the Norwegian Institute of Public Health has considered further use of the AstraZeneca vaccine in Norway, together with other experts.

"We now know significantly more about the association between the AstraZeneca vaccine and the rare but severe incidents with low platelet counts, blood clots and haemorrhages, than when Norway decided to pause use of the AstraZeneca-vaccine in March," says Geir Bukholm, Director of the Division of Infection Control and Environmental Health at the Norwegian Institute of Public Health.

"Based on this knowledge, we come with a recommendation to remove the AstraZeneca vaccine from the Coronavirus Immunisation Programme in Norway," says Bukholm.

Bukholm points out that this has not been an easy recommendation to make. It has a direct consequence for when the risk groups can receive a coronavirus vaccine, with subsequent protection, while also having an impact on when it will be possible to lift infection control measures.

Higher risk associated with AstraZeneca vaccine than from COVID-19 disease in Norway

Having come a long way in vaccinating the oldest citizens, Norway has reduced the risk of death for many of those most at risk. Since most of the elderly have either been vaccinated, or soon will be, this means that continued use of the vaccine would mainly be among the under-65 years age group if we were to use this vaccine in Norway.

Calculations have been performed based on Norwegian data where the risk of dying from COVID-19 disease among the different age groups is compared with the risk of dying from the severe, but rare, condition with severe blood clots observed after AstraZeneca vaccination.

"Since there are few people who die from COVID-19 in Norway, the risk of dying after vaccination with the AstraZeneca vaccine would be higher than the risk of dying from the disease, particularly for younger people," says Bukholm.

In addition, there is reason to assume that there is scepticism about using the AstraZeneca vaccine in Norway, and it is uncertain how many people would have accepted an offer of this vaccine now.

April 23, 2021 Reported Covid-19 Vaccine Side Effects USA GOVERNMENT COVID VACCINE ADVERSE EVENTS REPORTING SYSTEM (VAERS) (courtesy of openvaers.com)

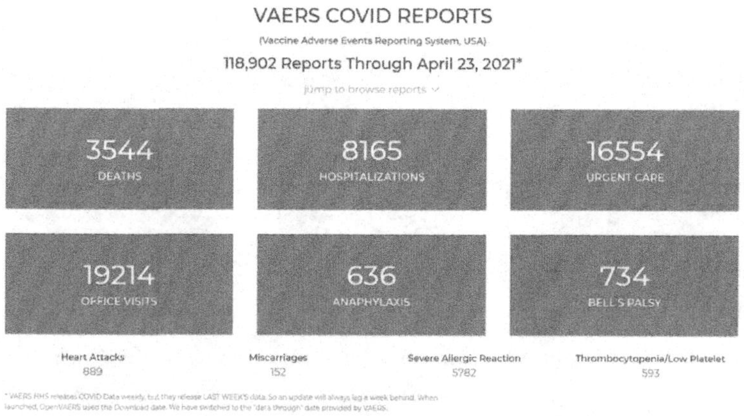

APRIL 2021 YOUR TV IS THE VIRUS (UNKNOWN PHOTOGRAPHER)

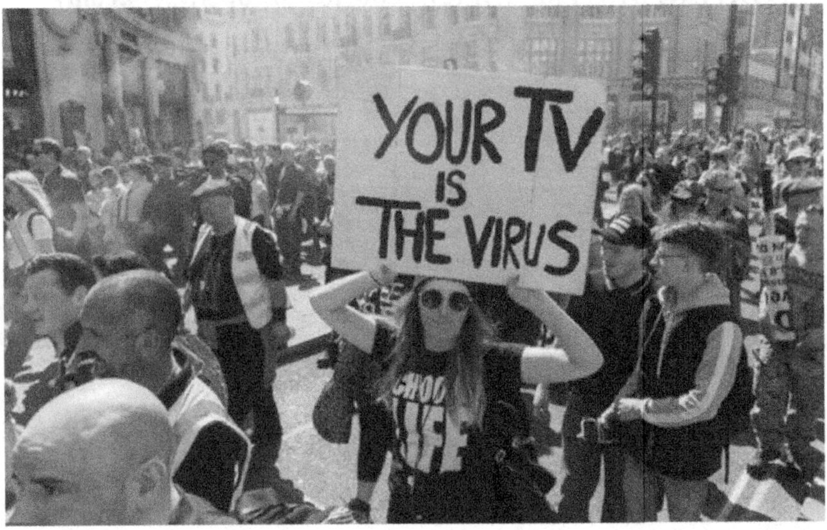

April 25, 2021 Bethel Park mother left paralyzed after getting first dose of Pfizer vaccine, doctors say nervous system played a part

https://www.wpxi.com/news/top-stories/bethel-park-woman-paralyzed-12-hours-after-getting-first-dose-pfizer-vaccine-doctors-searching-answers/ZSYTEX4H4FHKDFVSPGS3ILJZUI/

By Jillian Hartmann, WPXI-TV

BETHEL PARK, Pa. — There have been some negative side effects reported worldwide from the Pfizer, Moderna and Johnson & Johnson COVID-19 vaccines, but a Bethel Park woman told Channel 11 she has been affected by something that hadn't been seen at all yet: paralysis.

Doctors at Allegheny General Hospital ran a bunch of tests but then Rachael Cecere, 33, from Bethel Park was moved to the Cleveland Clinic a few days ago.

She spoke exclusively with Channel 11 from her hospital bed at the clinic. She received her first shot of the Pfizer vaccine last week at Rite Aid in Caste Village.

Twelve hours later, Cecere said almost her entire body was paralyzed.

"It was the scariest thing in the world to go to sleep completely fine (and walking), to wake up 1:30 in the morning and not be able to move at all," the woman said. "I'm literally counting on my daughter to hand me my phone to call to get help."

Paramedics came and rushed her to Jefferson Hospital. In the coming days, she was moved to Allegheny General Hospital in the Northside and then the Cleveland Clinic — as doctors ran a multitude of tests to figure out how and why this happened. An MRI and spinal tap were clear, and her blood work all came back negative, ruling out any rare diseases or disorders.

April 30, 2021 Salk Institute – The novel coronavirus' spike protein plays additional key role in illness

https://www.salk.edu/news-release/the-novel-coronavirus-spike-protein-plays-additional-key-role-in-illness/

The novel coronavirus' spike protein plays additional key role in illness

Salk researchers and collaborators show how the protein damages cells, confirming COVID-19 as a primarily vascular disease

LA JOLLA—Scientists have known for a while that SARS-CoV-2's distinctive "spike" proteins help the virus infect its host by latching on to healthy cells. Now, a major new study shows that they also play a key role in the disease itself.

The paper, published on April 30, 2021, in Circulation Research, also shows conclusively that COVID-19 is a vascular disease, demonstrating exactly how the SARS-CoV-2 virus damages and attacks the vascular system on a cellular level. The findings help explain COVID-19's wide variety of seemingly unconnected complications, and could open the door for new research into more effective therapies.

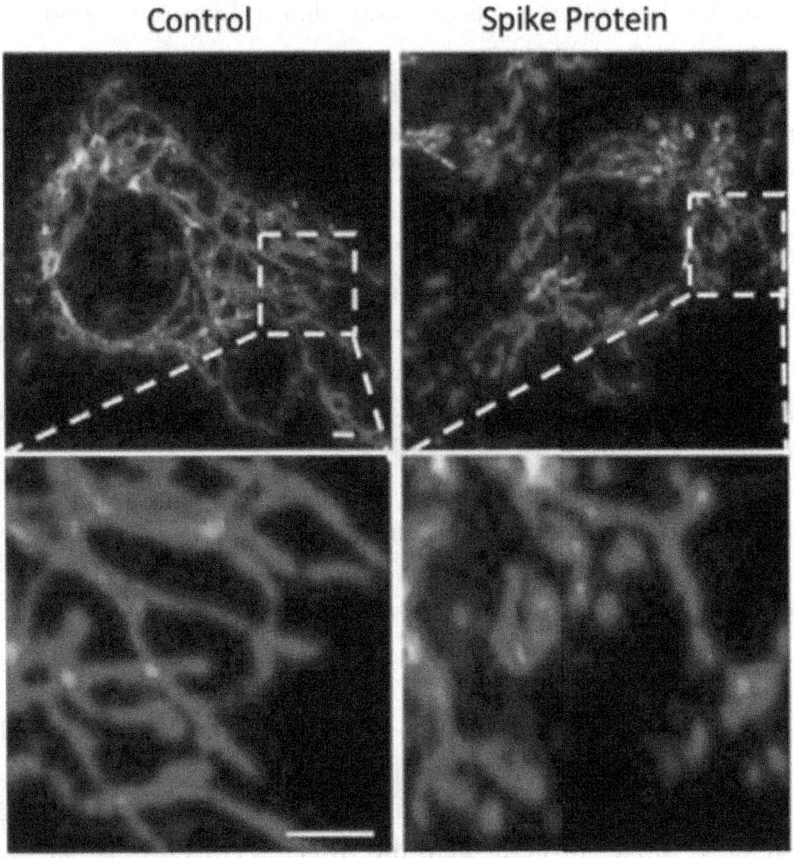

Representative images of vascular endothelial control cells (left) and cells treated with the SARS-CoV-2 Spike protein (right) show that the spike protein causes increased mitochondrial fragmentation in vascular cells.

Click here for a high-resolution image.

Credit: Salk Institute

"A lot of people think of it as a respiratory disease, but it's really a vascular disease," says Assistant Research Professor *Uri Manor*, who is co-senior author of the study. "That could explain why some people have strokes, and why some people have issues in other parts of the body. The commonality between them is that they all have vascular underpinnings."

Salk researchers collaborated with scientists at the University of California San Diego on the paper, including co-first author Jiao Zhang and co-senior author John Shyy, among others.

While the findings themselves aren't entirely a surprise, the paper provides clear confirmation and a detailed explanation of the mechanism through which the protein damages vascular cells for the first time. There's been a growing consensus that SARS-CoV-2 affects the vascular system, but exactly how it did so was not understood. Similarly, scientists studying other coronaviruses have long suspected that the spike protein contributed to damaging vascular endothelial cells, but this is the first time the process has been documented.

May 2, 2021 – Chart showing Declining Covid-19 Cases in Countries with < 3% vaccination rates in the European Union

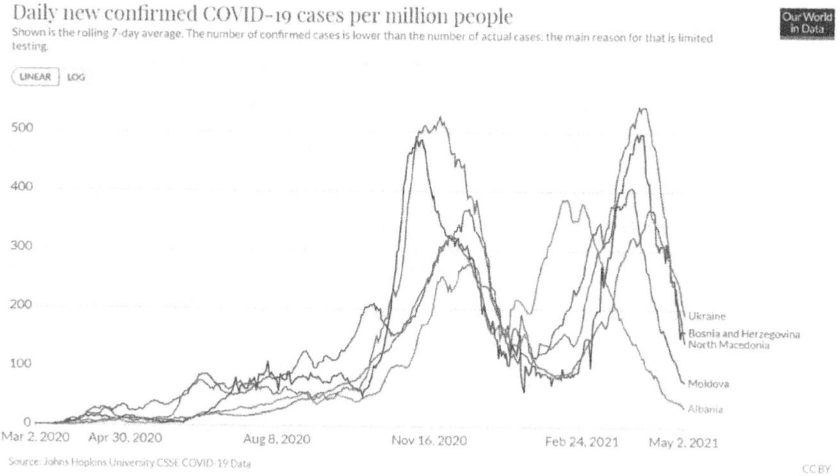

May 2, 2021 – Covid Vaccines: Already Close to 10,000 Post-Vaccination Deaths from Swiss Policy Research https://swprs.org/covid-rna-vaccines-deaths/ (Swiss Policy Research has consistently

been one of the best globally aggregated compilation of fully referenced data sources on Covid-19 since the beginning of the "pandemic")

Data from vaccine adverse event reporting systems in the US (VAERS), the EU (EUDRA) and the UK (MHRA) indicates that covid vaccinations have already been associated with **close to 10,000 deaths** *and several thousand non-trivial 'adverse events', including anaphylactic shocks, neurological and cardiovascular disorders, and miscarriages. These figures may be an underestimate, as vaccine reporting systems typically cover only a fraction of adverse events.*

Some post-vaccination deaths may be **unrelated** *to the vaccination. However, in the US, about 50% of post-vaccination deaths occurred in people who became ill within 48 hours of being vaccinated. In addition, in the US and Europe combined, several hundred cases of blindness, deafness, and spontaneous abortions have been reported shortly after covid vaccinations.*

Compared to the **hundreds of millions of covid vaccinations** *already performed, these numbers are small. Compared to the amount of covid deaths, too, these numbers are small. But compared to the standards for safe medical products, these numbers are certainly significant. Moreover, little is still known about the long-term safety profile of covid vaccines. Back in 2009/2010, it took one year for the public to learn about neurological damages caused by swine flu vaccine adjuvants.*

US physician **Dr. J. Patrick Whelan** *had warned the US FDA already in early December 2020 that vaccines based on the coronavirus spike protein may themselves trigger symptoms of severe systemic covid, including blood clots, pulmonary embolism and brain inflammation, even in children and young adults, who normally fight off a coronavirus infection in its early stages. In April 2021, this effect was confirmed ("SARS-CoV-2 spike protein alone may cause lung damage").*

Regarding **vaccine effectiveness**, *real-world studies indicate that after the second vaccine dose, effectiveness reaches about 90% in people up to 60 years old, but only about 65% in people over 80 years old. About one third of people over 80 do not develop neutralizing antibodies.*

As New York attorney Aaron Siri pointed out in an article on StatNews, neither governments nor employers are currently permitted to require covid vaccinations, as covid vaccines are ***experimental vaccines*** *that have not yet been licensed: they only received an "emergency use authorization" in the US and a "conditional marketing authorisation" in the EU. Indeed, the US FDA specifically notes that covid vaccines are "investigational vaccines not licensed for any indication."*

Additional Information

Case reports: *To study verified case reports of post-vaccination victims (deaths and injuries), see The Covid Blog (USA), The Defender (USA), Nashville et al. (USA), and Corona Blog (Germany).*

Data sources: *Reporting systems OpenVAERS (USA), EUDRA (EU), MHRA (UK).*

Critique: *Anti-Vaxxers Misuse Federal Data to Falsely Claim COVID Vaccines Are Dangerous (VN)*

Updates

Israel: *Increase in all-cause mortality and reports of a "murky wave of heart attacks". More.*

AstraZeneca vaccine: *Suspended in several countries due to 'rare blood clots'. Read more.*

Johnson and Johnson vaccine: *Suspended in the US due to 'rare blood clots'. Read more.*

April 2021 AstraZeneca Covid Vaccine: *The Norwegian Institute of Public Health stopped Covid-19 vaccinations with the AstraZeneca vaccine, arguing that "the risk of dying after vaccination with the AstraZeneca vaccine would be higher than the risk of dying from the disease, particularly for younger people."*

Cerebral blood clots: *Comparing the risks after covid and after vaccination. Read more.*

Israel: *Unexplained increase in 65+* all-cause *mortality after vaccination campaign:*

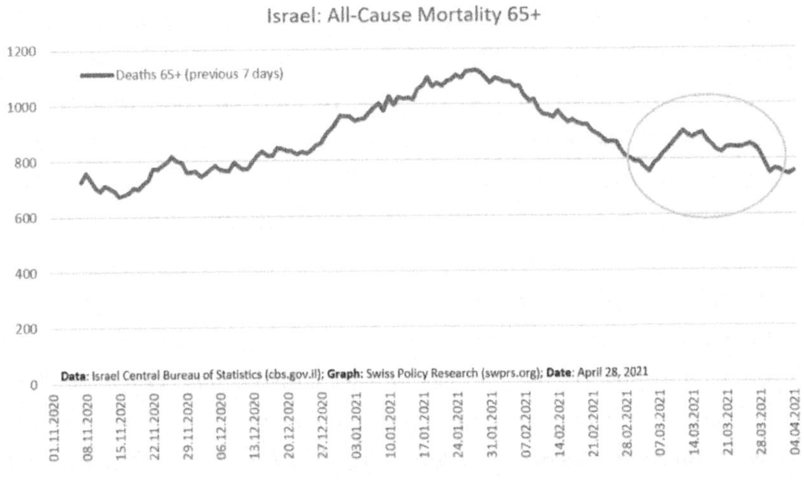

All-cause deaths 65+, previous 7 days (Data: Israel CBS). Read more.

July 2021 THE HILL – Officials probing if Moderna vaccine linked to higher risk of heart inflammation in young adults: report https://thehill.com/policy/healthcare/568710-health-officials-probing-possibility-moderna-vaccine-linked-with-higher

Federal health officials are conducting an investigation into the effects of the Moderna COVID-19 vaccine following new research that showed it may be linked to a higher risk of heart inflammation in young adults than previously though, according to a report from The Washington Post.

July 2021 BBC Headline: Heart inflammation link to Pfizer and Moderna jabs By James Gallagher Health and science correspondent https://www.bbc.com/news/health-57781637

The European Medicines Agency said the side-effects were more common in younger men. The medicines safety body said the benefits of Covid vaccines continue to far outweigh any risks. But doctors and patients have been advised to be aware of the symptoms of heart inflammation. UK approves Pfizer jab for 12 to 15-year-olds Mixing Covid jabs has good immune response, study finds These include chest pain, a feeling of breathlessness and a pounding or fluttering heartbeat. Anyone with these symptoms should see a doctor. Two conditions were linked to the vaccines – inflammation of the heart muscle itself, known as myocarditis, and inflammation of the fluid-filled sac the heart sits in, known as pericarditis.

September 2021 MSN News: Iceland suspends use of Moderna's Covid vaccine due to heart-inflammation fears https://www.msn.com/en-in/news/world/iceland-suspends-use-of-modernas-covid-vaccine-due-to-heart-inflammation-fears/ar-AAPiwLg

Iceland has decided to suspend Moderna's coronavirus vaccine citing concerns of increased risks of cardiac inflammation.

OCTOBER 8 2021 THE SUBURBAN – Five Scandinavian countries limit or halt Moderna https://www.thesuburban.com/news/covid_19/five-scandinavian-countries-limit-or-halt-moderna/article_7ac39fac-fae7-5937-acd1-6f94ac576e39.html

Finland has joined Sweden, Denmark and Norway in either banning or discouraging young adults or teens from getting the Moderna COVID-19 vaccine, because of the increased risk of myocarditis — heart inflammation. Dr. Hanna Nohynek, chief physician at the Finnish Institute for Health and Welfare, had told the media a decision was coming down Thursday. Finland's health authorities announced that men under 30 will not get the Moderna shot, and should get the Pfizer vaccine instead. Sweden banned Moderna for people under the age of 30, and Denmark did the same for people under 18. Instead of issuing a ban, Norway is urging people under 30 to choose Pfizer rather than Moderna. And on Friday, Iceland halted distribution of Moderna in general.

Oct 26, 2021 Chicago Tribune Judge to rule Friday in federal lawsuit by Chicago workers challenging vaccine mandates Jason Meisner, Chicago Tribune https://www.msn.com/en-us/news/crime/judge-to-rule-friday-in-federal-lawsuit-by-chicago-workers-challenging-vaccine-mandates/ar-AAPZezs CHICAGO — A federal judge on Tuesday said he was "puzzled" by an emergency request by more than 100 Chicago firefighters and other city employees seeking a freeze on vaccine mandate orders by Mayor Lori Lightfoot and Gov. J.B. Pritzker. The 130 plaintiffs named in the federal suit, mostly Chicago firefighters and paramedics, are asking U.S. District Judge John Lee for a temporary restraining order that would halt the city's requirement that all city workers report their vaccination status or risk being put on no-pay status. Protests mandates Europe

NOVEMBER 1, 2021 Americans who received the one-dose Johnson & Johnson COVID-19 vaccine were 3.5 times as likely to develop rare blood clots compared to the general population, study finds By MANSUR SHAHEEN U.S. DEPUTY HEALTH EDITOR FOR DAILYMAIL.COM PUBLISHED: 15:00 GMT, 1 November 2021 | https://www.dailymail.co.uk/health/article-10152723/Americans-received-one-dose-J-J-Covid-vaccine-3-5-times-likely-develop-blood-clots.html

Johnson & Johnson's COVID-19 vaccine increases a person's risk of developing rare blood clots, a new study suggests. Researchers from the Mayo Clinic in Rochester, Minnesota, compared data from the general population before the pandemic to data gathered from reported vaccine side-effects suffered by Americans. They found that a person who received the vaccine was 3.5 times as likely to develop brain blood clots as an average person before the pandemic. Blood clotting, and specifically cerebral venous sinus thrombosis (CVST) is a well known side-effect of the J&J vaccine, and the discovery of this risk was the reason usage of the vaccine was paused in April.

November 10, 2021 Australian Therapeutics Goods Administration requests information from Pfizer after medical journal alleges contractor 'falsified' safety data An investigation by a respected medical journal has alleged serious issues with Pfizer's vaccine safety trials, including claims of "falsified data". https://www.news.com.au/

technology/science/human-body/tga-requests-information-from-pfizer-after-medical-journal-alleges-contractor-falsified-safety-data/news-story/342806323e802035bb1d810e561977f4

EXCLUSIVE Australia's medicines regulator has sought additional information from Pfizer after an investigation by the British Medical Journal alleged serious issues with a small number of its vaccine safety trials, including claims of "falsified data" and slowness following up on adverse reactions. The Therapeutic Goods Administration (TGA) has stressed that Pfizer's vaccine is "highly safe and effective", and that Australians "should not be concerned about the issues raised in the article". The BMJ's report, published last week, centred on a former employee of Ventavia Research Group, a Texas-based contractor involved in the phase-three trials for Pfizer's Covid vaccine last year. According to Brook Jackson, a former regional director at Ventavia, the company "falsified data, unblinded patients, employed inadequately trained vaccinators, and was slow to follow up on adverse events", the BMJ reported. The whistleblower, who provided the BMJ with "dozens of internal company documents, photos, audio recordings and emails", recounted that she repeatedly notified the company of the problems before finally emailing a complaint to the US Food and Drug Administration on September 25, 2020.

November 10, 2021 International Business Times Moderna Vaccine Warning: France, Germany Caution Of Cardiac Inflammation Risks For People Under 30 https://www.ibtimes.com/moderna-vaccine-warning-france-germany-caution-cardiac-inflammation-risks-people-3335189

France and Germany are the latest European countries to issue warnings about the Moderna (MRNA) COVID vaccine for people under the age of 30 because of a "very rare" risk linked to myocarditis or heart inflammation. France's public health authority published its recommendation on Monday, saying "within the population aged under 30, this risk appears to be around five times lesser with Pfizer's Comirnaty jab compared to Moderna's Spikevax jab," Reuters reported. Germany issued its warning for citizens on Wednesday after its vaccine advisory committee, STIKO, received new safety data from the Paul Ehrlich Institute, Reuters said.

November 21, 2021 Violent protests break out in Europe over vaccine mandates, lockdowns By Jackie Salo https://nypost.com/2021/11/21/europes-covid-19-vaccine-mandates-spark-violent-protests/

Violent protests have broken out against COVID-19 vaccine mandates and lockdowns across Europe amid new tough rules to curb winter waves of the virus. Demonstrators angry about the new measures gathered in Austria, Croatia, Italy, Northern Ireland, the French territory of Guadeloupe and the Netherlands to protest the moves. In the Netherlands, a second night of riots broke out Saturday over a partial lockdown, one day after police opened fire on people protesting the rules in Rotterdam. Protesters hurled fireworks at police and set fire to bicycles in The Hague, as cops used horses, dogs and batons to chase the crowds away, the BBC reported.

JANUARY 11 2022 EU drug regulator expresses doubt on need for fourth booster dose https://www.reuters.com/business/healthcare-pharmaceuticals/eu-drug-regulator-says-more-data-needed-impact-omicron-vaccines-2022-01-11/ *Jan 11 (Reuters) – The European Union's drug regulator on Tuesday expressed doubts about the need for a fourth booster dose of COVID-19 vaccine and said there is currently no data to support this approach as it seeks more data on the fast-spreading Omicron variant. "While use of additional boosters can be part of contingency plans, repeated vaccinations within short intervals would not represent a sustainable long-term strategy," the European Medicines Agency's Head of Vaccines Strategy, Marco Cavaleri, told a media briefing. The EMA official raised concerns that a strategy of giving boosters every four months hypothetically poses the risk of overloading people's immune systems and leading to fatigue in the population.*

January 13 2022 Supreme Court blocks nationwide vaccine and testing mandate for large businesses, allows health care worker vaccine mandate to take effect https://edition.cnn.com/2022/01/13/politics/supreme-court-vaccine-mandate-covid-19/index.html

(CNN)The Supreme Court on Thursday blocked President Joe Biden's vaccine and testing requirement aimed at large businesses, but it allowed a vaccine mandate for certain health care workers to go into effect nationwide. The decision is a huge hit to Biden's attempts to use the power of the federal government to fight the Covid-19 pandemic. The President has emphasized the necessity of getting vaccinated against the virus for months and eventually decided to use the mandate on large employers as his main vehicle for convincing hesitant Americans to get their shots. In freezing a lower court opinion that allowed the regulation to go into effect nationwide, the majority sent a clear message the Occupational Safety and Health Administration, charged with protecting workplace safety, overstepped its authority. In contrast, the justices said that a separate agency could issue a rule to protect the health and safety of Medicare and Medicaid patients.

January 2022 Speech Therapist: 364% Surge In Baby And Toddler Referrals Thanks To Mask Wearing https://www.zerohedge.com/political/speech-therapist-364-surge-baby-and-toddler-referrals-thanks-mask-wearing *Jaclyn Theek told WPBF News that before the pandemic, only 5 per cent of patients were babies and toddlers, but this has soared to 20 per cent. Parents are describing their children's speech problems as "COVID delayed," with face coverings the primary cause of their speaking skills being seriously impaired. As young as 8 months old, babies start learning how to speak by reading lips, a thankless task if parents and carers smother themselves with masks to comply with mandates. A speech therapist says her clinic has seen a "364% increase in patient referrals of babies and toddlers". "It's very important kids do see your face to learn, so they're watching your mouth." What the hell have we done?!*

Feb 14, 2022 Moderna Stock Crash: Losses Top $140 Billion As Insiders Sell Millions Of Dollars In Shares https://www.forbes.com/sites/jonathanponciano/2022/02/14/moderna-stock-crash-losses-top-140-billion-as-insiders-sell-millions-of-dollars-in-shares/?sh=730291eb106b

Shares of Moderna plummeted Monday as Covid-19 vaccine-makers led a turbulent market decline, pushing the stock to its lowest level in nearly a year

after disappointing study results and a slew of sales from the firm's top executives added to concerns that have made one of last year's top-performing stocks crash more than 70%.

January 29, 2022 BBC: Freedom Convoy: Why Canadian truckers are protesting in Ottawa By Jessica Murphy https://www.bbc.co.uk/news/world-us-canada-60164561

After a week-long drive across Canada, a convoy of big rigs has arrived in the national capital to protest vaccine mandates and Covid-19 measures. Organisers insist it will be peaceful, but police say they're prepared for trouble. It's been dubbed the Freedom Convoy, and it's got the country talking. The movement was sparked by a vaccine mandate for truckers crossing the US-Canada border, implemented by Prime Minister Justin Trudeau's Liberal government earlier this month. Upset with the new measure that would require unvaccinated Canadian truckers crossing the two nations' boundary to quarantine once they've returned home, a loose coalition of truckers and conservative groups began to organise the cross-country drive that began in western Canada. It picked up steam and gathered support as it drove east. Many supporters, already opposed to Mr Trudeau and his politics, have grown frustrated with pandemic measures they see as political overreach. Social media and news footage showed trucks and companion vehicles snaking along highways, cheered on by people gathered on roadsides and overpasses, often waving Canadian flags and signs disparaging Mr Trudeau.

January 30, 2022 All Cause Mortality in the United States During 2021 By Gilbert G. Berdine, M.D https://www.aier.org/article/all-cause-mortality-in-the-united-states-during-2021/

The CEO of the OneAmerica insurance company recently disclosed that mortality in the 18-64 age group was 40 percent higher during the 3rd and 4th quarters of 2021 than during pre-pandemic levels. For reference, the CEO indicated that a 10 percent increase would have been a 1-in-200-year event. Furthermore, most of the deaths were not attributed to Covid.

February 6, 2022 Protests spread to more Canadian cities as Ottawa churches close their doors https://www.ctvnews.ca/canada/protests-spread-to-more-canadian-cities-as-ottawa-churches-close-their-doors-1.5769948

The so-called Freedom Convoy rolled into the nation's capital last weekend, and while some people went home over the course of the week, participation surged anew, with police estimating that thousands were part of the weekend crowd. Similar scenes played out in other parts of the country on Sunday, though on a smaller scale than the day before when thousands of people opposed to pandemic-related restrictions congregated in cities from coast to coast. Halifax police Const. John MacLeod said hundreds of trucks and cars made their way through the downtown core Sunday and caused quite a backlog, but officers were working to clear that out. He said the situation has been peaceful with no incidents to report. Ontario Provincial Police closed part of Highway 402 running to the border crossing between Sarnia and Port Huron, Mich., as a safety precaution because of pedestrians on the highway near a convoy of trucks and tractors. Ontario's solicitor-general praised police's handling of thousands of protesters in Toronto, but noted in a statement that Ottawa police "continue to express concerns about their ability to manage the ongoing occupation in their city." Ontario Premier Doug Ford also weighed in, saying the province has backed Ottawa during the nine-day protests that critics have branded an occupation.

February 10, 2022 New York Times: Protesters Opposing Covid Vaccine Pass Head to Paris By Storyful and Reuters https://www.nytimes.com/video/world/europe/100000008202463/france-protest-convoy-vaccine-pass-paris.html

Truckers and drivers departed from across France with the goal of converging as a convoy in Paris to protest the country's vaccination pass program. The effort was directly inspired by Canada's trucker-led movement.

FEB 14, 2022, 11:04 AM SGT Protest convoy against Covid-19 vaccine pass heads for banned Brussels rally https://www.straitstimes.

com/world/europe/protest-convoy-against-covid-19-vaccine-pass-heads-for-banned-brussels-rally

BRUSSELS (AFP) – Hundreds of cars, campervans and trucks taking part in a Canada-style protest convoy against Covid-19 regulations were preparing to enter Brussels on Monday (Feb 14) where Belgian officials have already banned a demonstration following a weekend attempt in Paris. Around 1,300 vehicles from across France had arrived near the French border town of Lille by late Sunday, according to police. The protest is one of several worldwide inspired by the truckers' standoff with authorities in Canada. Camped at a parking lot near Lille, protesters brandished French flags and chanted "We won't give up" and "Freedom, freedom". "We'll go to Brussels to try to block it, to fight against this policy of permanent control," said Mr Jean-Pierre Schmit, an unemployed 58-year-old who came from Toulouse. For Sandrine, 45, who came from Lyon, the government's response to the Covid-19 crisis had revealed that "we're losing our freedoms bit by bit, in an insidious way".

Friday Feb 25, 2022 German insurance data reveals COVID vaccine adverse events are 10 times higher than government reports:

https://www.lifesitenews.com/news/german-insurance-data-reveals-covid-vaccine-adverse-events-are-10-times-higher-than-govt-reports/

"The data available to our company gives us reason to believe that there is a very considerable under-recording of suspected cases of vaccination side effects after [patients] received the [COVID-19] vaccine,' wrote board member Andreas Schöfbeck. By: Patrick Delaney Fri Feb 25, 2022 – 6:15 pm EST (LifeSiteNews) – A large German health insurer has raised concerns over what its data shows to be an excessive underreporting by government authorities of adverse events after experimental COVID-19 gene-based vaccine injections. Andreas Schöfbeck, a board member of BKK ProVita (one of the largest German insurance companies), addressed the company's findings in a formal letter to the government's Paul Ehrlich Institute (PEI), which had reported earlier this year that there were 244,576 suspected cases of side effects from the gene-based injections in the calendar year 2021. Speaking to this figure, Schöfbeck wrote, "The data available to our company

gives us reason to believe that there is a very considerable under-recording of suspected cases of vaccination side effects after [patients] received the [COVID-19] vaccine." Explaining that their sample includes 10,937,716 insured clients, with available data covering only the first 7½ months of 2021, their company had already logged 216,695 cases of adverse reactions for COVID-19 gene-based injections. Extending this rate for the full year, and then applying it to the full population of Germany (around 83 million), one can estimate that likely 2.5 million to 3 million individuals in the nation were treated by medical professionals for such adverse events. "According to our calculations, we consider 400,000 visits to the doctor by our policyholders because of vaccination complications to be realistic to this day. Extrapolated to the total population, this value would be three million," Schöfbeck told WELT news. This is a "significant alarm signal," he said in his letter, as it "means around 4-5% of the vaccinated were under medical treatment for side effects," a rate about 10 times higher than the government's reported numbers. In commenting on his disclosure, Schöfbeck told WELT, "The numbers that resulted from our analysis are very far away from the publicly announced numbers. It would be unethical not to talk about it."

March 1, 2022 Epoch Times: By Meiling Lee – Pfizer's COVID-19 Vaccine Goes Into Liver Cells and Is Converted to DNA: Study
https://www.theepochtimes.com/pfizers-covid-19-vaccine-goes-into-liver-cells-and-is-converted-to-dna-study_4307594.html

The messenger RNA (mRNA) from Pfizer's COVID-19 vaccine is able to enter human liver cells and is converted into DNA, according to Swedish researchers at Lund University. The researchers found that when the mRNA vaccine enters the human liver cells, it triggers the cell's DNA, which is inside the nucleus, to increase the production of the LINE-1 gene expression to make mRNA.

March 4 2022 US FEDERAL GOVERNMENT COVID-19 VACCINE ADVERSE EVENT REPORTING SYSTEM SUMMARY DATA REPORT PULLED FROM https://vaers.hhs.gov/data.html (Summary Graphic Courtesy of www.OpenVaers.com)

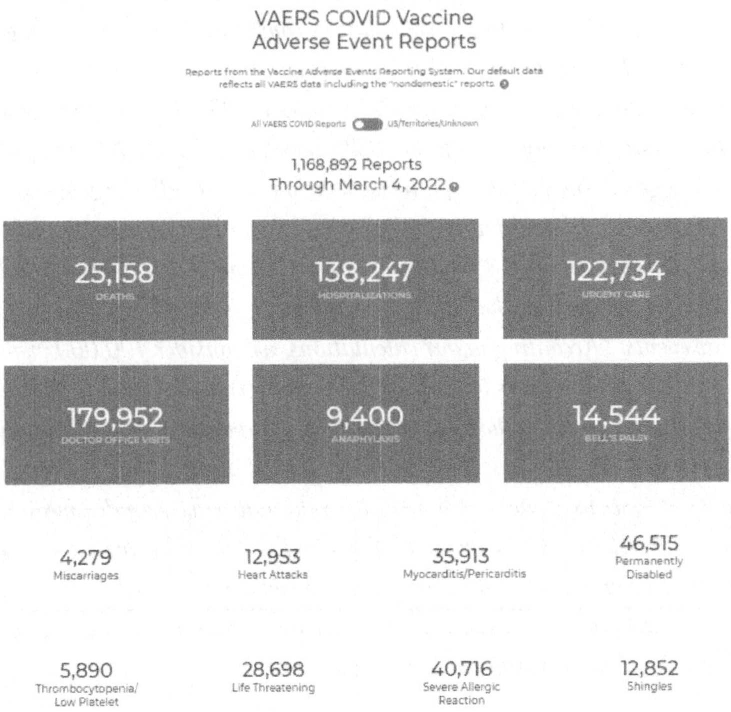

FINAL THOUGHTS ON COVID-19 VACCINES AND ISSUES WITH LAB TESTS

FLU VACCINES ARE KNOWN TO INCREASE CORONAVIRUS INFECTIONS BY 30% ACCORDING TO A 2019 STUDY BY THE ARMY

The US Pentagon study shared earlier shows the increased incidence of pneumonia and lung challenges among those people who had flu vaccines. For example, a variety of vaccine trials when vaccines were mandated for the first time were thought to have ignited, for example, the "Great Spanish Flu" epidemic of 1918 that followed the first mandatory vaccinations of soldiers in WW1, which was chronicled to have radiated out from the bases into the general population: The

Hidden Dangers in Polio Vaccine (Chapter 10 of Poisoned needle, by Eleanor McBean).

Some of these vaccine-associated epidemics may also have culled millions in the United States and other countries, along with many other iatrogenic (medical system caused) associated mass campaigns temporally associated with epidemics and increasing endemic disease frequencies. The widespread use of amphetamines for instance, such as Ritalin and Adderall and our growing population of young methamphetamine addicts is exploding. This generation of kids received their childhood meth baptisms between the ages of 8-13, when they "couldn't just sit still in school and play well with others," The psychologists now armed with drugs and the PHS reasoned that the tools now existed to manage the energetic nature of childhood, so they needed to be DRUGGED and learn to take their "MEDS!"

AIDS vaccines, MMR vaccines, and other vaccine trials highlight the insanity of the continued tacit acceptance of the Jennerian paradigm of vaccination and serve to underscore the insanity of the hypothesized viral cause of Acquired Immune Deficiency Syndromes(s) or the trumped but discredited Fauci-claimed benefits bestowed by "HIV/AIDS" vaccines, or vaccinations in any historical context. Indeed, a positive "HIV" test result brings us to its most egregious and glaring medical and biological paradox and contradiction and serves to underscore the current irrational conundrums of what "experts" are now claiming their testing for COVID-19 means. Such insanity brings these contradictions to new heights, especially regarding the principle of vaccination as a means to evoke immunity from foreign potentially harmful microbes or toxins, or in establishing the mythical state of artificially acquired herd immunity.

If a person tests "HIV" or COVID-19 positive among which there were said to have been 33 Million in the world HIV positives a decade ago, and now some 2 million, 7 hundred thousand COVID-19 initially nucleic acid sequence positive Covid-19 positive "bat-persons" who are on the verge of being condemned to quarantine, they will be asked to submit to an experimental COVID-19 vaccine that has not even been tested for safety on rats. Within a few months and already in a few places these COVID-19 vaccines are being proposed, and governments will ask that citizens receive this world's most toxic vaccine ever devised, according to Paul Offit. This warning of Paul Offit is important to notice because it was, he who ga**ve us and our children the rotavirus vaccine (until it was immediately recalled for causing intestinal intussusception in children a few weeks after it was released).**

The same failed "scientists" and public health leaders that attempted to bring us a failed AIDS vaccine are attempting to fast-track and bring us what will turn out to be a failed Covid vaccine, at great financial waste to the US taxpayers and great threat to public health and ethics and common sense. The same failed testing paradigm that inflated HIV case statistics has been used to inflate SARS-COVID-19 statistics counting positive tests as cases instead of actual atypical pneumonias or deaths. These tests give off a majority of false positives and include both tests using the same testing package fine print available to doctors administering the tests that these tests are not intended to accurately diagnose either HIV or SARS COVID-19.

Why were not any previous potentially large-scale "epidemics" accompanied by global lock-downs or quarantines to the extent warranted today during COVID-19? The declaration of a global pandemic and global lock-down as we are currently experiencing because of a "mutated enteric CoV-2 virus" commonly found in the intestines of the family dog, bats, pangolins, ferrets, people from Wuhan, China is unprecedented in history.

What if any link is there between recent flu and hepatitis c vaccination campaigns and hospitalizations of elderly people and especially beginning in September 2019, among Northern Italians that had received several hundred thousand doses of an H1N1 vaccine followed a few months later by a somewhat less mandated and less distributed "hepatitis C" vaccine?

We also hear about these multiple hail-storms of vaccinations which have occurred recently throughout the world such as the

H1N1 mandate last Fall in Italy that was "rolled out" to hundreds of thousands of Italians, followed before years end with a "Hepatitis C" roll-out to tens of thousands of Italians again in the areas that were first most stricken with pneumonia-associated COVID influenza in December 2019. Yet from other "experts" we are told about bats, fish markets, and ferrets and other critters from which the virus "jumped" to human beings without mention of the vaccine crusades that efficiently introduced vile pathogens into hundreds of thousands and indeed in some cases millions of arms and buttocks in places like Italy, that preceded the current outbreaks, and others in recent times. By the same token and regarding COVID's and CoV-2's origins, we have heard about bats, and camels in the Middle East who became blamed as the animal vectors for MERS (Middle Eastern Respiratory SARS).

How many of the elderly people in nursing homes who died from lung problems that were blamed on Covid-19 had recent flu vaccines in the United States? Given the recent US Pentagon study proving that flu vaccines are linked to increased incidences of pneumonia where is the accountability at? We have also heard about CoV-2 vaccines trials that were deployed during the 2002-3 epidemic, and trials of COVID-19-directed vaccines last November, 2019, and about the horrendous vaccine-induced "enhancement" syndrome, which occurs when anti-CoV-2 vaccine(s) (and others) inflame or enhance the physical harm in the lungs (or other organs such as the intestines). Worse, these same injuries are associated with the natural C0V-2 infections when no vaccine is given to symptomatic individuals, but when they do occur in asymptomatic carriers, they are blamed on the illness instead of the vaccine. Such reactions as enhancement of respiratory disease occurs because of plausible immunological mechanisms evoked by vaccinations that are known as eosinophil infiltrates in the lungs, or enhanced pneumonia virulence, and a host of other side effects too long to list including death.

We have heard about asymptomatics that "carry" "the virus" and who therefore are expressing antibodies which supposedly currently protect the positive asymptomatic "victim" and will continue to be expressed as evidence of past infection, but which also as antibodies are erroneously interpreted as potentially active viruses that can erupt as many as 60 years later to cause such things as cancer of the liver, as first concluded by many studies during the 1970's hepatitis B vaccine crusade eras following Baruck Blumberg's Au antigens and liver cancers, or attributed to other disease lacking any validated pathogen such as the so-called prion diseases launched by D. Carlton Gajducek, and which provided some of the justification for the debacle known as "the AIDS" era, along with its missing virus. A few years later, we also have learned from other accounts dismissed by the "experts: as "conspiracy," that documented evidence that a new virus containing an insertion of a new nucleotides attached to C0V-2 was being prepared as early as 2016 in Chinese labs who obtained 10% of their funding from Anthony Fauci, and we even have the delusions of the person, Luc Montagnier, who gave us "HIV" to give his blessings to this claim!

The repetitive failure of both human and animal vaccination experiments is clearly revealed and evident in the somewhat randomly chosen chronological history, and which show that it is almost a certainty that most vaccine campaigns can and do frequently predict when and where small epidemics will occur and endemic syndromes and diseases will increase in frequency, concomitantly with the vaccination campaigns themselves.

GENETIC DETERMINISM IN PART HAS MADE POSSIBLE THE CURRENT COVID-19 CRISIS AND THE ORWELLIAN LOCKDOWN EXPERIENCE IT HAS ENGENDERED MUST BE ABANDONED AND REPLACED WITH AN APPRECIATION OF THE DYNAMIC RECIPROCITY TAKING PLACE IN LIVING SYSTEMS

Almost as much as the imprisonment of reason and of human beings has continued through the Centuries interrupted because of the transition from sorcery, witchcraft, religious dogma, and the view of human beings as inherently sinful to the modern world view which sees humans as inherently sick by the Church of Modern Medicine, the biological scientists and their followers who have worshiped genetic determinism have long ago thrown away the key to that prison.

Causal arguments are an inevitable consequence of misapplied statistics that happen at low frequency that are thought to cause something to happen. Let me give a real example, rather than with birds, and in the context of another so-called retrovirus, "HIV." In 2004, the American Red Cross reported that even after repeated "HIV" testing using different test kit types, that "low-risk" populations, such as blood donors (or military recruits or nuns) will typically yield 12 (PCR) positive or 2 (ELISA) positive results out of 37,000,000 million units of blood, which means that 10 out of 12 were false positives (see Footnote 14). In a follow-up analysis of this Red Cross study, it was then claimed that 6 of the 12 PCR-positive subjects tests seroconverted within several months, thereby obtaining a "HIV" molecular signature in 8/12 cases, out of 37 million negatives.

Again, these numbers could represent statistical artifact, or the several who seroconverted may represent the detection of some kind of autoimmune condition in those who test positive, like psoriasis, arthritis, physiological stress, pregnancy, or a genetic polymorphism. Multifactorial singularities like these arise and become institutionalized as causal forces or processes despite the contradiction of simple logic: if a virus X causes cancer in 1 in a million who also have that virus or its markers, then 999,999 times out of a million it does not cause cancer.

Therefore, virus X causes cancer. In simple language, a multifactorial singularity is "a cause" confounded by many factors that influence statistics. Although they frequently employ math and numerical data, multifactorial singularies have no predictive power. Sciences such as Newton's science "works," and we can fly airplanes or spaceships, or predict where a bullet or an intercontinental ballistic hydrogen bomb will land in advance, after accounting for all or most of the variables like whether, masses of objects, and the rest.

In this context, because the forces are known and measurable, it does not matter that we are still seeking "the cause" of gravity, which becomes irrelevant. 14. Stramer et al. "Detection of HIV-1 and HCV Infections among Antibody-Negative Blood Donors by Nucleic Acid Amplification Testing. New England Journal of Medicine, Volume 351:760-768, August 19, Number 8, 2004. 33 When multifactorial singularities like "HPV and cancer, or "HBV and cancer" or "HIV/AIDS" arise, and their "forces" or pathogenesis is unknown, all that becomes relevant is the imagined cause, and everyone is unequivocally assured that it is deterministic or causal that "HIV" causes AIDS, except of course, in the minds of the hypotheses' initial framers, like Rous. Luc Montagnier.

For instance, Luc Montagnier said in a recent documentary following his Nobel acceptance that: "you can catch it ("HIV") many times and if your immune system is strong you can get rid of it" no problem! (This specific interview with the Nobelist, Luc Montagnier, discoverer of "HIV" can be watched online

https://vimeo.com/29599455

Here is how that interview unfolded:

Luc Montagnier: "...I believe HIV, we can be exposed to HIV many times without being chronically infected. Our immune system will get rid of the virus in a few weeks, if you have a good immune system; and this is also the problem with African pepople; their nutrition is not very equilibrated, they are in oxidative stress, even if they are not infected with HIV, so their immune system does not work well already, so it is prone, you know, to allow HIV to get in and persist. So, there are many ways, not the vaccine, many ways to decrease the transmission, just by simple measures of nutrition, giving anti-oxidants, proper anti-oxidants-hygiene measures, fighting the other infections."

Interviewer: "If you have a good immune system, then your body can naturally get rid of HIV?" Luc Montagnier: "**Yes**."

How should such realizations and revelations impeach genetic determinism that believes that the primary sequence controls and can predict the course of a pathological disease state, especially when, in the case of SARS-COVID-19, there are far more asymptomatic individuals than there are victims reporting any symptoms. The primary sequences of SARS-CoV-2 is infecting both populations (the asymptomatic and the victims experiencing illness), and yet these statements are continually ignored by those whom we bestow science's highest Nobel awards. Yet we are repeatedly taught by the government and military-supported media campaigns such misinformation and fear. "Everyone is at risk," you can catch "it" through just one contact, you don't need co-factors, Africa's population is being decimated by a virus although it's population has doubled or increased by more people that live in the U.S. during the so-called 25 year AIDS pandemic, that an antibody positive test is something to fear, that sexually-transmitted viruses jumped from non-human primates to black persons because biologists ignore phylogenetic sequence homologies in favor of racist thinking backed by phony science, etc. But when you check the primary sources of various Nobel discoverers as they recount their glory, their hard-won hypotheses, and listen to them candidly discuss their caveats, however, it becomes clear that forces other than science and reason are at work in most if not all of our higher educational systems, medical schools, and indeed, even in elementary school science and health classes. Apparently, the views of Payton Rous, Luc Montagnier, and many others are worthy of some investigation and analysis and intense questioning, and for many of the reasons they themselves provided. With these Nobel prize-worthy suggestions, Dr. Montagnier also has in effect dusted off the Century-old argument of his own country's biomedical forerunners, Louis Pasteur, and Antoine Beuchamp, regarding the supremacy of soil or terrain versus the seed, microbe, or toxin in the development of clinically visible disease. Thus among a few biomedical researchers Like Dr. Montagnier at least, it is becoming ever more widely acknowledged even by the Nobelist who is credited with first discovering "The AIDS Virus" that the soil or terrain of the organism, and not the "seeds" or germs (or "HIV"), ultimately determines if and how much illness will result from any seed, imagined or real. 15. 34 And because Montagnier is now claiming that "we can be exposed to HIV many times without being chronically infected...because our immune system will get rid of the virus in a few weeks, if you have a good immune system," then clearly, Montagnier has sided with Antoine Beauchamp's argument, and not Pasteur's in the context of "HIV" and AIDS.

CHAPTER IV

IRRECONCILABLE DIFFERENCES AND HISTORICAL DISTORTIONS

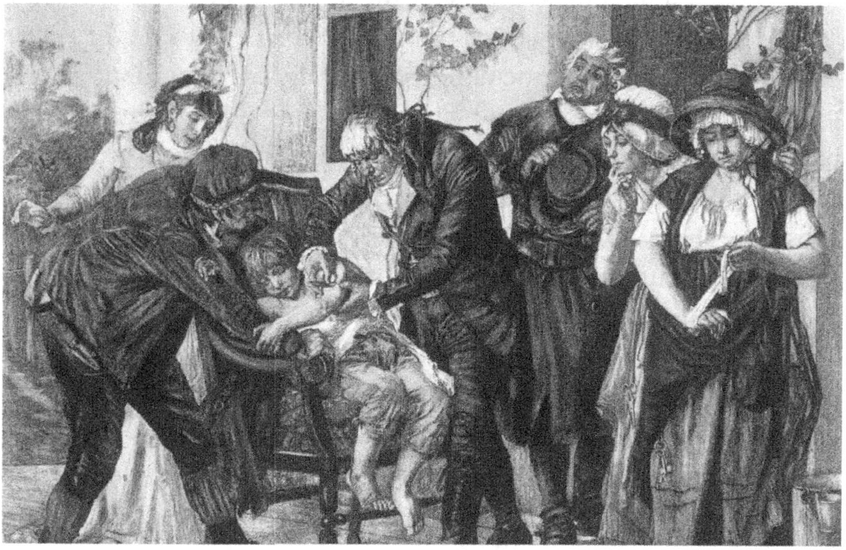

The Healthy Sick People

Living in an age of science and the intensive medicalization of our lives, it is easy to analyze things, and then criticize them, or the people and institutions with whom we associate the various pharmaceutical ads and products, or the social institutions in place that have created and maintain what we have today come to regard, trust, and react to, almost as if we were pious subjects of a religion, and this medical edifice was a kind of church.

Although it is easy to criticize consensus wisdom about illnesses and many of the therapeutic approaches that are in place as "standards of care" that are employed by medical professionals to try to deal with these maladies, it is far more difficult to fairly analyze a complex issue such as health or illness, or the therapeutic strategies and procedures in place used to maintain health and deal with sickness, and come up with good, workable, and successful solutions or viable alternatives.

For instance, as children, most of us experience vaccines as a moment of discomfort and pain we remember having experienced at the hands of a man or woman wearing a thin white robe, in a room smelling of disinfectant. Few of us then realize, or indeed ever appreciate that vaccines and inoculations are a kind of "operation" similar to the type that is done in a heart transplant, kidney transplant, or blood transfusion, albeit on a smaller scale. Similar to a transplant, we are subjected to an invasive intrusion to our systems, in which a substance that is foreign to the organism's molecular structure is introduced through a vaccine needle, and which is not "inspected" by the mucosal immune system, somewhat unlike an organ transplant where immune suppressive drugs such as cyclosporin's are used to prevent organ rejection. This simple similar relationship that vaccines share with organ transplants wreaked much pain and suffering early during the history of vaccinology due to a phenomenon that came to be known and feared called "graft-versus-host disease", a situation that would frequently occur where the infused lymph would end up rejecting the host's tissues, although in the case of vaccines, the organ that is transplanted is a soluble one (such as lymph or its components), and doesn't appear to be a solid tissue like a heart or kidney that is transplanted. Yet the surveillance mechanisms of the immune system don't care about quantity-it will react to a bee swing, mosquito bite, or spider bite using the same defenses as it would if an incompatible skin or organ were grafted or transplanted.

Introduction of foreign molecules into the body via vaccinations or inoculations is on a smaller scale than when a kidney transplant or heart transplant is carried out. When part of one's own body is transplanted elsewhere on your body, this is referred to technically as a homograft, and type of transplant from self to self typically does not cause the immune system to react to reject the graft. Xenographs (xeno is a Greek word which means "foreign" are transplants where the tissues of a different person are grafted (including blood transfusions because blood is a soluble tissue). The foreign substances introduced via vaccinates and inoculations are perceived somewhere between xenographs and homographs, but yet in some sensitive individuals, they can prove lethal, as if unmatched blood were transfused. So, in effect, substances introduced via vaccines effect a similar response on a smaller scale perhaps than transplanted organs or the transplantation of other body parts (like bone), yet they still are effectively an exposure of "non-self" to "self."

In most people, these "mini-soluble xenographs" only cause local inflammation and some pain at or around the injection site (as is always mentioned in vaccine ads), but in some "sensitive" people they can trigger massive immune responses, much as bee stings can in "bee venom-allergic people," such as anaphylaxis which can be life threatening. These soluble minigrafts also can wreak havoc in the long term, in ways that are only recently being understood.

Unmatched blood transfusions, or foreign bone grafts, or entire organ transplants also can be lethal, which is why these procedures usually require some kind of pre-treatment of the recipient of the transplant with an immune suppressive drug or procedure such as a preparatory blood transfusion. Blood transfusions also are known to effectively, if only transiently, depress the immune tissue rejection response in place of the use of cyclosporins, which are designed to repress the rejection response as long as the drug is consumed but which some studies have found to be directly carcinogenic.

When vaccines introduce foreign materials into the organism these foreign materials bypass the mucosal immune mechanisms that normally process the material and neutralize it or reject it. Whether the foreign material is bee venom, or a mosquito bite, or a heart or kidney transplant, skin graft, unmatched blood transfusion, or a vaccination or inoculation, host immune mechanisms (and there are many different mechanisms) only "care" about and react to the foreign substance if perceived as foreign by immune mechanisms, and whether it is only a small number of molecules introduced, or if it is a body part or an entire organ. If the material is perceived by the immune systems as "non-self," the immune system regards them as non-self and reacts, sometimes quite violently.

There even have been microinjection experiments using individual cells In Vitro, into which foreign cell cytoplasm is microinjected, and the recipient cells have been observed to encapsulate the microinjected foreign material and then cells will "spit" the foreign substance out (via exocytosis), or cells oxidizes the foreign material in lysosomes by exposing it to peroxide. At the tissue level and organ level, introduced foreign molecules, especially if they do not pass through the mucosal immunity systems in the portholes of the body that communicate directly with the outside world to process foreign materials (such as the lymph nodes), local histamine reactions in place are rapidly initiated (which is why vaccine makers state on their package inserts and commercials, that… "*side effects include pain and swelling at the injection site).*" These sort of reactions will occur in most recipients precisely because of this marvelous self-versus-non-self-recognition system, whereas the more severe reactions, which typically are less frequently encountered or recognized as reactions, seldom are causally linked to vaccinations, nor are they well understood or expected by most medical care givers or recipients of vaccines and inoculations, especially if they occur much later following the vaccination or inoculation, or in a place in the body at a distance from the adverse reactions occur far away from vaccine site, or much after the vaccine event. It would almost seem as if the organism always were aware of self-versus non-self, but as it turns out, it is not so simple as this, which will be discussed in some depth later.

When new vaccines or pharmaceuticals are marketed for diseases or conditions, we were not aware we had before we saw the commercials, instead of scientific discussion or a thorough medical appraisal of the potential harms (or potential long-term benefits, if any), we are presented with a suggestion: "Go ask your doctor if this vaccine is right for you." And now even your pharmacist has been given license to provide you with this or that new vaccine without accountability through a system of registration known as VAERS (the Vaccine Adverse Events Reporting System) for possible long-term vaccine side effects.

An underlying assumption from which these current advertisements and suggestions are advanced, is that human beings are no longer viewed by most modern persons **as inherently "sinful" by nature** as we were regarded before the era of Natural philosophy that gave rise to the mechanism of Natural Selection and what then followed: now, most modern humans have accepted the relentlessly and endlessly suggested notion that humans are **inherently "sick" from birth** when we are vaccinated before our immune systems are even fully functional, and remain inherently ill to the end of our lives when death usually arrives in a hospital.

The costumes and buildings of The Church have changed, but the belief systems have become even more malignant than in the past because communication has increased to such an exponential degree compared to what it used to be. Instead of crucifixes and black robes, and cathedrals of faith, these religious embellishments have been traded for stethoscopes that dangle about the necks of doctors, and the black robes traded for white robes, and the cathedrals upgraded to rebuild them into hospitals, now The Churches of Modern Medicine where the last rites are often performed with the instruments of iatrogenic-delivered disability and death. When the ear hears and then the mind comprehends these preemptive listed side effects, warnings, and contraindications during and especially at the end of the pharmaceutical ads, we are struck with the stark contradiction that what were supposed to have been "scientifically-proven" vaccines and drugs which are now being marketed and fed to millions of other "healthy inherently sick folks" like candy (who are not yet aware they are sick so they must be taught that they are by the commercial), these healthy sick folks must somehow in fact must be leading hopeful, happy lives despite their heavily drugged existence.

After intensively studying the historical record, it becomes clear that on occasion, if not frequently, that much of the imparted information about the etiology and transmission of any infectious agent associated with flu-like syndromes and many other infectious or communicable maladies contradicts itself. The virologists and others are constantly prophesying new "pandemic epidemics" we hear about daily in "breaking news" reports, and the prescription for any illness, infirmity, and aging itself, is typically pharmaceutical in nature. During almost every television show, on most networks, there is the constant clamor of unrelenting lawsuits and warnings about each drug's side-effects, while showing drug advertisements with hopeful pictures of what are advertised as extremely sick people climbing mountains or playing sports with children with smiles on their drug-managed faces, always followed, for purposes of liability, with that advertised drug's caveats. Also, this is often followed by sudden withdrawals and recalls of what were supposed to be "scientifically-proven" drugs that are marketed and fed to millions of other "healthy inherently sick folks" like candy (who are not yet aware they are sick so they must be taught that they are).

With all of this pharmaceutical and money-driven carnage that we have arrived at and have been asked to accept through most medical school training, and with the doctor's prescription pad, isn't it about time to give new promising approaches a fair chance?

The word "pharmaceutical" (φαρμακεια) or pharmacy derives from the Greek word "pharmakeia," which translates into "sorcery," or "witchcraft. Since ancient and through medieval times, potions, drugs, and other types of concoctions were associated with witches or sorcerers. Modern virologists and others are constantly prophesying about the emergence of new epidemics we hear about daily in "breaking news" reports, and the prescription for any illness, infirmity, and aging itself, now has become typically "pharmaceutical" of some kind or another. As we sit in a global "pandemic" lockdown the likes of which has never been seen and recorded to the extent and degree of uncertainty that it has currently expanded internationally, a unique opportunity has presented itself with the coming and the passing of this SARS COVID-19 global terrorist alert.

A new world view was forged after wide acceptance of the revolutionary insights of Alfred Russel Wallace, the co-discoverer of evolution via Natural Selection, and Charles Darwin regarding vaccination policies of the 1800's. With a growing acceptance of the insights provided by the book, Origin of Species and in other writings by others such as Malthus, and with the explosion of embryology and genetics that accompanied and followed this "golden" era of the life sciences, many human cultures began erecting new kinds of Churches, described best perhaps as clinics and hospital cathedrals.

The Eternal Life Prophets of the past, and their gold-painted cathedrals, staffed with their Cardinals, Bishops, Priests, and holy communions of the by-gone past slowly became transformed into the Public Health Service, physicians, insurance companies, and corporate Church of Modern Medicine. The traditions of the past were gradually merged into an unholy alliance to create new symbols of power.

The crucifixes dangling about the necks of black-robed priests of the past were now forged into stethoscopes to constantly remind of the afterlife, should our hearts suddenly stop pumping the four humors Aristotle had wrongly surmised comprise human consciousness. The black robes of the clergy were bleached white. This conveyed to the pious and the masses alike the impression of sterility, and purity.

In this unspeakable alliance, only the scenery, costumes, and communion rituals were changed. The potions and drugs concocted by biotechnology, biomedical researchers, and the Pharmaceutical witches and sorcerers were like the older potions as to their sources. They were blended from vile harmful extracts of puss and other putrid, rotting dead materials extracted from the diseased, and from fetal embryonic tissues, cadavers, and even the germs of human excrement as with the polio vaccines, and they began to be injected into small populations.

Among the newer vaccine potions in the 20th Century, highly purified tinctures called adjuvants were added along with long-lists of incomprehensible adverse reaction warning sheets accompanying each potion. The package inserts were even backed by Governments so The Priests and Cardinals and the new hospital cathedrals could avoid the dungeons of litigations, liability, and evade entire armies of "ambulance chasing" knights (lawyers) and their swift, terrifying horses (lawsuits). After all of this, Humans finally came to accept the new catechism: that humans must be inherently sick, but no longer so sinful perhaps as it was in the old times, and to have unshakable faith, allegiance, and devotion only to the Church of Modern Medicine. In the name of the Church, I pray.

PRO-VAXERS AND ANTI-VAXERS AND SEVEN OUTCOMES OF VACCINE CAMPAIGNS

The history of vaccines, and their relationship to the wellness or illness of populations is a complex issue that demands careful, scientific consideration. In some way vaccines have and will continue to touch all of our lives. The history of vaccines physically affects us as individuals, as families, and as a society. They have been associated also with severe cognitive, developmental, emotional impairments, countless autoimmune maladies, and cancers. Our pet dogs and cats suggest to us that vaccines are causally linked to cancer initiation at the sites of vaccines, and also systemic metastasis (spread). Regarding their influence on society as a whole, vaccines and the politics associated with their compulsory administrations have led to spiritual and financial devastation, and legal actions.

The evidence is indisputable that inoculations and vaccinations have had major impacts both on our physical health, as well as on our thinking and world views regarding disease resistance and disease avoidance. It is precisely for these reasons, the vaccine topic must be subjected to intense scientific investigation, instead of past and current appraisals which have been rooted in fear or dogma. An intensive study about the history of vaccines and epidemics and attempts to predict their effects on populations, or disease avoidance or attenuation (weakening of diseases) cannot be avoided any longer. Who could have foretold the coming of SARS-Co2 and COVID-19?

There are staunch proponents called pro-vaxers that advocate for universal mandatory vaccinations for every moving, breathing person, or animal in our world. There are rabid anti-vaxers who are at war with this idea, and both warring parties will sacrifice their careers, their friends, at times their legal freedom, and their entire futures to stop or promote the practice of vaccinations, and especially vaccine mandates. Anti-vaxers opposed to vaccines, have risked everything they hold dear, to have vaccinations stop. These folks sincerely believe that vaccinations and the people who promote them are ignorant or malevolent. I am one of them.

The anti-vaxers also believe that the pro-vaxers have ignored the complexity of the Human immune system, and if they did take the time to learn about it, they would see that vaccine-delivered alterations of the entire immune systems are a medical procedure to promote eugenic visions of social improvement. Vaccination is a concept hatched by Jenner so that humanity could be "immunologically-homogenized." Those doctors and Jennerian delusional believe that the responses of entire human populations can be controlled when confronted with new pathogens. In this context, biological diversity and immunological diversity are ignored while vague ideas of vaccine-acquired "herd immunity" have become advanced without critical discussion.

When the anti-vaxers regard pro-vaxers as malevolent because some pro-vaxers are clearly supporting ideas and efforts to deploy vaccines as human reproductive sterilization interventions on the scale of Nations and indeed on entire sections of the human population, it is perhaps a good time to have such a critical discussion.

When pro-vaxer arguments don't convince that vaccines can render some pathogen in the future harmless or not so harmful as it would be without vaccines, the anti-vaxers begin to beat the drums of personal freedom, and/or advocate that we make a last ditch effort to preserve what they perceived once as a sacred relationship between patients and physicians that shouldn't be interfered with by The Government. To ignore the relationship we have developed between our almost billion year-old evolving immune systems, and the universe of pathogens we live in is to deny the complexity of living systems.

Some of the delusional minds like Fauci's, Birx's, Gallo's, and Redfield's now promote the wearing of masks that cannot possibly impede the transmission of anything, not to mention an object 1,000-10,000 X smaller than the pores in the mask or the handles of the market stores that are opened, or from the shoes that you remove when you go by cheese at the grocery store.

Did these people never study micro? Or are they simple viral maniacs?

Pro-vaxers tend to operate primarily from a position of terror, in that they organize information and even political campaigns to spread the message that vaccine mandates should be in place to force vaccinations, and not to do so would risk the continuance of our entire species that could be wiped out by some deserved plague for our "sins" as was forecast prophetically in various stories and mythologies of Christianity and other religions, where deities are described, or perhaps fate itself, as having set into motion various plagues and pestilences on the people to wipe them out of some divine justice.

A new behavioral term that is now being used among pro-vaxers to describe a long-established trend and long hotly-debated issue they deem as dangerous, is gaining the support of a rather zealous following of "vaccine hesitancy watchers" and vaccine hesitancy "hit men." In recent years, this movement which began around 2016 and motivated by pro-vax groups in academia, increasingly have organized their efforts and unleashed their verbal and written assaults toward the abolition of any and all attempts to nurture "vaccine hesitancy," a term they coined to indict persons, especially parents who demand accountability and seek informed consent about what is in the vaccines that the giant pharmaceutical companies want to inject into their children, which essentially means the positing of questions or doubts about increasingly hostile mandates directed at school aged children, now seniors because of COVID-19, and everybody else. Great way to make a little extra cash at the autistic and allergy epidemics of our overly vaccinated children. Sign me up and I will vaccinate your grandma and your premature infant. A growing list or both peer-reviewed and non-peer reviewed publications describing the phenomenon and feared outcomes of vaccine hesitancy are listed in the National Library of Medicine's publication listings on MEDLINE (the on-line National Library of Medicine), which collectively describes the growing reluctance and trepidation of "vaccine-hesitant" parents to rush their kids or themselves off to their beloved physician, to the Walgreens pharmacist, or to their non-licensed or licensed apprentice, or to some other unaccountable vaccine provider such as emergency room admits, to get jabbed with the most recent, usually untested vaccine (even at times without permission). For example, the National Library of Medicine's free listings website PuBMed.Gov (https://pubmed.ncbi.nlm.nih.gov/?term=vaccine+hesitancy) has posted as of 12/01/ 2020, 1,300 results on the topic of vaccine hesitancy.

If this growing trend of **vaccine hesitancy** were allowed to go unchecked and to come into wide practice according to Medline-published pro-vaccine "logic," the outcome of hesitancy and resulting possibility of vaccine non-compliance or allowing opportunity for parental informed consent, could mean the extinction of humanity, due to vaccine-preventable mass plagues such as chickenpox, mumps or measles, or from diseases that strike 1 in 10,000 and of those which spontaneously resolve such as hepatitis B (more about this in a moment)

Here is the most recent Medline posting on vaccine hesitancy, which will become significant later in this analysis, because it was contributed by Italian authors who, since the mid-2000's, have increasingly been part of an Italian National effort to increasingly force vaccinations on their people, by issuing both legal and financial mandates and threats of incarceration as they have done here in the US for some time, and which in 2019 became one of the world's epicenters for COVID-19 following two mandated new vaccines given within 3 months of each other, between September 2020 (an H1N1 flu vaccine), and in late December, 2020 (a brand new never before tested "Hepatitis C" vaccine, which arguably never has been isolated and photographed. Here is that most recent posting on PUBMED:

Mattia Casua,[1] Frederico Toth.[2] The 2017 Italian reform on mandatory childhood vaccinations: Analysis of the policy process and early implementation. Health Policy doi: 10.1016/j. healthpol. 2020.11.004. Online ahead of print. Affiliations1. Ca' Foscari **University of Venice, Italy. 2. University of Bologna, Italy. DOI:10.1016/j.healthpol.2020.11.004**

Abstract

Background: ***The data on vaccination coverage*** *for the year 2016* ***were a cause of concern for the Italian government****. For some years, in fact, there has been a growing mistrust of vaccines in Italy, and consequently vaccination coverage rates have been decreasing. The number of cases of measles has been particularly high.*

Aim: *The purpose of this article is to examine the content and the preliminary outcomes of the Lorenzin* **Decree,** *which was passed in* ***2017*** (the authors of this article studied these data for 3 years). ***This reform embodies a 'hard' approach to the issue of childhood vaccinations, based on their mandatory nature and on the intensification of the sanctions against non-compliant subjects.***

Results: *The Lorenzin decree provides for* ***an increase in mandatory infant vaccines from four to ten****. Following the reform,* ***unvaccinated children are denied access to nurseries and kindergartens. Parents who do not have their children vaccinated are liable to pay a financial penalty****. Data on the preliminary outcomes of the reform show an increase in vaccination coverage.*

Conclusion: *The Italian experience provides some policy recommendations and* ***could be a source of inspiration for European countries that are tackling vaccine hesitancy and declining vaccination coverage rates. At least for the short term, the 'hard' approach adopted by the Italian government is, in fact, bearing fruit, having reversed the negative trend in vaccination coverage rates.***

Keywords: Childhood vaccination; Immunization coverage; Italy; Mandatory vaccinations; Policy Tools; Vaccine hesitancy.

Copyright © 2020 Elsevier B.V. All rights reserved. **Conflict of interest statement.** Declaration of Competing Interest The authors report no declarations of interest. Bull—–shit!

Yet a similar level of terror characterizes the anti-vaxers as well, as they see the "poisoned needle" they so loath as the harbinger of no other fate than disability and death linked to brain disorders, immunological disorders too long to list, and 2 out of 3 young children surviving to early adulthood as autistics, mental wrecks, and a prime reason that entire swaths of humanity have suffered and will continue suffering with a variety of behavioral disorders or worse, life-long issues with arthritis, Bell's palsy, epilepsy, and other severe afflictions that cannot all possibly be listed in something as large as an encyclopedia of thick medical books. The anti-vax propaganda continues to be vigilant to the predictions that vaccines cause epidemics and will eventually be seen to constitute the prime reason that 2 out of 3 children will be autism spectrum disorder or brain damage victims by 2030, or so certain projections have forecast.

Because this highly polarized and hateful schism has gone on for Centuries among equally naive yet dedicated and determined people, it is important to clearly state that the vaccine question is not a simple pro or con binary issue: the polarized pro-vax/ anti-vax

issue (a two-party system) must be approached much like Frederick Nietzsche's philosophy that he painstakingly described in his book, **Beyond Good and Evil** explains. Thinking about an issue as complex as epidemics and vaccines is far too complex to try to reduce it to "Good versus Evil," "right versus wrong," good versus bad, etc. Careful study of the history of vaccinology and epidemics and endemic diseases indicate that it is time that minds open up to new conceptual frameworks in the context of immunity, epidemics, natural versus artificially acquired resistance, beginning with at least seven possible distinguishable outcomes regarding the vaccine question that go way beyond the past and current pro-vax and anti-vax arguments (and "two party system) that has been in place since the early 1800's.

THE SEVEN OUTCOMES OF VACCINE CAMPAIGNS

It may surprise many to learn that the deontology associated with whether to allow vaccine mandates or not may not be a simple pro or con, for or against, decision, but may involve as many as an awareness of at *least* the 7 different individual and population-wide outcomes of vaccinations (and inoculations) that have been observed in the historical chronology of epidemics and vaccinations that will be presented in detail in Section II, and will be clearly revealed chronologically in the Great Vaccine timeline and Great Reset. The 7 vaccination outcomes are the following:

1. **vaccines and inoculations do nothing to most individuals in a population as if people were injected with a shot filled with water;**
2. **vaccines and inoculations do nothing to prevent diseases or future epidemics, yet the failure of predicted epidemics to arrive in the future is attributed to high vaccine compliance rates;**
3. **vaccines and inoculations cause disease definitions and disease classifications to change during or following vaccination**

or inoculation crusades. This outcome is typically seen when evidence for vaccine efficacy in preventing illness or epidemics is not observed (which usually is the case), or when instead of beneficial outcomes, substantial harm is immediately or within a short period of time following the vaccine roll-out observed in small groups or in populations (e.g. acute flaccid paralysis or polio was renamed and rep-classified as encephalitis following the acute flaccid paralysis explosion of acute infantile and childhood paralysis cases that occurred during and following the 1950's emergency Nation-wide response to rapidly withdraw the polio vaccines of Sabin and then Salk, following the failure of both the attenuated vaccine-delivered polio vaccine of Salk (which was withdrawn within weeks of its release-see Bookchin and Shoemaker's account of this period of the history of polio). For example, there is evidence that the oral polio vaccine currently of creating several small polio epidemics in India and in Nigeria as part of the WHO's and Gates Foundation's drives to promote polio vaccines in these Nations, which was followed by polio being renamed and reclassified as encephalitis. This same disease designation name change occurred also following the acute flaccid paralysis explosion of acute infantile and childhood paralysis cases that occurred during and following the 1950's emergency Nation-wide response to rapidly withdraw the polio vaccines of Sabin and then Salk's. (See Bookchin and Shoemaker's account of this period of the history of polio). Currently the Sabin oral polio vaccine is creating polio epidemics in India and in Nigeria as part of the WHO's and Gates Foundation's drives to promote polio vaccines in these Nations;

4. vaccines cause small outbreaks/harm small populations when the pathogens or toxins contained in the vaccine are not adequately attenuated or inactivated.
5. vaccines can spread the disease vaccinated against to people who either are or are not vaccinated: in other words,

vaccinated persons who acquire the illness against which they were vaccinated can spread the disease to others;

6. **vaccines cause different diseases in humans than vaccines are supposed to immunize against, and a review of the data presented in The Great Timeline and The Great Reset surrounding the smallpox, Great Influenza, and polio eras support this idea;**
7. **vaccines may alter the natural resistance of populations and thereby confound any and all efforts that are aimed at trying to scientifically acquire a better understanding the natural evolution of immunologic diversity.**

And I would like to suggest a new (#8) outcome which I experienced while raising my kids: vaccines increase the rate of allergies in young populations.

Regarding consequence 7 of vaccine campaigns, that if vaccines and inoculations IN THEORY artificially induce a population-wide state of resistance through vaccinations (and inoculations)-and a state erroneously known as vaccine-acquired herd immunity from a suspected pathogen is successfully achieved, why does this intervention fail every year in the context of the seasonal flu vaccines that are strongly mandated or strongly recommended (especially for school-aged children and the aged), and which is in some settings are required upon hire or military service. Navy crews that are confined to ships are 100% vaccinated and re-vaccinated as discussed earlier, and these small 100% vaccinated crews should achieved herd immunity, judging from how many times some of them are re-vaccinated, but sailors fall ill anyway, as reported quite faithfully by ship's physicians in their medical logs. And countries like Oman, or in other contexts which have on occasion achieved greater than 95% vaccine compliance such as Hawaii with smallpox vaccine, have shown that this artificial means of inducing immunity of the herd with vaccines or inoculations does not work, and outbreaks of the diseases vaccinated against always occur among the vaccinated.

The alteration of natural resistance of populations, is the most problematic and difficult to understand (**#7** on the previous page). The concept of naturally-acquired versus vaccine-acquired "herd immunity" present both real and theoretical conceptual conundrums about everything biologists and life scientists of all disciplines fundamentally agree with in the context of evolution and natural selection. The theory of herd immunity runs contrary to how it is thought that populations through geological time periods have survived without vaccines or inoculations.

The fields of evolutionary ecology and population genetics have both legitimately concluded for more than a Century, that a population's collective yet variable response against each previously encountered or never before encountered selective pressure depends on the population's diversity rather than its uniformity (in the case of immunology and vaccinology the selective pressure is a foreign pathogen or external foreign antigen, be it introduced through natural exposure or through vaccine-introduction). Variability and diversity of immunological response also is likely an important part of the diverse and ultimately robust immune response that Natur e Select s (at a population level of all potential immune responses, the fitness of that population to the environment), and which ultimately leads to health or disease in a universe swimming with pathogens encountered during the ontogeny and phylogeny of life of both individuals and populations of individuals among phylogenetic groups.

Agriculturalists and animal breeders have depended on for uncounted centuries that a little phenomenon called natural variation in populations and hybrid vigor are in almost every if not all populations observed, and which is present in all Kingdoms of living systems.

In biological systems and communities, it has been long appreciated that populations of plants or animals that are intentionally engineered or manipulated to generate either genetic and phenotypic uniformity or both in agriculture (or among animals that are exploited for food, breeding, or for imagined beneficial objectives sought after for increased usefulness via selective breeding in animal husbandry) are less apt to be robust or survive if and when an unanticipated or novel selective pressure should descend or arrive in a new bio-geographical area. Novel exposures of populations to selective forces which can in principle sicken or possibly become extinct precisely because there are not any variants among the population that will at random, be sufficiently different to be able to be unaffected by or resist that specific selective pressure assault, simply because they are all genotypically and phenotypically the same. One of the great examples of this fact was appreciated as far back as England during its industrial revolution.

VACCINES AS A SELECTIVE FORCE ON THE HUMAN IMMUNE SYSTEM

Vaccinologists, and pro-vaxers, whether they realize it or not, by proposing to jab 100's of millions of humans with the same antigen, or 4.9 Billion humans as the WHO proposed several years ago in response to what they believed was an "unstoppable H1N1 Pandemic about to strike, is in effect an attempt to "homogenize" the human immune response:

> ***"In 2009, Gregory Hartl, a spokesperson for the WHO Global Alert and Response initiative, and Dr. Marie-Paule Kieny, Director for Vaccine Research at the WHO organization said that H1N1 Pandemic is unstoppable and therefore all countries will need access to vaccines (funded by Bill and Melinda Gates) and that they want to vaccinate 4.9 billion people."***

In effect, perhaps a better way of appreciating the magnitude and importance of this issue is to review the evolutionary biological insight that was among the first to identify the plasticity of populations in response to an unequivocally newly encountered selective pressure.

The phenomenon became known among students of evolution as "industrial melanism. "Industrial melanism" was a name given to a novel phenomenon that was documented at the height of England's industrial revolution when there were enormous quantities of smoke being belched out of chimneys during their industrial revolution for the first time in human history. During this period of industrial growth, the population numbers of a species of white indigenous moths that was known by entomologists to populate and inhabit the birch trees in the British forests began to decline sharply. After the industrial revolution's waste began to accumulate and alter the environment, the naturalists noted that as the pollution and soot released by the newly built factories began to accumulate on the white bark-bearing birch trees, the trees began to turn a dingy gray from accumulating soot in the air, and the moth's natural bird predators had an enhanced ability to spot the white moths against the dingy-gray trees.

Over a period of several seasons, it was noticed that the moth population had drastically plunged to near extinction. As an indigenous species of pure white moths, thought to be long adapted in their pure-white coloring which concealed them against the white birch trees which were their home moths which concealed them from their avian predators, stood out like sore thumbs on the graying background as the industrial depositing of wastes and airborne soot increased. As a result, these moths became 'easy pickings' for birds their natural predators.

One observant entomologist, however, noted that a small subgroup of gray anatomically identical moths began to populate the graying birch trees and their population began to expand in numbers. This in effect was one of the first earlier and convincing confirmations of Darwin's and Wallace's Natural selection process by independent investigators who had been trying to solve an entirely different mystery than either Darwin or Wallace encountered on the voyages of The Beagle.

Although it is only theoretical, it is possible that vaccinations of entire populations are akin to industrial melanism in so far as the "soot" being deposited are the antigens in the vaccines, and if administered to entire populations, can run the risk of "selecting" a particular immune response among entire human populations. The selective force, being the vaccine antigens, and the vaccinologists and industrialists that unceasingly and carelessly promote them without evidence of safety or efficacy run the same risk that the white moths experienced on the newly and uniformly "soot-covered" birch trees. The universal vaccine advocates, if they are granted the power to enforce their vaccination mandates universally or among entire populations of countries, could theoretically disable the adaptive natural diverse collective population immunity that likely has been operational and in place before multicellular organisms and the specialization of tissues occurred in evolution due to naturally acquired, rather than artificially acquired presentation of antigens. Do they really have that right?

Perhaps the immunologist's and vaccinologist's intention was that by injecting the same identical antigen (molecularly foreign substance) directly into the tissues of every member of a vaccinated population, that a result being pursued could take form as a collectively uniform and thus predictable immune response of entire human populations which could therefore and somehow be uniformly protected, or made to process and respond to the introduced antigen in a stereotypical and predictable way and uniformly neutralize that antigen again or render it weaker, if it should appear in the future.

Yet this intention to direct or control the biological resistance of populations of living systems has been attempted many times in the context of vaccinations, and also in many different biological contexts. For example, in 1989, the country of Oman experienced a widespread paralysis outbreak six months after achieving **a complete vaccination rate**.

R. W. Sutter MD., A Patriarca MD., S. L. Cochi MD, et al. **Outbreak of paralytic poliomyelitis in Oman: evidence for widespread transmission among fully vaccinated children**. The Lancet Volume 338, Issue 8769, Pages 715-720, 21 September, 1991.

And again, it was reported a decade later in a report authored by some of the members of that same 1991 team group in an article entitled: Poliomyelitis in Oman. II. Toward eradication. Acta Tropica Volume 80, Issue 2, Pages 131-138 22 October, 2001 that:

> ***"In the past decade, the Sultanate of Oman has experienced three outbreaks of paralytic poliomyelitis—a widespread polio type 1 epidemic in 1988/1989, four cases of polio type 3 in three different regions in 1991, and a localized type 1 outbreak in 1993. The lessons learnt from each of these epidemics have guided us to modify and improve our polio eradication activities. Currently, these activities include administration of five primary and three booster doses of trivalent oral polio vaccine, yearly national immunization campaigns (NIDs) since 1995 with coverage of >90%, localized immunization campaigns, acute flaccid paralysis (AFP) surveillance which involves reporting of all cases by facsimile to the Department of Surveillance within 24 h of detecting a case and weekly zero reporting from 22 sentinel sites, and virological testing of stool specimens of all AFP cases and their close contacts at the national, World Health Organization accredited laboratory. The cumulative success of these activities has resulted in Oman being free from polio for the past 6 years. However, the possibility of importation of wild poliovirus, particularly from southern and western Asia still exists."***

This period of time spanning a decade of human vaccination experiments on the people of Oman does not support any theory that postulates that a stereotypical vaccine-provided theoretical protective response is something to strive for or desire in the first place or can be achieved. The "localized type 1 outbreak" in 1993 they reported occurred following 2 full years of immunizations (presumably between 1991-1993) which followed the claimed 1991 100% rate they reported may lend insights about the delusion (s) regarding herd immunity that will be discussed in some depth later on. Suffice it to say here regarding the decade-long experience in Oman, and despite its claimed 100% vaccine rate in in 1991 that resulted 2 years later in "a localized type 1 outbreak" in 1993, does not lend confidence in the protective efficacy of this (or any other) polio vaccine crusade.

In fact, in other countries, and during many times in the recorded histories of "local epidemics" and vaccine crusades, it has been noticed a number of times that ***the abatement or cessation of widespread (not necessarily universal) vaccinations resulted in an almost immediate and nearly complete eradication of normally-experienced disease cases that disappeared after the vaccine was discontinued.*** For example, in 1886-1892 in Australia when a few children died as a result of smallpox vaccinations, the government abolished compulsory vaccination in that country and smallpox suddenly declined to the vanishing point. Australia had only three cases of smallpox in 15 years as compared with Japan's record of **165,774** cases and **28,979** deaths from this cause in only 7 years **under compulsory vaccination and re-vaccination**.

Many in the biomedical community are mourning the fact that much of virology has been absolutely worthless and non-predictive of real events because they see the disconnect that is happening currently with the emerging and growing population of asymptomatics, compared to the vanishingly low death rates due to atypical pneumonias (SARS), which continue to hover at less than 1% in most places, to the point that an overall death rate of 0.6% was claimed by ER MDs in California. California's recent death toll numbers of 0.6% of persons who died ***with*** a SARS-CoV-2-positive test result (although they may have died by drowning or cardiovascular complications of diabetes complications or severe asthma because cases including asymptomatics who test positive). Of those who died ***because*** of an atypical pneumonia-associated cytokine storm (which they acquired only typically if they had 1, 2, or more pre-existing co-morbid conditions), in all likelihood, these victims most probably had received many compulsory vaccinations in our vaccination-happy and compliant culture, and/or they were physically extremely compromised, or more than 3 generations old.

The "reported" 0.6% SARS-CoV-2 cases linked to deaths in California means that the survival rate of persons exhibiting a positive SARS-CoV2 test is in the range of 99.4%, (**or higher**) which in some places in the US is safer than driving a car.

In other words, and despite all the rhetoric and hysteria and "end of life as we have known it" speak, I have not tripped over any dead SARS-C0V-2-infected corpses that died of atypical pneumonia or a hyper-immune reactive cytokine storm on my way to the grocery store to buy cheese or coffee since February of 2020, or sightings of a contagion that warrants a global lockdown, have you? Where are the funeral pyres we were shown pictures of which occurred during past European plagues?

As it appears to be the case with most if not all-natural self-limiting epidemics, it appears to be "the soil," and not "the seed" or "nasty pathogenic coronavirus" that needs most of our attention vigilance. Rather than all efforts to contain or "kill" or control in some way the suspected "perp," SARS-CoV-2," more attention needs to be directed at the "soil" of its target.

With the positive flow of information regarding a lack of COVID-19 "cases" in Japan, places in China, several states in the US such as Idaho, and in many other places currently keeping off the radar screens of the COVID-19 lockdown, social distancing, compulsory mask-mandate enforcers, and media attention, and who also haven't instituted mandatory social distancing, compulsory mask-wearing to enter stores or public spaces, or economy-destroying lockdowns, but instead have addressed the nutritional and overall health of their normal, asymptomatic, and COVID-19 symptomatic victims alike, and who have striven to implement increased vigilance and care for their over 75 year old negative-testing, positive-testing, and asymptomatic positive "carriers" and SARS-CoV-2 stricken populations alike.

Also, great efforts and strives have recently been made toward developing and implementing non-toxic approaches to combat COVID-19 with considerable if not 100% success rates such as vitamin C infusions which began in China several months ago, and in recent months, both in China and other countries, non-ventilator-applied therapies such as hyperbaric oxygen therapy (HBOT) with its nearly 100% rate of efficacy, and in most locations, reports have been coming forth from China, Florida, Iowa, and elsewhere about 100% complete and rapid recovery rates of even the sickest victims that are treated early with HBOT. Hyperbaric oxygen has been curative in the past for most if not all hypoxic conditions as the invention of HBOT follows the principles of Boyle's and Henry's gas pressure laws and relationships (which first quantified and then could predict how gases permeate solids when under increased pressure). HBOT also can be employed with or without enriched oxygen concentrations at 1.2 ATA pressures up to 2 ATA without risk of oxygen fire or explosion as HBT (Hyperbaric Therapy) alone has shown efficacy for reversal at normox pressures (21% O2 is normal atmospheric oxygen concentration). In fact, normox HBO was used as a control for 100% O2 at the same pressures in a recent clinical trial that treated cerebral palsy victims with objective evidence for improvement in both groups. Boyle's and Henry's gas laws assure that increased pressure will force gas penetration through solids and that simply providing this oxygen at normal concentrations is enough. Evidence has emerged recently, in addition, that both HBOT and HBT has been administered to large groups of people "dived" in bus-sized and even airplane-sized hyperbaric chambers, with 0 (zero) adverse events reported.

Contrary to recent reports and fears, ventilators being used for the sickest COVID-19 atypical pneumonia victims are NOT killing people per se. It is just since their first use in January, 2020, ventilators never have been able to provide enough O2 to the victims of SARS-CoV-2 atypical pneumonias (personal communication from Dr. William Maxfield, November 5, 2020. Dr. Maxfield is a Member, contributor, and C0-Director of The Florida ORCCA network (Oxygen Rescue Care Centers of America) of HBOT providers. Dr. Maxfield is a retired Chairman from Johns Hopkins Medical School's department of Radiation Oncology and has trained a generation of current HBOT providers who have collectively organized and run the Florida-based ORCCA network of HBOT providers, and also The American College of Hyperbaric Medicine in Wisconsin and throughout the nation.

It is becoming increasingly clear, in addition, that the topics associated with our overall state of health and therefore resistance of our population, and not the wraith-like existence and imagined horrors of the pathogen or seed, should consume most of our attention. We should no longer "fear the invisible," but conquer it by means of Nature's own free gifts. Consistent with this idea are the age breakdown categories of the elderly or people with preexisting conditions who are being most heavily affected by COVID-19. Despite the hyped propaganda that is broadcast about the occasional younger cases to compel us to accept, that similar to "HIV," and "AIDS," "everyone is at risk," this so-called "public health" propaganda simply is not true.

In fact, there is no longer scientific dispute that the pre-existing conditions like heart or vascular disease, diabetes, cancer, and respiratory illnesses bias the Covid-19 morbidity and mortality data statistics.

Consistent with all diseases, SARS-CoV-2 and COVID-19 has decidedly become, once again, an issue of "soil" and not the "seed" in explaining disease and vulnerability to disease (with the CoV-2 SARS virus being the seed, and the incredibly old or previously sick demographic being the principal "soil" of the "pandemic)." Despite this information, the principal final solution that is always repeatedly suggested and intensively propagandized and financially supported are vaccines and vaccine development.

CHAPTER V

CONCLUSION

Generalizations, and Predictions Diagnostics, Aetology, and Causation Regarding Our Present Crisis and the Futures of "The Healthy Sick People" and The Science of Vaccine Damage

It should be carefully considered if it makes biological sense to assume in the first place that this "pandemic" COVID-19 disease is attached to a flu-associated malady AND fatal pneumonia. It often has been suggested, without providing any evidence or history, that COVID-19 is essentially "a repeat" of the "Great Spanish Flu" epidemic of 1918-19. To address this groundless assertion and myth, the story of Pfeiffer's bacillus and the fruitless decade-long search by Rosenau and others to show the bacillus (bacterium) was the causative agent was an important chapter in the context of the current proposed CoV-2 test kits and highlights the failure for modern diagnosticians to employ routine electron microscopic verification of viremia, and corona-like viral particles.

In Rosenau's era, the electron microscopy technology that is the only technology we have that can clearly define and resolve coronavirus particles had not been invented yet. Therefore, the resolution to see a virus was not available to Rosenau and his colleagues. In fact, the first functional EM's were not available except as curiosities to physicists until the later 1930s, yet they have been in use in pathology labs at most major metropolitan centers world-wide for many decades since then. Pathologists had known that the term "pneumonia" is a term that describes a non-specific syndrome that has been linked to many causative factors-including biological, chemical, and physical, causes, and therefore it was a rational assumption of Rosenau's group to chase a bacterium. Yet 120 years later after Rosenau's findings had been published, and without the electron microscope's confirmation for each case or an occasional case, the likely causative agent remains unknown, other co-infecting microorganisms have been mentioned, and as a result, strategies to deal with that agent are operating " blind."

Pfeiffer's bacillus had been associated with melanomas prior to the 1918-19 "pandemic," Rosenau exhaustively pursued, and then published his non-findings and failure(s) to isolate the causative agent in a 1919 publication.

A few selected examples may reinforce some of these conclusions.

There exists an extensive peer reviewed literature beginning in the 1960's that presented detailed studies that demonstrated using electron microscopy, that there were crown-shaped viral particles on the scale of 120 nanometers in diameter and shaped like crowns which could be found in people with colds. Moreover, these particles were isolated and purified by centrifugal isolation into a single band of a certain molecular weight.

According to virus isolation protocols to demonstrate etiology, one subfraction of that purified band was placed on an electron microscope grid and photographed using an electron microscope which revealed a picture of all like-sized and same shaped particles, which is important, because only electron microscopes can generate the amplitudes and frequencies of electromagnetic light that can detect virus-sized particles which exist as cellular garbage essentially below the limits of visible light wavelengths, and the first functional electron microscopes that could see this cellular garbage called viruses arrived only in the later 1930's.

Typically, according to conventions of isolation and characterization procedures involving the visualization of the infectious agent or "perp" to use a criminal justice term designating guilt of a crime, which is in these cases thought to be infectious diseases, a fraction of that same electron microscope visualized band that was photographed to assure centrifuged-created homogeneity of an isolate having its own specific density in a sucrose gradient is segregated by centrifugal force and placed into another containment vessel, and when that fraction is re-injected back into human volunteers, they acquired mild "colds," as Tyrrell and Bynoe described in their 1996 paper entitled, "***Cultivation of viruses from a high proportion of patients with colds***" in The Lancet, in 1966. This work was repeated by a series of other highly reputable authors who repeated exactly the work Tyrrell and Bycoe had published and extended the volunteers they infected to a host of military volunteers, other volunteers from different walks of life, and even children.

Modern molecular biologists, however, who are currently modeling and generating grim predictions about the current COVID-19 "pandemic" using methods that exclusively can best described as "cloning" around without rigorous ultrastructural confirmation, have provided only several published reports that do not include these essential electron microscopic micrographs of a single "victim's" viral load in combination with rigorous isolation procedures to insure that the sequence data derived from tissue or lung homogenates contains viremia and clearly visible crown-shaped virus particles. One notable exception was a study published by Z Varga, A. Flammer, P. Steiger, M. Haberechker, R. Andermatt, A. S Zinkernagel, M. R. Mehra, R. Schuepbach, F. Ruschitzka, and H. Moch, in the May 2, 2020 issue of The Lancet (Vol 395, pps. 1417-18, and in an accompanying supplemental data article they provided on April 17, 2020 which provided more detailed information about the 3 individuals that were studied.

In 2002-3 during that SARS era, a paper written by R.A.M Fauchier et al. in the Netherlands (Nature Vol 423, 15 May 2003) was published claiming that the etiological agent that caused the respiratory illness and deaths during that "pandemic" had been identified according to Koch's postulates. These authors even went so far as to entitle their paper, "*Koch's postulates fulfilled for SARS virus.*"

In this primary research article, they provide one negative contrast 200,000 x electron micrograph (EM) of 3 crown-shaped spheres in the same field, which is claimed to have been derived from the lung of one of the two macaques they experimentally infected, and "which was identical to that inoculated" (identical to the appearance of the particles of the inoculum they do not show) although that inoculate isolate's EM is not provided in this paper.

When all is said and done, one EM micrograph showing 3 particles was presented, along with of course RT-PCR associated tests, which served to launch the entire SARS emergency back in 2003.

Perhaps this is because it was not fully realized that when dealing with viral agents associated with diseases, other standards must be addressed. This is because of the fact that viruses are obligate "parasites" that require living cells to propagate themselves, unlike mycoplasma, fungal, or bacterial pathogens. This is why modern methods of why virus isolation may have to satisfy additional caveats associated with establishing etiology that other living pathogens require to claim isolation has been achieved, because it had only been clearly explained and realized that until 2017, an accumulating body of information since SARS 2002-3 had suggested that In Vitro viral cultivation tends to severely attenuate viral virulence, and conversely, that passaging a viral strain in ovo or in small animal hosts can lead to an amplification of viral virulence, which was first clearly articulated to the general scientific audience in a publication written by J. Prescott, H. Feldmann, and D. Safronetz, in final edited form in Antiviral Research (January, 2017, pps. 1-9).

In this critical review article of Prescott et al., many key issues regarding viral vaccines, and vaccines in general become clear and are worth briefly reviewing here because once these facts are identified and appreciated, it becomes easier to draw conclusions about the changing nature of antigens of all kinds once they are in the hands of researchers, especially those involved in the production of vaccines.

Our companion animal friends, our beloved dogs and cats, are subjected to their yearly vaccination experiments each year, upon the threat to their owners of having to pay huge fines or even face incarceration, if their "tags" are not up to date, while they continue to develop cancers at or near the site of their vaccine injuries, or within brief time windows afterward and which the vaccine-induced malignancies systemically spread and killed them.

In a circular issued in 1884, and up to the time of the Royal Commission widely distributed with the approval of the Local Government Board it is stated that: "Soldiers who have been re-vaccinated can live in cities intensely affected by small-pox without themselves suffering to any appreciable degree from the disease." Wallace then goes on to state that: "I will now show you that this statement is absolutely false and presents the appropriate statistics to justify this conclusion.

At the end of this rather startling document, Wallace states on the bottom of Page 2 and 3 that: It is thus absolutely demonstrated that it is the exceptionally unvaccinated that possess the exceptional advantages, while the " exceptionally revaccinated " Army and Navy show quite exceptional disadvantages in a small-pox mortality during the same twenty years, more than four times as great as the exceptionally unvaccinated town of Leicester !

But the learned men of the Royal Commission never put these two facts side by side, so that the Government and the public might draw their own conclusions from them. So far as their Final Report shows, these gentlemen were ignorant or oblivious of the very existence of these facts, which conclusively prove that vaccination is not only a worthless but an injurious operation—a Gigantic Medical Imposture!

For the reasons now stated, we call upon voters of all parties to refuse support to every candidate who upholds the legal or other enforcement of vaccination, which, as we have shown, both spreads disease and increases mortality. No government has the right to order healthy infants to be blood-poisoned, under the pretense of protection against a danger that may never arise. The abolition of all laws enforcing or encouraging vaccination is therefore of more immediate and vital importance than any party dogma or any political programme. Note. (The evidence against vaccination and the mis-statements of doctors and officials are fully and clearly set forth in the author's pamphlet—" Vaccination a Delusion," to be obtained from the National Anti-Vaccination League, price 10|d., post free. ISSUED BY THE NATIONAL ANTI-VACCINATION LEAGUE, 50, Parliament Street, Westminster, London, S.W).

Natural Selection is important to address regarding the topic of pandemics, epidemics, and endemic disease, and also in the context of inoculations and the heavily publicized promoted "miracle cure" or dampening effect on Co-2 SARS vaccines in general, and COVI-Disease in particular.

A fundamental question raised is do we know or can we know if artificially acquired "herd immunity" is something that is desirable in the first place for a species, or might it be something to fear and avoid because it may antagonize Natural immunological diversity, or "species-wide heterogeneity," which has been a fundamental tenet that has insured our survival. The fundamental ideas of biology suggest that the continued evolution of all living systems depends upon variation, and a natural diversity.

In this same general context, and as the vaccine "immunization" and as the dream of an artificially acquired immunity envisions, if humans believe that vaccines protect them, then why should they insist on others being vaccinated if they believe they themselves are protected by the vaccine they received?

This would be akin to two next door neighbors living with their driveways adjacently positioned, and neighbor "A" believes that a wax coating he smears on his car will protect it from rust. If he believes the wax (vaccine) will protect his car from rusting, then why should he or she insist that neighbor "B" who lives next door, and whose car is parked only 6 feet away, refuses to wax their car? If the belief of neighbor "A" in wax's protective effect is justified, then is it logical that neighbor "A" should be imprisoned for 30-60 days, or fined $ 1000.00 or both, as Mayor DeBlasio threatened the Orthodox Jews in Brooklyn if they did not submit to a measles vaccine within 48 hours?

Also, the virologists mythical desired goal of artificially acquired "herd immunity" is a concept that is in direct violation of the benefits of natural variation known to occur in populations as has been time tested and found in a variety of contexts after the repeated observations that Wallace and Darwin originally described regarding natural variation of traits have been confirmed without exception, since these ideas were first proposed. It is also possible, for instance, that within a nearly 100% naturally immunized population that had perhaps acquired this immunity from past exposures, or perhaps not, a little property of all living systems to exhibit "resistance" for reasons that are not known (which of the many postulated theoretical specific immune reactions) may be responsible for this demonstrated refractoriness of the recipient to an infectious agent.

The theoretical population homogeneity of the virologists and vaccinologists envisions instead with this concept of artificially acquired herd immunity in place, is that a state of [immunological] sameness of exposure to some pathogen will protect against this pathogen if it is ever encountered, or when they hedge their theory, claim that the vaccine will lesson an infection when it strikes, and thwart its full infective potential, offering partial protection.

The virologists and vaccinologists propose that such a state of immunity happens naturally when immunological sameness rather than variation is sought through universal vaccine mandates and somehow becomes mysteriously established when immunological homogeneity is (theoretically) artificially induced via a universal vaccine crusade.

It may be worthwhile asking, when will these theorists begin to realize that every earthworm, snake, bird, whale, duck, artichoke, bacterium, skunk, pangolin, and any other organism you can think of that is still here living on earth, is a living shining example of herd immunity to the pathogens that have been here for about 1 billion years. Can some great hidden truth about human history's past or assumptions that is built on the quicksand and nameless mist of predictions and assumptions about human destiny be summoned to rescue this hundreds of year-long war from the ashes of perpetual waste? There must be some higher principle, some higher calling to understand our fate.

Yet the immunologists and vaccinologists somehow still want us to believe their twisted logic, that their mission to immunologically homogenize every human being on the planet with the same antigen will confer something they refer to as this mythical state of herd immunity. As this magical thinking is believed, for example, among vaccinologists and many microbiologists, "herd immunity" has existed as a natural indirect protection mechanism of all populations in all biological processes and situations that require the need to distinguish "self" from "non-self."

It is believed also and as an unproven and unsubstantiated idea, that unvaccinated individuals in the population who are in "hiding" from Pharma's vaccine needles, or who are too poor or uneducated to comply or be made to comply even through compulsory vaccination, will not threaten this magical state of herd immunity if a certain "threshold" of vaccinated or prior infected individuals exists, either naturally through past natural exposure, or through vaccination. This thinking provides a satisfying explanation, and also an epidemiological conundrum.

If the elderly aren't among a population of vaccinated, they are dismissed as having probably acquired immunity from some exposure to the current pathogen long ago, before any vaccines were invented. Based on this logic, it follows that if enough of a threshold of vaccine compliance is met, then any non-vaccinated folks (either who refused vaccines or lived in ghettos not accessible to government brow-beating to vaccinate) will be unlikely to either transmit a viable pathogen since the vaccinated will have somehow been magically protected, as if car wax had been smeared all over them before a rainstorm.

Yet these vaccine- recalcitrant refuseniks that remain unvaccinated will not be able to spread the pathogen to the majority of "the washed" who aren't "carriers," regardless of whether or not they have natural resistance, or have vaccine acquired resistance, since all of these groups will be immune, it is claimed after artificially acquired herd immunity of even 60%-80% antibody seropositivity is achieved through forced vaccination (depending on whose definition of herd immunity you accept…should we pick to run with the 59% compliance group, or the 62% vaccine-compliance group)?

THERE IS A SOLUTION: THE INVENTION OF THE TOILETS AND DEVELOPMENT OF THE CONCEPT OF HYGIENGE PROBABLY HAS BEEN MORE VALUABLE THAN VACCINES AND PROBABLY CONSTITUTES THE BEST PUBLIC HEALTH MEASURE YOU WILL EVER FIND ANYWHERE

There can be little doubt that there have been many hygienic, technological, and health-related improvements that have played the most significant and major roles in the prevention of both epidemic and endemic diseases, in recent history and during antiquity. The flushable toilets of the Greeks at Knossos Crete (2,000 BC), and the Roman aqueducts of Christ's era serve as two such examples of such technological advancements.

In this direction, if and when scientifically valid associations between vaccines, epidemics, and endemic disease are more fully understood, and as a consequence when harm is avoided, hopefully the conceptual advances this chronology delivers will serve to improve human health and well-being, and hopefully ward off tragedy due to misinformed thinking, irrational practices, fears, and eugenic ideas. Most importantly perhaps, the following information should raise the critical question: what is the evidence that even universal (100%) vaccination of a population will generate herd immunity, or are there perhaps better preventative measures that have been implemented already in the context of epidemics or even pandemics, or perhaps even better, rational ways already within our reach to increase natural resistance to avoid epidemics and lower endemic disease's consequences and suffering? What if debilitating syndromes such as autism spectrum disorders that are expected to affect 1 in

3 children by 2030 materialize as statistics predict with the current yearly increase rates, or other syndromes such as asthma, arthritis, cognitive disorders, and a plethora of other vaccine-associated illnesses materialize? What is the human and financial cost to our civilization? Can we afford to be complacent?

The vaccine issue is not polarized only between only pro-vaccine or anti-vaccine belief paths or belief systems, but at least seven other belief systems which are not often discussed or even recognized as therapeutic strategies or diagnostic criteria also have played critically important roles in what all of us come to believe about vaccines and the nature of human illnesses, or which strategy to deploy against them most successfully. Indeed, these more amorphous often bio-philosophical or epistemological issues have largely been neglected.

One good example of a relatively widely accepted and more or less non-controversial issue in most discussions about vaccines is the principle identified as herd immunity. Currently vaccine acquired immunity exploits the McFarlane Barnett idea of clonal selection, as opposed to some other theories of how the immune system and immune response operates. When carefully analyzed, these axioms of disease and therapeutics come with many conditions and caveats. For instance, the idea of herd immunity clashes with a broader biological concept that has been identified in many systems that are believed to maintain their existence precisely because of the diversity of individuals in a population.

Diversity insures that that variants will exist in a group of similar individuals and that because of this diversity variants will exist that are sufficiently different and that are more likely to withstand by virtue of that difference escape (unexpected, unknowable selective pressures forces that will by the nature of natural selection select the species as a group to persist that are most fit to carry on its kind as a population, while weeding out the population type less fit, or which by that species vulnerability, are "unfit" to carry on its kind over generations). The type of causality involved in this concept is a concept of efficient causes, not final causes or first causes, as has been discussed at some length in this indictment.

Yet, the apparent crisis that has justified global lock-downs and quarantines that are now attached to COVID-19 has never escalated into global planet-covering lock-downs or quarantines in most if not any of these other past (or present) declared epidemics. This may be because of a growing understanding of human physiology and how it interacts with the rest of the universe, including pathogens, or it could in part be due to the increased technological expansion of world-wide communication which also has been rapidly evolving even in our own life-times.

In fact, within the last 1000 years, the only epidemics on record that have described in terms epidemic and never with the word, pandemic, and which have justified local quarantines and lockdowns have been some of the plague epidemics, leprosy epidemics, small pox epidemics, and the several polio epidemics which occurred at different times-during the inoculation and then vaccine crusades of the late 1800's, early 1900's, and mid-1950's, that may have risen to the level of hysteria we see with COVID-19. The so-called polio epidemic distancing that did occur, however, were not as draconian as COVID-19: records show that people were temporarily banned from congregating in theaters and schools during the eras of paralysis "epidemics."

Perhaps it is no coincidence that we are faced with the same ethical and public health crisis policy conundrums today that Americans of the early decades of the late 1800's and early 1900's had to navigate through with the yellow fever epidemic in which blood-letting and mercury was still being applied for its victims, or the New England paralysis "epidemic" that later became associated with the late 1800's calcium arsenate poisonings of the tree orchards in New England and elsewhere. Calcium arsenate is an important environmental pollutant still today, and dominates much of the modern ground water pollution and contamination literature, because iron, lead, and calcium carbonate-rich rocks absorb arsenic, as do New Englanders who consumed a lot of fruit and developed paralysis. During the Great Spanish Flu epidemic of 1918 that followed the first mandatory vaccinations of WWI soldiers, or during the closing of many movie theaters and many schools during the 1950's and 1960's polio era during the height of the DDT era when the disease was believed to be spread by flies when DDT was being sprayed even in kitchens and on food why were not some or all of the same large-scale "epidemics" accompanied by global lock-downs as we are currently experiencing, or even culture-specific or country-wide lock-downs implemented during various National epidemics?

Some believe that these infertility inducers via vaccinations have been planned, but this is not a possibility that science can definitively solve. However, it may be worth noting that this possibility has not escaped the attention of many people, especially the parents of those children and relatives who have been vaccinated as claimed by the following report:

> **"A lowered probability of pregnancy in females in the USA aged 25–29 who received a human papillomavirus vaccine injection," by Gayle DeLong, *Journal of Toxicology and Environmental Health, Part A*, Volume 81, Issue 14, Pages 661-674, DOI 10.1080/15287394.2018.1477640 and which claimed...*Results suggest that females who received the HPV shot were less likely to have ever been pregnant than women in the same age group who did not receive the shot. If 100% of females in this study had received the HPV vaccine, data suggest the number of women having ever conceived would have fallen by 2 million. Further study into the influence of HPV vaccine on fertility is thus warranted."***

Yet the editors of the journal decided to retract the article after it was published because they claimed that:

> ***"Following review and publication of the article, we were alerted to concerns about the scientific validity of the study. As a result,***

> ***we sought advice on the methodology, analysis, and interpretation from a number of experts in the field...who did not like the "interpretation of the data in this paper,"***

and so, the editors felt it was best to take the following course:

> ***"and we have therefore taken the decision to retract it. The author has been notified of our decision. The retracted article will remain online to maintain the scholarly record, but it will be digitally watermarked on each page as "Retracted".***

This is simply just another example of what we academicians call "academic freedom."

SOURCES-Disease and History, by Frederick C. Cartwright, published by Sutton Publishing, 2014; Disease: The Story of Disease and Mankind's Continuing Struggle Against It, by Mary Dobson, published by Quercus, 2007;

-Encyclopedia of Pestilence, Pandemics, and Plagues, by Ed, Joseph P. Byrne, published by Greenwood Press, 2008; -Source Book of Medical History, Logan Clendening, published by Dover Publications, 1960.Article Title: Pandemics That Changed History. Editors: History.com https://www.history.com/topics/middle-ages/pandemics-timeline.

"LET THE FOOD BE THY MEDICINE" -SEIZURES CAN BE CONTROLLED

Our chronicle began with sanity, because insanity needs a point of reference that is not perceived by insanity. Sanity knows when insanity exists, but insanity is not aware of when sanity exists. Epidemic and endemic disease syndromes caused by vaccines in populations have been and are predictable to the extent that vaccine campaigns, epidemics, and chronic endemic maladies have been frequently linked and associated, as carefully kept military records have shown throughout history. Evidence from the 1800's in the Lancet and from elsewhere shows that the medical "professionals" of that century were clearly aware of the alarming relationship between inoculation, vaccination, and morbidity, and Dr. Alfred Russel Wallace led the charge, as widely acknowledged father of biogeography, and an author of one of the most read and famous books published in all of the 1800's, entitled, **The Malay Archipelago**, which described his extensive observations and findings that were mostly about differences among insects in Malaysia and Singapore, and later his observations included and were extended to include descriptions of all types of living systems of flora and fauna he encountered in Brazil's Amazon Rainforest, such as warning colorations on poisonous animals, and the transmutation of species or "Wallace Effect" as it is still called.

Alfred Russel Wallace's later named Wallace effect described how Natural Selection *"could contribute to speciation by encouraging barriers to hybridization,"* which in turn would provide barriers to trap variations and small changes geographically. Wallace's studies of natural variations among populations of organisms in a region of closely spaced islands with morphologically slightly different groups, along with Darwin's similar observations with finches and other groups of organisms that would be published years later in On the Origins of Species completed the first grand synthesis of the theory of Natural Selection, forming the basis of modern life sciences and molecular biology and genetics.

There is much evidence that Wallace was inspired by, and inspired many naturalists in different sciences, notably the critical geological pioneer, Charles Lyell. who wrote the landmark book, **Principles of Geology** that described how younger layers of earth were overlain upon older layers which became a central tenet of evolutionary biology? He also was influenced quite profoundly as were other evolutionary naturalists of his day by the thoughts and writings of population biologist, Thomas Malthus (creator of the Malthusian curve of population growth and demise, and author of the famous treatise entitled, "**An Essay on the Principle of Population**).

The geological and population biological insights of Lyell and Malthus shook the world of natural science, when he finally grasped the fact that his conclusions were nearly identical to Charles Darwin's who provided yet another central component to evolutionary theory, namely, the concept of how well populations (from Malthus) in competition became most "fit" to their environments (rather than the commonly held erroneous belief that biological fitness or "survival of the fittest" constituted a product of any apparent advantages of individuals within a population as the raw materials of selection. Many today still refer to and advocate this as a basis to explain how trunks of elephants have become extended, or how aggressive traits of predatory cats are "selected" by time as some still unfortunately believe.

Alfred Russel Wallace synthesized what Darwin wrote in his book, " Voyage of the Beagle," and was befriended and worked with Darwin. Alfred Russel Wallace then began to pursue, advocate, and then champion the theories of evolution by means of Natural Selection being the primary mechanism by which species diverge, but perhaps more important, how certain traits are conserved.

APPENDIX I

Reference List for Christine Johnson's Article, "Whose Antibodies are they Anyway?

References

1. Agbalika F, Ferchal F, Garnier J-P, et al. 1992. False-positive antigens related to emergence of a 25-30 kD protein detected in organ recipients. AIDS. 6:959-962.
2. Andrade V, Avelleira JC, Marques A, et al. 1991. Leprosy as a cause of false-positive results in serological assays for the detection of antibodies to HIV-1. Intl. J. Leprosy. 59:125.
3. Arnold NL, Slade RA, Jones MM, et al. 1994. Donors follow up of influenza vaccine-related multiple viral enzyme immunoassay reactivity. Vox Sanguinis. 67:191.
4. Ascher D, Roberts C. 1993. Determination of the etiology of seroreversals in HIV testing by antibody fingerprinting. AIDS. 6:241.
5. Barbacid M, Bolgnesi D, Aaronson S. 1980. Humans have antibodies capable of recognizing oncoviral glycoproteins: Demonstration that these antibodies are formed in response to cellular modification of glycoproteins rather than as consequence of exposure to virus. Proc. Natl. Acad. Sci. 77:1617-1621.

6. Biggar R, Melbye M, Sarin P, et al. 1985. ELISA HTLV retrovirus antibody reactivity associated with malaria and immune complexes in healthy Africans. Lancet. ii:520-543.
7. Blanton M, Balakrishnan K, Dumaswala U, et al. 1987. HLA antibodies in blood donors with reactive screening tests for antibody to the immunodeficiency virus. Transfusion. 27(1):118.
8. Blomberg J, Vincic E, Jonsson C, et al. 1990. Identification of regions of HIV-1 p24 reactive with sera which give "indeterminate" results in electrophoretic immunoblots with the help of long synthetic peptides. AIDS Res. Hum. Retro. 6:1363.
9. Burkhardt U, Mertens T, Eggers H. 1987. Comparison of two commercially available anti-HIV ELISA's: Abbott HTLV-III ELA and DuPont HTLV-III ELISA. J. Med. Vir. 23:217.
10. Bylund D, Ziegner U, Hooper D. 1992 Review of testing for human immunodeficiency virus. Clin. Lab. Med. 12:305-333.
11. Challakere K, Rapaport M. 1993. False-positive human immunodeficiency virus type 1 ELISA results in low-risk subjects. West. J. Med. 159(2):214-215.
12. Charmot G, Simon F. 1990. HIV infection and malaria. Revue du practicien. 40:2141.
13. Cordes R, Ryan M. 1995. Pitfalls in HIV testing. Postgraduate Medicine. 98:177.
14. Dock N, Lamberson H, O'Brien T, et al. 1988. Evaluation of atypical human immunodeficiency virus immunoblot reactivity in blood donors. Transfusion. 28:142.
15. Esteva M, Blasini A, Ogly D, et al. 1992. False positive results for antibody to HIV in two men with systemic lupus erythematosus. Ann. Rheum. Dis. 51:1071-1073.
16. Fassbinder W, Kuhni P, Neumayer H. et al. 1986. Prevalence of antibodies against LAV/HTLV-III [HIV] in patients with terminal renal insufficiency treated with hemodialysis and following renal transplantation. Deutsche Medizinische Wochenschrift. 111:1087.

17. Fleming D, Cochi S, Steece R. et al. 1987. Acquired immunodeficiency syndrome in low-incidence areas. JAMA. 258(6):785.
18. Gill MJ, Rachlis A, Anand C. 1991. Five cases of erroneously diagnosed HIV infection. Can. Med. Asso. J. 145(12):1593.
19. Healey D, Bolton W. 1993. Apparent HIV-1 glycoprotein reactivity on Western blot in uninfected blood donors. AIDS. 7:655-658.
20. Hisa J. 1993. False-positive ELISA for human immunodeficiency virus after influenza vaccination. JID. 167:989.
21. Isaacman S. 1989. Positive HIV antibody test results after treatment with hepatitis B immune globulin. JAMA. 262:209.
22. Jackson G, Rubenis M, Knigge M, et al. 1988. Passive immunoneutralisation of human immunodeficiency virus in patients with advanced AIDS. Lancet, Sept. 17:647.
23. Jindal R, Solomon M, Burrows L. 1993. False positive tests for HIV in a woman with lupus and renal failure. NEJM. 328:1281-1282.
24. Jungkind D, DiRenzo S, Young S. 1986. Effect of using heat-inactivated serum with the Abbott human T-cell lymphotropic virus type III [HIV] antibody test. J. Clin. Micro. 23:381.
25. Kashala O, Marlink R, Ilunga M. et al. 1994. Infection with human immunodeficiency virus type 1 (HIV-1) and human T-cell lymphotropic viruses among leprosy patients and contacts: correlation between HIV-1 cross-reactivity and antibodies to lipoarabionomanna. J. Infect. Dis. 169:296-304.
26. Lai-Goldman M, McBride J, Howanitz P, et al. 1987. Presence of HTLV-III [HIV] antibodies in immune serum globulin preparations. Am. J. Clin. Path. 87:635.
27. Langedijk J, Vos W, Doornum G, et al. 1992. Identification of cross-reactive epitopes recognized by HIV-1 false-positive sera. AIDS. 6:1547-1548.
28. Lee D, Eby W, Molinaro G. 1992. HIV false positivity after hepatitis B vaccination. Lancet. 339:1060.
29. Leo-Amador G, Ramirez-Rodriguez J, Galvan-Villegas F, et al. 1990. Antibodies against human immunodeficiency virus in

generalized lupus erythematosus. Salud Publica de Mexico. 32:15.

30. Mackenzie W, Davis J, Peterson D. et al. 1992. Multiple false-positive serologic tests for HIV, HTLV-1 and hepatitis C following influenza vaccination, 1991. JAMA. 268:1015-1017.
31. Mathe G. 1992. Is the AIDS virus responsible for the disease? Biomed & Pharmacother. 46:1-2.
32. Mendenhall C, Roselle G, Grossman C, et al. 1986. False-positive tests for HTLV-III [HIV] antibodies in alcoholic patients with hepatitis. NEJM. 314:921.
33. Moore J, Cone E, Alexander S. 1986. HTLV-III [HIV] seropositivity in 1971-1972 parenteral drug abusers – a case of false-positives or evidence of viral exposure? NEJM. 314:1387-1388.
34. Mortimer P, Mortimer J, Parry J. 1985. Which anti-HTLV-III/LAV [HIV] assays for screening and confirmatory testing? Lancet. Oct. 19, p873.
35. Neale T, Dagger J, Fong R, et al. 1985. False-positive anti-HTLV-III [HIV] serology. New Zealand Med. J. October 23.
36. Ng V. 1991. Serological diagnosis with recombinant peptides/proteins. Clin. Chem. 37:1667-1668.
37. Ozanne G, Fauvel M. 1988. Performance and reliability of five commercial enzyme-linked immunosorbent assay kits in screening for anti-human immunodeficiency virus antibody in high-risk subjects. J. Clin. Micro. 26:1496.
38. Papadopulos-Eleopulos E. 1988. Reappraisal of AIDS – Is the oxidation induced by the risk factors the primary cause? Med. Hypo. 25:151.
39. Papadopulos-Eleopulos E, Turner V, and Papadimitriou J. 1993. Is a positive Western blot proof of HIV infection? Bio/Technology. June 11:696-707.
40. Pearlman ES, Ballas SK. 1994. False-positive human immunodeficiency virus screening test related to rabies vaccination. Arch. Pathol. Lab. Med. 118-805.

41. Peternan T, Lang G, Mikos N, et al. Hemodialysis/renal failure. 1986. JAMA. 255:2324.
42. Piszkewicz D. 1987. HTLV-III [HIV] antibodies after immune globulin. JAMA. 257:316.
43. Profitt MR, Yen-Lieberman B. 1993. Laboratory diagnosis of human immunodeficiency virus infection. Inf. Dis. Clin. North Am. 7:203.
44. Ranki A, Kurki P, Reipponen S, et al. 1992. Antibodies to retroviral proteins in autoimmune connective tissue disease. Arthritis and Rheumatism. 35:1483.
45. Ribeiro T, Brites C, Moreira E, et al. 1993. Serologic validation of HIV infection in a tropical area. JAIDS. 6:319.
46. Sayers M, Beatty P, Hansen J. 1986. HLA antibodies as a cause of false-positive reactions in screening enzyme immunoassays for antibodies to human T-lymphotropic virus type III [HIV]. Transfusion. 26(1):114.
47. Sayre KR, Dodd RY, Tegtmeier G, et al. 1996. False-positive human immunodeficiency virus type 1 Western blot tests in non-infected blood donors. Transfusion. 36:45.
48. Schleupner CJ. Detection of HIV-1 infection. In: (Mandell GI, Douglas RG, Bennett JE, eds.) Principles and Practice of Infectious Diseases, 3rd ed. New York: Churchill Livingstone, 1990:1092.
49. Schochetman G, George J. 1992. Serologic tests for the detection of human immunodeficiency virus infection. In AIDS Testing Methodology and Management Issues, Springer-Verlag, New York.
50. Simonsen L, Buffington J, Shapiro C, et al. 1995. Multiple false reactions in viral antibody screening assays after influenza vaccination. Am. J. Epidem. 141-1089.
51. Smith D, Dewhurst S, Shepherd S, et al. 1987. False-positive enzyme-linked immunosorbent assay reactions for antibody to human immunodeficiency virus in a population of midwestern patients with congenital bleeding disorders. Transfusion. 127:112.

52. Snyder H, Fleissner E. 1980. Specificity of human antibodies to oncovirus glycoproteins; Recognition of antigen by natural antibodies directed against carbohydrate structures. Proc. Natl. Acad. Sci. 77:1622-1626.
53. Steckelberg JM, Cockerill F. 1988. Serologic testing for human immunodeficiency virus antibodies. Mayo Clin. Proc. 63:373.
54. Sungar C, Akpolat T, Ozkuyumcu C, et al. Alpha interferon therapy in hemodialysis patients. Nephron. 67:251.
55. Tribe D, Reed D, Lindell P, et al. 1988. Antibodies reactive with human immunodeficiency virus gag-coated antigens (gag reactive only) are a major cause of enzyme-linked immunosorbent assay reactivity in a bood donor population. J. Clin. Micro. April:641.
56. Ujhelyi E, Fust G, Illei G, et al. 1989. Different types of false positive anti-HIV reactions in patients on hemodialysis. Immun. Let. 22:35-40.
57. Van Beers D, Duys M, Maes M, et al. Heat inactivation of serum may interfere with tests for antibodies to LAV/HTLV-III [HIV]. J. Vir. Meth. 12:329.
58. Voevodin A. 1992. HIV screening in Russia. Lancet. 339:1548.
59. Weber B, Moshtaghi-Borojeni M, Brunner M, et al. 1995. Evaluation of the reliability of six current anti-HIV-1/HIV-2 enzyme immunoassays. J. Vir. Meth. 55:97.
60. Wood C, Williams A, McNamara J, et al. 1986. Antibody against the human immunodeficiency virus in commercial intravenous gamma globulin preparations. Ann. Int. Med. 105:536.
61. Yale S, Degroen P, Tooson J, et al. 1994. Unusual aspects of acute Q fever-associated hepatitis. Mayo Clin. Proc. 69:769.
62. Yoshida T, Matsui T, Kobayashi M, et al. 1987. Evaluation of passive particle agglutination test for antibody to human immunodeficiency virus. J. Clin. Micro. Aug:1433.
63. Yu S, Fong C, Landry M, et al. 1989. A false positive HIV antibody reaction due to transfusion-induced HLA-DR4 sensitization. NEJM.320:1495.
64. National Institute of Justice, AIDS Bulletin. Oct. 1988.

Made in United States
North Haven, CT
04 November 2026

21773569R00457